Breast Pathology

Breast Pathology

David J. Dabbs, MD
Professor and Chief of Pathology
Department of Pathology
Magee-Womens Hospital of UPMC
University of Pittsburgh School of Medicine
Pittsburgh, Pennsylvania

ELSEVIER
SAUNDERS

ELSEVIER
SAUNDERS

1600 John F. Kennedy Blvd.
Ste 1800
Philadelphia, PA 19103-2899

BREAST PATHOLOGY   ISBN: 978-1-4377-0604-8
Copyright © 2012 by Saunders, an imprint of Elsevier Inc.

Notice

Knowledge and best practice in this field are constantly changing. As new research and experience broaden our understanding, changes in research methods, professional practices, or medical treatment may become necessary.

Practitioners and researchers must always rely on their own experience and knowledge in evaluating and using any information, methods, compounds, or experiments described herein. In using such information or methods they should be mindful of their own safety and the safety of others, including parties for whom they have a professional responsibility.

With respect to any drug or pharmaceutical products identified, readers are advised to check the most current information provided (i) on procedures featured or (ii) by the manufacturer of each product to be administered, to verify the recommended dose or formula, the method and duration of administration, and contraindications. It is the responsibility of practitioners, relying on their own experience and knowledge of their patients, to make diagnoses, to determine dosages and the best treatment for each individual patient, and to take all appropriate safety precautions.

To the fullest extent of the law, neither the Publisher nor the authors, contributors, or editors, assume any liability for any injury and/or damage to persons or property as a matter of products liability, negligence or otherwise, or from any use or operation of any methods, products, instructions, or ideas contained in the material herein.

Library of Congress Cataloging-in-Publication Data

Dabbs, David J.
  Breast pathology / David J. Dabbs.
     p. ; cm.
  Includes bibliographical references and index.
  ISBN 978-1-4377-0604-8 (alk. paper)
  I. Title
  [DNLM: 1. Breast Neoplasms—pathology. 2. Breast—pathology. 3. Breast Diseases—pathology. WP 870]
  616.99449—dc23   2011039822

Executive Content Strategist: William R. Schmitt
Senior Content Development Specialist: Kathryn DeFrancesco
Publishing Services Manager: Pat Joiner-Myers
Senior Project Manager: Joy Moore
Designer: Louis Forgione

Printed in China

Last digit is the print number: 9 8 7 6 5 4 3 2 1

This Breast pathology textbook is dedicated to Breast pathologists across the globe who have contributed the abundance of information necessary to care for our patients.

This first edition is dedicated especially in honor of Edwin R. Fisher, MD, who passed away in March, 2008. Dr. Fisher was pathologist for the NSABP for nearly 50 years in Pittsburgh, Pennsylvania.

D. Craig Allred, MD
Professor, Department of Pathology and Immunology, Washington University School of Medicine, St. Louis, Missouri
Predictive and Prognostic Marker Testing in Breast Pathology: Immunophenotypic Subclasses of Disease

Sunil Badve, MD, FRCPath
Professor, Department of Pathology and Laboratory Medicine, Department of Internal Medicine, Indiana University School of Medicine, Indianapolis, Indiana
Sentinel Lymph Node Biopsy; Molecular-based Testing in Breast Disease for Therapeutic Decisions; Paget's Disease of the Breast

Frederick L. Baehner, MD
Assistant Professor of Clinical Pathology, Department of Pathology, University of California, San Francisco, San Francisco, California
Molecular-based Testing in Breast Disease for Therapeutic Decisions

Rohit Bhargava, MBBS
Associate Professor of Pathology, University of Pittsburgh; Co-Director of Surgical Pathology, Magee-Womens Hospital of UPMC, Pittsburgh, Pennsylvania
Predictive and Prognostic Marker Testing in Breast Pathology: Immunophenotypic Subclasses of Disease; Diagnostic Immunohistology of the Breast; Molecular Classification of Breast Carcinoma; Apocrine Carcinoma of the Breast; Pathology of Neoadjuvant Therapeutic Response of Breast Carcinoma

Werner Boecker, Dr.med.
Lecturer, Asklepius School of Medicine, Campus Hamburg Semmelweis University Budapest, Hamburg, Germany; Director Emeritus, Gerhard Domagk–Institute of Pathology, University of Müenster, Münster, North Rhine-Westphalia, Germany
Fibrocystic Change and Usual Epithelial Hyperplasia of Ductal Type

Mamatha Chivukula, MD
Associate Professor of Pathology, Department of Pathology, Magee-Womens Hospital of UPMC, Pittsburgh, Pennsylvania
Neoplasia of the Male Breast

Beth Z. Clark, MD
Assistant Professor of Pathology, Department of Pathology, Magee-Womens Hospital of UPMC, Pittsburgh, Pennsylvania
Adenosis and Microglandular Adenosis

David J. Dabbs, MD
Professor and Chief of Pathology, Department of Pathology, Magee-Womens Hospital of UPMC, University of Pittsburgh School of Medicine, Pittsburgh, Pennsylvania
Reactive and Inflammatory Conditions of the Breast; Patient Safety in Breast Pathology; Predictive and Prognostic Marker Testing in Breast Pathology: Immunophenotypic Subclasses of Disease; Diagnostic Immunohistology of the Breast; Adenosis and Microglandular Adenosis; Myoepithelial Lesions of the Breast; Fibrocystic Change and Usual Epithelial Hyperplasia of Ductal Type; Columnar Cell Alterations, Flat Epithelial Atypia, and Atypical Ductal Epithelial Hyperplasia; Lobular Neoplasia and Invasive Lobular Carcinoma; Metaplastic Breast Carcinoma; Pathology of Neoadjuvant Therapeutic Response of Breast Carcinoma; Neoplasia of the Male Breast

Ian O. Ellis, BM, BS, FRCPath
Professor of Cancer Pathology, Department of Histopathology, Nottingham City Hospital, Nottingham, United Kingdom
Ductal Carcinoma In Situ; Invasive Ductal Carcinoma of No Special Type and Histologic Grade

Nicole N. Esposito, MD
Assistant Professor, Department of Pathology and Cell Biology, University of South Florida College of Medicine; Chief of Breast and Gynecologic Pathology, James A. Haley Veterans Hospital, Tampa, Florida
Fibroepithelial Lesions; Papilloma and Papillary Lesions

Marie A. Ganott, MD
Associate Clinical Director, Breast Imaging, Department of Radiology, Magee-Womens Hospital of UPMC, Pittsburgh, Pennsylvania
Breast Imaging Modalities for Pathologists

Felipe C. Geyer, MD
Molecular Pathology Laboratory, The Breakthrough
Breast Cancer Research Centre, Institute of Cancer
Research, London, United Kingdom; Division
of Pathology, Hospital Israelita Albert Einstein,
Instituto de Ensino e Pesquisa Israelita Albert
Einstein, Sao Paulo, Brazil
*Lobular Neoplasia and Invasive Lobular Carcinoma;
Triple-Negative and Basal-like Carcinoma; Rare
Breast Carcinomas: Adenoid Cystic Carcinoma,
Neuroendocrine Carcinoma, Secretory Carcinoma,
Carcinoma with Osteoclast-like Giant Cells, Lipid-
Rich Carcinoma, and Glycogen-Rich Clear Cell
Carcinoma*

Christiane M. Hakim, MD
Associate Professor of Radiology, University of
Pittsburgh; Assistant Chief, General Radiology,
and Medical Director, Breast Imaging, Hillman
Cancer Center, Magee-Womens Hospital of UPMC,
Pittsburgh, Pennsylvania
Breast Imaging Modalities for Pathologists

Syed A. Hoda, MD
Professor, Weill Cornell Medical College; Attending
Pathologist, New York Presbyterian Hospital–Weill
Cornell Medical Center, New York, New York
Normal Breast and Developmental Disorders

Magali Lacroix-Triki, MD
Molecular Pathology Laboratory, The Breakthrough
Breast Cancer Research Centre, Institute of Cancer
Research, London, United Kingdom; Biology and
Pathology Department, Institut Claudius Regaud,
Toulouse, France
*Triple-Negative and Basal-like Carcinoma; Rare
Breast Carcinomas: Adenoid Cystic Carcinoma,
Neuroendocrine Carcinoma, Secretory Carcinoma,
Carcinoma with Osteoclast-like Giant Cells, Lipid-
Rich Carcinoma, and Glycogen-Rich Clear Cell
Carcinoma*

Shahla Masood, MD
Professor and Chair, Department of Pathology and
Laboratory Medicine, University of Florida College
of Medicine–Jacksonville; Medical Director and
Chief of Pathology, Shands Jacksonville Breast
Health Center, Jacksonville, Florida
Patient Safety in Breast Pathology

Syed K. Mohsin, MD
Pathologist, Department of Pathology, RMH
Pathology Associates, Inc.; Head of Breast Pathology
and Medical Director, Immunohistochemistry
Laboratory, Department of Pathology, Riverside
Methodist Hospital, Columbus, Ohio
Gross Examination of Breast Specimens; Radial Scar

Joseph T. Rabban, MD, MPH
Associate Professor and Assistant Director of Surgical
Pathology Service, Department of Pathology,
University of California, San Francisco, San
Francisco, California
Mesenchymal Neoplasms of the Breast

Emad A. Rakha, MD, PhD, FRCPath
Clinical Associate Professor, University of
Nottingham; Honorary Consultant Pathologist,
Nottingham University Hospitals NHS Trust,
Nottingham, United Kingdom
*Ductal Carcinoma In Situ; Invasive Ductal Carcinoma
of No Special Type and Histologic Grade*

Jorge S. Reis-Filho, MD, PhD, FRCPath
Professor of Molecular Pathology, Institute of Cancer
Research; Team Leader, Molecular Pathology Team,
The Breakthrough Breast Cancer Research Centre,
London, United Kingdom
*Lobular Neoplasia and Invasive Lobular Carcinoma;
Triple-Negative and Basal-like Carcinoma; Rare
Breast Carcinomas: Adenoid Cystic Carcinoma,
Neuroendocrine Carcinoma, Secretory Carcinoma,
Carcinoma with Osteoclast-like Giant Cells, Lipid-
Rich Carcinoma, and Glycogen-Rich Clear Cell
Carcinoma*

Christine G. Roth, MD
Assistant Professor, University of Pittsburgh School
of Medicine; Assistant Professor, Division of
Hematopathology, Department of Pathology,
University of Pittsburgh Medical Center, Pittsburgh,
Pennsylvania
Hematopoietic Tumors of the Breast

Reda S. Saad, MD, PhD, FRCPC
Associate Professor, Department of Laboratory
Medicine and Pathobiology, University of Toronto;
Staff Pathologist, Sunnybrook Health Sciences
Center, Toronto, Ontario, Canada
Metastatic Tumors in the Breast

Sunati Sahoo, MD
Associate Professor of Pathology, University of Texas
at Southwestern; Associate Professor, University of
Texas Southwestern Medical Center, Dallas, Texas
*Pathology of Neoadjuvant Therapeutic Response
of Breast Carcinoma; Special Types of Breast
Carcinoma: Tubular Carcinoma, Mucinous
Carcinoma, Cribriform Carcinoma, Invasive
Micropapillary Carcinoma, and Medullary
Carcinoma*

Sandra J. Shin, MD
Chief, Breast Pathology, and Associate Professor of
    Pathology and Laboratory Medicine, Weill Cornell
    Medical College; Attending Pathologist, New York
    Presbyterian Hospital, New York, New York
*Nipple Adenoma (Florid Papillomatosis of the Nipple);
Special Types of Breast Carcinoma: Tubular
Carcinoma, Mucinous Carcinoma, Cribriform
Carcinoma, Invasive Micropapillary Carcinoma, and
Medullary Carcinoma; Mesenchymal Neoplasms
of the Breast; Breast Tumors in Children and
Adolescents*

Jan F. Silverman, MD
Professor, Temple University School of Medicine;
    Professor, Drexel University College of Medicine;
    Chair and Director of Anatomic Pathology,
    Allegheny General Hospital, Pittsburgh,
    Pennsylvania
Metastatic Tumors in the Breast

Najwa Somani, MD, FRCPC
Assistant Professor, Department of Dermatology, and
    Associate Director of Dermatopathology, Indiana
    University School of Medicine; Staff Faculty, Indiana
    University Hospital, Indianapolis, Indiana
Paget's Disease of the Breast

Jules H. Sumkin, DO
Professor of Radiology, University of Pittsburgh; Chief,
    Radiology, Magee-Womens Hospital of UPMC,
    Pittsburgh, Pennsylvania
Breast Imaging Modalities for Pathologists

Steven H. Swerdlow, MD
Professor of Pathology, University of Pittsburgh
    School of Medicine; Director, Division of
    Hematopathology, University of Pittsburgh Medical
    Center–Presbyterian, Pittsburgh, Pennsylvania
Hematopoietic Tumors of the Breast

Victor G. Vogel, MD, MHS
Director, Cancer Institute, Geisinger Health System,
    Danville, Pennsylvania
Epidemiology of Breast Cancer

Amy Vogia, DO
Fellow in Breast Imaging, Department of Radiology,
    Magee-Womens Hospital of UPMC, Pittsburgh,
    Pennsylvania
Breast Imaging Modalities for Pathologists

Noel Weidner, MD
Senior Consulting Pathologist, Clarient Laboratories,
    Inc., Aliso Viejo, California
*Reactive and Inflammatory Conditions of the Breast;
Infections of the Breast; Myoepithelial Lesions of the
Breast; Metaplastic Breast Carcinoma*

Britta Weigelt, PhD
Postdoctoral Fellow, Cancer Research, UK London
    Research Institute, London, United Kingdom
Triple-Negative and Basal-like Carcinoma

Mark R. Wick, MD
Professor of Pathology, University of Virginia School of
    Medicine; Associate Director of Surgical Pathology,
    University of Virginia Health System, Charlottesville,
    Virginia
Tumors of the Mammary Skin

HOW TO USE THIS BOOK

This is the first comprehensive pathology textbook on breast pathology with multiple international authors in the United States. The intent of this book is to draw on the expertise of breast pathologists in the United States and across the world. The authors are all highly distinguished breast pathologists at the forefront of their areas of particular interests in academic medicine.

As a result, it has been somewhat challenging to maintain uniformity in format in this text. In addition to the lesion-based chapter approach of this textbook, there are specialty areas that are covered intensely.

Each lesion/entity-based chapter follows a format that includes an introduction, clinical presentation, clinical imaging, gross pathology, microscopic pathology, treatment and prognosis, and differential diagnosis. The specialty-titled chapters are more didactic, and these include chapters such as normal breast and developmental disorders, epidemiology and breast cancer risk, patient safety in breast pathology, the gross examination of breast specimens, sentinel lymph node pathology, breast imaging modalities for pathologists, immunohistology of the breast, and the molecular-based tests that address current issues in the study of breast pathology. The intent of each chapter is to integrate traditional gross and microscopic findings along with imaging studies and current molecular information and paradigms for classification.

We sincerely hope that you will enjoy this book and find it to be useful in your practice. As always, I appreciate feedback and suggestions; send to dabbsihc@gmail.com.

CONTENTS

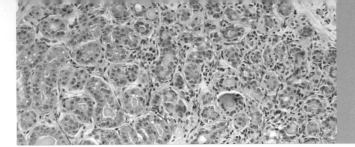

Normal Breast and Developmental Disorders

Syed A. Hoda

NORMAL BREAST

The breasts are the distinguishing feature of mammals and have evolved as milk-producing organs to provide appropriate nourishment to their offspring. There are other purported benefits of nursing. Physiologically, this act serves to help involute the uterus; psychologically, it helps to "bond" the mother and its offspring.[1] Other than the aforementioned functions of the breast, its intrinsic epigamic value cannot be overemphasized.

Embryology

Breast development in utero starts in the first trimester of gestation with multiple bilateral thickenings of the ectoderm on the ventral aspect of the fetus. This thickened ridge extends in a linear manner from the axilla to the groin, forming the so-called milk line (Figure 1-1). As fetal development proceeds, all except a pair of these thickenings, one on each side of the pectoral region, regress.[2–5]

In its earliest stages, the aforementioned thickening is caused by condensed mesenchymal tissue around an epithelial bud. Solid epithelial cord–like columns develop from the bud. Portions of dermis increasingly envelop the epithelial columns and develop into the connective tissue of the breast. More fibrocollagenous elements of the dermis extend into the developing breast and much later form the **suspensory ligaments of Cooper** (named after Astley Cooper, the English anatomist and surgeon, who described these structures in the 19th century). Gradually, the epithelial columns branch, canalize, and transform into ducts (and eventually into lobules). Thus, each column ultimately gives rise to a lobe of the breast. A "pit" in the epidermis forms at the convergence of the major (lactiferous) ducts, and shortly thereafter, its eversion forms the protuberant nipple (Figure 1-2).[6] Occasionally, the nipple may not evert, and this results in an inverted (or permanently retracted) nipple. This deformity may cause considerable difficulty in suckling.

In the third trimester, the developing mammary glands are responsive to maternal hormones and exhibit mild secretory changes. Upon delivery, the withdrawal of maternal hormones stimulates prolactin release, which initiates **colostrum** ("witch's milk") secretion. This occurs, to some degree, in approximately 90% of infants of both genders in the first few days after birth. Colostrum is actually composed of water, fat, and debris; it dissipates within a month or so of birth. During this time, and for a period of a few weeks thereafter, the breast is palpably enlarged. Until puberty, the breast tissue consists almost exclusively of major ducts.[7]

Gross Anatomy

The female breasts are rounded protuberances on either side of the anterior chest wall. The organ is present in rudimentary form in prepubertal girls, boys, and adult males. The bulk of female breast tissue overlies the pectoralis major muscle from the second to the sixth rib in the vertical axis and from the sternal edge to the midaxilla in the horizontal axis. Breast glandular tissue usually extends beyond these arbitrary boundaries. The

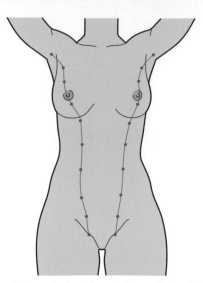

FIGURE 1-1 Schematic depiction of "the milk line." The milk line extends from the axilla to the inguinal region in the adult. Supernumerary nipples and/or breast tissue may persist anywhere along these lines.

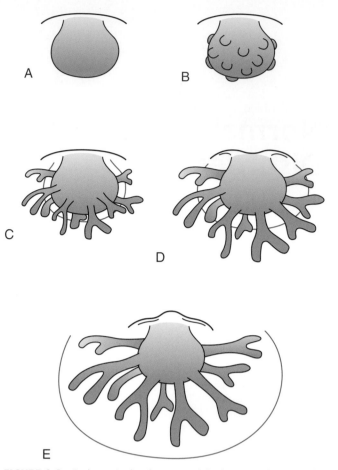

FIGURE 1-2 Embryonic development of the breast. Schematic depiction of developing mammary bud from that in a 6-week embryo to birth: epithelial primordium **(A)**, incipient duct formation **(B)**, early duct formation **(C)**, inverted nipple stage **(D)**, and elongation of ducts and eversion of nipple **(E)**. Area outlined in green depicts progressively growing connective tissue.

extension of breast tissue from the upper-outer quadrant into the axilla is eponymously referred to as the **tail of Spence** (after James Spence, a Scot surgeon of the 19th century). This "tail" can be difficult to envision on routine mammograms—and in earlier times, the patient was routinely placed in the so-called Cleopatra pose to allow such visualization.[8]

The breast is enveloped by fascial tissues. Anteriorly, there is superficial pectoral fascia. Posteriorly, there is deep pectoral fascia. These two layers of fascia blend with the cervical fascia superiorly and with that overlying the abdomen inferiorly. Fibrous bands (the aforementioned Cooper's ligaments), more numerous in the superior half of the breast, connect these two fascial layers. A "space" filled with loose connective tissue lies between the deep boundary of the breast and the fascia of underlying skeletal muscle. This retromammary space allows the breast some degree of movement over the underlying pectoral fascia. The fascia overlying the chest wall sometimes harbors breast glandular units. The glands rarely extend beyond this fascia into bands of underlying skeletal muscle. Such extension of breast glandular tissue into these deep structures is a normal anatomic feature that has clinical implications, for example, in modified radical mastectomies, which strive to remove as much of the breast glandular tissue as possible. Most mastectomies (short of the draconian radical mastectomies) are successful in removing no more than 90% of breast glandular tissue.

The **shape and size** of the breast depends not only upon genetic and racial factors but also upon age, diet, parity, and menopausal status of the individual. The breast can appear hemispherical, conical, pendulous, piriform, or thinned and flattened; however, typically, the breast is oval and hemispherical, with the long axis diagonally aligned over the chest. There is a distinct flattening of the superficial contour of the breast superior to the nipple.

The normal mature nonlactating female breast weighs approximately 200 g (±100 g).[9] The typical lactating breast may weigh more than 500 g. The average adult breast measures 12 cm in diameter and 6 cm in thickness. In a study of breast volume in 55 women, Smith and coworkers[10] found that the right breast was less voluminous: the mean for the right breast was 275 mL and that for the left breast was 290 mL. This discrepancy has been correlated to handedness. There is no correlation between breast mass and cancer risk because large breasts do not necessarily contain more glandular parenchyma.

The **nipple** being centrally located, and typically elevated from the surrounding areola, is the focal point of the skin of the breast. Its level in the thorax varies widely but, typically, overlies the fourth intercostal space in younger women. Both nipple and areola are pink, light brown, or darker (depending upon the general pigmentation of the body). These two structures are somewhat less pigmented in the nulliparous and become increasingly pigmented starting in the second month of pregnancy. The tinctorial change after pregnancy is irreversible.

Twelve to 20 minute rounded protuberances, representing prominent sebaceous gland units usually associated with a lactiferous duct, in the dermis, are present on the surface of the areola.[11] These protuberances are generally referred to as **Montgomery tubercles** (after Dr. William Montgomery, a 19th-century Irish obstetrician who described these structures, although it is possible that Morgagni, the 18th-century Italian anatomist, detailed the same structures much earlier). Montgomery's tubercles become prominent during pregnancy and lactation, reflecting the need for keeping the areola moist during feeding. The tubercles regress after menopause. Apocrine and sweat glands are also present in this area. Hair follicles are present at the edge of the areola. The presence of these glands and hair follicles may be involved in the pathogenesis of persistent subareolar abscesses.

Skin incisions for breast surgery are generally based on the knowledge of natural orientation of collagen fibers in the epidermis and dermis along the lines first described by Karl Langer, the 19th-century Austrian anatomist. Adherence to Langer's lines of skin orientation in making surgical incisions ensures minimal scarring and better cosmetic outcome.[12] These lines are based on mechanical principles rather than on any specific anatomic structures and are actually founded on the somewhat macabre premise of the direction in which the human cadaver's skin of a particular area will split if struck by a spike!

In the current TNM (tumor-node-metastasis) staging system, breast tumor of any size with direct extension to the chest wall and/or to the overlying skin with presence of nodules or ulceration is staged as T4. Invasion of the dermis by tumor does not qualify as T4.

Structure and Histology

Several collecting ducts, each of which drains a **mammary lobe,** open in the nipple. The lobes are arranged around the breast in a radial (spokelike) manner (Figure 1-3). Three-dimensional depictions of the breast lobe appear as cones—with its apex at the nipple and its base in the region of the deep fascia where most lobules reside.[13-16] Despite such depictions of mammary lobes in anatomy and pathology textbooks as discrete anatomic territories within the breast, the lobes grow intricately into one another around their edges and do not constitute distinct grossly identifiable entities. Thus, the lobes cannot be visually dissected during surgery. Notably, each duct system has a different anatomic extent: the larger ones may extend beyond a quadrant and the smaller may occupy much less than a quadrant. The lobes are independent systems; however, it is possible that a few lobes may interconnect at some level via ducts—although the evidence for this is rather dubious. Intraductal carcinoma extends in the long axis of the lobe along the duct system, utilizing the latter as a scaffold. Interlobar anastomosis, if it were to exist, could potentially allow intraductal carcinoma to spread beyond the primarily afflicted duct.

The nipple and areola are covered with **stratified squamous epithelium,** which is continuous with the surrounding skin over the breast. The opening of the collecting ducts at the nipple is typically plugged by keratinous

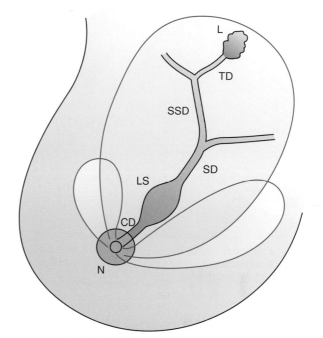

FIGURE 1-3 Sagittal section through the adult female breast. Three lobes are depicted in this diagram (all outlined in *green*). The central lobe shows its basic structure from the nipple (N). Depicted herein are collecting duct (CD), lactiferous sinus (LS), segmental duct (SD), subsegmental duct (SSD), terminal duct (TD), and lobule (L).

debris in the nonlactating breast. The squamous epithelium of the collecting ducts undergoes gradual transition to pseudostratified columnar epithelium and, finally, to cuboidal or low-columnar epithelium (Figure 1-4).

Approximately 20 **orifices of collecting ducts,** each representing a lobe of the breast, are present in the nipple. These orifices, which may be as few as 8 and as many as 24, are generally arranged as a central group and a peripheral group.[17] The deeper portion of the collecting ducts has a characteristically serrated contour for a variable distance before opening into its terminal portion. The latter portion has a relatively less convoluted and smoother profile. The lactiferous ducts in the nipple are surrounded by bundles of smooth muscle. The muscle fiber arrangement is principally circular, but some fibers are also arranged vertically, interlacing among collecting and lactiferous ducts. The circular muscle fibers cause nipple erection, readying it for suckling. By cyclic contraction, the vertically arrayed muscle bundles empty the lactiferous sinuses. There is virtually no adipose tissue immediately beneath the nipple and areola.

The portion of the **duct system** immediately below the collecting duct is the lactiferous sinus in which milk accumulates during lactation. This sinus communicates directly with segmental duct, which subdivides into subsegmental ducts, which in turn, subdivide into terminal ducts. The latter structures drain the lobule. Each lobe contains 20 to 40 lobules. The lobule is composed of groups of small glandular structures, the acini. The latter are the terminal portion of the duct system. The serially and dichotomously branching structure of the mammary gland, from the tubular-like collecting

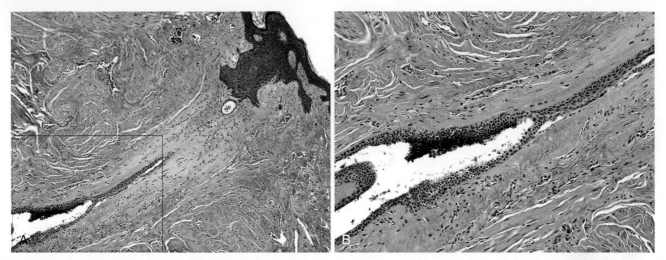

FIGURE 1-4   Vertical section through the nipple. **A,** A collecting duct is shown approaching the surface of the nipple (area in box is magnified in **B**). **B,** Squamous epithelium of the orifice undergoes gradual transition to the columnar epithelium of the collecting duct. **A** and **B,** Hematoxylin and eosin (H&E).

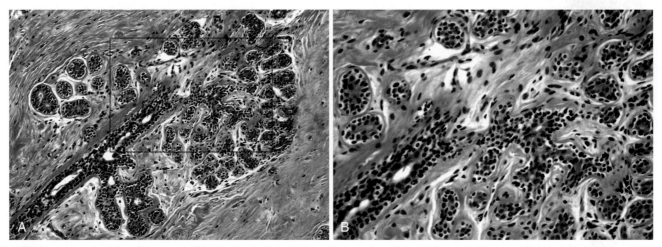

FIGURE 1-5   Terminal duct lobular unit (TDLU). **A,** The lobule is composed of multiple acini. Acini are on the right (area in box is magnified in **B**). **B,** The terminal duct on the left is seen exiting the lobule. Note inner epithelial layer (with denser cytoplasm) and outer myoepithelial layer (with clearer cytoplasm). **A** and **B,** H&E.

duct to the terminal acini, leads to its classification as a compound tubuloacinar (or tubulolobular) gland (Figure 1-5).

The **lobule** is inapparent to the naked eye on cut sections of breast tissue. However, with the aid of a magnifying lens, the lobules resemble minute drops of dew, and ducts may appear as linear streaks. The size of the "normal" lobule is extremely variable, as are the number of acini in each lobule. Each lobule consists of 10 to 100 (range 8–200) acini. The intralobular stroma consists of loose connective tissue and may also be populated by a mixed inflammatory cell infiltrate particularly in the secretory phase of the menstrual cycle. The lobule undergoes a variety of morphologic changes under various physiologic influences (Figure 1-6).

The fundamental glandular unit of the breast, and its most actively proliferating part, is the **terminal duct lobular unit** (**TDLU**). This unit comprises the lobule and its paired terminal duct. During pregnancy and lactation, the epithelial cells of the terminal ducts and

lobules undergo secretory changes; and most disease processes of the breast arise from the TDLUs (including cysts, which may be the consequence of the "unfolding" of the terminal ducts and lobular units). Indeed, the only common lesion believed to be strictly of ductal origin may be the larger solitary intraductal papilloma (Table 1-1).

Except for the terminal portion of the collecting ducts, **low-columnar to cuboidal epithelium** lines almost the entire duct system of the breast; including the segmental ducts, subsegmental ducts, terminal ducts, and acini. This lining epithelium is supported on its basal surface by a distinct layer of myoepithelial cells. The basement membrane or basal lamina lies under the myoepithelial cells. External to the basement membrane is connective tissue.

Myoepithelial cells facilitate milk secretion via their contractile property, which is largely under the influence of oxytocin. Oxytocin receptors have been detected on the surface of myoepithelial cells,[18] and this hormone

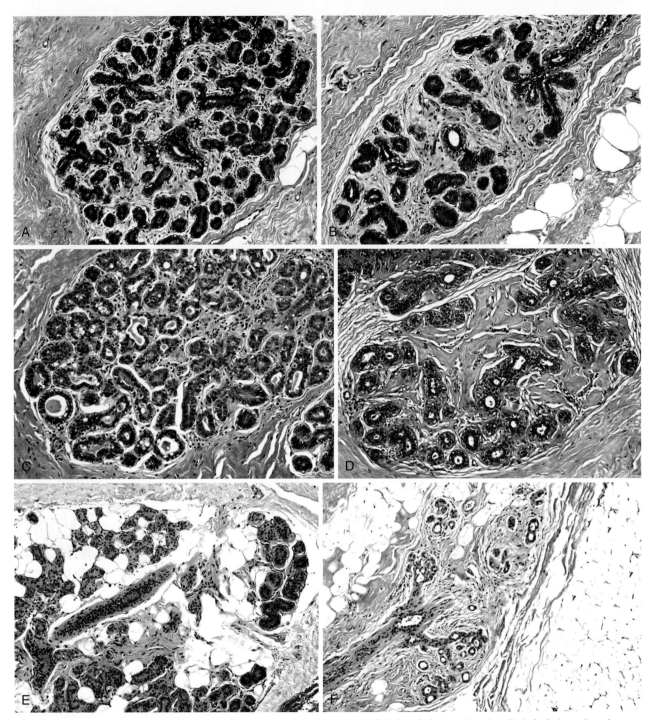

FIGURE 1-6 Mammary lobule at various physiologic stages. **A,** Lobule in an adult female breast, inactive. **B,** Lobule in early puberty; note the incipient development of the lobule. **C,** Lobule in the secretory phase of the menstrual cycle; note secretions in the glands. **D,** Lobule after menopause, with intralobular fibrosis. **E,** Lobule after menopause, with intralobular adipocytes. **F,** Lobule in the elderly; note glandular atrophy and relative prominence of myoepithelial cells. **A-F,** H&E.

is primarily responsible for the release of milk—a phenomenon called *milk let-down*.[19]

The myoepithelial cell layer is generally regarded as being spindle-shaped with usually inapparent cytoplasm. Indeed, in fine-needle aspiration cytology preparations, myoepithelial cells appear to be entirely devoid of cytoplasm (i.e., "naked"). The thin and compressed ("**bipolar**") nuclei of these cells are oriented perpendicular to the long axis of the duct. Myoepithelial cells extend from collecting ducts to the tip of the acini and may occasionally appear prominent either de novo (Figure 1-7) or in certain physiologic (e.g., atrophy) and pathologic (postradiation, adenomyoepithelioma) situations. Myoepithelial cells are inapparent in certain lesions (e.g., in macrocysts, in which these cells get particularly stretched).

A variety of immunohistochemical stains can be used to demonstrate the presence of myoepithelium around

TABLE 1-1	Histologic Alterations in Breast Glands and Stroma during Various Phases of the Menstrual Cycle*

Proliferative Phase (Days 3–7)

Epithelial cells are small with dark, centrally located nuclei and eosinophilic cytoplasm.
Myoepithelial cells are small.
Glandular lumens are nondilated without secretions.
Stroma is relatively dense.
No epithelial mitoses are present.

Luteal Phase (Days 8–14)

Epithelial cells are larger with apical snouts.
Rare epithelial mitoses are present.
Glandular lumens are enlarged.
Myoepithelial cells appear minimally vacuolated.
Luminal secretions become evident.
Stroma is edematous.
Blood vessels are congested.
Proliferation rate (as evidenced by Ki-67) is higher than in proliferative phase.

Secretory/Menstrual Phase (Days 15–22)

Epithelial cells have a high nuclear-to-cytoplasm ratio, with minute apical snouts.
Epithelial mitoses are rare.
Glandular lumens become smaller.
Luminal secretions become less evident.
Myoepithelial cells are highly vacuolated.
Stroma is densely compact.
Apoptotic figures are most numerous on day 28.
Size of the lobule almost doubles from that in the early proliferative phase (from ~1 mm to nearly 2 mm).

*Histologic changes may vary widely within the breast, its quadrants, and even within lobules.

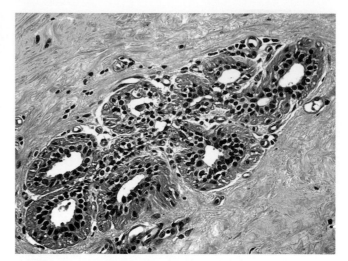

FIGURE 1-7 Prominent myoepithelial cells. The myoepithelial cells lie external to the epithelial cells and may occasionally appear prominent (myoid hyperplasia). H&E.

TABLE 1-2	Sites of Origin of Common Diseases in the Breast

From the Nipple

Paget's disease, florid papillomatosis of nipple (i.e., nipple adenoma)

From the Lactiferous Ducts

Subsclerosing duct hyperplasia, duct ectasia

From Segmental and Subsegmental Ducts

Solitary intraductal papilloma, duct ectasia

From the Terminal Duct Lobular Units

Cysts, epithelial hyperplasia, noninvasive and invasive carcinoma

ducts (Table 1-2 and Figure 1-8). The lack of myoepithelial cell layer around neoplastic glands is generally considered to be diagnostic of invasive carcinoma, barring special situations such as that encountered in microglandular adenosis[20,21] and solid-papillary carcinoma with smooth peripheral contours. Absence of myoepithelial cell layer has also been reported in some, but not all, apocrine cysts.[22] The use of double (or triple) immunolabeling with combinations of epithelial and myoepithelial immunostains is helpful in confirming early invasive carcinoma of breast (Figure 1-9).[23]

The **basement membrane,** composed of a relatively attenuated basal lamina, lies immediately outside of the myoepithelial cell layer and divides the glands from the stroma. The basement membrane can be highlighted using appropriate immunostains (e.g., laminin and collagen 4) or histochemical stains (reticulin and periodic acid–Schiff) (Figure 1-10). Stromal tissue lies beyond the basement membrane.

The mammary ducts and lobules are embedded within a variable **fibrous and fatty stroma.** The relative portions of glands and fibrous and adipose tissue vary with age and body habitus; however, stromal tissues make up the bulk of the breast in adult nonlactating and nonpregnant women. Adipose tissue is typically present in the interlobar stroma and not among lobules (at least not until atrophy ensues). The fibrous tissue assists in the mechanical coherence of the gland. The fibroblastic and myofibroblastic elements in the stroma of the breast often display a vaguely angiomatous appearance (hence, the term *pseudoangiomatous stromal hyperplasia*) (Figure 1-11). The volume-fraction of collagen-rich fibrous tissue is greater in younger adult women and accounts for the greater mammographic density therein.[24–26]

Apocrine cells are normal constituents of the glands of the breast in adult women, suggesting that this finding is a physiologic phenomenon (i.e., a normal line of metaplastic differentiation) rather than a pathologic finding.[27] The apocrine cells are typically pink and appear cuboidal or columnar and may exhibit a stubby apical snout (Figure 1-12).[28] Rarely, prominent apocrine granules may become evident—particularly at the apical portions of the cells (Figure 1-13). Cysts lined with apocrine epithelia typically bear calcium oxalate crystals, which may need polarizing microscopy to be

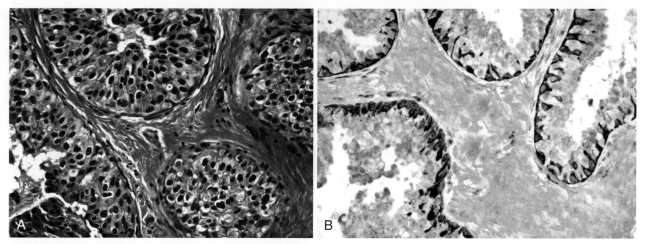

FIGURE 1-8   Myoepithelial immunostain (calponin) in ductal carcinoma in situ (DCIS). **A,** DCIS of solid and micropapillary types. H&E. **B,** Calponin immunostain demonstrates complete myoepithelial envelope around the neoplastic cells.

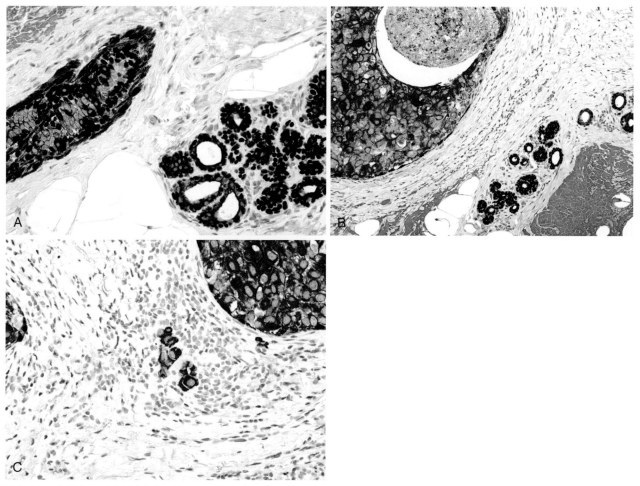

FIGURE 1-9   "Triple stain" highlights the myoepithelium and epithelium of mammary glands. The mammary ductal-lobular system is lined by a dual cell population: an inner epithelial cell layer and an outer myoepithelial cell layer. Red cytoplasmic immunostaining is seen in epithelial cells with cytokeratin. Brown cytoplasmic staining is observed in myoepithelial cells with myosin. Brown nuclear staining in myoepithelial cells is with p63. Shown here is a duct and an inactive lobule **(A),** ductal carcinoma in situ **(B),** and microinvasive carcinoma **(C center).** Note absence of myoepithelium around the cells of the microinvasive carcinoma. **A-C,** Triple immunostain: CK AE1/3 + myosin + p63.

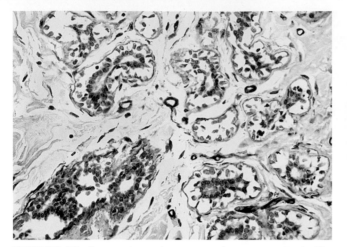

FIGURE 1-10 Basement membrane around mammary glands. The basement membrane around these inactive acini and terminal ducts is highlighted with collagen IV immunostain. Laminin immunostain and periodic acid–Schiff (PAS) or reticulin histochemical stain may also be used for this purpose. Collagen IV immunostain.

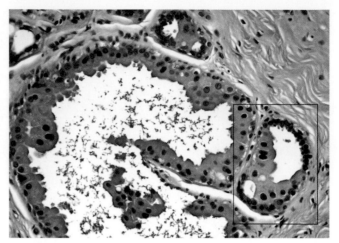

FIGURE 1-12 Apocrine metaplasia. The "pink" apocrine cells show bland round to ovoid nuclei. Transition of the normal cuboidal epithelium to the metaplastic apocrine epithelium is evident in the box. H&E.

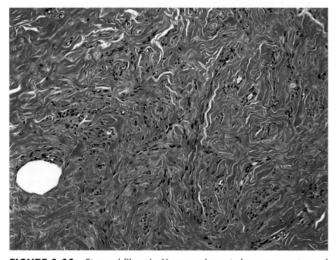

FIGURE 1-11 Stromal fibrosis. Younger breasts have more stromal (mainly fibrous) component. Occasionally, the fibroblastic and myofibroblastic proliferation displays a vaguely angiomatous appearance (hence, the term *pseudoangiomatous stromal hyperplasia*). H&E.

visualized (Figure 1-14).[29] Apocrine cells are almost always negative for both estrogen (ER) and progesterone (PgR) receptors and are strongly positive for epithelial membrane antigen (EMA), gross cystic disease fluid protein-15 (GCDFP-15), and androgen receptors (ARs).

Under certain influences, as yet unknown, **clear cell change** can occur in epithelial cells (of both ducts and lobules) as well as myoepithelial cells (Figure 1-15).[30–32] In epithelial cells, clear cell change can be commonly seen in association with apocrine metaplasia and following cytoplasmic accumulation of glycogen. In myoepithelial cells, clear cell change can occur either spontaneously or sporadically and may be seen in association with adenomyoepitheliosis and adenomyoepithelioma (Figure 1-16). Such change in either type of tissue does not appear to be related to any preneoplastic process.

Foam cells are normally found within glands (typically, those that are cystically dilated) and in stroma (Figure 1-17). Some of these foam cells are polygonal (and thus clearly histiocytic) in appearance; others may have either an epithelioid or spindle cell appearance.[33] **Pigment-laden histiocytes** appear in periductal connective tissue of approximately 15% of breasts (Figure 1-18).[34] These relatively large cells with low nuclear-to-cytoplasmic ratio contain pale yellow to dark brown pigment. The pigment seems to have the staining qualities of lipofuscin, being positive for periodic acid–Schiff (but diastase-resistant), weakly positive for acid-fast stain, and negative for iron. **Multinucleated stromal giant cells** may be present in the interlobular stroma (Figure 1-19). These giant cells are often present amid myofibroblast-dominant areas and have no known clinical significance.[35]

A framework of **elastic tissue** is present along the length of the duct system from the nipple to the subsegmental ducts. TDLUs are surrounded by a cuff of myxoid-appearing connective tissue that contains virtually no elastic tissue. The larger ducts have sparse specialized connective tissue and possess relatively more abundant elastic tissue. Abundant bundles of elastic tissue are present in the periductal stroma of approximately 50% of women over the age of 50 (Figure 1-20). **Elastosis** implies an excess of elastic fibers over normal, although the baseline level of elastic tissue in the female breast remains undefined.[36]

Two types of benign **clear cells** are present in the nipple among the stratified squamous epithelium. These are the so-called cellules claires and the Toker cells.[37] The more common **cellules claire** ("clear cells" in French) type (seen in about a third of the nipples) has clear cytoplasm and a semilunar nucleus that is compressed to the edge (Figure 1-21). The clarity of the cytoplasm is likely the result of hydropic change. These clear cells are typically numerous and scattered throughout the full thickness of the epidermis. The clear portion of the cytoplasm of cellules claires is nonreactive for various cytokeratins, EMA, carcinoembryonic antigen, and papillomavirus markers. The second type of clear cells (so-called

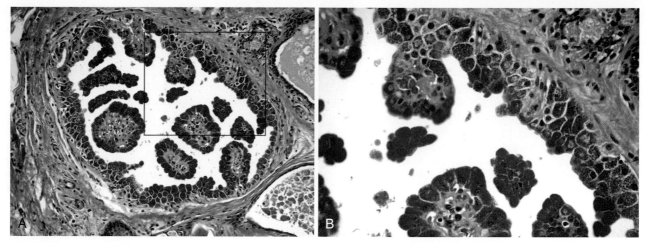

FIGURE 1-13   Cystic papillary apocrine hyperplasia with prominent apocrine granules. **A,** The apocrine type of metaplastic cells bear bright orange-red intracytoplasmic granules (area in box is magnified in **B). A** and **B,** H&E.

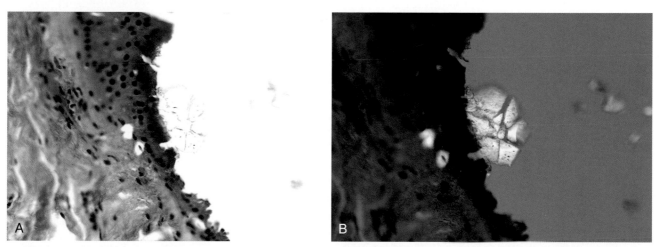

FIGURE 1-14   Cystic apocrine metaplasia with oxalate crystals. **A,** The apocrine cysts contain barely visible calcium oxalate crystals. **B,** The crystals can be better visualized under polarizing microscopy. **A** and **B,** H&E.

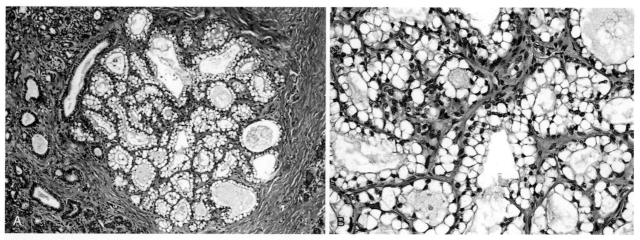

FIGURE 1-15   Clear cell metaplasia. **A** and **B,** Acini in a lobule show cells with abundant clear cytoplasm and bland nuclei. Note unaffected glands in the vicinity. **A** and **B,** H&E.

Toker cells) is more clinically significant because it can be mistaken for Paget's disease of nipple. These cells, first detailed by Cyril Toker, a pathologist in New York City, are "smaller in size than typical Paget cells" and "larger than their squamous neighbors."[38] Toker cells are either extensions of mammary duct epithelial cells into the epidermal surface of the nipple or remnants of the embryonic nipple bud (see earlier). These cells have round and cytologically insipid nucleus and cytoplasm that is pale and appear most numerous at the openings of lactiferous ducts.[39] Toker cells occur either singly or in aggregates of a few cells; they are most commonly encountered near the basal layer but may also be found in the more superficial layers. It is helpful in the differential diagnosis to know that Toker cells can appear dendritic or stellate on cytokeratin-7 (CK7) immunoreaction (Figure 1-22).

Paget's disease of nipple (named after Sir James Paget, the 19th-century British surgeon and pathologist) is the ascending extension of carcinoma cells, along the preexisting scaffold of the duct system of the breast, to the epidermis of the nipple.[40] Occasionally, these Paget cells form ductal structures. Except for *HER2*/neu immunostain (which is strongly positive in > 90% of Paget cells), immunohistochemistry is generally unhelpful in the differential diagnosis of Toker and Paget cells because both cell types are reactive for various cytokeratins (including cell adhesion molecule [CAM] 5.2 and CK7) and EMA and are nonreactive for CK20 and S-100 protein (Figure 1-23).[41–43]

Nipple-sparing mastectomy has lately become a popular option for those for whom mastectomy is mandated or preferable for any reason. This procedure, which spares the nipple-areolar complex, provides a reconstructed breast with cosmetically better outcome with the added possibility of retention of (at least some) sensation in the nipple. These advantages have to be weighed against the risks of leaving microscopic tumor in the nipple or the threat of the development of carcinoma in residual ductal or lobular tissue in the "spared" nipple.[44] In a study of 316 therapeutic nipple-sparing mastectomies, Brachtel and colleagues[45] found that 71% of nipples showed no abnormality, 21% had either ductal carcinoma in situ, invasive breast carcinoma, or lymphovascular channel involvement by tumor, and 8% had lobular carcinoma in situ. Lobules are present in 17% of normal nipples.[46]

Ultrastructure

On electron microscopy, the inactive luminal cells that line the entire length of the duct and lobular system of the breast contain mitochondria, rough endoplasmic reticulum, and secretory granules. Surface specialization is present with microvilli projecting into the extracellular lumen. Desmosomes are present along the lateral interface with neighboring epithelial cells. Presence of the secretory granules and droplets toward the apical pole of the cells depends upon the physiologic state of the organ. A seemingly continuous layer of myoepithelial cells lies under the epithelial cells. This layer is oriented at right angles to the epithelial cells. Contractile actin filaments are seen in myoepithelial cells that appear more electron-dense and contain intacytoplasmic myofibrils

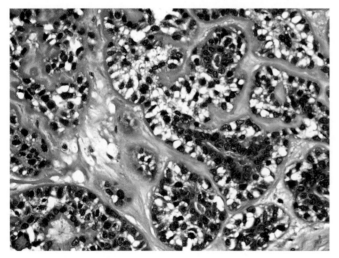

FIGURE 1-16   Clear cell cytoplasmic change in myoepithelial cells. Clear cell change in myoepithelia can appear pronounced. If the myoepithelial cells appear to be equal in number to the epithelial cells, the term *adeonomyoepitheliosis* may be used. H&E.

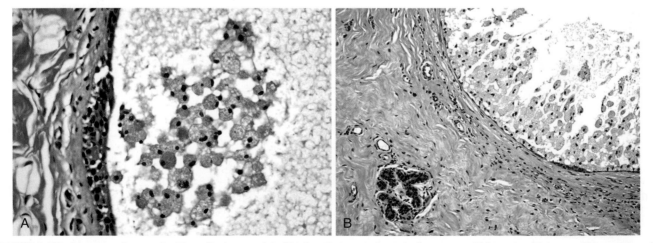

FIGURE 1-17   Mammary foam cells. These finely vacuolated histiocytic-type cells typically appear within cysts which may **(A)** or may only focally **(B)** be lined by epithelial cells. The derivation of foam cells (epithelial or histiocytic) had been controversial in the past. **A** and **B**, H&E.

with dense bodies and pinocytotic vesicles. The myoepithelial cells are attached to the underlying basement membrane (basal lamina) via hemidesmosomes. The epithelial cells appear to rest directly on the basal lamina wherever there is a gap between myoepithelial cells.[47,48]

Arterial Supply

The principal arterial supply to the breast is via the internal mammary artery, which caters to its central and medial portion. Somewhat confusing to the uninitiated is the fact that "internal mammary artery" and "internal thoracic artery" refer to the same arterial vessel.[49] Necrosis of breast tissue after coronary artery bypass graft with segments of internal mammary artery is a rarer complication than one could expect—especially because this vessel is so commonly utilized for this purpose.[50] The lateral thoracic artery supplies the upper and outer portions of the breast. Numerous other arterial vessels contribute to the arterial supply of the breast. These include various intercostals (mainly the second to

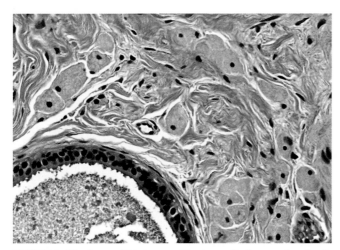

FIGURE 1-18 Stromal histiocytes. The large, finely vacuolated cells with minute nuclei are typically seen around cystically dilated ducts. H&E.

fourth), lateral thoracic, subscapular, thoracoacromial, and thoracodorsal arteries and branches thereof.[51,52]

Arteries in the breast normally exhibit sclerotic changes and intramural calcifications of the type seen in so-called Monckeberg's medial calcific arterial sclerosis (named after the eponymous German pathologist). Such calcified deposits are largely an aging change similar to that observed in other organs (Figure 1-24). Up to 9% of breasts in postmenopausal women exhibit arterial calcifications detectable on screening mammograms and such findings are not predictive of coronary heart disease at coronary angiography.[53]

Given the relatively rich arterial network in the breast, it is not surprising that the vessels get traumatized by invasive procedures such as needle core biopsies. A number of cases of arterial pseudoaneurysm formation after core biopsies (even with relatively thin needles) have been reported.[54]

Venous Drainage

In general, the venous drainage system of the breast follows the arterial system. However, the veins of the breast are much more variable than its arteries. The superficial venous system of the breast drains into the internal thoracic vein. The deep venous system drains into the perforating branches of the internal thoracic vein, lateral thoracic, axillary vein, and upper intercostal veins. A circular venous plexus lies around the areola.

Lymphatic System and Regional Lymph Nodes

The bulk (>75%) of the lymph drained from the breast enters the axilla.[55] Most of the remainder of lymph from the organ drains into the internal mammary nodes. There are also some minor lymphatic channels that lead to the interpectoral, internal thoracic, supraclavicular, and infraclavicular (and possibly even intramammary lymph nodes). Lymphatic channels of the breast follow a more or less direct path to the axillary or internal

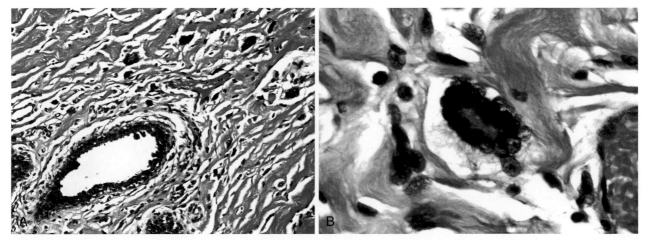

FIGURE 1-19 Multinucleated stromal giant cells in the breast. **A,** Stromal giant cells (of mesenchymal phenotype) are seen here in association with pseudoangiomatous stromal hyperplasia. **B,** Cell detail. **A** and **B,** H&E.

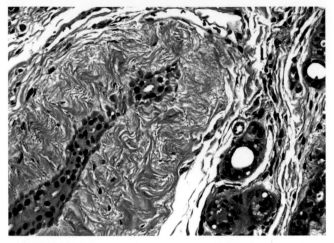

FIGURE 1-20 Stromal elastosis. Periductal stromal elastosis in an 85-year-old woman. Note the characteristic absence of stromal elastosis around the lobules. H&E.

mammary nodes without involving the rich subareolar lymphatic plexus.[56]

The **axillary lymph nodes** that lie along the axillary vein and its tributaries are usually divided into three levels: level 1 nodes lie in the low-axilla, lateral to the axillary border of pectoralis minor muscle; level 2 nodes lie in the mid-axilla, between the medial and the lateral borders of the pectoralis minor muscle; and level 3 nodes lie in the apex of the axilla, medial to the cranial margin of the pectoralis minor muscle and inferior to the clavicle.[57] The **Rotter's lymph nodes** (described by Josef Rotter, a 19th-century German surgeon), lie between the pectoralis major and pectoralis minor muscle, belong to the level 2 group, and may comprise up to four nodes. Level 3 lymph nodes are also known as *apical* or *infraclavicular nodes* (Figure 1-25). Metastases to the latter group of lymph nodes portend a worse prognosis. Rotter's nodes are characteristically involved in breast cancers that arise from the upper-central and upper-outer

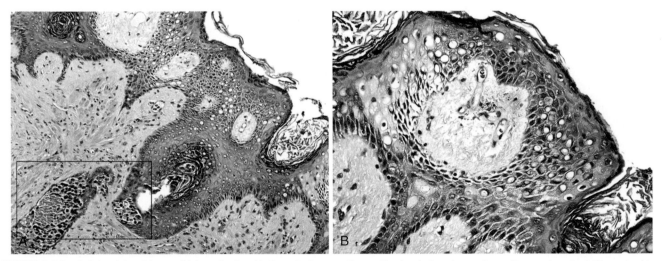

FIGURE 1-21 *Cellules claires* (clear cells) in a nipple with Paget's disease. Clear cells, simulating signet-ring cells, are abundant. The cytoplasm of these cells appears empty, and the nuclei are pushed to the edge. **A,** Note intraductal carcinoma in underlying collecting duct that extends into the epidermis of the nipple as Paget's disease (area in box is magnified in **B**). A and B, H&E.

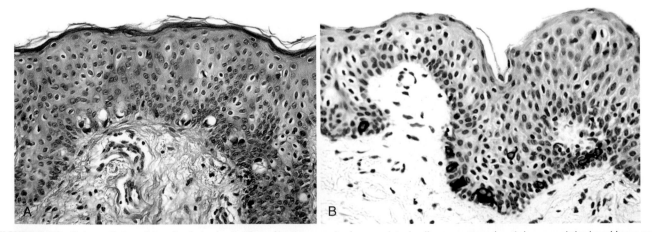

FIGURE 1-22 Toker cells in epidermis of nipple. **A,** These benign seemingly vacuolated cells are scattered mainly around the basal layer and possess more abundant cytoplasm and are paler than adjacent keratinocytes. H&E. **B,** Cytokeratin-7 immunostain highlights Toker cells and imparts a dendritic appearance to these cells.

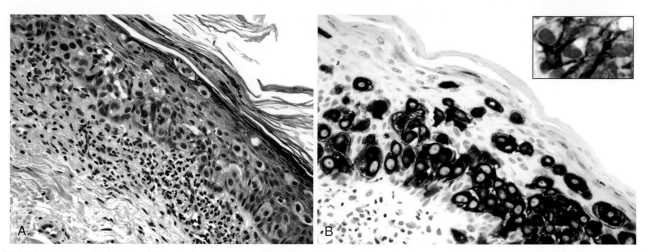

FIGURE 1-23 Paget's disease of the nipple. **A,** The much larger and paler malignant cells are evident amid the native squamous epithelium of the nipple. H&E. **B,** Cytokeratin-7 immunostain highlights the presence of Paget's cells. *HER2*/neu immunostain displays 3+ (on a scale of 0 to 3+) cytoplasmic membrane reactivity in Paget's cells *(inset)*.

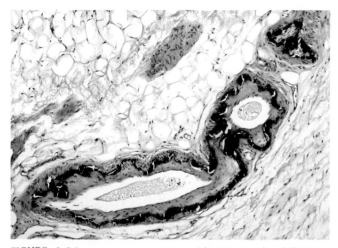

FIGURE 1-24 A mammary artery with intramural calcification. Annular intramural deposit of calcification is evident in the manner of Monckeberg's medial calcific sclerosis. H&E.

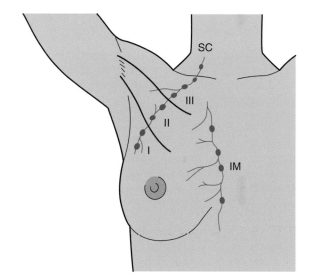

FIGURE 1-25 Lymphatic drainage of the breast. Schematic depiction of the breast and regional lymph nodes: axillary lymph nodes at levels I, II, and III (I, II, and III, respectively), supraclavicular lymph nodes (SC), and internal mammary lymph nodes (IM). The pectoralis minor muscle demarcates the various levels of axillary lymph nodes.

regions of the breast.[58] Axillary lymph nodes usually range from 20 to 30 in number, with an average of 24; however, up to 81 lymph nodes have been dissected from this group.[59] For years, conventional wisdom dictated that breast carcinoma involved the various levels of nodes in a stepwise fashion, progressing from levels 1 to 3. However, this traditional subdivision of axillary lymph nodes has been challenged by more recent studies that have studied the location of sentinel lymph nodes, that is, the first lymph nodes to receive lymphatic drainage from the breast.[60,61] Sentinel lymph nodes are seen at level 2 in up to 23% of patients, and metastases in level 3 lymph nodes only, skipping nodes at levels 1 and 2, are seen in about 2% to 3% of cases. Of note, sentinel lymph nodes are rarely found to be in extra-axillary locations and are generally encountered in cases in which the breast has been irradiated or prior axillary dissection has been undertaken.[62]

Intramammary lymph nodes, typically up to 1.5 cm in greatest extent, may be identified incidentally in breast biopsies or mastectomies performed for another

abnormality or may be identified as a density on mammogram.[63] In one series, intramammary lymph nodes were identified in 28% of mastectomies performed for operable breast carcinoma,[64] although in routine practice, these nodes are encountered in less than 1% of cases. Although up to 10% of these nodes can be positive for metastatic carcinoma, they may not be part of the usual lymphatic drainage system of the breast. Before diagnosing a positive intramammary lymph node, medullary carcinoma (with its prominent lymphoid response) must be considered in the differential diagnosis. A lymph node (regardless of its location) has a capsule, subcapsular sinus, and at least one well-formed lymphoid follicle. Intramammary lymph nodes are considered as axillary lymph nodes for staging purposes.

The **internal mammary lymph nodes** are located in the intercostal spaces, 2 to 3 cm from the edge of the

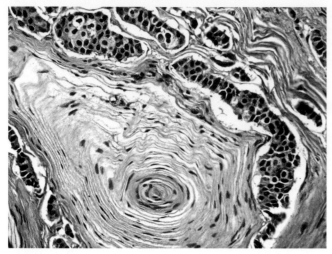

FIGURE 1-26 Pacinian corpuscle with invasive carcinoma. The onion-skin layering is characteristic of pacinian corpuscle (a type of mechanoreceptor nerve ending responsible for sensitivity to pain and pressure). Here, a receptor in the nipple is shown with invasive carcinoma surrounding it. H&E.

sternum in the endothoracic fascia—and are typically involved in carcinomas that are located in the upper-outer quadrant. **Supraclavicular lymph nodes** are classified as regional nodes and lie in the supraclavicular fossa, a triangle defined by the omohyoid muscle (laterally and superiorly), the internal jugular vein (medially), and the clavicle and subclavian vein (inferiorly). Involvement of the internal mammary nodes is staged as pN3b and that of the ipsilateral supraclavicular lymph nodes as pN3c. Lymphatic drainage to the contralateral breast has not been demonstrated, although metastases to contralateral axilla have been reported.

In the current staging system, N1 implies metastatic involvement of 1 to 3 lymph nodes; N2, 4 to 9 "positive" lymph nodes; and N3, 10 or more "positive" lymph nodes. As such, a lymph node dissection with a harvest of more than 10 lymph nodes should be considered to be adequate for staging purposes.

Nerve Supply

Nerve supply of the breast is derived from the anterior and lateral branches of the second to sixth intercostal (T2–6) nerves, which convey sensory and sympathetic efferent fibers. The nerve supply of the nipple is complex and is mainly from the anterior branch of the lateral cutaneous ramus of T4.[65] Most sensory fibers terminate close to the epidermis as free endings, serving to signal the process of suckling to the central nervous system. Despite its well-deserved reputation as being extremely "sensitive," relatively few nerves and nerve endings, including Meissner's light touch receptors (named after the 19th-century German physiologist) and Pacini's pressure corpuscles (named after the 19th-century Italian anatomist) are histologically identifiable in routinely prepared sections of the nipple. Rarely, these structures can exhibit tumoral involvement (Figure 1-26). Secretory activities of the breast are mainly under hormonal control rather than via efferent motor fibers.

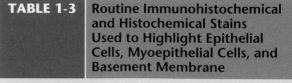

TABLE 1-3 Routine Immunohistochemical and Histochemical Stains Used to Highlight Epithelial Cells, Myoepithelial Cells, and Basement Membrane

Immunostains for Epithelial Cells

CKs 7, 8, 18, 19 (low-molecular-weight CKs).
CAM 5.2.
Alpha-lactalbumin (during secretory phase).
S-100 protein (sporadic).
bcl-2.
GCDFP-15, especially in apocrine metaplastic cells.
EMA reacts relatively strongly with apical region of active secretory cells.

Immunostains for Myoepithelial Cells

Smooth muscle actin.
SMM-HC.
Caldesmon.
Calponin.
CD10.
p63 (a p53 homologue with nuclear staining).
P-cadherin.
S-100 protein (variable reactivity).
Cytokeratins (CK5, CK5/6, CK14, CK17, 34betaE12: higher-molecular-weight cytokeratins).
14-3-3 sigma.
CK17 is usually positive in all *ductal* myoepithelial cells but is rarely positive in *lobular* myoepithelial cells.
ER, PgR, and AR are almost always negative in myoepithelial cells anywhere.

Immunostains for Basement Membrane (Basal Lamina)

Collagen IV.
Laminin.
Reticulin.

AR, androgen receptor; CAM, cell adhesion molecule; CK, cytokeratin; EMA, epithelial membrane antigen; ER, estrogen receptor; GCDFP, gross cystic disease fluid protein; PgR, progesterone receptor; SMM-HC, smooth muscle myosin–heavy chain.

Hormone Regulation

The breast is the target organ of a variety of hormones that are responsible for its physical development as well as the initiation and maintenance of lactation.[66–70]

Estrogen and progesterone production by the ovary at puberty influences the initial growth of the breast. Despite its predominant role, estrogen is unable to work independently of other hormones. Cyclic hormonal changes during each menstrual cycle alter the histology of mammary glands (Table 1-3). The breasts become swollen and somewhat "lumpy" in the latter half of the cycle. These changes are the physical manifestations of stromal edema and lobular proliferation. Strictly speaking, the use of the term "resting" breast in the premenopausal breast is incorrect because the breast is hardly ever entirely quiescent during these years. During pregnancy, the development of breast is further stimulated by the continuous production of estrogen and progesterone. In this period, the breast's growth is further influenced by prolactin, adrenal steroids, insulin, and growth hormone.

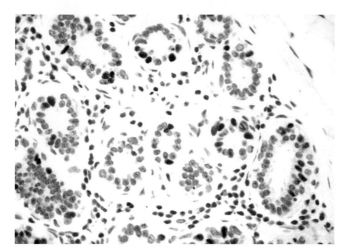

FIGURE 1-27 Estrogen receptor (ER) in a normal adult lobular unit. Approximately 15% of the glandular epithelial cells show ER reactivity, although there is slight variation in ER reactivity in various phases of the menstrual cycle. ER immunostain.

At delivery, the loss of placenta and degeneration of corpus luteum causes an abrupt drop in estrogen and progesterone levels. Milk production is then brought about by prolactin and adrenal cortical steroids. Suckling initiates impulses that act on the hypothalamus, resulting in the release of oxytocin in the posterior pituitary. Oxytocin stimulates the myoepithelial cells of the breast glands, causing them to contract and eject milk from the glands. Upon the cessation of feeding and end of the stimulation of suckling, secretion of milk ceases and the gland gradually reverts to an inactive state.

ER is positive in epithelial cells of mammary glands in 15% of cells, and PgR and AR are both sporadically positive in epithelial cells of ducts and lumen (Figure 1-27).[71] ER, PgR, and AR are almost always negative in myoepithelial cells. There is a higher frequency of ER-positivity in normal breast glandular cells during the proliferative phase of the menstrual cycle, and there is a higher frequency of PgR-positivity during the secretory phase. Oral contraceptive use decreases ER content of epithelial cells in the resting mammary epithelium.[72]

Two forms of ER, ER-α and ER-β, exist. ER-α can be demonstrated in nuclei of ductal and lobular epithelial cells; however, its expression varies with the phase of menstrual cycle and with the proliferative index. ER-β can be seen not only in ductal and lobular cells but also in myoepithelial and stromal cells. Relative levels of the two types of ER may have a potential, as yet unclear, role in breast carcinogenesis.[73]

Thelarche

The breast starts to develop upon the onset of puberty around the age of 11 years (range 9–14). This process of *thelarche* occurs mainly owing to the cyclic effect of estrogen and, to a lesser extent, of progesterone.[74] Other signs of puberty follow soon thereafter. During early adulthood, stromal growth is responsible for most of the increase in breast size. At puberty, the ducts lengthen and undergo repeated branching. The lobules,

and acini therein, proliferate. The connective tissue becomes denser, and adipose tissue starts to accumulate. Each menstrual cycle fosters progressive gland development, the individual glands not returning to the previous cycle's baseline. The gland proliferation continues until the mid-30s or so, and then plateaus until menopause, unless pregnancy ensues. The previously mentioned changes parallel the transformation of the physical contours of the breast (Figure 1-28).

Pregnancy and Lactation

Among mammals, human beings are unique in the relatively large size of their quiescent breast; however, as in other species, the ultimate structural maturation and functional activity of the human breast occur after the completion of pregnancy with the establishment of lactation.

The total weight gain of each breast during pregnancy is approximately 300 g. The principal changes in the breast in pregnancy are the hyperplasia and hypertrophy of alveoli in each lobule (Figure 1-29). The peak proliferative activity in glandular cells is observed during the first half of the pregnancy. The second half involves the maturation of the gland into a functional organ of lactation. With progression of pregnancy, the glandular cells become more vacuolated and secretions become evident in lumens of glands. The interglandular stroma becomes relatively attenuated. By the beginning of the third trimester, the lobules form grapelike clusters.[75,76]

With the onset of lactation, typically within 1 to 4 days after parturition, the epithelial cells appear vacuolated with a "hobnail" appearance (Figure 1-30). Luminal accumulation of secretions becomes readily evident. Milk production averages 1 to 2 mL/g of breast tissue per day. The rate of lactation is constant for the first 6 months after its onset. Lactation can continue for as long as 3½ years, as long as frequent suckling is maintained. Upon cessation of lactation, the process of involution takes a few (typically 3–4) months, although residual signs of lactation may be encountered for several months thereafter (Figure 1-31). The process of involution affects the individual acini and lobules at different rates. After lactation ends, the breasts tend to become pendulous as the parenchyma shrinks within the erstwhile stretched skin.

Microscopic foci of lactational-like changes in nonlactating and nonpregnant women can be encountered in up to 3% of breast biopsies.[77] The changes resemble those seen in the truly lactating breasts, except for the absence of abundant secretions in acinar lumen (Figure 1-32). Such lactational-like changes are typically uneven and only some acini in a lobule may be affected.

Milk

Human milk is a complex fluid, composed largely of water (88%), lactose (7%), fat (4%), protein (1%, chiefly casein and lactalbumin), and various minerals including potassium, calcium, sodium, and magnesium. Vitamins and antibodies (mainly immunoglobulin A [IgA]) are also present. Colostrum (milk of early lactation) is relatively richer in its antibody content.[78]

Menopause

The female breast undergoes gradual regression starting at the end of the fourth decade. The changes are much more evident in the terminal duct lobular unit. There is progressive lobular atrophy. Ducts become variably ecstatic and there is an increase in stromal fat deposition. The regressive process continues until menopause (which typically occurs some 10 yr later) and beyond.[79] The morphologic pattern in the elderly may ultimately resemble the male breast; however, most menopausal women produce enough endogenous estrogen to maintain some remnants of lobules.

Male Breast

The adult male breast consists mainly of large ducts without lobule formation. The ducts, which generally do not extend beyond the central subareolar portion of

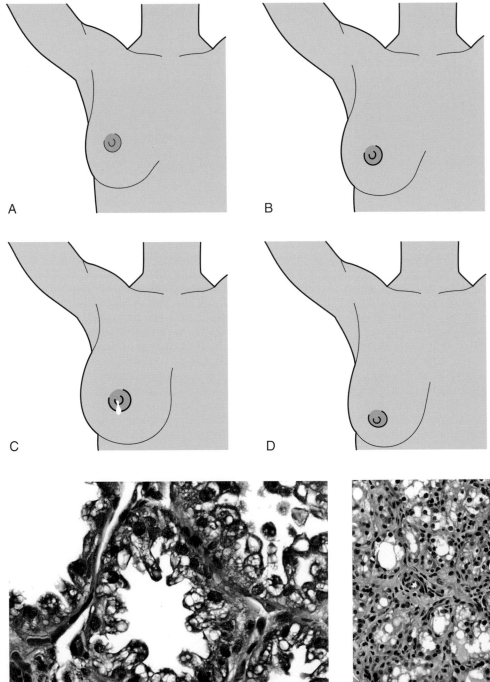

A

B

C

D

FIGURE 1-28 Changes in contour of breast at various phases. Schematic drawing illustrates contour of the breast in a typical adult **(A)**, fuller contour in midpregnancy **(B)**, rounded contour in lactation **(C)**, and droop contour in postmenopause **(D)**.

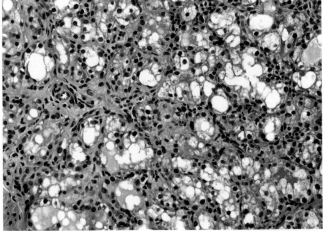

FIGURE 1-29 Breast in midpregnancy. Acinar cells have a hobnail appearance with vacuolated cytoplasm. Note the absence of luminal secretions. H&E.

FIGURE 1-30 Lactating breast. The acini are expanded with accumulation of secretions. Acinar epithelia appear finely vacuolated. H&E.

the male breast, are embedded amid varying amounts of fibrous stroma and adipose tissue. The ducts are lined by a single layer of low cuboidal epithelium that lies on an inconspicuous myoepithelial cell layer. Lobule formation is only rarely encountered in male breasts.

Slight physiologic enlargement occurs at puberty, and in the elderly, due to androgen-estrogenic imbalance. Gynecomastia at puberty is common and affects the majority of boys.

DEVELOPMENTAL DISORDERS

A variety of developmental anomalies affect the breast. Some of these abnormalities preclude functioning of the breast (e.g., amastia), others hamper its optimal functioning (e.g., inverted nipple), whereas some merely pose a cosmetic problem (e.g., polythelia and asymmetry). A variety of morphologic abnormalities, without any functional deficit, may be considered to be deformities. These include the so-called Snoopy-nose breast or tubular breast in which the breast resembles the shape of a tuberous plant root.

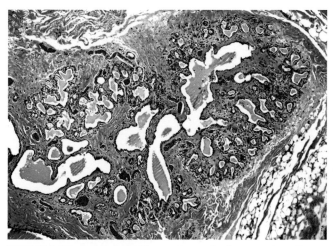

FIGURE 1-31 Involution of breast 1 month after cessation of lactation. Acini are dilated with accumulation of secretions. H&E.

Some degree of physiologic breast asymmetry is the rule rather than the exception. Asymmetry is common during breast growth and may persist into adulthood in approximately 5% of cases.[80,81] Asymmetry may be related to handedness. The left breast is usually larger than the right. A number of conditions, including developmental disorders, surgery, radiation, and trauma, may produce asymmetry. In states of extreme malnutrition or emaciation, the breasts may reduce in size, and such reductions in size are not always symmetrical. Abnormalities of development account for most cases of obvious breast asymmetry. Threshold for acceptance of asymmetry differs with each woman. Biopsy of either of the asymmetrical breasts should not be undertaken for cosmetic reasons alone, until full development has been achieved, because of the likelihood of permanent breast damage.[82] Differences in size or length of its extension into the axilla are regarded as variations and not disorders. True disorders of breast include those instances in which breast tissue is absent or hypoplastic or where there are accessory breasts or nipples.

Amastia

Amastia is an extremely rare condition in which the normal growth of the breast and nipple does not occur following the complete failure of mammary line development at around 6 weeks in utero.[83] This disorder has been literally known since biblical times, and its first recorded reference is in Song of Solomon "We have a little sister, and she hath no breasts" (VIII:8).

Amastia is the complete failure of the breast to develop. This is an exceedingly uncommon abnormality and may be accompanied by a variety of developmental defects including those of shoulder and chest. Amastia has also been reported in association with skeletal (mainly of the ulnar rays of the hand) and renal defects and is known to occur in siblings.[84,85]

Ulnar mammary syndrome (UMS) is a rare pleiotropic autosomal disorder characterized by the classical findings of ulnar defects, mammary and apocrine gland hypoplasia, and genital abnormalities. Having mapped

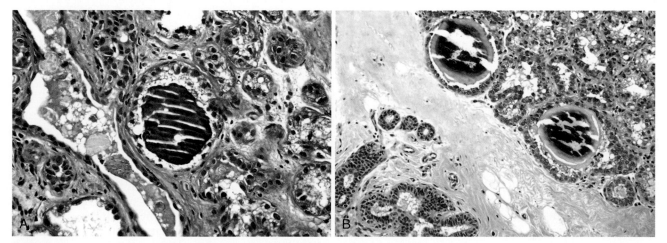

FIGURE 1-32 Focal lactational and pregnancy-like change in a nonpregnant nonlactating woman. Secretory changes are present in a lobule with acinar cells appearing variably vacuolated. **A,** Characteristic laminated calcifications are present. **B,** Adjacent lobule is inactive. H&E.

the UMS locus in one kindred to 12q23-24.1, Bamishad and associates[86] identified the *TBX3* as the causal gene for UMS. *TBX3* is a member of the T-box gene family. The products of the latter are transcription factors that have been shown to be crucial in embryologic development of various organs including the pituitary gland and the heart with obvious implications for their appropriate morphogenesis.

Poland sequence, a usually sporadic and unilateral condition, represents the major differential diagnosis of isolated amastia. The two conditions can be clinically confused unless the absence of pectoralis major muscle is identified via ultrasound examination. Athelia tends to occur unilaterally as part of the Poland sequence and bilaterally in certain types of ectodermal dysplasias. Isolated absence of the breast could be related to a vascular disruption sequence as suggested by Bianca and coworkers.[87]

Hypoplasia

Hypoplasia refers to a major difference in breast size relative to the other, beyond the slight asymmetry that occurs normally. Hypoplasia of breast can be unilateral or bilateral, and it can occur as a congenital defect or it may[88] be associated with carcinoma.[89]

Congenital mammary hypoplasia is associated with hypoplasia of the ipsilateral pectoral muscle in 90% of cases. *Acquired mammary hypoplasia* has been commonly encountered in patients who had been irradiated in the mammary region before puberty for cutaneous hemangiomas (and also in the distant past for secretion of witch's milk!). Generally, the degree of mammary hypoplasia correlates with the radiation dose.[90,91] Surgical excision of the developing mammary gland should be performed only in rare cases in which a neoplasm is highly suspected.

Appropriate caution should be exercised to avoid the breast area in surgical incisions on the chest of female children undergoing corrective surgery for congenital heart defects.[92] Other types of injury or trauma, including those related to dog bites,[93] burns, and seat belts, have resulted in restricted breast growth. A wide range of nipple and breast abnormalities can be associated with Becker's hairy pigmented nevus.[94]

That trauma to the breast before thelarche resulted in failure of the breast to develop was apparently known to the fictional Amazonian (*a maz* meaning "without breast") nation. This nation was composed of independent women who had trauma inflicted to the right breast at a tender age to retard its development in order to gain competitive advantage in combat, mainly archery.

Polymastia

The "milk line" (see earlier) usually undergoes regression in fetal life. Persistence of portions of accessory mammary glandular tissue along the milk line (polymastia) is encountered in up to 3% of adult women (and exists in more than one location in about one third of these cases). Polymastia is most commonly identified in the axilla. Other common locations include the inframammary fold and the vulva.[95] There appears to be a left-sided preponderance.

The entire spectrum of breast diseases from fibrocystic changes to carcinoma can occur in the accessory breast tissue in these locations.[96,97] The most common presentation of polymastia is an axillary lump with pain or tenderness (particularly premenstrual). Occasionally, bulky polymastia can cause a significant cosmetic problem. Polymastia when associated with a nipple may function during pregnancy.[98] Polymastia is reportedly more common in people of Asian ancestry and was noted to occur in 5.2% of Japanese women more than a century ago.[99]

Supernumerary Nipple

Supernumerary or accessory nipple (polythelia) is the most common mammary anomaly to be identified in either gender. It occurs along the milk line and has been found in up to 2.4% of neonates.[100,101]

Owing to deeper pigmentation, accessory nipples are not always recognized for what they are and are commonly mistaken for nevi, achrochordon, or cutaneous fibroma. Accessory nipples are most commonly encountered below the breast on the left chest. Multiple nipples have been reported to occur within one areola.[102] They may occasionally enlarge during pregnancy or lactation. Histologically, the supernumerary nipples may show any or all of the features typically observed in the area of nipple including epidermal thickening, pilosebaceous units, smooth muscle, and mammary ducts.[103]

Aberrant Breast

The presence of mammary glandular parenchyma beyond the usual anatomic extent of the breast or of the milk line is referred to as *aberrant breast*. Neither nipple nor areola is formed in the aberrant tissue, and the tissue remains clinically inapparent unless it become the site of a physiologic (hypertrophic and/or hyperplastic) or pathologic process. The mammary glands in aberrant breast tissue are histologically indistinguishable from that of the native breast and may undergo changes similar to those encountered in the orthotopic organ, including almost all physiologic and pathologic changes. The extremely rare occurrence of aberrant breast tissue within axillary lymph nodes may be mistaken for metastatic carcinoma.[104]

Macromastia

Macromastia refers to inappropriate excessive growth of the breast. It can occur in adolescence, in pregnancy, or in an iatrogenic (i.e., medication) setting.

Adolescent macromastia occurs, as the name implies, at puberty. The breasts undergo a massive increase in size over several months. This is a bilateral disease and is usually (but not always) symmetrical. Histologically, the breast tissue shows mainly increase in stromal tissue with pseudoangiomatous stromal hyperplasia (PASH) and may also show some degree of epithelial hyperplasia.

Gravid macromastia most commonly occurs in early pregnancy and usually affects women in their first pregnancy. This is a rare disease, occurring in 1 in 10,000 pregnant women.[105] Obviously related to the hormonal gush that occurs in early pregnancy (and possibly related to inordinate sensitivity of breast tissue to this surge), both breasts undergo quick enlargement. Extremely rapid enlargement of breast tissue may erode the overlying skin—a clinical scenario that may require mastectomy for local control. Gravid macromastia may recur in subsequent pregnancies. The chance of recurrence is reduced by reduction mammoplasty that is best performed between pregnancies. Histologically, the breast tissue shows mainly increased dense stromal tissue with PASH.

Iatrogenic macromastia is the excessive growth of breast tissue related to medications. Two drugs that have been most often related to macromastia are penicillamine (mainly used in rheumatoid arthritis) and indinavir (an antiretroviral medication used for the treatment of human immunodeficiency virus infection). Use of cyclosporine, marijuana, and cimetidine may also lead to unilateral or bilateral breast enlargement.

Other Disorders of the Breast

Premature thelarche is breast development before puberty. *Precocious puberty* is breast development accompanied by other signs of puberty. *Adolescent* or *juvenile hypertrophy* is the postpubertal continuation of unilateral or bilateral breast development in which the gland undergoes massive enlargement (≤8 kg each). Instances of *accessory nipples occurring in a familial setting* have been reported.[106–108] *Inverted nipple* is a developmental disorder that results in a permanently retracted nipple that causes difficulty in suckling. *Athelia* is the least commonly encountered mammary anomaly. *Amazia* is a term used when breast tissue is absent but the nipple is present.

Multiple physiologic abnormalities (some due to anatomic causes), including delayed onset and galactorrhea, may occur during lactation. *Delayed onset of lactation* may be due to lack of suckling, obesity, or hormonal problems (including increased progesterone levels due to retained placenta). *Galactorrhea* is generally defined as inappropriate secretion of milk in the absence of pregnancy or feeding for a period of 6 months (a pituitary prolactinoma is the usual primary suspect in such cases).

Occasional reports of seemingly inexplicable mammary abnormalities such as presence of ectopic breast tissue in the posterior thigh of a male, "mammae erraticae," have been reported.[109]

SUMMARY

A variety of glandular and stromal alterations, including stromal fibrosis and cyst formation, which were previously referred to as fibrocystic "disease," overlap with normal physiologic adjustments or adaptations in morphology. These "changes" lie at the borderline of pathologic states. In recent years, appropriately enough, there has been a diminished emphasis on the word "disease" in the context of such alterations.[110] Thus, histology of the "normal" breast, in some respects, is a relative term.

The normal histology of the breast has, thus far, been largely defined via routinely prepared hematoxylin and eosin–stained sections and selected immunohistochemical stains. This is bound to change as molecular techniques (including laser capture microdissection) are increasingly used to study "normal" and abnormal breast tissue. Already, there is cumulative evidence that histologically inactive breast tissue can exhibit abnormal genotype either by virtue of loss of heterozygosity or allelic imbalance.[111–114] Studies of "normal" breast tissue may also elucidate the presence of the hitherto elusive progenitor stem cells, which could lead to understanding of its role in various physiologic processes and pathologic conditions of the breast.[115,116]

Several recent evolutionary changes in surgical practice have influenced the practice of surgical pathology. These include sentinel lymph node biopsy, high-definition surgery with magnified three-dimensional view of the operative field,[117] and nipple-sparing mastectomy. These changes require that the surgical pathologist possesses an intimate knowledge of normal anatomy and histology of the breast.

There is scant evidence to support the oft-repeated (and perhaps oversimplified) contention that "the breast is a modified sweat gland."[118] In a forceful rebuttal, Ackerman and colleagues[119] took the contrary view that the breast is a distinctive region of the skin and subcutaneous tissue stating that "one thing is certain: the breast is not a sweat gland or a modified sweat gland, as should be apparent both intellectually and esthetically." Be that as it may, the breast is a specialized organ that is quite unique, histologically and in many other respects.

REFERENCES

1. Winberg J. Mother and newborn baby: mutual regulation of physiology and behavior—a selective review. Dev Psychobiol 2005;47:217-229.
2. Anbazhagan R, Osin PP, Bartkova J, et al. The development of epithelial phenotypes in the human fetal and infant breast. J Pathol 1998;184:197-206.
3. Hovey RC, Trott JF. Morphogenesis of mammary gland development. Adv Exp Med Biol 2004;554:219-228.
4. Osborne MP. Breast anatomy and development. In Harris JR, Lippman ME, Morrow M, eds. Diseases of the Breast. Philadelphia: Lippincott Williams & Wilkins; 2010; pp. 3-13.
5. Osin PP, Anbazhagan R, Bartkova J, et al. Breast development gives insights into breast disease. Histopathology 1998;33:275-283.
6. Sternlicht MD. Key stages in mammary gland development. The cues that regulate ductal branching morphogenesis. Breast Cancer Res 2006;8:201-212.
7. Anderson TJ. Normal breast. Myths, realities, and prospects. Mod Pathol 1998;11:115-119.
8. Goodrich WA Jr. The Cleopatra view in xeromammography: a semi-reclining position for the tail of the breast. Radiology 1978;128:811-812.
9. Kent JC, Mitoulas L, Cox DB, et al. Breast volume and milk production during extended lactation in women. Exp Physiol 1989;84:435-440.
10. Smith DJ, Palin WE, Katch VL, Bennett JE. Breast volume and anthropomorphic measurements: normal values. Plast Reconstr Surg 1986;78:331-335.

11. Smith DM Jr, Peters TG, Donegan WI. Montgomery's areolar tubercle. A light microscopic study. Arch Pathol Lab Med 1982;106:60-63.

12. Cady B. How to perform adequate local excision of mammographically detected lesions. Surg Oncol Clin North Am 1997;6:315-334.

13. Going JJ, Moffat DF. Escaping from the flat land: clinical and biological aspects of human mammary duct anatomy in three dimensions. J Pathol 2004;203:538-544.

14. Moffat DF, Going JJ. Three dimensional anatomy of complete duct systems in human breast: pathological and developmental implications. J Clin Pathol 1996;49:48-52.

15. Ohtake T, Kimjima I, Fukushima T, et al. Computer-assisted complete three-dimensional reconstruction of the mammary ductal/lobular systems. Cancer 2001;91:2263-2272.

16. Wellings SR, Jensen HM, Marcum RG. An atlas of subgross pathology of the human breast with special reference to possible precancerous lesions. J Natl Cancer Inst 1975;55:231-273.

17. Love SM, Barsky SH. Anatomy of the nipple and breast ducts revisited. Cancer 2004;101:1947-1957.

18. Bussolati G, Cassoni P, Ghisolfi G, et al. Immunolocalization and gene expression of oxytocin receptors in carcinomas and non-neoplastic tissues of the breast. Am J Pathol 1996;148:1895-1903.

19. Adriance MC, Inman JL, Petersen OW, Bissell MJ. Myoepithelial cells: good fences make good neighbors. Breast Cancer Res 2005;7:190-197.

20. Clement PB, Azzopardi JG. Microglandular adenosis of the breast—a lesion simulating tubular carcinoma. Histopathology 1983;7:169-180.

21. Rosen PP. Microglandular adenosis: a benign lesion simulating invasive mammary carcinoma. Am J Surg Pathol 1983;7:137-144.

22. Cserni G. Lack of myoepithelium in apocrine glands of the breast does not necessarily imply malignancy. Histopathology 2008;52:253-254.

23. Prasad ML, Hyjek E, Giri DD, et al. Double immunolabelling with cytokeratin and smooth muscle actin in confirming early invasive carcinoma of breast. Am J Surg Pathol 1999;23:176-181.

24. Gram IT, Funkhouser E, Tabar L. The Tabar classification of mammographic parenchymal patterns. Eur J Radiol 1997;24:131-136.

25. Wellings SR, Wolfe JN. Correlative studies of the histological and radiographic appearance of the breast parenchyma. Radiology 1978;129:299-306.

26. White E, Velentgas P, Mandelson MT, et al: Variation in mammographic breast density by time in menstrual cycle among women aged 40-49. J Natl Cancer Inst 1998;90:906-910.

27. Eusebi V, Damiani S, Losi L, Millis RR. Apocrine differentiation in breast epithelium. Adv Anat Pathol 1997;4:139-155.

28. Lendrum AC. On the "pink" epithelium of the cystic breast and staining of its granules. Pathol Bacteriol 1945;57:267-272.

29. Tornos C, Silva E, el-Naggar A, Pritzker KP. Calcium oxalate crystals in breast biopsies. The missing microcalcifications. Am J Surg Pathol 1990;14:961-968.

30. Barwick K, Kashgarian M, Rosen PP. Clear cell change within duct and lobular epithelium of the human breast. Pathol Annu 1982;17:319-328.

31. Tavassoli FA, Yeh IT. Lactational and clear cell changes of the breast in nonlactating, nonpregnant women. Am J Clin Pathol 1987;87:23-29.

32. Vina M, Wells CA. Clear cell metaplasia of the breast: a lesion showing eccrine differentiation. Histopathology 1989;15:85-92.

33. Damiani S, Cattani MG, Buonamici L, Eusebi V. Mammary foam cells. Characterization by immunohistochemistry and in situ hybridization. Virchows Arch 1998;432:433-440.

34. Avies JD. Pigmented periductal cells (ochrocytes) in mammary dysplasias: their nature and significance. J Pathol 1974;114:205-218.

35. Rosen PP. Multinucleated mammary stromal giant cells: a benign lesion that simulates invasive carcinoma. Cancer 1979;44:1305–1308.

36. Farahmand S, Cowan DF. Elastosis in the normal aging breast. Arch Pathol Lab Med 1991;115:1241-1246.

37. Garijo MF, Val D, Val-Bernal JF. An overview of the pale and clear cells of the nipple epidermis. Histol Histopathol 2009;24:367-376.

38. Toker C. Clear cells of the nipple epidermis. Cancer 1970;25:601-610.

39. Nofech-Mozes S, Hanna W. Toker cells revisited. Breast J 2009;15:394-398.

40. Kohler S, Rouse RV, Smoller BR. The differential diagnosis of pagetoid cells in the epidermis. Mod Pathol 1998;11:79-92.

41. Lundquist K, Kohler S, Rouse RV: Intraepidermal cytokeratin 7 expression is not restricted to Paget cells but is also seen in Toker cells and Merkel cells. Am J Surg Pathol 1999;23:212-219.

42. Yao DX, Hoda SA, Chiu A, et al: Intraepidermal cytokeratin-7 immunoreactive cells in the non-neoplastic nipple may represent intraepithelial extension of lactiferous duct cells. Histopathology 2002;40:230-236.

43. Zeng Z, Melamed J, Symmans PJ, et al: Benign proliferative nipple duct lesions frequently contain CAM 5.2 and anti-cytokeratin 7 immunoreactive cells in the overlying epidermis. Am J Surg Pathol 1999;23:1349-1355.

44. Schnitt SJ, Goldwyn RM, Slavin SA. Mammary ducts in the areola: implications for patients undergoing surgery of the breast. Plast Reconstr Surg 1993;92:1290-1293.

45. Brachtel EF, Rusby JE, Michaelson JS, et al. Occult nipple involvement in breast cancer: clinicopathologic findings in 316 consecutive mastectomy specimens. J Clin Oncol 2009;27:4948-4954.

46. Rosen PP, Tench W. Lobules in the nipple. Pathol Annu 1985;20:317-322.

47. Rosen PP: Anatomy and physiologic morphology. In Rosen PP, ed. Rosen's Breast Pathology. 3rd ed. Phildelphia: Lippincott Williams & Wilkins; 2009:1-21.

48. Tannenbaum M, Weiss M, Marx AJ. Ultrastructure of the human mammary ductule. Cancer 1969;23:958-978.

49. Van Deventer PV, Page BJ, Graewe FR. Vascular anatomy of the breast and nipple-areola complex. Plast Reconstr Surg 2008;121:1861-1862.

50. Wong MS, Kim J, Yeung C, Williams SH. Breast necrosis following left internal mammary artery harvest: a case series and a comprehensive review of the literature. Ann Plast Surg 2008;61:368-374.

51. Naccarato AG, Viacava P, Bocci G, et al. Definition of the microvascular pattern of the normal human adult mammary gland. J Anat 2003;203:599-603.

52. Cunningham L. The anatomy of the arteries and veins of the breast. J Surg Oncol 1997;9:71-85.

53. Zgheib MH, Buchbinder SS, Abi Rafeh N, et al. Breast arterial calcifications on mammograms do not predict coronary heart disease at coronary angiography. Radiology 2010;254:367-373.

54. McNamara MP, Boden T. Pseudoaneurysm of the breast related to 18G core biopsy: successful repair using thrombin injection. AJR Am J Roentgenol 2002;179:924-926.

55. Entourgie SH, Niewig OE, Valdes Olmos RA, et al. Lymphatic drainage patterns from the breast. Ann Surg 2004;239:232-237.

56. Tanis PJ, Niewig OE, Olmos RAV, Kroon BBR. Anatomy and physiology of lymphatic drainage of the breast from the perspective of sentinel node biopsy. J Am Coll Surg 2001;192:399-409.

57. Berg JW. The significance of axillary node levels in the study of breast carcinoma. Cancer 1955;8:776-778.

58. Chandawarkar RY, Shinde SR. Interpectoral nodes in carcinoma of the breast: requiem or resurrection. J Surg Oncol 1996;62:158-161.

59. Fisher B, Slack NH. Number of lymph nodes examined and the prognosis of breast carcinoma. Surg Gynecol Obstet 1970;131:79-88.

60. Lee AH, Ellis IO, Pinder SE, et al. Pathological assessment of sentinel lymph node biopsies in patients with breast cancer. Virchows Arch 2000;436:97-101.

61. McMasters KM, Giuliano AE, Ross MI, et al. Sentinel lymph node biopsy for breast cancer—not yet standard of care. N Engl J Med 1998;339:990-995.

62. Cody HS 3rd. Clinical significance and management of extra-axillary sentinel lymph nodes: worthwhile or irrelevant? Surg Oncol Clin North Am 2010;19:507-517.

63. Jadusingh IH. Intramammary lymph nodes. J Clin Pathol 1992;45:1023-1026.
64. Egan RL, McSweeney MB. Intramammary lymph nodes. Cancer 1983;51:1838-1842.
65. Jaspers JJP, Posma AN, van Immerseel AAH, Gittenberger-de Groot AC: The cutaneous innervations of the female breast and nipple-areola complex: implications for surgery. Br J Plast Surg 1997;50:249-259.
66. Fanager H, Ree HJ. Cyclic changes of human mammary gland epithelium in relation to the menstrual cycle–an ultrastructural study. Cancer 1974;34:574-585.
67. Longacre TA, Bartow SA. A correlative morphologic study of human breast and endometrium in the menstrual cycle. Am J Pathol 1981;104:23-34.
68. Olsson H, Jernstrom H, Alm P, et al: Proliferation of the breast epithelium in relation to menstrual cycle phase, hormonal use, and reproductive factors. Breast Cancer Res Treat 1996;40:187-196.
69. Ramakrishnan R, Khan SA, Badve S. Morphological changes in breast tissue with menstrual cycle. Mod Pathol 2002;15:1348-1356.
70. Vogel PM, Georgiade NC, Fetter BE, et al. The correlation of histologic changes in the human breast with the menstrual cycle. Am J Pathol 1981;104:23-34.
71. Shoker BS, Jarvis C, Sibson DR, et al. Oestrogen receptor expression in the normal and precancerous breast. J Pathol 1999;188:237-244.
72. Williams G, Anderson E, Howell A, et al. Oral contraceptive (OCP) use increases proliferation and decreases oestrogen receptor content of epithelial cells in the normal human breast. Int J Cancer 1991;48:206-210.
73. Shaaban AM, O'Neill PA, Davies MP, et al. Declining estrogen receptor-beta expression defines malignant progression of human breast neoplasia. Am J Surg Pathol 2003;27:1502-1512.
74. Monaghan P, Perusinghe NP, Cowen P, Gusterson BA. Peripubertal human breast development. Anat Rec 1990;226:501-508.
75. Battersby S, Anderson TJ. Proliferative and secretory activity in the pregnant and lactating human breast. Virchows Arch (A) 1988;413:189-196.
76. Battersby S, Anderson TJ. Histological changes in breast tissue that characterize recent pregnancy. Histopathology 1989;15:415-433.
77. Kiaer HW, Andersen JA. Focal pregnancy-like changes in the breast. Acta Pathol Microbiol Scand 1977;85:931-941.
78. Walker A. Breast milk as the gold standard for protective nutrients. J Pediatr 2010;156(2 Suppl):S3-S7.
79. Cowan DF, Herbert TA. Involution of the breast in women aged 50-104 years: a histopathologic study of 102 cases. Surg Pathol 1989;2:323-324.
80. Pitanguy I. Surgical treatment of breast hypertrophy. Br J Plast Surg 1967;20:78-85.
81. Rees TD. Mammary asymmetry. Clin Plast Surg 1975;2:371-374.
82. Simon BE, Hoffman S, Kahn S. Treatment of asymmetry of the breasts. Clin Plast Surg 1975;2:375-390.
83. Trier WC. Complete breast absence. Case report and review of the literature. Plast Reconstr Surg 1965;36:430-439.
84. Kowlessar M, Orti E. Complete breast absence in siblings. Am J Dis Child 1968;115:9-92.
85. Linden H, Williams R, King J, Blair E, Kini U. Ulnar mammary syndrome and TBX3: expanding the phenotype. Am Med Genet Part A 2010;149A:2809-2812.
86. Bamishad M, Lin RC, Law DJ, et al. Mutations in human TBX3 alter limb, apocrine and genital development in ulnar-mammary syndrome. Nat Genet 1997;16:311-315.
87. Bianca S, Licciardello M, Barrano B, Ettore G. Isolated congenital amastia: a subclavian artery supply disruption sequence. Am J Med Genet Part A 2010;152A:792-794.
88. Haramis HT, Collins RE. Unilateral breast atrophy. Plast Reconstr Surg 1995;95:916-919.
89. Funicello A, De Sandre R, Salloum L, et al. Infiltrating ductal carcinoma of the hypomastic breast: a case report. Am Surg 1998;64:1037-1039.
90. Furst CJ, Ludell M, Ahlback SO, Holm LE. Breast hypoplasia following irradiation of the female breast in infancy and early childhood. Acta Oncol 1989;28:519-523.
91. Kolar J, Bek V, Vrabec R. Hypoplasia of the growing breast after contact x-ray therapy for cutaneous angiomas. Arch Dermatol 1967;96:427-430.
92. Cherup LL, Siewers RD, Futrell SW. Breast and pectoral muscle maldevelopment after anterolateral and posterolateral thoracotomies I children. Ann Thorac Surg 1986;41:492-497.
93. Miyata N, Abe S. Dog-bite injuries to the breast in children: deformities to secondary sex characteristics and their repair in an extended follow-up. Ann Plast Surg 1999;43:542-545.
94. Urbani CE, Betti R. Polythelia with Becker's nevus. Dermatology 1998;196:251-252.
95. Levin N, Diener RL. Bilateral ectopic breast of the vulva. Report of a case. Obstet Gynecol 1968;32:274-276.
96. Levin M, Pakarakas HA, Chang M, et al. Primary breast carcinoma of the vulva. A case report and review of the literature. Gynecol Oncol 1995;56:448-451.
97. Page RN, Dittrich L, King R, et al. Syringomatous adenoma of the nipple occurring within a supernumerary breast: a case report. J Cutan Pathol 2009;36:1206-1209.
98. Viera AJ. Breast feeding with ectopic axillary breast tissue. Mayo Clin Proc 1999;74:1021-1022.
99. Iwai T. A statistical study on the polymastia of the Japanese. Lancet 1907;2:753-759.
100. DeCholnoky T. Supernumerary breast. Arch Surg 1939;39:926-941.
101. Kenny RD, Filippo JK, Black EB. Supernumerary nipples and anomalies in neonates. Am J Dis Child 1987;141:987-988.
102. Abramson DT. Bilateral intraareolar polythelia. Arch Surg 1975;110:1255.
103. Mehregan AH. Supernumerary nipple. A histologic study. J Cutan Pathol 1981;8:96-104.
104. Kadowaki M, Nagashima T, Sakata H, et al. Ectopic breast tissue in axillary lymph node. Breast Cancer 2007;14:425-428.
105. Beischer NA, Hueston JH, Pepperell RJ. Massive hypertrophy of the breasts in pregnancy: report of 3 cases and review of literature. Obstet Gynecol Surv 1989;44:234-243.
106. Toumbis-Ioannou E, Cohen PR. Familial polythelia. J Am Acad Dermatol 1994;30:667-668.
107. Cellini A, Offidavi A. Familial supernumerary nipples and breasts. Dermatology 1992;185:56-58.
108. Benmously-Mlika R, Deghais S, Bchetnia M, et al. Supernumerary nipples in association with Hailey-Hailey disease in a Tunisian family. Dermatol Online J 2008;14:15.
109. Camisa C. Accessory breast on the posterior thigh of a man. J Am Acad Dermatol 1980;3:467-469.
110. Love SM, Gelman RS, Silen W. Fibrocystic "disease" of the breast—a nondisease? N Engl J Med 1982;307:1010-1014.
111. Lakhani SR, Chaggar R, Davies S, et al. Genetic alterations in "normal" luminal and myoepithelial cells of the breast. J Pathol 1999;189:496-503.
112. Deng G, Lu Y, Zlotnikov G, et al. Loss of heterozygosity in normal tissue adjacent to breast carcinomas. Science 1996;274:2057-2059.
113. Larson PS, de las Morenas A, Bennett SR, et al. Loss of heterozygosity or allelic imbalance in histologically normal breast epithelium is distinct from loss of heterozygosity or allele imbalance in coexisting carcinomas. Am J Pathol 2002;161:283-290.
114. Perou CM, Jeffrey SS, van de Rijn M, et al. Distinctive gene expression patterns in human mammary epithelial cells and breast cancers. Proc Natl Acad Sci U S A 1999;96:9212-9217.
115. Bocker W, Moll R, Poremba C. Common adult stem cells in the human breast give rise to glandular and myoepithelial cell lineages: a new cell biological concept. Lab Invest 2002;82:737-746.
116. Hiclakivi-Clarke L, de Assis S. Fetal origins of breast cancer. Trends Endocrinol Metab 2006;17:340-348.
117. Lim SM, Kum CK, Lam FL. Nerve-sparing axillary dissection using the da Vinci Surgical System. World J Surg 2005;29:1352-1355.
118. Rosai J. Breast. In Rosai J, ed. Ackerman's Surgical Pathology. 8th ed. Philadephia: Mosby; 1996; p. 1565.
119. Ackermann AB, Kessler G, Gyorfi T, et al. Contrary view. The breast is not an organ per se, but a distinctive region of skin and subcutaneous tissue. Am J Dermatopathol 2007;29:211-218.

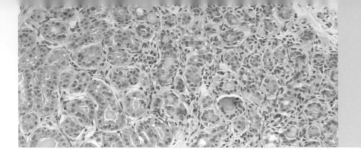

2

Reactive and Inflammatory Conditions of the Breast

Noel Weidner • David J. Dabbs

INTRODUCTION

Benign, reactive and inflammatory tumorous conditions of the breast are the most common reasons why patients undergo breast biopsies. Benign conditions account for the majority of breast biopsies, and reactive or inflammatory conditions comprise the majority of pathologic findings in this category. Inflammatory related changes and reactive changes that mimic neoplasia are commonly seen in fibrocystic changes (FCC), but FCC is discussed in Chapter 18. Conditions discussed here are less common than FCC, but nevertheless are often seen in daily practice, even in general surgical pathology services. It is important to recognize the gross and microscopic versions of these lesions to effect appropriate treatment and avoid the pitfalls of these lesions that may mimic neoplasia.

MAMMARY DUCT ECTASIA

Clinical Presentation

Mammary duct ectasia has been reported under many descriptors (e.g., varicocele tumor, comedomastitis, periductal mastitis, plasma cell mastitis, stale-milk mastitis, chemical mastitis, granulomatous mastitis, and mas obliterans) (Figure 2-1).[1]

Most cases occur in premenopausal parous women, possibly caused by duct obstruction and/or triggered by different components of stagnant colostrum. It may produce retraction or inversion of the nipple, and nipple discharge is present in approximately 20% of patients.

> **KEY CLINICAL FEATURES**
> ***Mammary Duct Ectasia***
>
> - Usually occurs in premenopausal parous women.
> - Likely caused by duct obstruction and/or stagnant colostrum.
> - Produces nipple retraction, inversion, or discharge in approximately 20% of patients.

Microscopic Pathology

This is a disorder that affects large ducts of the breast, so there is ectasia of large ducts, with accumulation of detritus in the lumen and fibrous thickening of the wall, which contains an increased amount of elastic fibers. Calcification is common, producing tubular, annular, and linear shadows on the mammogram. There is no epithelial hyperplasia or apocrine metaplasia. If there is epithelial denudation, the luminal material may escape from the duct, and a florid inflammatory reaction results, which is rich in macrophages and plasma cells.

In advanced stages of mammary duct ectasia, fibrous obliteration of the ducts can occur. Indeed, ductitis obliterans or mastitis obliterans is a rare late manifestation of mammary ductal ectasia. Indeed, Wang and coworkers[2] reported a long-term diabetic patient who presented with bilateral bloody nipple discharge and poorly defined nodularities around the nipple of both breasts. The ductography showed multiple segments of irregular ductal narrowing and intraluminal filling defects in both breasts. The bilateral resection of the subareolar portion of the breast showed exuberant fibrous obliteration of the large- and medium-sized ducts by granulation tissue associated with few histiocytes. Ductal dilatation and intraductal accumulation of histiocytes were also present. This represents a late and florid form of mammary ductal ectasia.

Treatment and Prognosis

Excision biopsy should be curative. Recurrence is uncommon.

Differential Diagnosis

Differential diagnostic considerations include fibrocystic changes, diabetic sclerosing lymphocytic lobulitis, idiopathic granulomatous lobular mastitis, and periareolar abscess (Zuska's disease). Accurate diagnosis can help avoid or limit radical surgeries in this group of patients. Mammary duct ectasia is likely unrelated to fibrocystic disease, but duct ectasia may be related to breast abscesses, which usually result from rupture of mammary ducts. They most often occur during lactation but also independently from it.[3,4] Abscesses may also be located deep within the parenchyma or periareolar region.[5] Microscopically, a central cavity filled with neutrophils and secretion is surrounded by inflamed and eventually

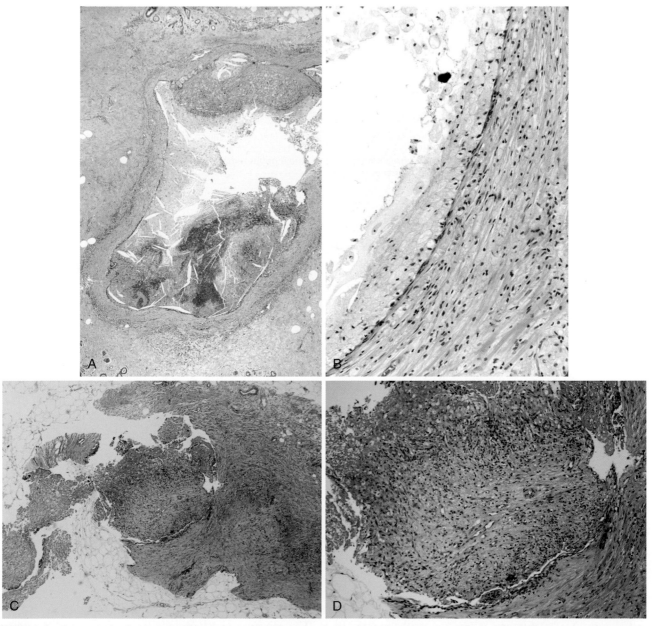

FIGURE 2-1 Duct ectasia. **A,** Note the dilated duct with inflamed wall, intraluminal secretions, and hemorrhage. **B,** Attenuated ectatic duct wall is shown with numerous foamy histiocytes. **C,** Mastitis obliterans at low power; the duct is filled with granulation tissue. **D,** Higher magnification of **C** shows the duct wall and nodule of granulation tissue filling the duct lumen.

Continued

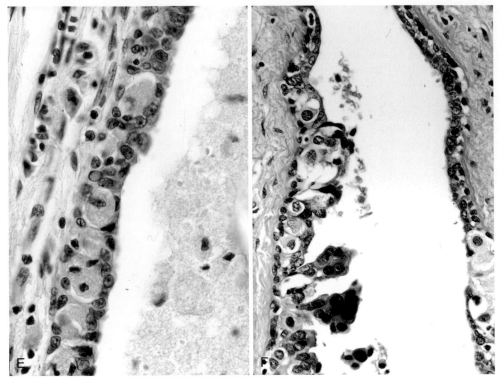

FIGURE 2-1, cont'd Duct ectasia. **E,** Sometimes, intraepithelial foamy histiocytes are present mimicking pagetoid spread of carcinoma. A helpful feature pointing toward intraepithelial histiocytes is the concomitant presence of luminal histiocytes. **F,** Shown here is true pagetoid spread of carcinoma cells down the duct epithelial lining. Note the atypia, and if doubt remains, consider using a keratin and CD68 immunostain to make the distinction between histiocytes and carcinoma cells.

fibrotic breast parenchyma with obliteration of the lobular pattern. Clinically, a localized abscess may simulate carcinoma. Periareolar abscess associated with squamous metaplasia of lactiferous ducts (SMOLDering breast disease) is referred to as *Zuska's disease*.[6,7] SMOLDering breast disease requires surgical excision to effect cure.

KEY PATHOLOGIC FEATURES

Mammary Duct Ectasia

- Ectasia of large ducts with detritus in the lumen.
- Fibrous thickening of the wall, calcification common.
- No epithelial hyperplasia or apocrine metaplasia.
- Periductal florid inflammatory reaction rich in macrophages and plasma cells.
- Fibrous obliteration of the ducts can occur (ductitis obliterans or mastitis obliterans).

FAT NECROSIS

Clinical Presentation

Clinically significant fat necrosis is most likely of traumatic origin, and it often involves the superficial subcutaneous tissue rather than the breast parenchyma itself (Figure 2-2). A history of trauma can be elicited in about half of the cases, usually 1 to 2 weeks before the time of diagnosis. Cases of mammary fat necrosis have

also been reported after radiation therapy and as a local manifestation of Weber-Christian disease.[8]

KEY CLINICAL FEATURES

Fat Necrosis

- Simulates carcinoma; skin retraction and stellate scar–like nature.
- Likely traumatic origin (~50% of cases).
- Trauma history elicited in about half, 1 to 2 weeks before diagnosis.
- Often involves superficial subcutaneous tissue rather than deep breast.
- Can occur after radiation therapy or in Weber-Christian disease.

GROSS PATHOLOGY

The disease can simulate carcinoma because of skin retraction and the scirrhous (stellate scar–like) nature of the reparative response. The lesions may be gray-white or orange-brown, depending upon the deposition of hemoglobin-derived pigments.

Microscopic Pathology

The microscopic diagnosis is usually easy, but the frozen section may cause some difficulty. Traumatic fat necrosis shows variable and irregular stellate fibrosis,

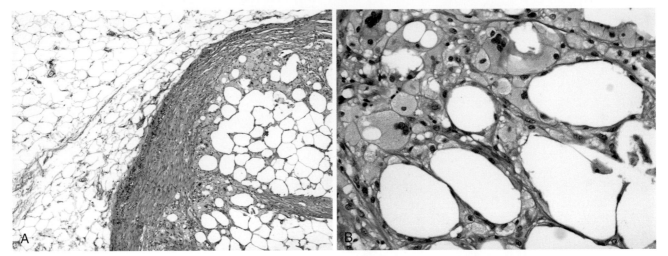

FIGURE 2-2 Fat necrosis. **A,** Note the relatively circumscribed area of organizing fat necrosis. **B,** Note foamy histiocytes and pooled fat vacuoles characteristic of fat necrosis.

occurring around areas of necrotic, variably vacuolated fat with abundant admixed foamy macrophages.

Treatment and Prognosis

Fat necrosis is a benign disease, which should be cured by excision.

Differential Diagnosis

Foamy macrophages are uncommon in carcinoma, and they are the clue to the correct diagnosis. Cytokeratin immunocytochemistry stains should help in difficult cases. Rare histiocyte-like variants of lobular carcinoma occur and should be ruled out.

KEY PATHOLOGIC FEATURES

Fat Necrosis

- Lesions may be gray-white or orange-brown.
- Microscopic diagnosis usually easy, but frozen section may be difficult.
- Traumatic fat necrosis shows irregular stellate fibrosis around necrotic, variably vacuolated, fat with admixed foamy macrophages.

GRANULOMATOUS LOBULAR MASTITIS

Clinical Presentation

Granulomatous lobular mastitis causes a breast mass, sometimes mimicking carcinoma, in women of child-bearing age. It is characterized by multiple, chronic-active, necrotizing, granulomatous abscesses centered on the segmental ducts and attached lobules yielding a lobulocentric disease pattern (Figures 2-3 and 2-4). Women with granulomatous lobular mastitis are usually parous (often within 5 yr of pregnancy) or on oral contraceptive therapy.[9–11]

KEY CLINICAL FEATURES

Granulomatous Lobular Mastitis

- Causes a breast mass, sometimes mimicking carcinoma.
- Women of child-bearing age.
- Women usually parous (often within 5 yr of pregnancy).
- Patient may be on oral contraceptive therapy.

Gross Pathology

It presents as a gray-tan mass lesion, which is irregular, that often mimics invasive carcinoma.

Microscopic Pathology

The inflammatory changes are characterized by destructive, necrotizing, granulomatous inflammation involving numerous polymorphonuclear leukocytes, multinucleated giant cells, and focal lipogranuloma-like changes. Lobulocentric abscesses develop in adjacent segmental ducts and terminal duct lobular units with relative sparing of interlobular stroma.

Treatment and Prognosis

There is a strong tendency for persistence or recurrence in over half of the cases, and the cause remains unknown, but obstruction and/or hypersensitivity reaction have been suggested.[12] Awareness of this condition is important, because surgical therapy is suboptimal for recurrent disease, which requires antibiotics and even corticosteroids before resolution occurs. In fact, resolution may require several years of therapy.

Differential Diagnosis

Granulomatous lobular mastitis is distinct from variants of duct ectasia or periductal mastitis, which involve dilated large ducts rather than lobules. Yet, infection must always be considered with necrotizing

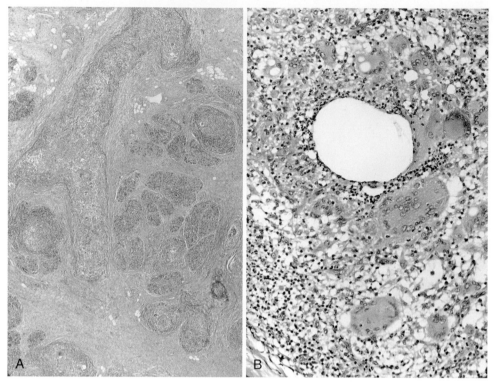

FIGURE 2-3 Granulomatous lobular mastitis. **A,** Note the lobulocentric pattern of inflammation. **B,** Note a lobule essentially destroyed by the granulomatous lobular mastitis containing an "empty" (i.e., formerly pooled lipid-containing) vacuole surrounded by multinucleated giant cells and abundant neutrophils.

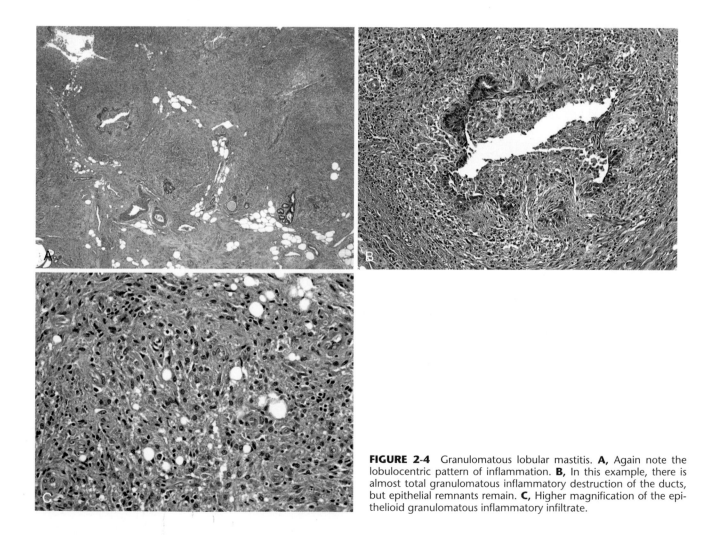

FIGURE 2-4 Granulomatous lobular mastitis. **A,** Again note the lobulocentric pattern of inflammation. **B,** In this example, there is almost total granulomatous inflammatory destruction of the ducts, but epithelial remnants remain. **C,** Higher magnification of the epithelioid granulomatous inflammatory infiltrate.

granulomatous disease. Indeed, histoplasmosis has been shown to cause a granulomatous lobular mastitis–like pattern of inflammation.[13] Mycobacterial, fungal, parasitic, and cat-scratch disease should also be considered and ruled out with appropriate stains.[13]

Ogura and colleagues[14] offer new insight into the nature of granulomatous lobular mastitis. Recently, this group examined 18 cases of "diffuse or lobulocentric mastitis" to clarify its clinicopathologic features. All cases were categorized into three types: nonspecific mastitis with neutrophilic infiltration (n = 7), nonspecific mastitis with lymphoplasmacytic infiltration (n = 9), and granulomatous lobular mastitis (n = 2). The three types of mastitis presented similar ultrasound findings and shared certain histologic features including fibrosis and diffuse or lobulocentric inflammation. Granulomatous lobular mastitis showed specific clinicopathologic features including lobulocentric inflammation with giant cells, diffuse immunoglobulin G4+ (IgG4+) plasma cells, and also a high level of serum IgG4. They concluded that granulomatous lobular mastitis could be categorized into IgG4-related and non–IgG4-related granulomatous lobular mastitis. IgG4 immunohistochemistry and serum IgG4 might be useful for diagnosis of IgG4-related granulomatous lobular mastitis and could help to avoid overtreatment such as wide excision.

IgG4-related sclerosing disease is a recently described syndrome characterized by mass-forming lesions in various organs due to dense lymphoplasmacytic infiltrates and stromal sclerosis, elevated serum IgG4 titer, increased tissue IgG4 plasma cells, and favorable clinical outcome. Cheuk and associates[15] describe four patients with IgG4-related sclerosing mastitis, which may also be related to granulomatous lobular mastitis as implicated by the immediately prior discussion. All patients were female with a mean age of 47.5 years, presenting with painless masses in one or both breasts. One patient had concurrent IgG4-related lymphadenopathy, and another had eyelid swelling of undetermined cause. The serum IgG4 titer was elevated in one tested patient, and circulating autoantibodies were found in three tested patients. All patients were well with no recurrence after excision or biopsy of the mass. Histologically, the breast masses featured dense lymphoplasmacytic infiltrates, prominent stromal sclerosis, and loss of breast lobules. Phlebitis was present in one case. IgG4 cells ranged from 272 to 495 per high-power field, constituting 49% to 85% of all IgG cells. IgG4 cells were scarce in nine of nine cases of lymphocytic mastitis and six of seven cases of granulomatous mastitis studied as controls. Thus, IgG4-related sclerosing mastitis appears to be a distinctive form of mastitis, sometimes accompanied by other components of IgG4-related sclerosing disease, and shows a favorable clinical outcome.

Sarcoidosis can involve the breast, but it does not contain the necrosis and polymorphous inflammatory infiltrate of granulomatous lobular mastitis.[3,16] A peculiar lesion called *granulomatous angiopanniculitis of the breast* has been described.[17] This lesion contains multiple, non-necrotic, noncaseous granulomas with a giant cell component and lymphocytic angiitis, which predominantly involves the subcutis but can extend into the breast tissue without affecting lobules or ducts.[17] This pattern is quite distinct from granulomatous lobular mastitis. Moreover, giant cell arteritis, localized polyarteritis nodosa, and Wegener's granulomatosis can involve the breast, causing a large-vessel necrotizing arteritis or a necrotizing granulomatous angiitis with necrosis.[18-20] Vasculitis is not a usual component of granulomatous lobular mastitis. Finally, foreign body reaction to polyvinyl plastic or silicone used for mammoplasty can result in tumor-like masses, granulomas, and sinus tracts.

Also in the differential diagnosis of granulomatous breast disease is breast carcinoma with osteoclastic giant cells (OGCs), which is characterized by multinucleated OGCs. Often, these tumors display inflammatory hypervascular stroma. OGCs may derive from tumor-associated macrophages, but their nature remains controversial. In one report, two cases are described, in which OGCs appear in common microenvironment despite different tumoral histology (Figure 2-5).[21] One case was a 44-year-old woman who had OGCs accompanying invasive ductal carcinoma, and the second was an 83-year-old woman with carcinosarcoma. Immunohistochemically, in both cases, tumoral and nontumoral cells strongly expressed vascular endothelial growth factor (VEGF) and matrix metalloproteinase-12 (MMP-12), which promote macrophage migration and angiogenesis. The Chalkley count on CD31-stained sections revealed elevated angiogenesis in both cases. The OGCs expressed bone-osteoclast markers (MMP-9, tartrate-resistant acid phosphatase [TRAP], cathepsin K) and a histiocyte marker (CD68), but not a major histocompatibility complex (MHC) class II antigen, human leukocyte antigen-DR (HLA-DR). The results indicated a pathogenesis, regardless of tumoral histology, that OGCs derive from macrophages, likely in response to hypervascular microenvironments with secretion of common cytokines. The OGCs had acquired bone-osteoclast–like characteristics, but lost antigen presentation abilities as an anticancer defense. The authors concluded that the appearance of OGCs may not be antitumoral immunologic reactions, but rather protumoral differentiation of macrophage responding to hypervascular microenvironments induced by breast cancer.

To be included in the differential with any granulomatous process is Rosai-Dorfman disease, which can occur in the breast. Morkowski and coworkers[22] recently reported an additional three cases and reviewed the literature. Rosai-Dorfman disease (also known as *sinus histiocytosis with massive lymphadenopathy*) is an uncommon, idiopathic, benign histiocytic lesion. It usually involves the cervical lymph nodes and, less commonly, extranodal sites. Involvement of the breast is rare, with only 17 cases reported in the English literature to date. These authors described three new patients with extranodal Rosai-Dorfman disease in the breast. All three patients—aged 45, 53, and 54 years—presented with solid breast lesions that were detected on screening mammography and had no clinical history of Rosai-Dorfman disease or radiographic evidence of extramammary involvement. Initial diagnoses were accomplished by needle core biopsy in one case

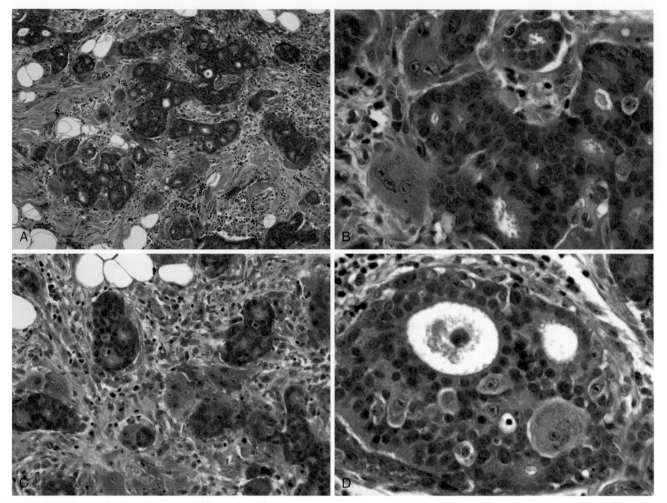

FIGURE 2-5   Osteoclast-like giant cell reaction to invasive breast carcinoma. **A,** Invasive cribriform carcinoma with granulomatous/osteoclast-like giant cell stromal reaction. **B** and **C,** Note the intimate association of the osteoclast-like giant cells with the tumor cells. **D,** Some osteoclast-like giant cells appear to infiltrate tumor cell nests.

KEY PATHOLOGIC FEATURES

Granulomatous Lobular Mastitis

- Gray-tan mass lesion; irregular; mimicking invasive carcinoma.
- Lobulocentric pattern with relative sparing of interlobular stroma.
- Necrotizing, granulomatous abscesses centered on segmental ducts and lobules.
- Also polymorphonuclear leukocytes, giant cells, lipogranuloma-like changes.

and excisional biopsy in the other two. Because Rosai-Dorfman disease frequently mimics invasive breast carcinoma in its clinical presentation and radiographic appearance—and can mimic other benign or malignant histiocytic lesions microscopically—awareness and appropriate diagnosis of this entity are essential for proper treatment. An important note in this discussion is that granular cell tumor and invasive lobular carcinoma (histiocytoid variant) can have lesional cells with histiocytic qualities—it is important not to miss these lesions (Figures 2-6 and 2-7).

SCLEROSING LYMPHOCYTIC LOBULITIS

Clinical Presentation

Sclerosing lymphocytic lobulitis of the breast is an inflammatory breast lesion thought to be of autoimmune origin, much like Sjögren's syndrome, Hashimoto's thyroiditis, and pancreatic insulinitis.[23] A very similar, if not identical, lesion was initially reported by Soler and Khardori[24] as fibrous disease of the breast. Subsequent reports emphasized the association of sclerosing lymphocytic lobulitis with diabetes (i.e., diabetic mastopathy)[25–27]; but Schwartz and Strauchen[28] and Lammie and colleagues[23] reported very similar pathologic features in nondiabetic patients, but often with other evidence of autoimmune disease (Hashimoto's thyroiditis or circulating autoantibodies). Diabetic patients with sclerosing lymphocytic lobulitis have early-onset, long-standing, insulin-dependent diabetes, which developed premenopausally.

Gross Pathology

The breasts contain hard, painless, irregularly contorted, movable, fibrotic, gray-tan masses, which are often bilateral, but may be solitary. Mammography reveals dense

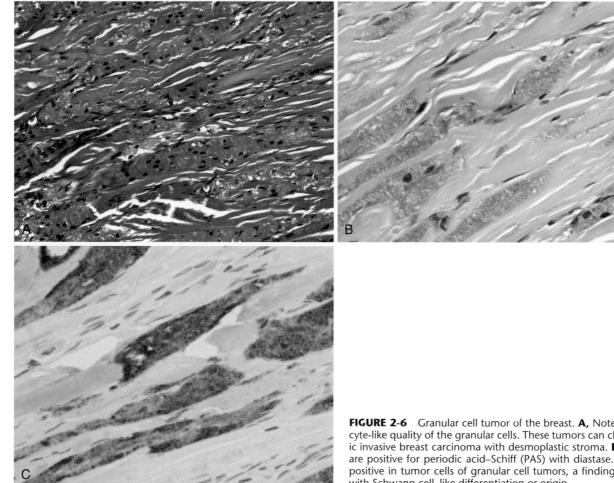

FIGURE 2-6 Granular cell tumor of the breast. **A,** Note the histiocyte-like quality of the granular cells. These tumors can closely mimic invasive breast carcinoma with desmoplastic stroma. **B,** Granules are positive for periodic acid–Schiff (PAS) with diastase. **C,** S100 is positive in tumor cells of granular cell tumors, a finding consistent with Schwann cell–like differentiation or origin.

KEY CLINICAL FEATURES

Sclerosing Lymphocytic Lobulitis

- Hard, painless, irregularly contorted, movable, fibrotic, gray-tan masses.
- Masses often bilateral, but may be solitary.
- Fine-needle aspiration yields insufficient material in about 50%.
- Inflammatory mass lesion likely of autoimmune origin.
- Often associated with diabetes (i.e., diabetic mastopathy).
- Very similar lesions occur in nondiabetic patients.
- May be other autoimmune diseases (e.g., Hashimoto's thyroiditis or circulating autoantibodies).
- Diabetic patients have early-onset, long-standing, insulin-dependent diabetes.

tissue suggestive of malignancy. Fine-needle aspiration (FNA) biopsy of these hard masses yields insufficient material for diagnosis in approximately 50% of cases.

Microscopic Pathology

Histologically, the masses show lymphocytic lobulitis (mature lymphocytes and plasma cells surrounding acini and invading across basement membranes), lymphocytic

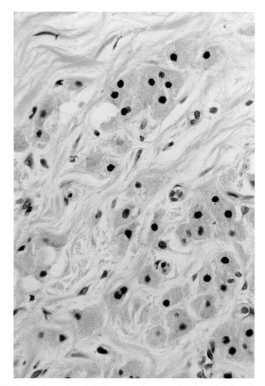

FIGURE 2-7 Invasive lobular carcinoma, histiocytoid cell variant. Note the close resemblance to histiocytes. These cells will be keratin-positive.

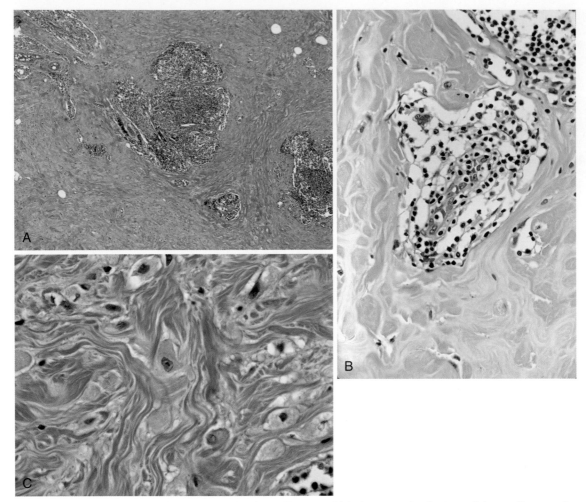

FIGURE 2-8 Sclerosing lymphocytic lobulitis. **A,** Note the dense fibrosis and lobulocentric distributions of the small mature lymphocytes. Often, the lymphocytes extend into the ducts epithelial cells. **B,** Also note that the lymphocytes can closely "hug" small vessels, simulating a "lymphocytic vasculitis." **C,** Some cases contain large epithelioid fibrocytes, simulating invasive carcinoma cells.

vasculitis (mature lymphocytes surrounding a small venule), and dense keloid-like fibrosis, which, in 75% of cases, contains peculiar epithelioid cells embedded in the dense fibrous tissue (Figure 2-8).[27] According to Tomaszewski and associates,[27] the lobulitis and vasculitis can be found in nondiabetic patients, but the epithelioid fibroblasts appear to be unique to the diabetic condition. Fong and coworkers[29] recently reported on an interesting case of diabetic (lymphocytic) mastopathy with a granulomatous component. They reported a case of a 66-year-old woman who presented with multiple painless masses in both breasts. Prior bilateral biopsies were misdiagnosed as Rosai-Dorfman disease. A recent lumpectomy specimen revealed a gray-white, smooth-cut surface with a discrete masslike lesion. The histopathology demonstrated a fibrotic breast parenchyma with foci of dense fibrosis and scattered inconspicuous breast epithelium surrounded by lymphocytes that formed aggregates and follicles with germinal centers. The inflammation was in a periductal, perilobular, and perivascular distribution. In addition, an exuberant inflammatory response with histiocytes and fibroblasts was present. This inflammatory response focally surrounded areas of fat necrosis and formed noncaseating granulomas with

rare multinucleated giant cells. This process had infiltrative, ill-defined edges and involved the subcutaneous tissues. The overlying epidermis was normal. The final diagnosis was diabetic mastopathy with an exuberant lymphohistiocytic response. Immunohistochemical studies and flow cytometry confirmed the polyclonal nature of the lymphoid infiltrate. After the histologic evaluation, they inquired whether the patient had a history of diabetes mellitus, and learned that she did have type 2 non–insulin-dependent diabetes mellitus. It is important that pathologists may not be provided with a history of diabetes mellitus, but the characteristic fibrosis, lymphocytic ductitis/lobulitis, and sclerosing lobulitis with perilobular and perivascular lymphocytic infiltrates should provide clues for an accurate diagnosis, even when an exuberant and an unusual lymphohistiocytic response is present. A timely, accurate diagnosis can help limit repeat surgeries in this vulnerable group of patients.

Immunologic studies of sclerosing lymphocytic lobulitis show a predominance of B lymphocytes in the vast majority of cases and expression of HLA-DR antigen in involved lobular epithelium. These immunologic features are very much like those found in benign lymphoepithelial lesions of salivary gland and in Hashimoto's

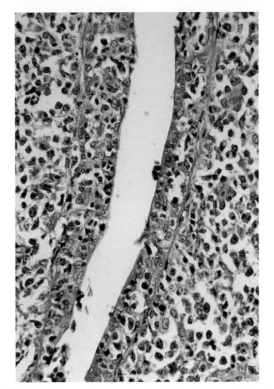

FIGURE 2-9 Primary low-grade B-cell lymphoma of the breast. Note the numerous clustered multicellular aggregates of intraepithelial lymphocytes (i.e., lymphoepithelial lesions).

thyroiditis. Five of seven patients studied by Lammie and colleagues[23] had the HLA-DR 3, 4, or 5 phenotype, which is associated with a higher incidence of autoimmune disease (type 1 diabetes and Hashimoto's thyroiditis).

Treatment and Prognosis

Sclerosing lymphocytic lobulitis is a benign lesion. Excision is curative, although recurrence is possible, though unlikely.

Differential Diagnosis

Lymphocytic lobulitis needs to be differentiated from lymphoma, especially marginal zone type with lympho-epithelial lesions, presenting in the breast (Figure 2-9). The differential diagnosis also includes Rosai-Dorfman disease, inflammatory myofibroblastic tumor, granulomatous mastitis, sclerosing lipogranulomatous response/sclerosing lipogranuloma, breast infarct, Mondor's disease, vasculitis, lupus panniculitis, and rheumatoid nodules.

Schwartz and Strauchen[28] speculated about a possible association of sclerosing lymphocytic lobulitis with an increased incidence of lymphoma development, much like that observed with Sjögren's syndrome and Hashimoto's thyroiditis. The resulting lymphomas are thought to be related to mucosa-associated lymphoid tissue (MALT). However, with insufficient follow-up, these authors were unable to reach a conclusion. Aozasa and colleagues,[30] Lamovec and Jancar,[31] Hugh and associates,[32] and Mattia and coworkers[33] all concluded that primary breast lymphomas may show features characteristic of MALT lymphomas (i.e., presence of lymphoepithelial lesions, tendency to remain localized or recur at other MALT sites, low-grade cytology, and indolent behavior) arising from other organs, such as the stomach, salivary glands, and thyroid. Moreover, Aozasa and colleagues[30] found enough histologic and immunologic evidence to suggest that most mammary lymphomas are B-cell tumors and are associated with coexisting or antecedent lymphocytic mastopathy. In fact, histologic evidence of lymphocytic mastopathy in mammary tissue apart from lymphomas could be evaluated in 11 of 19 patients, and evidence of lymphocytic mastopathy was confirmed in 10 of the 11 patients (>90%). The so-called lymphoepithelial lesion, a characteristic finding for MALT lymphomas, was observed in 42% of their breast lymphomas. However, other observers have not been able to document MALT features in breast lymphoma.[34,35]

When rare primary breast lymphomas develop, they are most commonly of the diffuse, large cell type with B-cell differentiation,[36] but virtually any of the morphologic types defined by the "Working Formulation" can occur. This author has observed a diffuse, small, cleaved lymphoma of the breast that presented with numerous spindle forms and sclerosis, which closely mimicked a primary sarcoma. Also, lymphomas can infiltrate in a single-file pattern like infiltrating lobular carcinoma, and the lymphoepithelial lesion–like spread can mimic pagetoid spread of a breast carcinoma. Breast lymphomas can mimic solid variants of infiltrating lobular carcinoma, and likewise metastatic lobular carcinoma in lymph nodes can simulate primary lymphoma.

A variety of pseudolymphomas (lymphoid hyperplasias) of the breast have been reported, but they may actually represent either florid cases of sclerosing lymphocytic lobulitis or undetected examples of early, low-grade, B-cell, MALT lymphomas.[33,37,38] Indeed, Lin and colleagues[38] concluded their report of five pseudolymphomas of the breast by stating that "the microscopic picture of pseudolymphoma of the breast greatly resembles that seen in the salivary gland in Sjögren's syndrome." Yet, none of their cases actually had Sjögren's syndrome.

There are additional studies focusing on primary breast lymphoma (PBL) that increase our insight. Martinelli and associates[39] reviewed patients with histologically proven, previously untreated follicular or marginal-zone primary breast lymphoma (MZL PBL) of the breast diagnosed from 1980 to 2003. Major end points were progression-free survival (PFS), overall survival (OS), and potential prognostic factors. They collected data on 60 cases of PBL (36 follicular and 24 MZL). Stage was I(E) or II(E) in 57 patients and IVE in 3 patients owing to bilateral breast involvement. Surgery, chemotherapy, and radiotherapy (RT), alone or in combination, were used as first-line treatments in 67%, 42%, and 52% of patients, respectively. Overall response rate was 98%, with a 93% complete response rate. Five-year PFS were 56% for MZL and 49% for follicular PBL ($P = .62$). Relapses were mostly in distant sites (18 of 23 cases); no patients relapsed within RT fields. Their data showed an indolent behavior of MZL PBL, comparable with that of other primary extranodal MZL. Conversely, patients with follicular PBL had inferior PFS and OS when compared with limited-stage nodal follicular non-Hodgkin's lymphomas, suggesting an adverse prognostic role of primary breast localization in this histologic subgroup.

Moreover, Cao and coworkers[40] studied the clinical records of 27 PBL patients treated at the Cancer Center of Sun Yat-sen University (China) from 1976 to 2005. Of the 27 patients, 26 were women and 1 was a man, with the age ranging from 12 to 84; 18 were at stage IE, 6 at stage IIE, and 3 at stage III/IVE. According to the World Health Organization (WHO) 2001 lymphoma classification system, 22 had B-cell lymphoma (including 17 cases of diffuse large B-cell lymphoma, 2 cases of MALT lymphoma, 1 case of MZL, and 2 cases of unclassified B-cell lymphoma), 3 had peripheral T-cell lymphoma, and 2 had unclassified lymphoma. Of the 27 patients, 8 received mastectomy and chemotherapy, 12 received excision of the breast lesion and chemotherapy (the 5-year overall survival rates were 23% and 58%, $P = .006$), 5 received chemotherapy alone, and 2 received lesion excision alone; 24 achieved complete remission (CR) after scheduled treatment, 1 achieved partial remission (PR), and 2 patients had progressive disease (PD). With a follow-up of 10 years and median 38 months, the 5-year overall and disease-free survival rates of the 27 patients were 47% and 23%, respectively. As to the 20 patients with high- or moderate-grade disease (diffuse large B-cell lymphoma and peripheral T-cell lymphoma), the 5-year overall and disease-free survival rates were 48% and 27%, respectively. Sixteen patients had tumor relapse during the follow-up in the ipsilateral breast (6 cases), contralateral breast (4 cases), central nervous system (CNS) (3 cases), bone marrow (1 case), and lymph nodes (2 cases). In this series, the main subtypes of PBL were diffuse large B-cell lymphoma and peripheral T-cell lymphoma. The effect of radical operation was limited in PBL; the optimal sequence appeared to be lumpectomy followed by standard anthracycline-based regimens and RT. PBL tends to relapse to the CNS, therefore, computed tomography (CT) or magnetic resonance imaging (MRI) of the CNS is necessary during follow-up.

Because sclerosing lymphocytic mastitis "ends" with lobular atrophy and sclerosis, so-called megalomastia should be considered in the differential diagnosis.[41] Megalomastia is a rare entity characterized by enlargement of one or both breasts. Most cases occur in children and there is often a family history of the disease. The main histologic features are isolated, small, atrophic lobules embedded in abundant, hypocellular collagenous stroma. Some of these fibrotic breasts may show so-called juvenile units, which are composed of branching ducts without lobules surrounded by a rim of myxomatous, alcian blue–positive stroma. Juvenile units resemble mammary tissue during early breast development.

Sometimes, the epithelioid stromal cells in sclerosing lymphocytic lobulitis can be so prominent and abundant that the possibility of an infiltrating carcinoma or granular cell tumor can be seriously considered.[42] Ashton and colleagues[42] reported that the stromal cells have features of myofibroblasts, reacting with antiactin. These cells were negative for antibodies to keratin (AE1/3), S100, desmin, Mac 287, Factor XIIIa, CD20 (L26), and CD45RO (UCHL-1); but they reacted with anti-CD68 (Kp-1), suggesting some lysosome formation. These stains are important, because rarely, lymphoepithelioma-like carcinoma of the breast occurs, wherein the lymphoid infiltrate could simulate lymphocytic lobulitis and obscure the underlying carcinoma.[43]

Breast infarct can complicate a large variety of conditions, including intraductal papilloma, fibroadenoma, phyllodes tumor, hyperplastic lobules during pregnancy, syphilis, and Wegener's granulomatosis.[44–48] Infarct can also occur in association with anticoagulant therapy, postpartum abscess and gangrene, thrombophlebitis migrans disseminata, and mitral stenosis with heart failure.[5]

Mondor's disease is a thrombophlebitis with thrombosis involving the breast and contiguous thoracoabdominal wall.[11,23] It may simulate neoplasm, often has a sudden onset, and appears as a firm, slightly nodular cord beneath the skin. Ecchymosis may be present. Mondor's disease may be related to mechanical injury and in about one half of cases the disease occurs after mastectomy and is associated with breast carcinomas.[49] The condition is self-limited and practically never recurs.

Rheumatoid nodules and periarteritis nodosa may present as single or multiple breast masses.[49–51] Abscess of the breast usually results from rupture of mammary ducts, often but not always with pregnancy.[3,4] A localized abscess may simulate carcinoma. Although rare in North America, tuberculosis of the breast may be secondary to bloodstream dissemination or to extension from an adjacent tuberculous process. Likewise, actinomycosis, coccidioidomycosis, and histoplasmosis of the breast can cause necrotizing cranulomatous masses (sometimes with sinus tracts)—mass lesions that may be mistaken for breast carcinoma. Moreover, the regional nodes may be involved; occasionally, these nodes are intramammary.[31] Sarcoidosis can begin in the breast and remain localized in this organ for long periods.[3,52] Foreign body reaction to polyvinyl plastic or silicone used for mammoplasty can cause masses and sinus tracts.[49,53] Breast infarct can develop within fibroadenoma, intraductal papilloma, phyllodes tumor, hyperplastic lobules during pregnancy, and in breasts involved with syphilis and Wegener's granulomatosis.[44–48] Also, infarct can occur in association with anticoagulant therapy.[5]

KEY PATHOLOGIC FEATURES

Sclerosing Lymphocytic Lobulitis

- Masses have lymphocytic lobulitis, lymphocytic vasculitis, and dense keloid-like fibrosis.
- Approximately 75% contain epithelioid fibroblasts in dense fibrous tissue
- Epithelioid cells can mimic invasive carcinoma cells.
- Rarely, diabetic mastopathy has exuberant lymphohistiocytic response.

SUMMARY

Reactive and inflammatory conditions of the breast comprise a heterogeneous group of lesions that are characterized by specific gross and microscopic findings.

The role of the pathologist is to correctly identify the lesion, infer the proper etiology, and separate the neoplastic entities that are encountered in the differential diagnosis.

REFERENCES

1. Haagensen CD. Mammary-duct ectasia. A disease that may simulate carcinoma. Cancer 1951;4:749-761.
2. Wang Z, Leonard Jr MH, Khamapirad T, Castro CY. Bilateral extensive ductitis obliterans manifested by bloody nipple discharge in a patient with long-term diabetes mellitus. Breast J 2007;13:599-602.
3. Banik S, Bishop PW, Ormerod LP, O'Brien TE. Sarcoidosis of the breast. J Clin Pathol 1986;39:446-448.
4. Scholefield JH, Duncan JL, Rogers K. Review of a hospital experience of breast abscesses. Br J Surg 1987;74:469-470.
5. Robitaille Y, Seemayer TA, Melmo WL, Cumberlidge MC. Infarction of the mammary region mimicking carcinoma of the breast. Cancer 1974;33:1183-1189.
6. Sebek B. Periareolar abscess associated with squamous metaplasia of the lactiferous ducts (Zuska's disease). Lab Invest 1988;58:83A.
7. Watt-Boolsen S, Rasmussen NR, Blichert-Toft M. Primary periareolar abscess in the nonlactating breast. Risk of recurrence. Am J Surg 1987;153:571-573.
8. Clarke D, Curtis JL, Martinez A, et al. Fat necrosis of the breast simulating recurrent carcinoma after primary radiotherapy in the management of early stage breast carcinoma. Cancer 1983;53:442-445.
9. Kessler E, Wollach Y. Granulomatous mastitis. A lesion clinically simulating carcinoma. Am J Clin Pathol 1972;58:642-646.
10. Going JJ, Anderson TJ, Wilkinson S, Chetty U. Granulomatous lobular mastitis. J Clin Pathol 1987;40:535-540.
11. Brown KL, Tang PH. Postlactational tumoral granulomatous mastitis: a localized immune phenomenon. Am J Surg 1979;138:326-329.
12. Murthy MSN. Granulomatous mastitis and lipogranuloma of the breast. Am J Clin Pathol 1973;60:432-433.
13. Osborne BM. Granulomatous mastitis caused by histoplasma and mimicking inflammatory breast carcinoma. Hum Pathol 1989;20:47-52.
14. Ogura K, Matsumoto T, Aoki Y, et al. IgG4-related tumour-forming mastitis with histological appearances of granulomatous lobular mastitis: comparison with other types of tumour-forming mastitis. Histopathology 2010;57:39-45.
15. Cheuk W, Chan AC, Lam WL, et al. IgG4-related sclerosing mastitis: description of a new member of the IgG4-related sclerosing diseases. Am J Surg Pathol 2009;33:1058-1064.
16. Gansler TS, Wheeler JE. Mammary sarcoidosis. Two cases and literature review. Arch Pathol Lab Med 1984;108:673-675.
17. Wargotz ES, Lefkowitz M. Granulomatous angiopanniculitis of the breast. Hum Pathol 1989;20:1084-1088.
18. Clement PB, Senges H, How AR. Giant cell arteritis of the breast: case report and literature review. Hum Pathol 1987;18:1186-1190.
19. Pambakian H, Tighe JR. Breast involvement in Wegener's granulomatosis. J Clin Pathol 1971;24:343-349.
20. Ng WF, Chow LTC, Lam PWY. Localized polyarteritis nodosa of the breast: report of two cases and a review of the literature. Histopathology 1993;23:535-539.
21. Shishido-Hara Y, Kurata A, Fujiwara M, et al. Two cases of breast carcinoma with osteoclastic giant cells: are the osteoclastic giant cells pro-tumoural differentiation of macrophages? Diagn Pathol 2010;5:55.
22. Morkowski JJ, Nguyen CV, Lin P, et al. Rosai-Dorfman disease confined to the breast. Ann Diagn Pathol 2010;14:81-87.
23. Lammie GA, Bobrow LG, Staunton MDM, et al. Sclerosing lymphocytic lobulitis of the breast—evidence for an autoimmune pathogenesis. Histopathology 1991;19:13-20.
24. Soler NG, Khardori R. Fibrous disease of the breast, thyroiditis and cheiroarthropathy in type 1 diabetes mellitus. Lancet 1984;1:193-194.
25. Byrd BF, Harmann WH, Graham LS, Hogle HH. Mastopathy in insulin-dependent diabetics. Ann Surg 1987;205:529-532.
26. Logan WW, Hoffmann NY. Diabetic fibrous breast disease. Radiology 1989;172:667-670.
27. Tomaszewski JE, Brooks JS, Hicks D, Livolsi VA. Diabetic mastopathy: a distinctive clinicopathologic entity. Hum Pathol 1992;23:780-786.
28. Schwartz IS, Strauchen JA. Lymphocytic mastopathy. An autoimmune disease of the breast? Am J Clin Pathol 1990;93:725-730.
29. Fong D, Lann MA, Finlayson C, et al. Diabetic (lymphocytic) mastopathy with exuberant lymphohistiocytic and granulomatous response: a case report with review of the literature. Am J Surg Pathol 2006;30:1330-1336.
30. Aozasa K, Ohsawa M, Saeki K, et al. Malignant lymphoma of the breast. Immunologic type and association with lymphocytic mastopathy. Am J Clin Pathol 1992;97:699-704.
31. Lamovec J, Jancar J. Primary malignant lymphoma of the breast. Lymphoma of the mucosa-associated lymphoid tissue. Cancer 1987;60:3033-3041.
32. Hugh JC, Jackson FI, Hanson J, Poppema S. Primary breast lymphoma. An immunohistologic study of 20 new cases. Cancer 1990;66:2602-2611.
33. Mattia AR, Ferry JA, Harris NL. Breast lymphoma: A B-cell spectrum including the low grade B-cell lymphoma of mucosa associated with lymphoid tissue. Am J Surg Pathol 1993;17:574-587.
34. Bobrow LG, Richards MA, Happerfield LC, et al. Breast lymphomas: a clinicopathologic review. Hum Pathol 1993;24:274-278.
35. Arber DA, Simpson JF, Weiss LM, Rappaport H. Non-Hodgkin's lymphoma involving the breast. Am J Surg Pathol 1994;18:288-295.
36. Brustein S, Filippa DA, Kimmel M, et al. Malignant lymphoma of the breast. A study of 53 cases. Ann Surg 1987;205:144-150.
37. Fisher ER, Palekar AS, Paulson JD, Golinger R. Pseudolymphoma of breast. Cancer 1979;44:258-263.
38. Lin JJ, Farha GJ, Taylor RJ. Pseudolymphoma of the breast. I. In a study of 8,654 consecutive tylectomies and mastectomies. Cancer 1980;45:973-978.
39. Martinelli G, Ryan G, Seymour JF, et al. Primary follicular and marginal-zone lymphoma of the breast: clinical features, prognostic factors and outcome: a study by the International Extranodal Lymphoma Study Group. Ann Oncol 2009;20:1993-1999.
40. Cao YB, Wang SS, Huang HQ, et al. Primary breast lymphoma—a report of 27 cases with literature review. Ai Zheng 2007;26:84-89.
41. Anastassiades OT, Choreftaki T, Ioannovich J, et al. Megalomastia: histological, histochemical and immunohistochemical study. Virchows Arch A 1992;420:337-344.
42. Ashton MA, Lefkowitz M, Tavassoli FA. Epithelioid stromal cells in lymphocytic mastitis: a source of confusion with invasive carcinoma. Mod Pathol 1994;7:49-54.
43. Kumar S, Kumar C. Lymphoepithelioma-like carcinoma of the breast. Mod Pathol 1994;7:129-131.
44. Elsner B, Harper FB. Disseminated Wegener's granulomatosis with breast involvement. Report of a case. Arch Pathol 1969;87:544-547.
45. Jordan JM, Rowe WT, Allen NB. Wegener's granulomatosis involving the breast. Report of three cases and review of the literature. Am J Med 1987;83:159-164.
46. Lucey JJ. Spontaneous infarction of the breast. I. Clin Pathol 1975;28:937-943.
47. Morgan MC, Weaver MG, Crowe JP, Abdul-Karim FW. Diabetic niastopathy. A clinicopathologic study in palpable and nonpalpable breast lesions. Mod Pathol 1995;8:349-354.
48. Rickert RR, Rajan S. Localized breast infarcts associated with pregnancy. Arch Pathol 1974;97:159-161.
49. Herrmann JB. Thrombophlebitis of breast and contiguous thoracoabdominal wall (Mondor's disease). N Y State J Med 1966;66:3146-3152.
50. Cooper NE. Rheumatoid nodule in the breast. Histopathology 1991;19:193-194.
51. Coyne JD, Baildam AD, Asbury D. Lymphocytic mastopathy associated with ductal carcinoma in situ of the breast. Histopathology 1995;26:579-580.
52. Fitzgibbons PL, Smiley DF, Kem WH. Sarcoidosis presenting initially as breast mass. Report of two cases. Hum Pathol 1985;16:851-852.
53. Symmers WS. Silicone mastitis in "topless" waitress and some other varieties of foreign-body mastitis. Br Med J 1968;3:19-22.

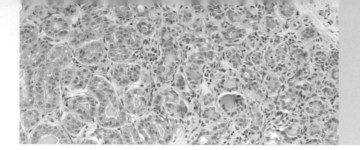

3

Infections of the Breast

Noel Weidner

INTRODUCTION

Breast infection is uncommon in the United States, yet it still occurs, even in neonates. It usually affects women between 18 and 50 years. Breast infections in adults can be divided into two basic types: lactational and nonlactational infection.[1] The breast infection can extend to the skin overlying the breast or it may be secondary to a primary skin infection such as a ruptured keratinous cyst or to an underlying condition such as hidradenitis suppurativa. Whatever the cause and the circumstances, breast infections should be treated early and aggressively. First, appropriate antibiotics should be given early to reduce formation of abscesses. Second, hospital referral is indicated if the infection does not settle rapidly with antibiotics. Third, if an abscess is suspected, it should be confirmed by aspiration before it is drained surgically. Finally, breast cancer should be excluded in patients with an inflammatory lesion that is solid on aspiration or that does not settle despite apparently adequate treatment.

Neonatal breast infection is most common in the first few weeks of life when the breast bud is enlarged. *Staphylococcus aureus* is the usual organism, but occasionally *Escherichia coli* is the cause. If an abscess develops, the incision to drain the pus should be placed as peripheral as possible to avoid damaging the breast bud, because damage to the breast bud will impair normal breast growth and development.

Neonatal breast infections are not the only concern for the neonate. Infectious disease is a leading cause of morbidity and hospitalization for infants and children. During infancy, breastfeeding protects against infectious diseases, particularly respiratory infections, gastrointestinal infections, and otitis media. Little is known, however, about the longer-term impact of breastfeeding on infectious disease in children. Tarrant and coworkers[2] investigated the relationship between infant feeding and childhood hospitalizations from respiratory and gastrointestinal infections in a population-based birth cohort of 8327 children born in 1997 and followed for 8 years. These investigators found that giving breast milk and no formula for at least 3 months substantially reduced hospital admissions for many infectious diseases in the first 6 months of life, when children are most vulnerable. Beyond 6 months of age, there was no association between breastfeeding status at 3 months and hospitalization for infectious disease.

In spite of this positive effect of breastfeeding, some worry that breastfeeding itself may lead to systemic neonatal infections. Indeed, mother-to-child transmission of hepatitis B virus (HBV) is among the most important causes of chronic HBV infection and is the most common mode of transmission worldwide.[3] The presence of hepatitis B surface antigen (HBsAg), hepatitis B early antigen (HBeAg), and HBV DNA in breast milk has been confirmed, but several studies have reported that breastfeeding carries no additional risk that might lead to vertical transmission.[3] Beyond some limitations, the surveys thus far have not demonstrated any differences in HBV transmission rate regarding feeding practices in early childhood.

Furthermore, breastfeeding remains a common practice in parts of the world where the burden of human immunodeficiency virus (HIV) is highest and the fewest alternative feeding options exist.[4] Thus, HIV-positive mothers are faced with the dilemma of whether or not to breastfeed their infants. This is in keeping with regional cultural norms, but in doing so, the mother risks transmitting the virus through breast milk. Furthermore, subclinical mastitis is common in HIV-infected women and is a contributing risk factor for mother-to-child transmission of HIV.[5] The alternative is to pursue formula feeding, which reduces transmission of HIV but comes with its own set of risks, including a higher rate of infant mortality from diarrheal illnesses. Treatment of mothers and/or their infants with antiretroviral (ART) drugs is a strategy that has been employed for several decades to reduce HIV transmission through pregnancy and delivery, but the effect of these agents when taken during breastfeeding is incompletely studied. Exclusive breastfeeding is much safer than mixed feeding (i.e., the supplementation of breastfeeding with other foods) and should be encouraged even in settings where ART for either the mother or the infant is not readily available. The research published regarding maternal treatment with highly active antiretroviral therapy (HAART) during pregnancy and the breastfeeding period has all been nonrandomized with relatively little statistical power but suggests maternal HAART can drastically reduce the risk of transmission of HIV.[4] Infant prophylaxis has been intensively studied in several trials and has been shown to be as effective as maternal treatment with antiretrovirals, reducing the transmission rate after 6 weeks to as low as 1.2%.[4] There is hope that perinatal HIV transmission may be greatly reduced in breastfeeding populations worldwide through a combination of behavioral interventions that encourage exclusive breastfeeding and pharmacologic interventions with ART for mothers and/or their infants.

LACTATING BREAST INFECTION

Clinical Presentation

Abscess of the breast usually results from rupture of mammary ducts, often but not always with pregnancy and lactation.[6,7] These abscesses present as swollen, often erythematous and painful breast masses, which may simulate carcinoma. Lactation-related breast infection is most frequently seen within the first 6 weeks of breastfeeding, although some women develop it with weaning, and the lactating infection presents with pain, swelling, and tenderness. There is usually a history of a cracked nipple or skin abrasion. *S. aureus* is the most common organism responsible, but *S. epidermidis* and streptococci are occasionally cultured.

Gross Pathology

The typical abscess causes an edematous pink-red mass, which is cavitated centrally and filled with yellow viscous fluid (pus).

Microscopic Pathology

Breast tissue is displaced by chronic-active inflammation with numerous neutrophils, mixed with scattered plasma cells and histiocytes (Figure 3-1). Special stains may demonstrate causative organisms.

Treatment and Prognosis

All abscesses in the breast can be managed by repeated aspiration or incision and drainage. Few breast abscesses require drainage under general anesthesia, except those in children, and placement of a drain after incision and drainage is unnecessary. Better maternal and infant hygiene and early treatment with antibiotics have considerably reduced the incidence of abscess formation during lactation. Dener and Inan[8] assessed contributing factors in developing puerperal breast abscess and evaluated the treatment options. During the 4-year study period, 128 nursing women with breast infection were followed. Of these, 102 had mastitis (80%) and 26 had breast abscess (20%). All mastitis patients were treated with antibiotics and none developed an abscess. Ten abscesses were aspirated, and 16 abscesses were treated by incision and drainage. Healing times were similar. There was no significant difference between the mastitis and the abscess groups regarding age, parity, localization of breast infection, cracked nipples, positive milk cultures, or mean lactation time. Duration of symptoms and healing were longer in cases of abscess. Multivariate analyses showed that duration of symptoms was the only independent variable for abscess development. Recurrent mastitis developed in 13 patients (10.2%) within a median of 24 weeks of follow-up. The authors found that delayed treatment of mastitis can lead to abscess formation and that it can be prevented by early antibiotic therapy. Ultrasonography was helpful for detecting abscess formation, and in selected cases, the abscess can be drained with needle aspiration with excellent cosmesis.

Drainage of milk from the affected segment should be encouraged and is best achieved by continuing breastfeeding. Tetracycline, ciprofloxacin, and chloramphenicol should not be used to treat lactating breast infection because they may enter breast milk and can harm the baby. If the inflammation or an associated mass lesion still persists, further investigations are required to exclude an underlying carcinoma. An established

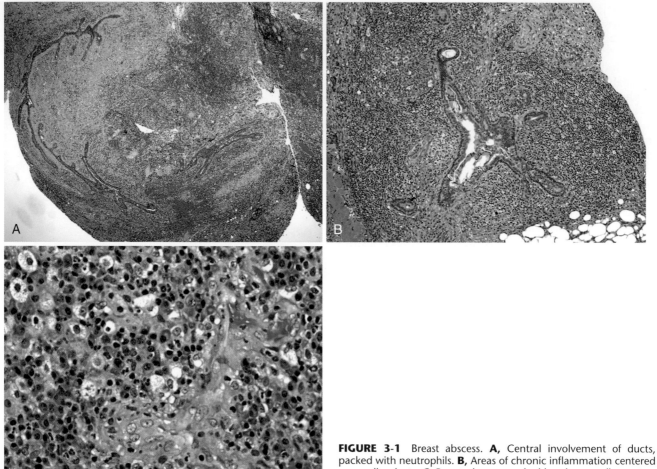

FIGURE 3-1 Breast abscess. **A,** Central involvement of ducts, packed with neutrophils. **B,** Areas of chronic inflammation centered on smaller ducts. **C,** Breast abscess marked by plasma cells, neutrophils, and histiocytes.

abscess should be treated by either recurrent aspiration or incision and drainage. Many women wish to continue to breastfeed, and they should be encouraged to do so.

Differential Diagnosis

Putative "abscesses" that have solid areas or do not respond to therapy should be considered potential carcinomas, and tissue biopsy should be taken to rule out this possibility. Finally, not all that appears to be abscess in these patient groups are abscesses.[9] Galactoceles, noninfected milk-filled cysts, present as tender masses; aspiration is both diagnostic and curative. Benign fibroadenomas occasionally enlarge significantly or infarct during pregnancy. A physiologic nipple discharge is common during pregnancy and may be bloody. Rare cases of massive breast hypertrophy during pregnancy have been reported. The mortality of breast cancer during pregnancy is related to delay: compared stage-for-stage with nonpregnant controls, the prognosis is similar. As a general rule, the cancer should be treated surgically and the pregnancy may be allowed to progress.

In this vein, primary squamous cell carcinoma (SCC) of the breast is a very rare neoplasm, with fewer than 100 cases reported in the English-language literature. However, primary breast SCC seems to have a propensity to mimic breast abscess, and these patients can be misdiagnosed and initially treated for breast abscess. There may be skin erythema associated with an underlying mass, and an infectious cause is often considered in these cases. These tumors unfortunately tend to be large (in the 4- to 5-cm range) and diagnosed at an advanced stage. For this reason, breast biopsy should be considered in cases of breast abscess, especially if there are any atypical features. Treatment of primary SCC of the breast is similar to that of more common types of breast cancer (i.e., breast conservation is possible and lymph node dissection is recommended). Because metastasis to the breast from other primary tumor sites has been reported (lung, cervix, skin, and esophagus), patients with pure SCC should undergo evaluation to exclude this possibility.

KEY PATHOLOGIC FEATURES
Lactating Breast Infections

- Cause edematous pink-red, variably firm masses.
- May be cavitated centrally and filled with yellow viscous fluid (pus).
- Chronic-active inflammation with neutrophils, mixed with plasma cells.
- Special stains may demonstrate causative organisms.

NONLACTATING BREAST INFECTION

Clinical Presentation

Nonlactating infections can be separated into those occurring centrally in the periareolar region and those affecting the peripheral breast tissue. Periareolar infection is most commonly seen in young women in their early 30s.

Histologically, there is active inflammation around nondilated subareolar breast ducts—a condition termed by some as *periductal mastitis*. This condition has been confused with and called "duct ectasia," but duct ectasia is a separate condition affecting an older age group that is characterized by subareolar duct dilatation with less pronounced and less active periductal inflammation. Current evidence suggests that smoking is an important factor in the cause of periductal mastitis but not in duct ectasia. About 90% of women who get periductal mastitis or its complications smoke cigarettes compared with 38% of the same age group in the general population.

The importance of smoking was recently underscored in a study by Gollapalli and colleagues.[10] This group investigated risk factors that predispose to the development of primary breast abscesses and subsequent recurrence. It was a case-control study of patients with a primary or recurrent breast abscess, with recurrence defined by the need for repeated drainage within 6 months. Sixty-eight patients with a primary breast abscess were identified. Univariate analysis indicated that smoking, obesity, diabetes mellitus, and nipple piercing were significant risk factors for development of primary breast abscess. Multivariate logistic regression analysis confirmed smoking as a significant risk factor for the development of primary breast abscess, and in the subtype of subareolar breast abscess, nipple piercing was identified as a risk factor in addition to smoking. Recurrent breast abscess occurred in 36 (53%) patients.

A second study points toward not only smoking but also other contributing factors. Bharat and associates[11] investigated the patients' and microbiologic risk factors that predispose to the development of primary breast abscesses and subsequent recurrence. Recurrent breast abscess was defined by the need for repeated drainage within 6 months. Patient characteristics were compared with the general population and between groups. A total of 89 patients with a primary breast abscess were identified; 12 (14%) were lactational and 77 (86%) were nonlactational. None of the lactational abscesses recurred, whereas 43 (57%) of the nonlactational abscesses did so. Compared with the general population, patients with a primary breast abscess were predominantly African American (64% vs. 12%), had higher rates of obesity (body mass index > 30: 43% vs. 22%), and were tobacco smokers (45% vs. 23%). The only factor significantly associated with recurrence in the multivariate logistic regression analysis was tobacco smoking. Compared with patients who did not have a recurrence, patients with recurrent breast abscesses had a higher incidence of mixed bacteria (20.5% vs. 8.9%), anaerobes (4.5% vs. 0%), and *Proteus* (9.1% vs. 4.4%) but a lower incidence of *Staphylococcus* (4.6% vs. 24.4%). Risk factors for developing a primary breast abscess include African American race, obesity, and tobacco smoking. Patients with recurrent breast abscesses are more likely to be smokers and have mixed bacterial and anaerobic infections. Broader antibiotic coverage should be considered for the higher-risk groups.

Apparently, substances in cigarette smoke may either directly or indirectly damage the wall of the subareolar breast ducts. The damaged tissues then become infected by either aerobic or anaerobic organisms. Initial presentation may be with periareolar inflammation (with or without an associated mass) or with an established abscess. Associated features include central breast pain, nipple retraction at the site of the diseased duct, and nipple discharge.

KEY CLINICAL FEATURES
Nonlactating Breast Infection

- Causes an edematous pink-red lump.
- Can be separated into central periareolar and peripheral types.
- Periareolar infection is common in women in their early 30s.
- Smoking and nipple piercing are significant risk factors for periareolar abscesses.
- May be complicated by mammary duct fistula between skin and abscess.
- Peripheral abscesses often associated with diabetes, rheumatoid arthritis, steroid treatment, granulomatous lobular mastitis, and trauma.

Gross Pathology

The typical abscess causes an edematous pink-red mass, which is cavitated centrally and filled with yellow viscous fluid (pus). A mammary duct fistula is a communication between the skin usually in the periareolar region and a major subareolar breast duct. A fistula can develop after incision and drainage of a nonlactating abscess, it can follow spontaneous discharge of a periareolar inflammatory mass, or it can result from biopsy of a periductal inflammatory mass. Treatment is by excision of the fistula and diseased duct or ducts under antibiotic cover. Recurrence is common after surgery, and the lowest rates of recurrence and best cosmetic results have been achieved in specialist breast units. Operation performed through a circumareolar incision gives excellent cosmetic results.

Microscopic Pathology

Breast tissue is displaced by chronic-active inflammation with numerous neutrophils, mixed with scattered plasma cells and histiocytes. Special stains may demonstrate causative organisms.

Treatment and Prognosis

A periareolar inflammatory mass should be treated with a course of appropriate antibiotics, and abscesses should be managed by aspiration or incision and drainage. Care should be taken to exclude an underlying neoplasm if the mass or inflammation does not resolve after appropriate treatment. But abscesses associated with periductal mastitis commonly recur because treatment by incision or aspiration does not remove the underlying diseased duct. Up to a third of patients develop a mammary duct fistula after drainage of a nonlactating periareolar abscess. Recurrent episodes of periareolar sepsis should be treated by excision of the diseased duct by an experienced breast surgeon under antibiotic cover.

The majority of reports concerning nonpuerperal breast abscess (NPBA) identify aerobic and facultative bacterial isolates as the predominant flora in this disease, and nonpuerperal breast abscess are often caused by mixed flora. Walker and coworkers[12] nicely showed this with a fine-needle aspiration (FNA) study. In this study, FNA was performed in 29 women with NPBA; 12 (41%) of the patients had a history of chronic NPBA. The mean age of patients was 39.2 years. The aspirated material was cultured both anaerobically and aerobically. A total of 108 bacterial strains were recovered from 32 specimens; 2 specimens yielded no bacterial growth. A mean of 3.6 different bacteria were recovered from each culture-positive specimen. Anaerobic recovery outweighed aerobic-facultative recovery by a factor of 2:1. Significantly, 37 strains (5 aerobes and 32 anaerobes) were harvested only from enriched broth subcultured for 4 to 14 days after initial culture processing. Coagulase-negative staphylococci (60% of total aerobes) and peptostreptococcal (47% of total anaerobes) were the predominant bacterial isolates. These findings indicated that NPBA is due to a mixed flora with a major anaerobic component. Furthermore, the results suggested that routine cultures often overlook the involvement of anaerobes in these infections.

Differential Diagnosis

Putative "abscesses" that have solid areas or do not respond to therapy should be considered potential carcinomas, and tissue biopsy taken to rule this possibility out. Another consideration is so-called Zuska's (SMOLDering) breast disease, which is discussed in the next section.

KEY PATHOLOGIC FEATURES
Nonlactating Breast Infection

- Mass with central cavity filled with yellow viscous fluid (pus).
- Chronic-active inflammation with neutrophils, scattered plasma cells, and histiocytes.
- Active inflammation around subareolar breast ducts ("periductal mastitis").
- Duct ectasia is a separate condition affecting an older age group.

ZUSKA'S (SMOLDERING) BREAST DISEASE

Clinical Presentation

Today, almost 90% of nonpuerperal breast abscesses are subareolar breast abscesses. Zuska first described this distinct entity in 1951 as "fistulas of lactiferous ducts."[13] Subareolar breast abscesses are located in the retro- and periareolar areas. These abscesses occur as a result of obstruction of the lactiferous ducts by squamous metaplasia of their epithelium (so-called squamous metaplasia of lactiferous ducts [SMOLDering] breast disease). Subsequent inflammatory reaction and infection produce local and general symptoms. Nipple retraction, recurrent episodes of erysipelas, and presence of painful nodules under the areola in a nonlactating woman are possible signs and symptoms. The presence of a milky draining sinus in the areola is characteristic.

KEY CLINICAL FEATURES
Zuska's (SMOLDering) Breast Disease

- Zuska first described the entity in 1951 as "fistulas of lactiferous ducts."
- Edematous pink-red and indurated nipple.
- Result of obstruction of lactiferous ducts by squamous metaplasia.
- Squamous metaplasia of lactiferous ducts [SMOLDering] breast disease.
- Nipple retraction, recurrent erysipelas, painful nodules, nonlactating woman.
- Milky draining sinus in the areola is characteristic.
- Surgical excision is necessary for cure.

Gross Pathology

Zuska's disease causes an edematous pink-red and indurated nipple, which may have a cavitated central masslike lesion filled with yellow viscous fluid (pus). A mammary duct fistula may develop between the involved subareolar ducts and the skin surface.

Microscopic Pathology

Subareolar lactiferous ducts are mildly ectatic, filled with and surrounded by chronic-active inflammation and fibrosis. Level sections usually reveal squamous metaplasia of the lactiferous ducts (Figure 3-2).

Treatment and Prognosis

Subareolar breast abscesses are troublesome and have a tendency to recur and to form extended fistulas. Treatment with antibiotics in the acute and chronic phase is mandatory; surgical removal of abscess and duct is sometimes curative. Meguid and colleagues[14] reviewed patients with subareolar abscesses and documented the need for surgery to effect cure. They noted that when a subareolar breast abscess (SBA) is incised and drained, an

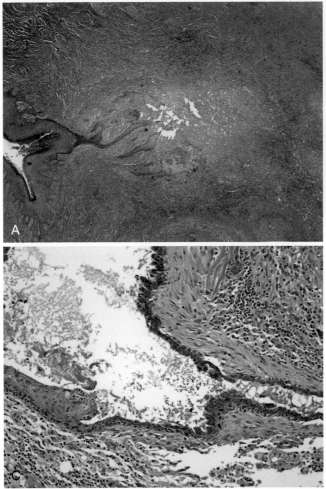

FIGURE 3-2 Zuska's disease or SMOLDering (squamous metaplasia of lactiferous ducts) breast disease. **A,** A lactiferous duct near the nipple, which is filled by chronic-active inflammatory cells with marked periductal reaction. **B,** Higher magnification of the inflamed lactiferous duct with focal squamous metaplasia. **C,** Squamous metaplasia is clearly present within the lactiferous duct.

extraordinarily high frequency of recurrence is noted. To develop a pathogenesis-based treatment plan, 24 women with a total of 84 abscesses were monitored. In 9 women, SBA was under the left areola, under the right in 7, and in 8, the SBA occurred either simultaneously or sequentially under both areolae. In 11 of 24 patients, a chronic lactiferous duct fistula also existed. In 4 of 24 patients, 4 SBAs were treated with antibiotics alone; all recurred. In 16 of 24 patients, initial treatment was incision and drainage plus antibiotics; all recurred. When the abscess plus the plugged lactiferous duct was excised, there were no recurrences; however, in 4 patients, a new abscess in a different duct occurred. This was treated by en bloc resection of all subareolar ampullae, without further recurrence. Patients with a fistulous tract had the fistula, its feeding abscess, and its plugged lactiferous duct excised, without recurrence. In first-time SBA, the organism was usually staphylococcus; in recurrences, mixed flora was isolated. Pathologic findings ranged from squamous metaplasia with keratinization of lactiferous ducts to chronic abscess. The cause of SBA is plugging of the lactiferous duct within the nipple by keratin. To prevent recurrence, the abscessed ampulla with its plugged proximal duct needs to be excised.

These findings were further underscored by Versluijs-Ossewaarde and associates,[15] who also found an association of SMOLD with smoking. This group described the characteristics of SBAs and analyzed the results of surgical treatment in relation to the prevention of recurrences. Almost 70% of patients smoked more than 10 cigarettes a day. The recurrence rate after excision of the lactiferous ducts was 28%, and after management without excision of the lactiferous ducts was 79%. Gram-positive bacteria were isolated more frequently in primary SBAs (not significant). Anaerobic microorganisms were more frequently cultured in recurring SBAs. Definitive treatment of SBAs should consist of excision of the affected lactiferous ducts.

Differential Diagnosis

The diagnostic challenge is to differentiate this benign condition from a breast cancer.

KEY PATHOLOGIC FEATURES
Zuska's (SMOLDering) Breast Disease

- Subareolar lactiferous ducts mildly ectatic, filled, and surrounded by chronic-active inflammation and periductal inflammation and fibrosis.

- Sections reveal squamous metaplasia of the lactiferous ducts (see Figure 3-2).

- Mammary duct fistula between subareolar ducts and skin surface.

MISCELLANEOUS BREAST INFECTIONS

Peripheral Nonlactating Breast Abscesses

These are less common than periareolar abscesses and are often associated with an underlying condition such as diabetes, rheumatoid arthritis, steroid treatment, granulomatous lobular mastitis, and trauma. Pilonidal abscesses in sheep shearers and barbers have been reported to occur in the breast. Infection associated with granulomatous lobular mastitis can be a particular problem. This condition affects young parous women, who may develop large areas of infection with multiple simultaneous peripheral abscesses. There is a strong tendency for this condition to persist and recur after surgery. Large incisions and extensive surgery should, therefore, be avoided in this condition. Steroids have been tried but with limited success. Peripheral breast abscesses should be treated by recurrent aspiration or incision and drainage.

Skin-Associated Infection

Primary infection of the skin of the breast, which can present as cellulitis or an abscess, most commonly affects the skin of the lower half of the breast. These infections are often recurrent in women who are overweight, have large breasts, or have poor personal hygiene. Cellulitis most commonly affects the skin of the breast after surgery or radiotherapy. *S. aureus* is the usual causative organism, although fungal infections have been reported.

Treatment of acute bacterial infection is with antibiotics and drainage or aspiration of abscesses. Women with recurrent infections should be advised about weight reduction and keeping the area as clean and dry as possible (this includes careful washing of the area up to twice a day, avoiding skin creams and talcum powder, and wearing either a cotton bra or a cotton T-shirt or vest worn inside the bra).

Sebaceous cysts are common in the skin of the breast and may become infected. Some recurrent infections in the inframammary fold are due to hidradenitis suppurativa. In this condition, the infection should first be controlled by a combination of appropriate antibiotics and drainage of any pus (the same organisms are found in hidradenitis as in nonlactating infection). Conservative excision of the affected skin is effective at stopping further infection in about half of patients; the remainder have further episodes of infection despite surgery.

Infections following Breast Surgery or Manipulation

Breast abscess can occur after the treatment of breast cancer. In a retrospective review of 112 patients undergoing lumpectomy and radiation therapy, Keidan and coworkers[16] found a 6% incidence of delayed breast abscess (time to onset ranging from 1.5–8 mo, median 5 mo). Prophylactic antibiotics, postoperative chemotherapy, primary versus re-excisional lumpectomy, and different surgeons were not associated with increased risk of delayed abscess. The size of the lumpectomy cavity correlated with the incidence of infection. Because 6 of 7 abscess cultures grew staphylococci (coagulase-negative 3 cases, coagulase-positive 3 cases), and 4 of these patients experienced prior biopsy site infection, skin necrosis, or repeated seroma aspirations, a skin source for contamination was suggested. Treatment of the abscesses with antibiotics and immediate drainage produced acceptable but inferior cosmesis.

There is also risk that breast implants might develop periprosthetic infection followed by device exposure and extrusion. Spear and colleagues[17] reviewed patients with periprosthetic infection or threatened or actual device exposure. Twenty-four patients encompassing 26 affected prostheses were available and were classified into seven groups based on initial presentation as follows: group 1, mild infection (*n* = 8); group 2, severe infection (*n* = 4); group 3, threatened exposure without infection (*n* = 3); group 4, threatened exposure with mild infection (*n* = 3); group 5, threatened exposure with severe infection (*n* = 1); group 6, actual exposure without clinical infection (*n* = 5); and group 7, actual exposure with infection (*n* = 2). To salvage the prosthesis in these patients, various treatment strategies were utilized. All patients with a suspected infection or device exposure were started immediately on appropriate antibiotic therapy (oral antibiotics for mild infections and parenteral antibiotics for severe infections). Salvage methods included one or more of the following: antibiotic therapy, débridement, curettage, pulse lavage, capsulectomy, device exchange, primary closure, and/or flap coverage. Twenty (76.9%) of 26 threatened implants with infection or threatened or actual prosthesis exposure were salvaged after aggressive intervention. The presence of severe infection adversely affected the salvage rate in this series. A statistically significant difference exists among those patients without infection or with mild infection only (groups 1, 3, 4, and 6); successful salvage was achieved in 18 (94.7%) of 19 patients, whereas only 2 of 7 of those implants with severe infection (groups 2, 5, and 7) were salvaged (*P* = .0017). Ten (90.9%) of 11 devices with threatened or actual exposure, not complicated by severe infection (groups 3, 4, and 6), were salvaged. Several treatment strategies were developed for periprosthetic infection and for threatened or actual implant exposure. Patients with infection were placed on oral or intravenous antibiotics; those who responded completely required no further treatment. For persistent mild infection or threatened or actual exposure, operative intervention was required, including some or all of the following steps: implant removal, pocket curettage, partial or total capsulectomy, débridement, site change, placement of a new implant, and/or flap coverage; the menu of options varied with the precise circumstances. No immediate salvage was attempted in 5 cases, owing to either severe infection, nonresponding infection with gross purulence, marginal tissues, or lack of options for healthy tissue coverage. Based on the authors' experience, salvage attempts for periprosthetic infection and prosthesis exposure may be successful, except in cases of overwhelming infection or deficient soft tissue coverage. Although an attempt at implant salvage may be offered to a patient, device removal and delayed reinsertion will always remain a more conservative and predictable option.

Breast infections have also been reported after reduction mammaplasty and nipple piercing. Boettcher and associates[18] reported two cases of breast infections with *Mycobacterium fortuitum* and one with *M. chelonei* after bilateral reduction mammaplasty. Reduction mammaplasty is one of the most common plastic surgery procedures performed in the United States, with the goal of correcting symptomatic macromastia. More than 70,000 cases were performed in 2009, with few complications and low infection rates. Infection with atypical myobacterium is exceptionally rare after breast surgery in the absence of a prosthetic implant. All of the patients had a delayed presentation after complete wound healing and were refractory to first-line antibiotic therapy. All three required long-term antibiotics in consultation with an infectious disease specialist. The patients all required surgical drainage, and two patients also required formal operative débridement. Nonetheless, all three patients eventually went on to complete wound healing.

Piercing is a growing fashion trend among young people, and as might be expected, cases of breast abscess after nipple piercing are now being reported, with some patients requiring hospitalization. However, the risk for breast infection is, on the one hand, underestimated by the women and, on the other hand, played down by piercing studios. Healing of the initial wound channel varies and can take up to 6 to 12 months. The risk for infection is approximately 10% to 20%, often months after the procedure. Most patients are 25 to 35 years old and the time from piercing to infection ranges from 5 to 12 months. Treatment includes various combinations of incision, abscess cavity removal, placement of irrigation tubing, and intravenous antibiotics postoperatively. Hospital stays can be up to 9 days. Relapse sometimes occurs and may result in additional surgery. Causal agents have been atypical mycobacteria, coagulase-negative staphylococcus, group B streptococcus, and microaerophilic staphylococcus. Of additional interest, Lewis and coworkers[19] reported a rare breast infection occurring 4 months after nipple piercing. Clinical examination suggested carcinoma and *M. fortuitum* was eventually isolated after surgical biopsy and débridement. Antibiotic therapy was initiated intravenously using two drugs and oral therapy was continued for 6 months. A contralateral mycobacterial lesion emerged and was excised along with a residual fibrotic nodule at the original biopsy site. The authors suggest that when adequate sampling of a complex and suspicious breast mass is benign and initial bacterial cultures are sterile, mycobacterial infection should be considered, particularly when there is a history of previous nipple piercing procedures.

Unusual Breast Infections and Other Infections and Conditions

Rarely, infection of the breast with actinomycosis, coccidioidomycosis, and histoplasmosis can cause necrotizing granulomatous masses (sometimes with sinus tracts); these mass lesions can be mistaken for breast carcinoma.[20,21] Moreover, the regional nodes may be involved; occasionally, these nodes are intramammary.

Although rare in North America, tuberculosis of the breast may be secondary to bloodstream dissemination or to extension from an adjacent tuberculous process. Clues to its diagnosis include the presence of a breast or axillary sinus in up to half of patients. The most common presentation of tuberculosis nowadays is with an abscess resulting from infection of a tuberculous cavity by an acute pyogenic organism such as *S. aureus*. An open biopsy is often required to establish the diagnosis. Treatment is by a combination of surgery and antituberculous chemotherapy. Syphilis, actinomycosis, and mycotic, helminthic, and viral infections occasionally affect the breast but are rare. Berger and colleagues[22] report a 42-year-old woman who developed severe, recurrent breast abscesses caused by *Corynebacterium minutissimum*. Prior reports of *C. minutissimum* infection have been limited to erythrasma, a minor dermatosis.

Lesions That Can Mimic Breast Infection

Sarcoidosis can begin in the breast and remain localized in this organ for long periods.[6,23] Foreign body reaction to polyvinyl plastic or silicone used for mammoplasty can cause masses and sinus tracts.[24,25] Breast infarct can develop within fibroadenoma, intraductal papilloma, phylloides tumor, hyperplastic lobules during pregnancy, and in breasts involved with syphilis and Wegener's granulomatosis.[26–30] Infarct can also occur in association with anticoagulant therapy.[31]

Worth noting here is that pyoderma gangrenosum (PG) can involve the breast and mimic infection. Indeed, Davis and associates[31] report that PG may occur in unusual sites and not be readily recognized. Delays in diagnosis and appropriate treatment may result in extensive ulcerations and scarring. They documented two patients with PG involving the breasts after breast operation and note that delays in diagnosis can result in extensive ulcerations and scarring of the breasts. PG is a noninfectious purulent ulcerative disease triggered mainly by chronic inflammatory bowel disease, monoclonal gammapathy, polyarthritis, and hematologic malignancies; exceptionally, it can be triggered by surgery alone. When PG is associated with fever, it can mimic infectious cellulitis. When it is located on the breast, unnecessary and deleterious surgical débridement may be performed. Several elements help to make the diagnosis: nipples are little affected by PG, often symmetrical lesions on both breasts, other similar lesions elsewhere on the body, resistance to wide-spectrum antibiotherapy, blood count abnormalities (leukemia), and negativity of bacterial culture.

Another lesion that could be mistaken for infection, especially parasitic infections, is so-called eosinophilic mastitis.[32,33] Eosinophilic mastitis is an extremely rare condition characterized by heavy eosinophilic infiltrates around ducts and lobules. Sometimes, the patients have peripheral eosinophilia secondary to a systemic syndrome with peripheral eosinophilia such as asthma,

Churg-Strauss syndrome, or hypereosinophilic syndrome.[34,35] Peripheral eosinophilia may also be associated with other allergic or atopic diseases, collagen vascular diseases, and parasitic infection. In addition, tissue eosinophilia has been described in association with several malignancies, but this affects breast carcinomas only rarely. In the differential is granulomatous mastitis, in which significant eosinophilic infiltrates can occur.

Other cases of so-called eosinophilic mastitis occur with no known peripheral eosinophilia (Figure 3-3). In these cases, the pathogenesis is unknown, but it could reflect a local reaction to intraluminal substances. The presence of heavy eosinophilic infiltrates in this entity may represent a form of allergic reaction. Local excision is recommended to exclude an underlying malignant disease, but these lesions can recur, sometimes years later. Indeed, recurrence despite excision with negative margins may indicate that control of the eosinophilia—and possibly the underlying disorder—is just as important in preventing further recurrences.

Factitial Disease

Artifactual or factitial diseases are created by the patient, often through complicated or repetitive actions. Such patients may undergo many investigations and operations before the nature of the disease is recognized. Often, patients inject foreign material into the breast, which causes a foreign body giant cell reaction to the material (Figure 3-4). The diagnosis is difficult to establish but should be considered when the clinical

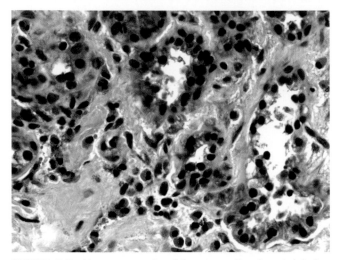

FIGURE 3-3 Numerous eosinophils surrounding breast lobules. There were associated features of duct ectasia, but the patient did not have eosinophilia or other conditions known to be associated with prominent eosinophilic response. This appears to be a case of idiopathic "eosinophilic mastitis."

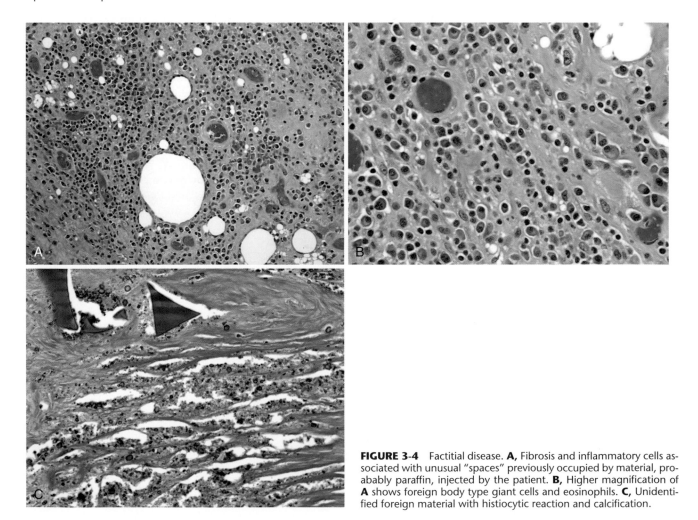

FIGURE 3-4 Factitial disease. **A,** Fibrosis and inflammatory cells associated with unusual "spaces" previously occupied by material, probably paraffin, injected by the patient. **B,** Higher magnification of **A** shows foreign body type giant cells and eosinophils. **C,** Unidentified foreign material with histiocytic reaction and calcification.

situation does not conform to common appearances or pathologic processes.

SUMMARY

Breast inflammatory processes, whether infectious or not, command attention to detail by both clinician and pathologist. The etiology of infectious processes needs to be discovered and pathogenesis determined. Cancer is always in the differential diagnosis, both clinically and pathologically.

REFERENCES

1. Dixon JM. ABC of breast diseases: Breast infection. BMJ 1994;309:946-949.
2. Tarrant M, Kwok MK, Lam TH, et al. Breast-feeding and childhood hospitalizations for infections. Epidemiology 2010;21:847-854.
3. Petrova M, Kamburov V. Breastfeeding and chronic HBV infection: clinical and social implications. World J Gastroenterol 2010;16:5042-5046.
4. Slater M, Stringer EM, Stringer JS. Breast feeding in HIV-positive women: what can be recommended? Paediatr Drugs 2010;12:1-9.
5. Arsenault JE, Aboud S, Manji KP, et al. Vitamin supplementation increases risk of subclinical mastitis in HIV-infected women. J Nutr 2010;140:1788-1792.
6. Banik S, Bishop PW, Ormerod LP, O'Brien TE: Sarcoidosis of the breast. J Clin Pathol 1986;39:446-448.
7. Scholefield JH, Duncan JL, Rogers K. Review of a hospital experience of breast abscesses. Br J Surg 1987;74:469-470.
8. Dener C, İnan A. Breast abscesses in lactating women. World J Surg 2003;27:130-133.
9. Scott-Conner CE, Schorr SJ. The diagnosis and management of breast problems during pregnancy and lactation. Am J Surg 1995;170:401-405.
10. Gollapalli V, Liao J, Dudakovic A, et al. Risk factors for development and recurrence of primary breast abscesses. J Am Coll Surg 2010;211:41-48.
11. Bharat A, Gao F, Aft RL, et al. Predictors of primary breast abscesses and recurrence. World J Surg 2009;33:2582-2586.
12. Walker AP, Edmiston CE, Krepel CJ, Condon RE. A prospective study of the microflora of nonpuerperal breast abscess. Arch Surg 1988;123:908-911.
13. Guadagni M, Nazzari G. Zuska's disease. G Ital Dermatol Venereol 2008;143:157-160.
14. Meguid MM, Oler A, Numann PJ, Khan S. Pathogenesis-based treatment of recurring subareolar breast abscesses. Surgery 1995;118:775-782.
15. Versluijs-Ossewaarde FNL, Roumen RMH, Goris RJA. Subareolar breast abscesses: characteristics and results of surgical treatment. Breast J 2005;11:179-182.
16. Keidan RD, Hoffman JP, Weese JL, et al. Delayed breast abscesses after lumpectomy and radiation therapy. Am Surg 1990;56:440-444.
17. Spear SL, Howard MA, Boehmler JH, et al. The infected or exposed breast implant: management and treatment strategies. Plast Reconstr Surg 2004;113:1634-1644.
18. Boettcher AK, Bengtson BP, Farber ST, Ford RD. Breast infections with atypical mycobacteria following reduction mammoplasty. Aesthetic Surg J 2010;30:542-548.
19. Lewis CG, Wells MK, Jennings WC. *Mycobacterium fortuitum* breast infection following nipple-piercing, mimicking carcinoma. Breast J 2004;10:363-365.
20. Bocian JJ, Fahmy RN, Michas CA. A rare case of coccidioidoma of the breast. Arch Pathol Lab Med 1991;115:1064-1067.
21. Tesh RB, Schneidau JD. Primary cutaneous histoplasmosis. N Engl J Med 1966;275:597-599.
22. Berger SA, Gorea A, Stadler J, et al. Recurrent breast abscesses caused by *Corynebacterium minutissimum*. J Clin Microbiol 1984;20:1219-1220.
23. Fitzgibbons PL, Smiley DF, Kem WH. Sarcoidosis presenting initially as breast mass. Report of two cases. Hum Pathol 1985;16:851-852.
24. Herrmann JB. Thrombophlebitis of breast and contiguous thoracicoabdominal wall (Mondor's disease). N Y State J Med 1966;66:3146-3152.
25. Symmers WS. Silicone mastitis in "topless" waitress and some other varieties of foreign-body mastitis. Br Med J 1968;3:19-22.
26. Elsner B, Harper FB. Disseminated Wegener's granulomatosis with breast involvement. Report of a case. Arch Pathol 1969;87:544-547.
27. Jordan JM, Rowe WT, Allen NB. Wegener's granulomatosis involving the breast. Report of three cases and review of the literature. Am J Med 1987;83:159-164.
28. Lucey JJ. Spontaneous infarction of the breast. Clin Pathol 1975;28:937-943.
29. Morgan MC, Weaver MG, Crowe JP, Abdul-Karim FW. Diabetic niastopathy. A clinicopathologic study in palpable and nonpalpable breast lesions. Mod Pathol 1995;8:349-354.
30. Rickert RR, Rajan S. Localized breast infarcts associated with pregnancy. Arch Pathol 1974;97:159-161.
31. Davis MDP, Alexander JL, Prawer SE. Pyoderma gangrenosum of the breasts precipitated by breast surgery. J Am Acad Dermatol 2006;55:317-320.
32. Komenaka IK, Schnabel FR, Cohen JA, et al. Recurrent eosinophilic mastitis. Am Surg 2003;69:620-623.
33. Bolca Topal N, Topal U, Golkalp G, Saraydaroglu O. Eosinophilic mastitis. JBR-BTR 2007;90:170-171.
34. Villalba-Nuño V, Sabaté JM, Gómez A, et al. Churg-Strauss syndrome involving the breast: a rare cause of eosinophilic mastitis. Eur Radiol 2002;12:646-649.
35. Thompson AB, Barron MM, Lapp NL. The hypereosinophilic syndrome presenting with eosinophilic mastitis. Arch Intern Med 1985;145:564-565.

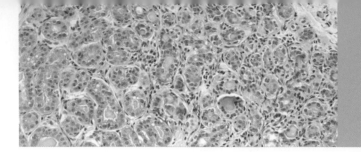

4

Epidemiology of Breast Cancer

Victor G. Vogel

INTRODUCTION

More than 192,000 American women were diagnosed with invasive breast cancer in 2009.[1] In addition, there were 62,000 cases of in situ disease, and more than 40,000 deaths. Breast cancer is the most commonly diagnosed cancer among women in the United States and accounts for 26% of all female cancers (excluding nonmelanoma skin cancers and in situ cancers). Although breast cancer may occur in men, it is rare. Among U.S. females, breast cancer ranks second to lung cancer in terms of cancer mortality, with 41,000 female breast cancer deaths annually. These deaths account for 15% of the burden of cancer mortality among female Americans. Fortunately, mortality from breast cancer has decreased in recent years due to early detection and improved treatment of the disease. Data from the National Cancer Institute's (NCI) Surveillance Epidemiology and End Results (SEER) program show that the breast cancer mortality rate declined 2.3% each year between 1990 and 2003.[2] The percentage of women surviving at least 5 years after diagnosis has risen to 88%, and 5-year survival is 98% for women diagnosed with localized disease.[2,3]

RISK FACTORS FOR BREAST CANCER

Age, Race, and Ethnicity

Breast cancer incidence rises sharply with age (Figure 4-1 and Tables 4-1 and 4-2).[4] The overall incidence rate of breast cancer is low at younger ages (e.g., 1.4 per 100,000 women ages 20–24).[4] As women begin to transition through menopause, the rates of breast cancer increase substantially; data from SEER show that, between 1999 and 2003, the incidence rate of breast cancer was 119.3 per 100,000 for women ages 40 to 44, 249.0 per 100,000 for women ages 50 to 54, and 388.3 for women ages 60 to 64. The highest rate of breast cancer is observed among women ages 75 to 79, in whom about 490 incident cases of breast cancer are diagnosed for every 100,000 women in this age group.

Breast cancer rates also differ by race and ethnicity. Although African American women have a lower overall incidence of breast cancer than white women, African Americans have a higher incidence of breast cancer before age 35, as shown in Figure 4-1.[4] Although breast cancer incidence is higher in black women than in white women among women younger than 40 years, the reverse is true among those aged 40 years or older. In the NCI SEER database, there are qualitative interactions between age and race.[4] Age-specific incidence rates overall (expressed as number of breast cancers per 100,000 women-yr) are higher among black women than among white women younger than 40 years (15.5 vs. 13.1), and then, age-specific rates crossed with rates higher among white women (281.3) than among black women (239.5) aged 40 years or older. The black-to-white incidence rate crossover is observed for all tumor characteristics than for high-risk tumor characteristics.

In addition, breast cancer mortality is substantially greater at all ages among African Americans than it is among whites (34 vs. 25 deaths per 100,000 women, respectively; Figure 4-2).[5] Estimates of the prevalence of breast cancer risk factors indicate that African American

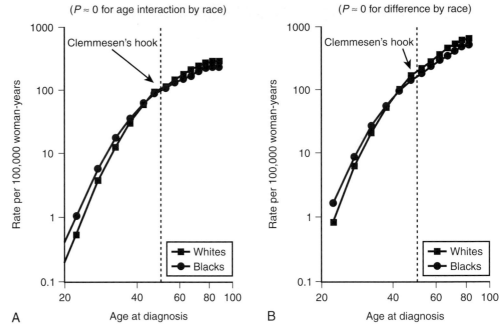

FIGURE 4-1 Age-specific incidence rates for breast cancer among white and black women in the National Cancer Institute (NCI) Surveillance Epidemiology and End Results (SEER) 9 Registries database from 1975 through 2004. **A,** Age-specific incidence rates. **B,** Age-specific incidence rate curves from the age-period–cohort-fitted model adjusted for calendar period and birth cohort effects. *Data from Anderson WF, Rosenberg PS, Menashe I, et al. Age-related crossover in breast cancer incidence rates between black and white ethnic groups. J Natl Cancer Inst 2008;100:1804-1814.*

TABLE 4-1	Traditional Risk Factors for Breast Cancer
Risk Factor	**Relative Increase in Risk (Absence of the Factor Compared with the Greatest Risk Category)**
Age at menarche	1.3
Age at first live birth	1.9
Age at menopause	1.5
Family history of breast cancer in first-degree relatives (mother, sisters, daughters)	1.7 (mother) 5.0 (two first-degree relatives)
Proliferative benign breast disease	2.0 5.0 (atypical hyperplasia)
Lobular carcinoma in situ	10
Birthplace/ethnicity	1.5–2.5

and white women differ in terms of their ages at menarche, menstrual cycle patterns, birth rates, lactation histories, patterns of oral contraceptive use, levels of obesity, frequency of menopausal hormone use, physical activity patterns, and alcohol intake.[6] In the 1970s, the percentage of breast cancer patients with an early age at onset was much higher among white women than among black women, but by the 1990s, the relationship had reversed, as shown in Figure 4-3. By 2000, and in the years since, a greater proportion of black than white women are diagnosed with breast cancer before age 45 years. The reasons for this secular change are not yet clear.[4]

Both incidence and mortality rates among Hispanics, Native Americans, Asians and Pacific Islanders, and Alaskan Natives are lower than for whites and African Americans.[3]

Benign Breast Disease

In some women, ductal cells proliferate, resulting in intraductal hyperplasia. Among these women, some may progress to atypia, and a smaller proportion progress to develop lobular or ductal carcinoma in situ. Some, but not all, of these women eventually develop invasive malignancy. Benign breast lesions can be classified according to their histologic appearance. Benign breast lesions thought to impart no increased risk of breast cancer include adenosis, duct ectasia, simple fibroadenoma, fibrosis, mastitis, mild hyperplasia, cysts, and metaplasia of the apocrine or squamous types.[7,8] Lesions associated with a slight increase in the subsequent risk of developing invasive breast cancer include complex fibroadenoma, moderate or florid hyperplasia with or without atypia, sclerosing adenosis, and papilloma. Atypical hyperplasia of either the ductal or the lobular type is associated with a 4- to 5-fold increased risk of developing subsequent breast cancer, and this risk increases to approximately 10-fold if it is also associated with a family history of invasive breast cancer in a first-degree relative.

There is an excess risk of invasive breast cancer with the diagnosis of proliferative disease without and with atypia, particularly among premenopausal women.[9–11] Women with nonproliferative benign conditions of the breast and no or remote family history of breast cancer do not experience an excess incidence of breast cancer; however, for women with the same diagnosis but with a first-degree family history of breast cancer, the risk of a subsequent invasive breast cancer increases by about two thirds. Among women with a diagnosis of proliferative diseases without atypia, this risk was increased by

TABLE 4-2	Newer Epidemiologic Risk Factors for Breast Cancer

Characteristic	Menopausal Status*	Comparison Category	Risk Category	Estimate of Effect†
Demographic Factors				
Age (yr)	Both	40–44	50–54	IRR 2.09
	Both	40–44	75–79	IRR 4.11
Race	Both	African American	White	IRR 1.16
	Both	Asian/Pacific Islander	White	IRR 1.42
	Both	Hispanic	White	IRR 1.57
Genetic Factors				
BRCA1 mutation	Both	No mutation	Mutation present in gene	Lifetime risk 50–73% by age 50 and 65–87% by age 70
BRCA2 mutation	Both	No mutation	Mutation present in gene	Lifetime risk 59% by age 50 and 82% by age 70
Hormonal Factors				
Oral contraceptive use	Both	Never users	Current users	RR 1.24 (1.15–1.33)
	Both	Never users	≥10 yr since last use	RR 1.01 (0.96–1.05)
Postmenopausal hormone therapy use	Postmenopausal	Nonusers with an intact uterus	Estrogen + progestin users	HR 1.24 (1.01–1.54)
	Postmenopausal	Nonusers with a hysterectomy	Estrogen users	HR 0.80 (0.62–1.04)
Circulating estradiol	Premenopausal	Lowest quartile	Highest quartile	OR 1.00 (0.66–1.52)
	Postmenopausal	Lowest quintile	Highest quintile	RR 2.00 (1.47–2.71)
Circulating estrone	Premenopausal	Lowest quartile	Highest quartile	OR 1.16 (1.48–3.22)
	Postmenopausal	Lowest quintile	Highest quintile	RR 2.19 (1.48–3.22)
Testosterone	Premenopausal	<1.13 nmol/L	≥2.04 nmol/L	OR 1.73 (1.16–2.57)
	Postmenopausal	Lowest quintile	Highest quintile	RR 2.22 (1.59-3.10)
Other Biologic Factors				
Mammographic breast density	Both	<5% density	≥75% density	RR 4.64 (3.64–5.91)
Bone mineral density	Postmenopausal	Lowest quartile at each of three skeletal sites	Highest quartile at each of three skeletal sites	RR 2.70 (1.4–5.3)
Circulating IGF-1	Premenopausal	25th percentile	75th percentile	OR 1.93 (1.38–2.69)
	Postmenopausal	25th percentile	75th percentile	OR 0.95 (0.62–1.33)
Circulating IGFBP-3	Premenopausal	25th percentile	75th percentile	OR 1.96 (1.28–2.99)
	Postmenopausal	25th percentile	75th percentile	OR 0.97 (0.53–1.77)
Behavioral Factors				
Body mass index	Postmenopausal	<21.0 kg/m^2	≥33.0 kg/m^2	RR 1.27 (1.03–1.55)
Height	Premenopausal	<1.60 cm	≥1.75 cm	RR 1.42 (0.95–2.12)
	Postmenopausal	<1.60 cm	≥1.75 cm	RR 1.28 (0.94–1.76)
Weight	Postmenopausal	<60.0 kg	≥80.0 kg	RR 1.25 (1.02–1.52)
Alcohol use	Both	Never drinkers	>12 g/day	RR 1.10 (1.06–1.14)
Smoking	Postmenopausal	Never smokers	Smoked > 40 yr	RR 1.5 (1.2–1.9)
Night work	Both	No nightshift work	Any nightshift work	OR 1.48 (1.36–1.61)
Dietary Factors				
Total fat intake	Both	Lowest quartile	Highest quartile	OR 1.13 (1.03–1.25)
Saturated fat intake	Both	Lowest quartile	Highest quartile	OR 1.19 (1.06–1.35)
Meat intake	Both	Lowest quartile	Highest quartile	OR 1.17 (1.06–1.29)

TABLE 4-2	Newer Epidemiologic Risk Factors for Breast Cancer (Continued)			
Characteristic	Menopausal Status*	Comparison Category	Risk Category	Estimate of Effect†
Environmental Factors				
Ionizing radiation	Both	0–0.09 Gy exposure to Nagasaki or Hiroshima atomic bomb	≥0.50 Gy exposure to Nagasaki or Hiroshima atomic bomb	RR varies depending on age at exposure: RR = 9 at age 0–4; RR = 2 at age 35–39

*Menopausal status at the time of diagnosis.
†95% confidence intervals are given in parentheses.
HR, hazard ratio; IGF-1, insulin-like growth factor-1; IGFBP-3, insulin-like growth factor-1 receptor binding protein-3; IRR, incidence rate ratio; OR, odds ratio; RR, relative risk.
From Gierach G, Vogel V. Epidemiology of breast cancer. In Singletary SE, Robb GL, Hortobagyi GN, eds. Advanced Therapy of Breast Disease. 2nd ed. Hamilton, Ontario: BC Decker; 2004; pp. 58-83.

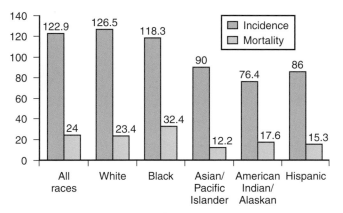

FIGURE 4-2 Breast cancer incidence and mortality by racial/ethnic group in the United States. The age-adjusted incidence rate was 122.9 per 100,000 women per year. These rates are based on cases diagnosed in 2003 to 2007 from 17 SEER geographic areas. *From Howlader N, Noone AM, Krapcho M, et al (eds). SEER Cancer Statistics Review, 1975-2008. Bethesda, MD: National Cancer Institute, 2010.*

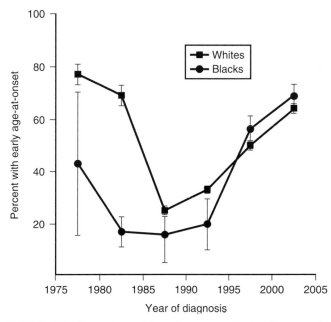

FIGURE 4-3 Percentage of breast cancer patients with an early age at onset by race in the NCI SEER 9 Registries database from 1975 through 2004. *Data from Anderson WF, Rosenberg PS, Menashe I, et al. Age-related crossover in breast cancer incidence rates between black and white ethnic groups. J Natl Cancer Inst 2008;100:1804-1814.*

80% if there is a remote family history of breast cancer and by more than twofold for those with first-degree family history of breast cancer.

Family History

Women having a first-degree relative with a history of breast cancer are at increased risk of the disease themselves.[12] The risk conferred by family history is further increased if the affected family member was diagnosed with the disease at a younger age. For example, a woman with a first-degree relative diagnosed with breast cancer before age 40 has a nearly sixfold increased risk of being diagnosed with breast cancer before she is 40 compared with a woman of the same age but without a family history of breast cancer.[13] Two genes, *BRCA1* and *BRCA2*, have been implicated in familial breast cancer, but these account for less than 10% of all breast cancer cases.[14] *BRCA* mutations are most strongly related to breast cancer occurring in younger, premenopausal women. Among women diagnosed with breast cancer before age 40, 9% have a *BRCA* mutation, compared with only 2% of women of any age diagnosed with breast cancer.[15] Additional genes such as *TP53, PTEN, ATM,* and the Lynch syndromes play a minor role in familial breast cancer syndromes.

Reproductive Factors

Early age at menarche and late age at menopause have been found to elevate breast cancer risk, whereas premenopausal oophorectomy reduces risk. Late age at first and possibly last full-term pregnancy (e.g., >30 yr) have been associated with an elevated risk, and breast cancer risk decreases with increasing parity.[16] The timing of the initiation of the carcinogenic process is an important consideration when studying the effect of reproductive factors on breast cancer risk.[17] Risk of premenopausal breast cancer decreases about 9% for each 1 year increase in age at menarche, whereas risk of postmenopausal breast cancer decreases only about 4% for each 1 year increase in age at menarche. Breast cancer risk increases with increasing age at first full-term pregnancy by 5% per year for breast cancer diagnosed before menopause and by 3% for cancers diagnosed

TABLE 4-3	Possible Protective Factors for Breast Cancer			
Characteristic	Menopausal Status*	Reference Group	Comparison Group	Estimate of Effect†
	Postmenopausal	Lowest quintile	Highest quintile	RR 0.66 (0.43–1.00)
Other Biologic Factors				
Bone fracture	Postmenopausal	No fracture in past 5 yr	History of fracture	OR 0.80 (0.68–0.94)
Behavioral Factors				
Body mass index	Premenopausal	<21.0 kg/m^2	≥33.0 kg/m^2	RR 0.58 (0.34–1.00)
Physical activity	Premenopausal	<9.1 hr/wk	≥20.8 hr/wk	OR 0.74 (0.52–1.05)
	Postmenopausal	Not currently active	>40 metabolic-equivalent hr/wk	RR 0.78 (0.62–1.00)
NSAID use	Both	Nonusers	Current user of any NSAID	OR 0.80 (0.73–0.87)
Dietary Factors				
Calcium (dietary)	Postmenopausal	≤500 mg/day	>1250 mg/day	RR 0.80 (0.67–0.95)
Folate (total)	Both	150–299 µg/day	≥600 µg/day	RR 0.93 (0.83–1.03)
Soy	Premenopausal	Low intake	High intake	OR 0.70 (0.58–0.85)
	Postmenopausal	Low intake	High intake	OR 0.77 (0.60–0.98)
Vitamin D (total)	Postmenopausal	<400 IU	≥800 IU	RR 0.89 (0.77–1.03)

*Menopausal status at the time of diagnosis.
†95% confidence intervals are given in parentheses.
NSAID, nonsteroidal anti-inflammatory drug; OR, odds ratio; RR, relative risk.
Data from Gierach G, Vogel V. Epidemiology of breast cancer. In Singletary SE, Robb GL, Hortobagyi GN, eds. Advanced Therapy of Breast Disease. 2nd ed. Hamilton, Ontario: BC Decker; 2004; pp. 58-83.

after menopause. Each full-term pregnancy is associated with a 3% reduction in breast cancer risk diagnosed before menopause, whereas the reduction was 12% for breast cancer diagnosed later.

Breastfeeding

In addition to a protective effect of parity on breast cancer, breastfeeding appears to contribute to a reduced risk as well. As duration of breastfeeding increases, the risk of breast cancer decreases, although parity may be a confounding factor. Hypothesized mechanisms for the protective effect of breastfeeding include the decline in estrogen production related to the suppression of ovulatory cycles and an increased secretion of prolactin.[18] The relative risk of breast cancer decreases by approximately 4% for every 12 months of breastfeeding and decreases by 7% for each birth. The size of the decline in the risk of breast cancer does not differ significantly for women in developed and developing countries and does not vary significantly by age, menopausal status, ethnic origin, the number of births a woman had, or her age at her first child's birth. The cumulative incidence of breast cancer in developed countries would be reduced by more than half if women had the average number of births (6.5 vs. 2.5) and lifetime duration of breastfeeding (24 vs. 3 mo per child) that had been prevalent in developing countries until recently. Strong epidemiologic evidence does not exist for a relationship between being breastfed in infancy and breast cancer incidence in adult life.[19]

Obesity

Obesity has emerged as a significant risk factor for postmenopausal breast cancer and is possibly a protective factor for premenopausal breast cancer. Further, adjustment for measures of obesity attenuates, but does not eliminate, the racial difference in stage at breast cancer diagnosis.[20,21] The most frequently used measure of obesity is the body mass index (BMI) (Table 4-3). BMI is a measure of weight for height and is calculated as weight in kilograms divided by the square of height in meters (kg/m^2). Among postmenopausal women, some studies report either no association or only a weak association between BMI and breast cancer risk,[22,23] whereas the vast majority report that increased BMI significantly raises the risk of breast cancer[24-26] (e.g., a 4% increase in the odds of postmenopausal breast cancer for every 1 kg/m^2 increase in current BMI[25]). The risk of breast cancer increases 7% with each 4 kg/m^2 increase in BMI among postmenopausal women.[24] Some studies have reported that the positive association between BMI and postmenopausal breast cancer risk occurs only or more strongly among women with certain other risk factors, such as a family history of breast cancer[27] or older age.[28] A consistent finding is that elevated BMI increases the risk of postmenopausal breast cancer only among women who have never used postmenopausal hormone therapy.[26,29-31]

Central adiposity, commonly measured by waist circumference or waist-to-hip ratio, has been positively associated with postmenopausal breast cancer,[32,33] and this effect is stronger in women who never used hormone replacement therapy.[34] Finally, multiple studies have reported that weight gain during adulthood increases postmenopausal breast cancer risk[35] whereas weight loss can reduce this risk.[32,36]

Obesity appears to have an opposite effect on breast cancer risk among premenopausal women. Few studies report either a positive association[37] or no association[35] between BMI and premenopausal breast cancer, and BMI may be inversely associated with premenopausal or early-age breast cancer risk,[24,38,39] with an 11% reduction in risk for every 4 kg/m^2 increase in BMI.[24] The effect of BMI on premenopausal breast cancer risk may vary by race, with one study reporting a negative association among white women but no association among African American women.[22]

Similar relationships between obesity and premenopausal breast cancer risk are observed when other anthropometric measures are considered. Weight may either be negatively associated[24,32] or not associated[40,41] with premenopausal breast cancer. One study reported a positive association between waist-to-hip ratio and risk of premenopausal breast cancer,[33] whereas another reported no association.[34] The effect of weight gain on premenopausal breast cancer may also vary by race, with studies of white women reporting either no[42,43] or a negative association,[35] whereas a study of Hispanic women reported a nonsignificant positive association.[43] Overall, the totality of the current evidence suggests that obesity reduces the risk of premenopausal breast cancer.

Endogenous Hormones

The mechanisms through which estrogens contribute to the carcinogenic process are complex; however, evidence exists confirming estrogens cause both normal and malignant breast cell proliferation.[44] Many established breast cancer risk factors can be attributed to some means of elevated estrogen exposure. For example, both an early age of menarche and a late age of menopause are related to prolonged exposure to the high levels of estrogen that occur during the menstrual cycle, and both are associated with increased breast cancer risk.[45,46] Surgical menopause, which results in an abrupt arrest of estrogen secretion by the ovaries, is protective against breast cancer.[47] Moreover, the rate of age-specific breast cancer slows around the time of menopause, a time when estrogen levels decline.[3] Increased bone mineral density, a potential reflection of cumulative estrogen exposure, is associated with increased breast cancer development in menopausal women and obesity, which is positively correlated with circulating estrogen levels, is associated with postmenopausal breast cancer risk.[24,48]

Numerous studies have consistently demonstrated that increased levels of endogenous estrogen are related to increased risk of breast cancer in postmenopausal women.[49,50] Nine prospective studies examining hormone levels in relation to postmenopausal breast cancer reported a twofold increase in risk of breast cancer for women in the highest quintile of estradiol (E2) compared with those in the lowest quintile.[50]

In addition to the observational studies linking circulating estradiol concentrations and breast cancer risk, convincing data from large clinical trials show that drugs that block the action of estrogen reduce breast cancer incidence. The risk reduction is more pronounced in women with higher estrogen levels than in those with lower levels; thus further strengthening the evidence that estrogen exposure is associated with the development of breast cancer.[51,52] In the Multiple Outcomes of Raloxifene Evaluation (MORE) trial, it was found that postmenopausal women with the highest E2 levels had a twofold risk of breast cancer in comparison with women with the lowest levels of E2.[53] Women in the placebo arm of the trial had nearly seven times the risk of developing breast cancer than women with E2 levels lower (0.6%/yr) than the assays detection limit, and women with circulating levels of estradiol greater than 10 pmol/L in the raloxifene group had a breast cancer rate 76% lower than women with similar levels of E2 in the placebo group. Inhibiting the action of estrogen plays an obvious role in the risk reduction of breast cancer.[51,54,55]

Estrogen Metabolism

Although the evidence linking estrogen and breast cancer is compelling, there is growing evidence that the way estrogen is metabolized is associated with the risk of breast cancer.[56-59] E2 metabolism is predominantly oxidative. E2 is first (reversibly) converted to estrone, which is irreversibly converted to either 2- or 16α-hydroxyestrone in order to eliminate it from the body. Both 16-OH estrone and 16-OH estradiol strongly activate the classic estrogen receptor and, similar to E2, can stimulate uterine tissue growth.[56] Conversely, the 2-OH metabolites do not appear to promote cellular proliferation and may even have antiestrogenic effects.[59] Because the 2-OH and 16-OH metabolites compete for a limited substrate pool, a rise in one pathway will reduce the amount of product in the competing pathway. However, the relative activity of these two metabolic pathways (2:16-OH) may be an endocrine biomarker for breast cancer risk. Despite the biologic evidence, however, epidemiologic support is lacking. Only a handful of studies have explored the association between breast cancer risk and 2:16-OHE1 ratio, with mixed results.[59-64]

Possible explanations for these disparate findings include small sample sizes, retrospective study designs, and the use of prevalent breast cancer cases. Metabolite levels in women with breast cancer may not reflect the hormonal milieu during the etiologically relevant time period. Moreover, the use of prevalent cases may mask any association because estrogen metabolism may be altered by treatment.[65] Notably, the only two prospective studies to date have found a decreased risk associated with high urinary 2:16-OH ratio[62,64]; however, in neither study was the results statistically significant. Moreover, in one study the association was limited to premenopausal women only.[64]

Dietary Fat and Serum Estradiol

Varying levels of fat consumption may influence the incidence of hormonally dependent breast cancer by modifying levels of circulating estrogens.[66-68] In fact, free fatty acids added to plasma can significantly increase levels of E2 in vitro.[69,70] A meta-analysis found serum E2 levels to be 23% lower in healthy postmenopausal women consuming the least amount of dietary fat than in women with the highest fat intake.[66] The Diet and Androgens (DIANA) Randomized Trial found a nonsignificant reduction in serum estradiol (18.0% reduction vs. 5.5% reduction) among postmenopausal women consuming a low–animal fat and high–omega-3 diet.[67] However, not all studies evaluating dietary fat and estrogen levels have observed reductions in circulating E2 levels; it has been hypothesized that inadequate dietary assessment may be one cause of this contradiction.

Oral Contraceptives and Postmenopausal Hormone Therapy

Exposure to exogenous estrogen has been related to breast cancer risk. In the general population, oral contraceptive use is weakly associated with breast cancer risk. In 1996, the Collaborative Group on Hormonal Factors in Breast Cancer analyzed the worldwide epidemiologic evidence on the relation between breast cancer risk and use of hormonal contraceptives.[71] Women had a slight but significant increased risk of breast cancer while taking oral contraceptives compared with the risk among nonusers. Reassuringly, the risk diminished steadily after cessation of use, with no increase in the risk 10 years after cessation of oral contraceptives, irrespective of family history of breast cancer, reproductive history, geographic area of residence, ethnic background, differences in study designs, dose and type of hormone, and duration of use.

More recent population-based studies of the risk of breast cancer among former and current users of oral contraceptives do not suggest that these drugs increase risk.[72,73] Among women aged 35 to 64 years participating in a population-based, case-control study (The National Institute of Child Health and Human Development Women's Contraceptive and Reproductive Experiences [CARE] Study), current or former oral contraceptive use was not associated with a significantly increased risk of breast cancer.[73]

A retrospective cohort study evaluated the effect of oral contraceptives among women with a familial predisposition to breast cancer.[74] After accounting for age and birth cohort, ever having used oral contraceptives was significantly associated with a threefold increased risk of breast cancer among first-degree relatives only. The elevated risk among women with a first-degree family history of breast cancer was most evident for oral contraceptive use during or before 1975, when formulations were likely to contain higher dosages of estrogen and progestins.

In 1997, the Collaborative Group on Hormonal Factors in Breast Cancer[75] reanalyzed approximately 90% of the worldwide epidemiologic evidence on the relation between risk of breast cancer and use of postmenopausal hormone replacement therapy. Among current users of hormone replacement therapy, or those who ceased use 1 to 4 years previously, the risk of having breast cancer diagnosed increased by 2.3% for each year of use; the relative risk was 1.35 for women who had used hormone replacement therapy for 5 years or longer. A meta-analysis also found an increased risk of breast cancer risk associated with the use of hormone replacement therapy.[76]

The results of the Women's Health Initiative (WHI) showed that this increased risk may occur only among users of combined estrogen and progestin regimens[77] and not among women using unopposed estrogen.[78] The WHI conducted two separate randomized, controlled primary prevention trials of hormone replacement therapy use among postmenopausal women ages 50 to 79: (1) a trial of conjugated equine estrogens, 0.625 mg daily, plus medroxyprogesterone acetate, 2.5 mg daily, in a single tablet versus placebo among women with an intact uterus, and (2) a trial of conjugated equine estrogens, 0.625 mg daily versus placebo among women with a hysterectomy. Women randomized to take the combination of estrogen and progestin had a 24% increase in risk of invasive breast cancer compared with those randomized to placebo.[77] However, in the unopposed estrogen trial, women randomized to active treatment had a lower risk of invasive breast cancer compared with women randomized to placebo,[78] although the duration of follow-up in WHI may not have been long enough to observe an association between breast cancer and unopposed estrogen use. The Nurse's Health Study, an observational study of women's health, reported that breast cancer risk increased with the duration of unopposed estrogen use (10 yr relative risk = 1.06, 15 yr = 1.18, and 20 yr = 1.42).[79] The relationship was more notable among estrogen receptor–positive and progesterone receptor–positive tumors and became statistically significant after 15 years of use.

Preeclampsia

Preeclampsia, a common complication of pregnancy, may be a particularly sensitive marker for endogenous hormonal factors associated with the development of breast cancer. In a review of the connection between preeclampsia and breast cancer risk, the data suggest that both a personal and a maternal history of preeclampsia are inversely and independently associated with subsequent breast cancer risk.[80] Preeclampsia may be a novel marker of endogenous hormonal factors that are related to breast cancer development, including reduced levels of estrogens and insulin-like growth factor-1 (IGF-1), and elevated levels of progesterone, androgens, and IGF-1–binding protein. These factors may act both individually and synergistically to decrease breast cancer risk.

Induced Abortion

It has been hypothesized that an interrupted pregnancy might increase a woman's risk of breast cancer owing to proliferation of breast cells without the later protective effect of differentiation. In a cohort of 1.5 million women, induced abortion as determined by a national Danish registry was not associated with an increased risk of breast cancer. No increases in risk were found in subgroups defined according to age at abortion, parity, time since abortion, or age at diagnosis of breast cancer.[81] The relative risk of breast cancer increased with increasing gestational age of the fetus at the time of the most recent induced abortion, but induced abortions appear to have no overall effect on the risk of breast cancer.

Mammographic Breast Density

Mammographic breast density is determined by the relative proportions of fat and structural tissues in the breast as viewed on a mammogram. Both qualitative and quantitative methods of measuring breast density exist, although quantitative methods are typically used in contemporary studies. Breast density is most often measured as the percentage of the breast composed of dense tissue.

Numerous studies have investigated associations between breast density and breast cancer since Wolfe hypothesized such a relationship in the mid 1970s. A recent meta-analysis of such studies showed a high degree of consistency.[82] The combined relative risk from incidence studies of the general population using qualitative Wolfe patterns was 1.8 for P1 (prominent ducts in anterior quarter of breast subareolar) versus N1 (mostly fatty, no visible ducts), 3.0 for P2 versus N1, and nearly 4.0 for DY (diffuse or nodular densities) versus N1. Combined relative risk estimates of studies using the Breast Imaging Reporting and Data System (BIRADS) qualitative classification with fatty breast as the referent group were 2 for scattered density, less than 3 for heterogeneously dense, and 4 for extremely dense.

Similar combined estimates of relative risks using quantitative percent density assessments were also reported. Compared with having less than 5% breast density, incidence studies had combined relative risks of 1.8 for 5% to 24% density, 2.1 for 25% to 49% density, 3.0 for 50% to 74% density, and 4.6 for 75% or greater density. The combined relative risk estimates for prevalence studies were similar but slightly lower: 1.4 for 5% to 24% density, 2.2 for 25% to 49% density, 3.0 for 50% to 74% density, and 3.7 for 75% or greater density versus less than 5% density.[82]

Presence of masking bias would result in underestimated relative risks reported by prevalence studies, in which cancers were detected at the time of screening, and overestimated relative risks reported by incidence studies; this is consistent with the results of the previously mentioned meta-analysis. Breast density remains associated with breast cancer risk regardless of age, menopausal status, or race,[82] and mammographic breast density may be a stronger risk factor for postmenopausal breast cancer than for premenopausal breast cancer.[83,84]

Higher-percent breast density remains a strong risk factor for breast cancer among women with known *BRCA1/BRCA2* mutations.[85] The odds of breast cancer among mutation carriers with density of 50% or greater were twice that of mutation carriers with less than 50% density.[85]

Few studies have reported how changes in breast density relate to changes in breast cancer risk.[86] One study reported that women who consistently had high-risk Wolfe patterns (P2 or DY) had over twice the risk of breast cancer compared with women who consistently had low-risk Wolfe patterns (N1 or P1). Those women whose patterns on the first mammogram were either P2 or DY but then had a low-risk pattern on a subsequent mammogram had similar risk to women with consistently low-risk Wolfe patterns.[87] Although the ability of breast density to change in response to known risk factors for breast cancer, such as use of postmenopausal hormone therapy, has been established, it is unclear what these changes in breast density mean in terms of altering breast cancer risk.[88]

EXOGENOUS HORMONES AND MAMMOGRAPHIC DENSITY

Studies have repeatedly shown that increased breast density is related to hormone replacement therapy use.[89,90] The percent of women whose density changes after initiating hormone replacement therapy varies by type of hormone replacement therapy used, with increased density occurring more often in estrogen plus progestin regimens than with estrogen-alone regimens.[89–91] In the WHI, investigators reported that 75% of women on active treatment experienced an increase in breast density after 1 year. The mean change in percent density from baseline to year 1 was 6.0% in the treatment group compared with –0.9% in the placebo group.[91] Short-term cessation of hormone replacement therapy use before mammography results in a decrease in breast density[92] or less frequent increase in density compared with women who continue to take hormone replacement therapy,[90] and even months after cessation of therapy, there appears to be residual effects of hormone replacement therapy on breast density.[93]

Data on the effect of oral contraceptive use on breast density are limited, likely because the majority of women for whom screening mammography is recommended (age $\geq$ 40 yr) are postmenopausal and would not be currently using oral contraceptives. One study has reported, however, that use of oral contraceptives before first birth was not related to breast density later in life.[94]

Exercise and Physical Activity

Interest in physical activity as a means for reducing breast cancer risk is growing, although evidence for an association between physical activity and breast cancer is not entirely consistent. The strength of association between physical activity and breast cancer ranges from 0.3 to 1.6.[95,96] Thirty-two studies observed a reduction in breast cancer risk in women who were most physically active, and the risk reduction averaged between 30% and 40%. An inverse dose-response relationship between increasing activity levels and decreased breast cancer risk was found in 20 of 23 studies that examined this trend. Only 2 studies observed an opposite trend such that breast cancer risk increased with increasing physical activity levels; the remaining studies found no association at all.

Weight control may play a particularly important role owing to links between excess weight, central adiposity, and increased breast cancer risk. Some public health organizations have issued physical activity guidelines for cancer risk reduction. Based upon the results of the aforementioned observational studies, controlled, clinical trials are needed to elucidate the mechanisms by which physical activity may influence breast cancer risk.

Alcohol Consumption

Whereas the association of alcohol consumption with increased risk for breast cancer has been a consistent finding in the majority of epidemiologic studies since 1990, questions remain regarding the interactions between alcohol and other risk factors and the biologic mechanisms involved. Meta-analyses of epidemiologic studies have examined the dose-response relation and assessed whether effect estimates differed according to various study characteristics.[95,97] Overall, there is a monotonic increase in the relative risk of breast cancer with alcohol consumption, but the magnitude of the effect was small; in comparison with nondrinkers, women averaging 12 g/day of alcohol consumption (approximately one typical drink) had a relative risk of 1.10. Estimates of relative risk were 7% greater in hospital-based case-control studies than in cohort studies or community-based case-control studies, 3% greater in studies published before 1990 than in studies published later, and 5% greater in studies conducted outside of the United States than in U.S. studies. The findings of five U.S. cohort studies published since 1990 yielded no increased risk for consumers of 12 g/day, as compared with nondrinkers. Cohort studies with less than 10 years of follow-up gave estimates 11% higher than cohort studies with longer follow-up periods. No meaningful differences were seen by menopausal status or type of beverage consumed.

Alcohol-related breast cancer risk may be associated with endogenous hormone levels.[97] Results from the Nurses' Health Study are consistent with the hypothesis that the use of alcohol increases the risk for breast cancer through a hormonal mechanism.[98] Risk for breast cancer was about 30% higher in women who currently used postmenopausal hormones for 5 or more years and did not drink alcohol. Those who never used postmenopausal hormones but drank 1.5 to 2 drinks or more alcohol daily had a nonsignificantly increased risk of 28%. Current users of postmenopausal hormones for 5 years or longer who consumed 20 g or more of alcohol daily had a relative risk for breast cancer nearly twice that of nondrinking, nonusers of postmenopausal hormones. Women who are making decisions about alcohol and postmenopausal hormone use may want to consider the added risks associated with breast cancer.

Smoking

The role of active and passive smoking in breast cancer remains controversial, largely owing to the fact that breast cancer is hormone-dependent and cigarette smoking appears to have antiestrogenic effects in women.[99,100] Until recently, most reports demonstrated no association between smoking and breast cancer risk; however, many studies included passive smokers within the referent category, possibly diluting any true effect that active or passive smoking exposure might have on breast cancer risk. In a review addressing the epidemiologic evidence for a link between smoking and breast cancer, five studies found significantly increased risks for passive smokers compared with unexposed women, and six reported 40% increased risk for active smokers versus those unexposed, suggesting a similar strength of association for active or passive smoking and breast cancer risk.[101]

The risk of breast cancer is significantly higher (70%) in parous women who initiated smoking within 5 years postmenarche and in nulliparous women who smoked 20 or more cigarettes per day (sevenfold increase in risk) and for 20 or more cumulative pack-years.[102] On the contrary, postmenopausal women who began smoking after their first full-term pregnancy and whose BMI increased from age 18 had half the risk of breast cancer. Cigarette smoke appears to exert a dual action on the breast, with different effects in premenopausal and postmenopausal women, thus reinforcing the importance of smoking prevention. Further, the timing of exposure in relation to windows of susceptibility is extremely important in the design of studies to investigate relationships between cigarette smoke exposure and risk of breast cancer.

Some strong and biologically meaningful associations have been reported for carcinogen-metabolizing genes (e.g., NAT1, NAT2, and catechol-O-methyltransferase [COMT] genotypes).[101] In addition, low-penetrance genes may be associated with breast cancer risk with any certainty.[103]

Breast Implants

There is no convincing evidence for a causal association between breast implants and breast cancer. Scientific studies have consistently determined that, when compared with women without implants, women with breast implants are not at increased risk for breast cancer incidence or recurrence, are not diagnosed with later-stage breast malignancies, and do not have a decreased length of survival.[104]

Ionizing Radiation

There is a well-established relationship between exposure to ionizing radiation and the risk of developing breast cancer.[105,106] Excess breast cancer risk has been consistently observed in association with a variety of exposures, such as the Hiroshima or Nagasaki atomic explosions, fluoroscopy for tuberculosis, and radiation treatments for medical conditions (e.g., Hodgkin's disease). Although risk is inversely associated with age at radiation exposure, exposures past the menopausal age seem to carry a low risk. Although an estimate of the risk of breast cancer associated with medical radiology puts the figure at less than 1% of the total,[107] certain populations, such as AT (ataxia-telangiectasia) heterozygotes, may be at increased risk from usual sources of radiation exposure.[108]

Many women develop breast cancer after treatment for Hodgkin's lymphoma at a young age. A case-control study conducted within an international population-based cohort of 3817 female 1-year survivors of Hodgkin lymphoma diagnosed at age 30 years or younger computed cumulative absolute risks of breast cancer, using modified standardized incidence ratios to relate cohort breast cancer risks to those in the general population, enabling application of population-based breast cancer rates, and allowing for competing risks by using population-based mortality rates in female Hodgkin's lymphoma survivors. Cumulative absolute risks of breast cancer increased with age at end of follow-up, time since Hodgkin lymphoma diagnosis, and radiation dose. For a Hodgkin lymphoma survivor who was treated at age 25 years with a chest radiation dose of at least 40 Gy without alkylating agents, the cumulative absolute risks of breast cancer by age 35, 45, and 55 years were 1.4%, 11.1%, and 29.0%, respectively. Cumulative absolute risks are lower in women treated with alkylating agents. Thus, breast cancer projections varied considerably by type of Hodgkin's lymphoma therapy, time since Hodgkin's lymphoma diagnosis, and age at end of follow-up. These estimates are applicable to Hodgkin's lymphoma survivors treated with regimens of the past and can be used to counsel such patients and plan management and preventive strategies.[109]

Women with a history of benign breast disease (BBD) or a family history of breast cancer appear to have greater breast cancer risk following relatively low ionizing radiation exposure compared with other women.[110] Breast cancer risk is elevated among women exposed to medical radiation before age 20 versus unexposed women, and this increased risk is observed only among women with a history of BBD. Overall, risk is not associated with exposure to medical radiation after age 20 years, although among women with a positive family history of breast or ovarian cancer, exposed women have an increased risk. The elevated risks are attributable to exposures and radiation doses that are no longer common, hampering study generalizability to younger cohorts. In theory, breast cancer patients treated with lumpectomy and radiation therapy may be at increased risk for second breast or other malignancies compared with those treated by mastectomy. Outcome studies after a median follow-up of 15 years show no difference, however, in the risk of second malignancies.[111]

Environmental Toxins

Whether environmental contaminants increase breast cancer risk is unknown. The association between breast cancer with endogenous estrogen or hormonally related events has led to the hypothesis that exposures to exogenous estrogen agonists or antagonists in the environment may increase the risk of breast cancer.[112] Although a few studies support this hypothesis, the vast majority of epidemiologic studies do not. Several studies have sought to determine whether breast cancer risk is increased in relation to exposure to organochlorines, compounds (e.g., polychlorinated biphenyls [PCBs], dioxins, organochlorine pesticides [dichlorophenyltrichloroethane {DDT}], lindane, hexachlorobenzene) with known estrogenic characteristics that were extensively used in some areas of the United States until the 1970s. The few available studies of occupational exposure to PCBs and dioxin have not supported a causal association with breast cancer risk. Most studies have been conducted among white women in developed countries where heavy pesticide spraying is no longer in use. Overall, the evidence does not support an association between environmental exposure to organochlorines and breast cancer risk. Additional studies of recent and ongoing exposures do not support the hypothesis that organochlorine compounds increase breast cancer risk.[113,114]

SUMMARY

Epidemiologic studies are vital to our understanding of the etiology and pathogenesis of breast cancer. The central promoting agent of importance in breast carcinogensis is estrogen, and this is confirmed by the host of epidemiologic studies cited in this chapter. These data emphasize the importance of proper recognition of breast atypias and precursor breast lesions to optimize patient care and patient safety.

REFERENCES

1. American Cancer Society. Cancer Facts & Figures 2008. Atlanta: American Cancer Society; 2008.
2. American Cancer Society. Breast Cancer Facts & Figures 2005-2006. Atlanta: American Cancer Society; 2005.
3. Altekruse SF, Kosary CL, Krapcho M, et al. SEER Cancer Statistics Review, 1975-2007. Published 2009. Updated 2010. Available at http://seer.cancer.gov/csr/1975_2007/
4. Anderson WF, Rosenberg PS, Menashe I, et al. Age-related crossover in breast cancer incidence rates between black and white ethnic groups. J Natl Cancer Inst 2008;100:1804-1814.
5. National Cancer Institute. Surveillance, Epidemiology, and End Results (SEER) Program Stat Database: Mortality—All COD, Public-Use with State, Total U.S. for Expanded Races/Hispanics. Updated 200604/2006. Available at http://seer.cancer.gov/data/metadata.html
6. Bernstein L, Teal CR, Joslyn S, Wilson J. Ethnicity-related variation in breast cancer risk factors. Cancer 2003;97 (1 Suppl):222-229.
7. Vogel VG. Breast cancer risk factors and preventive approaches to breast cancer. In Kavanagh JSS, Einhorn N, DePetrillo AD, eds. Cancer in Women. 1st ed. Cambridge, MA: Blackwell Scientific Publications; 1998; pp. 58-91.
8. Fitzgibbons PL, Henson DE, Hutter RV. Benign breast changes and the risk for subsequent breast cancer: an update of the 1985 consensus statement. Cancer Committee of the College of American Pathologists. Arch Pathol Lab Med 1998;122:1053-1055.
9. Colditz GA, Rosner B. Cumulative risk of breast cancer to age 70 years according to risk factor status: data from the Nurses' Health Study. Am J Epidemiol 2000;152:950-964.
10. Marshall LM, Hunter DJ, Connolly JL, et al. Risk of breast cancer associated with atypical hyperplasia of lobular and ductal types. Cancer Epidemiol Biomarkers Prev 1997;6:297-301.
11. Hartmann LC, Sellers TA, Frost MH, et al. Benign breast disease and the risk of breast cancer. N Engl J Med 2005;353:229-237.
12. Loman N, Johannsson O, Kristoffersson U, et al. Family history of breast and ovarian cancers and BRCA1 and BRCA2 mutations in a population-based series of early-onset breast cancer. J Natl Cancer Inst 2001;93:1215-1223.
13. Collaborative Group on Hormonal Factors in Breast Cancer. Familial breast cancer: collaborative reanalysis of individual data from 52 epidemiological studies including 58,209 women with breast cancer and 101,986 women without the disease. Lancet 2001;358:1389-1399.

14. Hulka BS, Moorman PG. Breast cancer: hormones and other risk factors. Maturitas 2001;38:103-113; discussion 113–116.

15. National Cancer Institute. Genetics of Breast and Ovarian Cancer (PDQ). Health Professional Version. Published September 18, 2005. Bethesda, MD: National Cancer Institute; 2005.

16. Kelsey JL, Gammon MD, John EM. Reproductive factors and breast cancer. Epidemiol Rev 1993;15:36-47.

17. Clavel-Chapelon F, Gerber M. Reproductive factors and breast cancer risk. Do they differ according to age at diagnosis? Breast Cancer Res Treat 2002;72:107-115.

18. Tryggvadottir L, Tulinius H, Eyfjord JE, Sigurvinsson T. Breast-feeding and reduced risk of breast cancer in an Icelandic cohort study. Am J Epidemiol 2001;154:37-42.

19. Michels KB, Trichopoulos D, Rosner BA, et al. Being breast-fed in infancy and breast cancer incidence in adult life: results from the two nurses' health studies. Am J Epidemiol 2001;153:275-283.

20. Cui Y, Whiteman MK, Langenberg P, et al. Can obesity explain the racial difference in stage of breast cancer at diagnosis between black and white women?. J Womens Health Gend Based Med 2002;11:527-536.

21. Jones BA, Kasi SV, Curnen MG, et al. Severe obesity as an explanatory factor for the black/white difference in stage at diagnosis of breast cancer. Am J Epidemiol 1997;146:394-404.

22. Hall IJ, Newman B, Millikan RC, Moorman PG. Body size and breast cancer risk in black women and white women: the Carolina Breast Cancer Study. Am J Epidemiol 2000;151:754-764.

23. den Tonkelaar I, Seidell JC, Collette HJ, de Waard F. A prospective study on obesity and subcutaneous fat patterning in relation to breast cancer in post-menopausal women participating in the DOM project. Br J Cancer 1994;69:352-357.

24. van den Brandt PA, Spiegelman D, Yaun SS, et al. Pooled analysis of prospective cohort studies on height, weight, and breast cancer risk. Am J Epidemiol 2000;152:514-527.

25. Trentham-Dietz A, Newcomb PA, Egan KM, et al. Weight change and risk of postmenopausal breast cancer (United States). Cancer Causes Control 2000;11:533-542.

26. Key TJ, Appleby PN, Reeves GK, et al. Body mass index, serum sex hormones, and breast cancer risk in postmenopausal women. J Natl Cancer Inst 2003;95:1218-1226.

27. Carpenter CL, Ross RK, Paganini-Hill A, Bernstein L. Effect of family history, obesity and exercise on breast cancer risk among postmenopausal women. Int J Cancer 2003;106:96-102.

28. La Vecchia C, Negri E, Franceschi S, et al. Body mass index and post-menopausal breast cancer: an age-specific analysis. Br J Cancer 1997;75:441-444.

29. Lahmann PH, Lissner L, Gullberg B, et al. A prospective study of adiposity and postmenopausal breast cancer risk: the Malmo Diet and Cancer Study. Int J Cancer 2003;103:246-252.

30. Li CI, Malone KE, Daling JR. Interactions between body mass index and hormone therapy and postmenopausal breast cancer risk (United States). Cancer Causes Control 2006;17:695-703.

31. Morimoto LM, White E, Chen Z, et al. Obesity, body size, and risk of postmenopausal breast cancer: the Women's Health Initiative (United States). Cancer Causes Control 2002;13:741-751.

32. Harvie M, Howell A, Vierkant RA, et al. Association of gain and loss of weight before and after menopause with risk of postmenopausal breast cancer in the Iowa Women's Health Study. Cancer Epidemiol Biomarkers Prev 2005;14:656-661.

33. Connolly BS, Barnett C, Vogt KN, et al. A meta-analysis of published literature on waist-to-hip ratio and risk of breast cancer. Nutr Cancer 2002;44:127-138.

34. Huang Z, Willett WC, Colditz GA, et al. Waist circumference, waist:hip ratio, and risk of breast cancer in the Nurses' Health Study. Am J Epidemiol 1999;150:1316-1324.

35. Verla-Tebit E, Chang-Claude J. Anthropometric factors and the risk of premenopausal breast cancer in Germany. Eur J Cancer Prev 2005;14:419-426.

36. Parker ED, Folsom AR. Intentional weight loss and incidence of obesity-related cancers: the Iowa Women's Health Study. Int J Obes Relat Metab Disord 2003;27:1447-1452.

37. Chu SY, Lee NC, Wingo PA, et al. The relationship between body mass and breast cancer among women enrolled in the Cancer and Steroid Hormone Study. J Clin Epidemiol 1991;44:1197-1206.

38. Tehard B, Clavel-Chapelon F. Several anthropometric measurements and breast cancer risk: results of the E3N cohort study. Int J Obes (Lond) 2006;30:156-163.

39. Swanson CA, Coates RJ, Schoenberg JB, et al. Body size and breast cancer risk among women under age 45 years. Am J Epidemiol 1996;143:698-706.

40. Yoo K, Tajima K, Park S, et al. Postmenopausal obesity as a breast cancer risk factor according to estrogen and progesterone receptor status (Japan). Cancer Lett 2001;167:57-63.

41. Freni SC, Eberhardt MS, Turturro A, Hine RJ. Anthropometric measures and metabolic rate in association with risk of breast cancer (United States). Cancer Causes Control 1996;7:358-365.

42. Huang Z, Hankinson SE, Colditz GA, et al. Dual effects of weight and weight gain on breast cancer risk. JAMA 1997;278:1407-1411.

43. Wenten M, Gilliland FD, Baumgartner K, Samet JM. Associations of weight, weight change, and body mass with breast cancer risk in Hispanic and non-Hispanic white women. Ann Epidemiol 2002;12:435–440.

44. Williams G, Anderson E, Howell A, et al. Oral contraceptive (OCP) use increases proliferation and decreases oestrogen receptor content of epithelial cells in the normal human breast. Int J Cancer 1991;48:206-210.

45. Clavel-Chapelon F. E3N-EPIC Group. Differential effects of reproductive factors on the risk of pre- and postmenopausal breast cancer. Results from a large cohort of French women. Br J Cancer 2002;86:723-727.

46. Titus-Ernstoff L, Longnecker MP, Newcomb PA, et al. Menstrual factors in relation to breast cancer risk. Cancer Epidemiol Biomarkers Prev 1998;7:783-789.

47. Lilienfeld AM. The relationship of cancer of the female breast to artificial menopause and martial status. Cancer 1956;9:927-934.

48. Zmuda JM, Cauley JA, Ljung BM, et al. Bone mass and breast cancer risk in older women: differences by stage at diagnosis. J Natl Cancer Inst 2001;93:930-936.

49. Kaaks R, Rinaldi S, Key TJ, et al. Postmenopausal serum androgens, oestrogens and breast cancer risk: the European prospective investigation into cancer and nutrition. Endocr Relat Cancer 2005;12:1071-1082.

50. Key T, Appleby P, Barnes I, Reeves G. Endogenous Hormones and Breast Cancer Collaborative Group. Endogenous sex hormones and breast cancer in postmenopausal women: reanalysis of nine prospective studies. J Natl Cancer Inst 2002;94:606-616.

51. Cummings SR, Duong T, Kenyon E, et al. Serum estradiol level and risk of breast cancer during treatment with raloxifene. JAMA 2002;287:216-220.

52. Fisher B, Costantino JP, Wickerham DL, et al. Tamoxifen for prevention of breast cancer: report of the National Surgical Adjuvant Breast and Bowel Project P-1 Study. J Natl Cancer Inst 1998;90:1371-1388.

53. Lippman ME, Krueger KA, Eckert S, et al. Indicators of lifetime estrogen exposure: effect on breast cancer incidence and interaction with raloxifene therapy in the multiple outcomes of raloxifene evaluation study participants. J Clin Oncol 2001;19:3111-3116.

54. Vogel VG, Costantino JP, Wickerham DL, et al. Effects of tamoxifen vs raloxifene on the risk of developing invasive breast cancer and other disease outcomes: the NSABP Study of Tamoxifen and Raloxifene (STAR) P-2 trial. JAMA 2006;295:2727-2741.

55. Vogel VG, Costantino JP, Wickerham DL, et al. Update of the National Surgical Adjuvant Breast and Bowel Project Study of Tamoxifen and Raloxifene (STAR) P-2 Trial: preventing breast cancer. Cancer Prev Res (Phila) 2010;3:696-706.

56. Fishman J, Martucci C. Biological properties of 16 alpha-hydroxyestrone: implications in estrogen physiology and pathophysiology. J Clin Endocrinol Metab 1980;51:611-615.

57. Bradlow HL, Hershcopf R, Martucci C, Fishman J. 16 Alpha-hydroxylation of estradiol: a possible risk marker for breast cancer. Ann N Y Acad Sci 1986;464:138-151.

58. Schneider J, Huh MM, Bradlow HL, Fishman J. Antiestrogen action of 2-hydroxyestrone on MCF-7 human breast cancer cells. J Biol Chem 1984;259:4840-4845.

59. Schneider J, Kinne D, Fracchia A, et al. Abnormal oxidative metabolism of estradiol in women with breast cancer. Proc Natl Acad Sci U S A 1982;79:3047-3051.

60. Adlercreutz H, Fotsis T, Hockerstedt K, et al. Diet and urinary estrogen profile in premenopausal omnivorous and vegetarian women and in premenopausal women with breast cancer. J Steroid Biochem 1989;34:527-530.

61. Kabat GC, Chang CJ, Sparano JA, et al. Urinary estrogen metabolites and breast cancer: a case-control study. Cancer Epidemiol Biomarkers Prev 1997;6:505-509.

62. Meilahn EN, De Stavola B, Allen DS, et al. Do urinary oestrogen metabolites predict breast cancer? Guernsey III cohort follow-up. Br J Cancer 1998;78:1250-1255.

63. Ursin G, London S, Stanczyk FZ, et al. Urinary 2-hydroxyestrone/16alpha-hydroxyestrone ratio and risk of breast cancer in postmenopausal women. J Natl Cancer Inst 1999;91:1067-1072.

64. Muti P, Bradlow HL, Micheli A, et al. Estrogen metabolism and risk of breast cancer: a prospective study of the 2:16alpha-hydroxyestrone ratio in premenopausal and postmenopausal women. Epidemiology 2000;11:635-640.

65. Osborne MP, Telang NT, Kaur S, Bradlow HL. Influence of chemopreventive agents on estradiol metabolism and mammary preneoplasia in the C3H mouse. Steroids 1990;55:114-119.

66. Wu AH, Pike MC, Stram DO. Meta-analysis: dietary fat intake, serum estrogen levels, and the risk of breast cancer. J Natl Cancer Inst 1999;91:529-534.

67. Berrino F, Bellati C, Secreto G, et al. Reducing bioavailable sex hormones through a comprehensive change in diet: the diet and androgens (DIANA) randomized trial. Cancer Epidemiol Biomarkers Prev 2001;10:25-33.

68. Holmes MD, Spiegelman D, Willett WC, et al. Dietary fat intake and endogenous sex steroid hormone levels in postmenopausal women. J Clin Oncol 2000;18:3668-3676.

69. Bruning PF, Bonfrer JM. Free fatty acid concentrations correlated with the available fraction of estradiol in human plasma. Cancer Res 1986;46:2606-2609.

70. Reed MJ, Cheng RW, Beranek PA, et al. The regulation of the biologically available fractions of oestradiol and testosterone in plasma. J Steroid Biochem 1986;24:317-320.

71. Breast cancer and hormonal contraceptives: collaborative reanalysis of individual data on 53,297 women with breast cancer and 100,239 women without breast cancer from 54 epidemiological studies. Collaborative Group on Hormonal Factors in Breast Cancer. Lancet 1996;347:1713-1727.

72. Hankinson SE, Colditz GA, Manson JE, et al. A prospective study of oral contraceptive use and risk of breast cancer (Nurses' Health Study, United States). Cancer Causes Control 1997;8:65-72.

73. Marchbanks PA, McDonald JA, Wilson HG, et al. Oral contraceptives and the risk of breast cancer. N Engl J Med 2002;346:2025-2032.

74. Grabrick DM, Hartmann LC, Cerhan JR, et al. Risk of breast cancer with oral contraceptive use in women with a family history of breast cancer. JAMA 2000;284:1791-1798.

75. Breast cancer and hormone replacement therapy: collaborative reanalysis of data from 51 epidemiological studies of 52,705 women with breast cancer and 108,411 women without breast cancer. Collaborative Group on Hormonal Factors in Breast Cancer. Lancet 1997;350:1047-1059.

76. Beral V. Million Women Study Collaborators. Breast cancer and hormone-replacement therapy in the Million Women Study. Lancet 2003;362:419-427.

77. Chlebowski RT, Hendrix SL, Langer RD, et al. Influence of estrogen plus progestin on breast cancer and mammography in healthy postmenopausal women: the Women's Health Initiative Randomized Trial. JAMA 2003;289:3243-3253.

78. Stefanick ML, Anderson GL, Margolis KL, et al. Effects of conjugated equine estrogens on breast cancer and mammography screening in postmenopausal women with hysterectomy. JAMA 2006;295:1647-1657.

79. Chen WY, Manson JE, Hankinson SE, et al. Unopposed estrogen therapy and the risk of invasive breast cancer. Arch Intern Med 2006;166:1027-1032.

80. Innes KE, Byers TE. Preeclampsia and breast cancer risk. Epidemiology 1999;10:722-732.

81. Melbye M, Wohlfahrt J, Olsen JH, et al. Induced abortion and the risk of breast cancer. N Engl J Med 1997;336:81-85.

82. McCormack VA, dos Santos Silva I. Breast density and parenchymal patterns as markers of breast cancer risk: a meta-analysis. Cancer Epidemiol Biomarkers Prev 2006;15:1159-1169.

83. Byrne C, Schairer C, Wolfe J, et al. Mammographic features and breast cancer risk: effects with time, age, and menopause status. J Natl Cancer Inst 1995;87:1622-1629.

84. Boyd NF, Lockwood GA, Byng JW, et al. Mammographic densities and breast cancer risk. Cancer Epidemiol Biomarkers Prev 1998;7:1133 1144.

85. Mitchell G, Antoniou AC, Warren R, et al. Mammographic density and breast cancer risk in BRCA1 and BRCA2 mutation carriers. Cancer Res 2006;66:1866-1872.

86. Vachon CM, Pankratz VS, Scott CG, et al. Longitudinal trends in mammographic percent density and breast cancer risk. Cancer Epidemiol Biomarkers Prev 2007;16:921-928.

87. Salminen TM, Saarenmaa IE, Heikkila MM, Hakama M. Risk of breast cancer and changes in mammographic parenchymal patterns over time. Acta Oncol 1998;37:547-551.

88. Chlebowski RT, McTiernan A. Biological significance of interventions that change breast density. J Natl Cancer Inst 2003;95:4 5.

89. Greendale GA, Reboussin BA, Slone S, et al. Postmenopausal hormone therapy and change in mammographic density. J Natl Cancer Inst 2003;95:30-37.

90. Colacurci N, Fornaro F, De Franciscis P, et al. Effects of a short-term suspension of hormone replacement therapy on mammographic density. Fertil Steril 2001;76:451-455.

91. McTiernan A, Martin CF, Peck JD, et al. Estrogen-plus-progestin use and mammographic density in postmenopausal women: Women's Health Initiative randomized trial. J Natl Cancer Inst 2005;97:1366-1376.

92. Harvey JA, Pinkerton JV, Herman CR. Short-term cessation of hormone replacement therapy and improvement of mammographic specificity. J Natl Cancer Inst 1997;89:1623-1625.

93. Crandall C, Palla S, Reboussin BA, et al. Positive association between mammographic breast density and bone mineral density in the Postmenopausal Estrogen/Progestin Interventions Study. Breast Cancer Res 2005;7:R922-R928.

94. Jeffreys M, Warren R, Gunnell D, et al. Life course breast cancer risk factors and adult breast density (United Kingdom). Cancer Causes Control 2004;15:947-955.

95. Ellison RC, Zhang Y, McLennan CE, Rothman KJ. Exploring the relation of alcohol consumption to risk of breast cancer. Am J Epidemiol 2001;154:740-747.

96. Friedenreich CM, Orenstein MR. Physical activity and cancer prevention: etiologic evidence and biological mechanisms. J Nutr 2002;132(11 Suppl):3456S-3464S.

97. Singletary KW, Gapstur SM. Alcohol and breast cancer: review of epidemiologic and experimental evidence and potential mechanisms. JAMA 2001;286:2143-2151.

98. Summaries for patients. Alcohol, postmenopausal hormone therapy, and breast cancer. Ann Intern Med 2002;137:I43.

99. Egan KM, Stampfer MJ, Hunter D, et al. Active and passive smoking in breast cancer: prospective results from the Nurses' Health Study. Epidemiology 2002;13:138-145.

100. Russo IH. Cigarette smoking and risk of breast cancer in women. Lancet 2002;360:1033-1034.

101. Morabia A. Smoking (active and passive) and breast cancer: epidemiologic evidence up to June 2001. Environ Mol Mutagen 2002;39:89-95.

102. Band PR, Le ND, Fang R, Deschamps M. Carcinogenic and endocrine disrupting effects of cigarette smoke and risk of breast cancer. Lancet 2002;360:1044-1049.

103. Willett WC, Rockhill B, Hankinson SE, et al. Epidemiology and nongenetic causes of breast cancer. In: Osborne CK, ed. Diseases of the Breast. Philadelphia: Lippincott Williams & Wilkins; 2000; pp. 175-220.

104. Hoshaw SJ, Klein PJ, Clark BD, et al. Breast implants and cancer: causation, delayed detection, and survival. Plast Reconstr Surg 2001;107:1393-1407.

105. Boice Jr JD. Radiation and breast carcinogenesis. Med Pediatr Oncol 2001;36:508-513.

106. Tokunaga M, Land CE, Yamamoto T, et al. Incidence of female breast cancer among atomic bomb survivors, Hiroshima and Nagasaki, 1950-1980. Radiat Res 1987;112:243-272.

107. Evans JS, Wennberg JE, McNeil BJ. The influence of diagnostic radiography on the incidence of breast cancer and leukemia. N Engl J Med 1986;315:810-815.
108. Swift M, Morrell D, Massey RB, Chase CL. Incidence of cancer in 161 families affected by ataxia-telangiectasia. N Engl J Med 1991;325:1831-1836.
109. Travis LB, Hill D, Dores GM, et al. Cumulative absolute breast cancer risk for young women treated for Hodgkin lymphoma. J Natl Cancer Inst 2005;97:1428-1437.
110. Hill DA, Preston-Martin S, Ross RK, Bernstein L. Medical radiation, family history of cancer, and benign breast disease in relation to breast cancer risk in young women, USA. Cancer Causes Control 2002;13:711-718.
111. Obedian E, Fischer DB, Haffty BG. Second malignancies after treatment of early-stage breast cancer: lumpectomy and radiation therapy versus mastectomy. J Clin Oncol 2000;18:2406-2412.
112. Calle EE, Frumkin H, Henley SJ, et al. Organochlorines and breast cancer risk. CA Cancer J Clin 2002;52:301-309.
113. Gammon MD, Santella RM, Neugut AI, et al. Environmental toxins and breast cancer on Long Island. I. Polycyclic aromatic hydrocarbon DNA adducts. Cancer Epidemiol Biomarkers Prev 2002;11:677-685.
114. Gammon MD, Wolff MS, Neugut AI, et al. Environmental toxins and breast cancer on Long Island. II. Organochlorine compound levels in blood. Cancer Epidemiol Biomarkers Prev 2002;11:686-697.

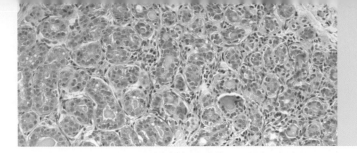

5

Patient Safety in Breast Pathology

Shahla Masood • David J. Dabbs

INTRODUCTION

Despite the long-standing worldwide attention given to the fight against breast cancer, this disease remains a serious illness, affecting not only the physical but also the emotional well-being of many individuals around the world. As a global public health problem, breast cancer is a heterogenous disease with a rather unpredictable outcome, ranging from an indolent tumor to a rapidly progressive disease with the ability to claim the life of an individual. Accurate diagnosis of breast cancer and reliable characterization of the biology of this tumor are critically important in treatment planning and predication of response to therapy and clinical outcome. Pathologists fulfill the critical role in setting the foundation of breast care for an individual patient. Breast pathology involves the morphologic and biologic recognition of abnormalities that are associated with the spectrum of changes seen in benign tissue, atypical proliferative disease, precursor lesions, and malignancy.

It is clear that pathologists carry a major responsibility of rendering diagnoses and providing prognostic and predictive information. Any mistake in this exercise is associated with serious consequences. If these tasks are not done properly, the clinicians are misled and the patients will subsequently suffer from an inappropriate treatment. This overview is designed to expand on the changing role of pathologists in the concept of promoting personalized breast health care and in securing patient safety. In addition, efforts are in place to outline the current challenges associated with the practice of breast pathology and to suggest strategies that may potentially minimize errors in breast pathology. Finally, it is our intent to illustrate practices that we have adopted that maximize patient safety while minimizing risk.

CHANGING ROLE OF PATHOLOGISTS IN BREAST CANCER DIAGNOSIS AND MANAGEMENT

Over the past few decades, substantial progress has been made in the diagnosis and treatment of breast cancer. Advances in breast imaging and emphasis on screening programs have led to the increased detection of in situ lesions and small breast carcinomas. Minimally invasive and cost-effective diagnostic sampling procedures such as fine-needle aspiration biopsy and core needle biopsy have replaced open surgical biopsies. Breast-conserving therapy and reconstructive surgery have enhanced cosmetic results, with a positive impact on the self-image and sexuality of patients with breast cancer.[1-5]

Sentinel lymph node biopsy provides a better alternative to the traditional axillary node dissection. The expanded role of radiotherapeutics and widespread use of neoadjuvant and adjuvant chemotherapy have contributed to improved patient outcomes. In addition, advances in molecular (biology) testing and recognition of predictive and prognostic factors have provided new opportunities for novel, effective, and individualized cancer therapy. Furthermore, the recent discovery of breast cancer susceptibility genes and the intensive efforts to identify risk factors may ultimately lead to the detection of precursor lesions and the prevention of breast cancer.

More importantly, enhanced public awareness of breast cancer has resulted in increased funding for biomedical research, behavioral science, education, screening, treatment, and survivorship programs.[6–15]

Above all, there has been a significant change in the fundamental concept of delivery of care to patients with breast cancer. Integrated care through a multidisciplinary approach has been widely advocated by different specialists involved in caring for patients with this disease. As a result, large numbers of multidisciplinary breast health centers have been established around the world.[16]

Pathologists have played a central role in the realization of this progress. In fact, pathologists have for many years been partners in the study and management of breast cancer. Aside from providing diagnostic information, pathologists have studied the characteristics of cancer, such as tumor size, lymph node metastasis, hormone receptor protein status, expression of oncogenes and tumor suppressor genes, and the rate of cellular proliferation, as well as other factors. This information has long been used clinically to identify those patients with both localized and metastatic breast cancer who are likely to respond to hormonal manipulation and/or chemotherapy.[17–21]

In addition, as more breast cancer treatments aimed at molecular targets (such as trastuzumab [Herceptin] therapy) become available, breast pathologists will continue to have a central role in the development, validation, implementation, and appropriate use of predictive and prognostic testing to better treat patients with breast cancer.[22–26]

CURRENT CHALLENGES IN THE PRACTICE OF BREAST PATHOLOGY

Public Perception about Pathologists

The importance of breast pathology has remained underrecognized among medical communities and the public. Pathologists, who make the ultimate determination of the nature of a disease and dictate the course of therapy for an individual patient, are often overshadowed by other members of the management team. Patients frequently do not understand the role of pathologists in their care and do not realize that inaccurate interpretation of pathology samples and test results may lead to inappropriate treatment. The issue of pathology becomes real when the patients become aware of a mistake in the diagnosis of their disease or there is significant discrepancy between the clinical presentation and the pathologic diagnosis. In these circumstances, the treating physicians are the ones who often initiate the review of the pathology materials.

The public should become fully aware of the complexity involved in the interpretation of difficult cases in breast pathology. Physicians engaged in the diagnosis and management of breast cancer can play a critical role in educating the public and in encouraging patients to understand the pathology of their disease and seek a second opinion about the accuracy of their pathology diagnosis.[27,28]

Diversity in Tissue Handling, Processing, and Reporting

Proper breast cancer therapy requires a clear understanding of the nature and extent of the disease. Pathologists are expected to provide complete information on specimen and tumor description, orientation and analysis of surgical margins, and full reporting of histologic features. Cancer committees of the College of American Pathologists and the Association of Directors of Anatomic and Surgical Pathologists have published practice synoptic protocols for the examination of surgical specimens from patients with breast cancer.[29,30] Similar protocols for assessment of hormone receptors and *HER-2/neu* oncogene have recently been developed.[31,32] The protocols have been designed to assist pathologists in various practice settings to follow a uniform approach in technical evaluation of breast samples and in interpretation of test results.

Synoptic guidelines are not widely used and there is extensive diversity in pathology reporting of factors that affect the treatment of breast cancer patients. This issue is best demonstrated by the study conducted by Wilkinson and coworkers[33] that reviewed the level of adherence to College of American Pathologists (CAP) guidelines in 100 breast cancer cases. They reported that CAP guidelines are not widely integrated in breast pathology. As an example, out of 100 cases reviewed, there was evidence of margin orientation in only 25% of cases. It is clear that mere recommendation of CAP practice guidelines might be insufficient to accomplish quality improvement in breast pathology reporting. Until more specific requirements for the mandatory use of guidelines is determined, the breast pathology reports may suffer from inconsistencies, which may have an adverse effect on patient care.[27]

The protocols for *HER2* and hormone receptor analysis[31,32] are intended to ensure the highest-quality test results. The protocols mandate compliance of the testing process to ensure that the preanalytic, analytic, and postanalytic components of the tests receive uniform attention.

Diagnostic Issues in Breast Pathology

Currently, there are no uniform guidelines to effectively measure the rate of diagnostic errors in academic and community medical centers. In addition, the fear of disclosure and medicolegal issues are factors that limit the reporting of diagnostic errors in breast pathology. Breast pathology is complex and there are many look-alikes, which are easy to misdiagnose as cancer if the pathologist is not experienced. These difficult cases include a variety of atypical proliferative lesions, low-grade ductal carcinoma in situ (DCIS), lobular neoplasia, papillary lesions, atypical sclerotic lesions, fibroepithelial tumors, mucinous lesions, and the status of microinvasion. Borderline proliferative breast disease continues to rank high among the breast pathology entities that pose a diagnostic challenge. These lesions are variably interpreted by community and academic pathologists alike.[27,34,35] There are no specific differentiating morphologic criteria or biologic markers that can reliably stratify these borderline breast lesions. The existing criteria are based, at times, on subjective opinion and are the result of retrospective studies that have proved not to be easily reproducible.[36] There are studies that have demonstrated that variability in diagnosis of breast cancer can be reduced after education and adoption of standard histologic criteria. However, the issue of concern is that the experts often do not agree on the standard criteria. It is not easy to force agreement and adherence to established criteria. Therefore, diagnostic variability remains an issue.[36,37]

The article published in the July 19, 2010, issue of *The New York Times* about a few patients who had undergone cancer therapy for overdiagnosis of DCIS brought international attention.[38] The story of each patient was real and the message was powerful. The patients spoke about a serious issue that had a major impact on their lives. Their stories brought to public attention an issue that has been known to the medical community for some time and yet we have no solutions to offer in resolving this issue. Several position papers from different societies were issued in an effort to restore the trust of the public and to minimize the associated anxiety. Meanwhile, discussions are taking place among the key opinion leaders and several organizations in an effort to explore possibilities for future direction.[39]

Distinction between atypical ductal hyperplasia (ADH) and low-grade DCIS remains a diagnostic challenge in the practice of breast pathology. Reported studies, including a highly cited article by Dr. Rosai in 1991,[34] continue to highlight the significant interobserver variability even among experienced breast pathologists. This issue is compounded by the increasing number of tissue sampling by core needle biopsy as a consequence of screening mammography. The small sample size of core needle biopsies and tissue fragmentation contribute to the complexity of an accurate diagnosis of DCIS. It is important to recognize that assessment of core needle biopsy is different from circumstances under which the various diagnostic criteria were originally defined by reviewing multiple histologic sections obtained from surgical excisions.[39]

The real challenge is how to minimize the occurrence of overdiagnosis of DCIS and how to balance the scope of therapy based on the biology and the extent of this disease. DCIS is a heterogeneous disease characterized by neoplastic proliferation of epithelial cells within a breast duct with no ability to metastasize. DCIS is considered a precursor lesion with a variable rate of progression into invasive breast cancer. Based on nuclear grade, presence or absence of necrosis, and the pattern of morphologic features, DCIS is stratified into different grades and types. High–nuclear grade lesions are associated with rapid growth, larger sizes, and early progression to an invasive cancer and generally are easier to diagnose.[40]

In contrast, low–nuclear grade lesions remain indolent, and even when they progress to invasive cancer, the tumor is frequently low grade and well differentiated. Low-grade DCIS and high-grade DCIS represent two genetically distinct entities that lead to different forms of invasive cancer. Low-grade DCIS shares similar morphologic and biologic features with ADH, which raises the question of whether these two lesions represent different spectrums of the same entity.[40,41]

Alternate terminologies of mammary intraepithelial neoplasia by Dr. Rosai and ductal intraepithelial neoplasia by Dr. Tavassoli have not been fully embraced by the pathology community.[34,35] This is despite the fact that the unifying concept of mammary intraepithelial neoplasia may eliminate the use of the term "in situ carcinoma" and may reduce the chances of overtreatment.[36,39]

Interestingly, in 1978, Haagensen and colleagues[42] proposed the term "lobular neoplasia," which is commonly used for the spectrum of lobular proliferations when they observed obvious overlapping features between atypical lobular hyperplasia and lobular carcinoma in situ. Their intention was to eliminate the term "lobular carcinoma in situ." Although the current follow-up management of patients with lobular carcinoma in situ is different from that of DCIS, the psychological impact on the patient of hearing the term "in situ carcinoma" may be the same.

There is no doubt that the term "carcinoma" carries a negative connotation for both patients and physicians. The fear of cancer paralyzes patients, particularly those who have a strong family history of cancer. The patients often give up too soon and resort to drastic therapeutic measures that may not be necessary. Similarly, the term "in situ cancer" may have a different significance for each physician based on the pattern of their clinical practice. This potentially may lead to overtreatment.[39]

Currently, there is no consensus about the terminology that should be used to define the biology of the spectrum of prognostically relevant proliferative change in breast pathology. There is no single morphologic criterion or biomarker that can reliably identify patients who may develop breast cancer. The currently used risk stratification models and statistics are only a reflection of the science of probabilities. The proposed concept of progression of normal mammary epithelial cells to hyperplasia, atypical hyperplasia, carcinoma in situ, and finally, an invasive cancer is truly an oversimplification of the complex process of tumorigenesis.[36,39]

In addition, designing well-controlled prospective studies to monitor the morphologic and biologic changes associated with progression of normal mammary epithelial cells into malignant lesions is unrealistic. It is incredibly difficult to convince a patient with a proven diagnosis of DCIS not to undergo the standard surgical therapy and to participate in a clinical trial or expect asymptomatic patients to undergo repeated tissue biopsy for the purpose of contribution to research. Therefore, it may be advisable to find another alternative to define the morphologic features of a breast lesion, correlate it with the finding of breast imaging, and make an effort to measure the extent of the tissue.[39]

We use the term "borderline breast disease" instead of "in situ carcinoma" to encompass the spectrum of ADH and low-grade DCIS. This change is particularly of the importance in assessment of tissue samples obtained by core needle biopsy. These patients can be followed up with complete surgical excision of the lesion and close surveillance. This alternative eliminates the fear and anxiety of the patient and provides a more balanced approach in monitoring the progression of the disease of each patient.[34,39,43]

Similarly, the variability in the results of prognostic/predictive factors in breast cancer has been a longstanding issue, which has been addressed periodically, and most recently, in 2010. Laboratory error rates approximating 20% for both estrogen receptor and *HER-2*/neu were the sentinel events that yielded the new American Society of Clinical Oncology (ASCO)/CAP recommendations for both testing venues.[31,32,44–46] These findings cross over many areas, which include patient safety and increased medical expenses. These facts are disappointing and are a reflection of our inability to standardize the technologies and our failure to foster a cost-effective strategy for breast health care. As molecular targeted therapy continues to result in more options, the magnitude of the cost associated with potential errors in the use of the emerging technologies will be more experienced, not to mention the side effects and the discomfort that each patient will experience.[27,35]

The Approach to Training and Education

The more important issue of concern is the general assumption that breast pathology is a component of general surgical pathology and does not require special training. This is in contrast to other areas such as neuropathology, dermatopathology, hematopathology, cytopathology, and molecular pathology that are recognized by the American Board of Pathology as subspecialties deserving of special certification. A few available breast pathology fellowships are currently funded by individual departments and are not officially considered Accreditation Council for Graduate Medical Education (ACGME)–accredited programs. Currently, breast pathology training for residents is limited to what is offered during their surgical pathology rotations. Aside from a few major academic institutions, pathology residents may not be fully familiar with the concept of integration of breast pathology into breast care and may not be aware of the value of the multidisciplinary approach to the diagnosis and management of breast cancer. Pathology residents find their way into medical centers and medical communities where the majority of breast cancer patients are treated and they continue the same trend of practice of breast pathology. The reticence against the concept of subspecialty status in breast pathology is not in the best interest of patient safety.[27,35,47]

The Issues Surrounding Financial Compensation and Communication of Test Results

Adequate tissue sampling, appropriate use of ancillary studies such as immunocytochemistry as diagnostic adjuncts, and implementation of well-controlled biomarker studies for prognostic/predictive factors require sufficient financial compensation. The current low reimbursement rate is a major barrier to the everyday practice of breast pathology. Conversely, the rush to introduce new technologies into clinical practice makes it difficult to assess the risk and benefits of these modalities for individual patients and limits our ability to find the right answers for many of our questions that directly affect patients. More importantly, the current practice of referral of pathology samples to commercial laboratories based on the insurance status of patients is a real barrier to direct communication between pathologists and other physicians involved in patient care.[35,37]

SUGGESTIONS TO MINIMIZE ERRORS IN BREAST PATHOLOGY

Acknowledgment of the Problem and Improvement of the Status of Training and Education

Overall, there is now sufficient evidence to suggest that there are serious shortcomings in the current practice of breast pathology that may adversely affect patient care. It is also critically important to realize that the majority of breast cancer cases are being managed in community medical centers, small cities, and rural areas where access to optimal practice of breast pathology may not always be possible. Pathology is the foundation of breast cancer care and requires serious attention. The time has come for the experts in breast pathology and leadership of pathology societies as well as other disciplines to join hands in an effort to understand the gravity of the problems associated with unresolved issues regarding breast pathology practices. The first step is to acknowledge the challenges associated with the current patterns of practice in breast pathology. Studies should be designed to appropriately analyze the problems and quantitate their impact on therapy, patient outcome, and health economy.[27]

The next step is to incorporate sufficient training in breast pathology and encourage accreditation of breast pathology fellowships. Breast care is no different from other organs and deserves to have the attention of subspecialty-trained physicians. It is promising that there are now fellowship positions available for breast surgery, breast imaging, and breast pathology across the country. By integrating the efforts of the scientific/medical community and establishing different thresholds for breast health care, we may be able to minimize the anxiety and the fear of our patients, reduce the cost associated with unnecessary medical procedures, and provide high-quality care to our patients. Meanwhile, encouragement of participation in some form of continuing medical education in breast pathology may assist the practicing pathologists to become more familiar with the new concepts in this discipline.[27,28]

The majority of breast pathology cases are diagnosed outside multidisciplinary breast centers and academic institutions. Breast cancer cases are often treated by physicians in group practices, who trust the information written in pathology reports as the guiding light to manage their patients. The idea of a second opinion and the review of pathology slides is still a foreign concept among the majority of patients and physicians. Therefore, the real challenge facing pathologists at large is how to prevent/minimize the occurrence and frequency of diagnostic errors in the everyday practice of breast pathology at a global level.[47]

Currently, there is no independent measure in our pathology training to determine the level of competency of our graduates in breast pathology. There is also no mechanism to correlate the competency with the follow-up performance. What may appear as a competent pathology resident who can differentiate a benign versus a malignant breast lesion in a palpable and locally advanced breast cancer may result in poor performance where he or she functions in an environment where the majority of breast lesions are composed of small image-detected lesions of borderline nature. To address this issue, we must begin to examine the competency of our graduating pathology residents in breast pathology and to also recognize the value of specialty fellowship training in this discipline.[27,28,47]

Integration of Breast Pathology into Clinical Practice of Breast Care

Currently, there is an increasing emphasis in delivery of optimal breast health care via an integrated and multidisciplinary approach. This changing trend in clinical practice provides a unique opportunity for pathologists to become fully engaged in treatment planning and management of breast cancer patients. Multidisciplinary case review of breast cancer cases with participation of pathologists has already shown an interpretative change of diagnosis up to 29% and change in surgical management of patients in 9% of cases.[48] In the area of increased rate of image-detected biopsies, there is a definite need for a comprehensive correlation of pathologic findings with breast imaging that requires effective communication among pathologists, radiologists, and surgeons.[49]

The discussion about the biology of tumor and molecular distinction among various types of abnormalities by the pathologists at breast tumor conferences is important for the design of individualized therapy. The value of active involvement of pathologists in breast health care has recently been demonstrated by National Accreditation Program for Breast Centers (NAPBC). This organization recognizes pathologists as an integral part of the multidisciplinary team of breast centers (Figure 5-1). The NAPBCs is a consortium of national professional organizations dedicated to the improvement of the quality of care and monitoring for outcome of patients with diseases of the breast. NAPBC is designed to improve the quality of care by setting standards and monitoring the continuity of an integrated care. Participation of pathologists in multidisciplinary breast tumor conferences is considered essential for the accreditation process and the adherence to standard pathology reporting and tumor staging is one of the required standards.[50]

Rendering a second opinion in difficult-to-diagnose cases should become a routine process among pathologists. Obtaining a second opinion is another safety net, which brings peace of mind for both physicians and patients and is worth the additional time and cost to the

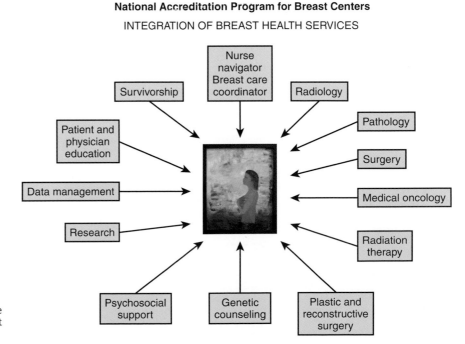

National Accreditation Program for Breast Centers

INTEGRATION OF BREAST HEALTH SERVICES

FIGURE 5-1 The proposed infrastructure for National Accreditation Program for Breast Centers (NAPBC)-accredited breast centers.

health care system. The benefit of a second opinion in breast pathology is now well established. Studies have shown that there is significant missing information in the original pathology report that can alter the management of the patient with breast cancer. The estimated rate of changes in the surgical therapy following a second opinion may be up to 7.5% of cases. In 40% of cases additional prognostic information may alter the outcome and the course of additional therapy.[51]

Establishment of Quality Assurance Measures

Establishment of quality indicators and monitoring of the status of compliance are critical steps in improving the quality of practice of breast pathology. This approach may require guidance and effective interaction.[52] In a well-designed study reported by Imperato and associates in 2008 in the *American Journal of Medical Quality*,[52] the authors demonstrated the value of educational intervention in improvement in breast pathology practice among Medicare patients undergoing unilateral extended simple mastectomy. The authors reported that the aggregate performance on quality indicators (presence of carcinomas, laterality of specimens, number of lymph nodes present, number of positive nodes, documentation of lymph nodes, histologic type, and largest dimension of the tumor) in 555 breast pathology reports was 83.7% whereas performance was 69.4% or less on 10 indicators (resection margin status, verification of tumor size, gross observation of the lesion, histologic grade, angiolymphatic invasion, nuclear grade, location of the tumor, mitotic rate, extent of tubule formation, and perineural invasion). There were also significant interhospital disparities in the performance levels for these quality indicators. The authors in this study demonstrated that, by focused educational intervention, in subsequent review of breast pathology cases from the same pathology groups, a statistically significant

improvement ($P < .0001$) occurred in all the quality indicators, ranging from 12.0% to 19.9%. Therefore, it is reasonable to assume that education plays an important role in changing the pattern of practice of breast pathology (Table 5-1).

There is no doubt that there is a need for standardization and establishment of uniform guidelines for the practice of breast pathology. Appropriate quality assurance and quality control measures should be integrated in anatomic pathology laboratories. Reporting of errors in cancer diagnosis and in the interpretation of prognostic/predictive factors is a critical step in improving patient safety. The review of outside pathology slides and reports by local pathologists before the initiation of any therapy is another measure to consider and is easy to implement in every institution.[27,34,48–53]

IMPLEMENTATION OF PATIENT SAFETY–CENTERED BREAST PATHOLOGY IN PRACTICE

Masood[27] and Perkins and coworkers[35] identified many of the key issues that affect quality practice in breast pathology, including diagnostic accuracy, reimbursement issues, tissue banking, pathologists' training, clinical team integration of the pathologists, and maintenance of the highest standards practiced through quality assurance.

The Magee-Women's Hospital of the University of Pittsburgh Medical Center (UPMC), an academic women's hospital practice, has implemented all of the facets described by these authors. The implementation of these measures at Magee-Women's Hospital of UPMC is a starting point for improvement of the standard of practice for breast pathology. It is not the standard of care, and it is not the only answer, nor is it the only model that will supply the intended outcomes. The descriptions that follow have been implemented into our practice.

TABLE 5-1	Comparative Performance on Eight Quality Indicators for Unilateral Extended Simple Mastectomy among Medicare Patients in New York State*		
Quality Indicator	**Baseline Percent Performance ($n = 555$)**	**Postintervention Percent Performance ($n = 297$)**	**Percent Improvement**
Histologic grade	59.1	75.8	16.7
Nuclear grade	44.3	61.3	17.0
Mitotic rate	22.5	42.4	19.9
Extent of tubule formation	19.6	37.7	18.1
Verification of tumor size	63.0	81.8	18.9
Angiolymphatic invasion	45.6	63.3	17.7
Documentation of lymph nodes	83.7	96.3	12.6
Resection margin status	69.4	82.8	13.4

*Baseline: January 1 to December 31, 1999; postintervention: December 1, 2001 to May 31, 2002.
Data from Imperato PJ, Waisman J, Wallen D, et al. Improvements in breast cancer pathology practices among Medicare patients undergoing unilateral extended simple mastectomy. Am J Med Qual 2003;18:164.

Tissue Handling, Processing, and Reporting

PREANALYTIC FACTORS

The preanalytic factors that are controlled include fixation of all specimens according to the recently published ASCO/CAP Guidelines for Hormone Receptor and Her2 testing.[31,32] At our institution, all specimens received a minimum of 8 hours exposure to 10% neutral phosphate buffered formalin, with a maximum of 72 hours. All breast core biopsy specimens as well as breast excision specimens are correlated with radiographic and imaging findings. The pathologist has desktop computer access to the radiology imaging system and electronic medical record in which the patient is searchable along with imaging findings and radiologic reports. Where possible, a radiologist places relevant information on the surgical pathology requisition. In most instances, the information the radiologist supplies is sufficient for the pathologist to correlate the morphologic findings.

Histologic processing is according to the ASCO/CAP guidelines, and the tissue core biopsy specimens are processed with five levels on each core biopsy according to the work of Renshaw.[54] Examination of five tissue levels in this manner maximizes the ability to uncover any significant atypia present on the biopsy. In this scheme, the tissue sections between cut levels that are stained are saved for immunohistochemistry (IHC) at each level in the event that immunostains for myoepithelial cells, hormone receptors, proliferation markers, or *HER2* are required.

Preanalytic handling of breast excision specimens begins in the frozen section area where fresh specimens from the operating rooms are received. The day before patients' surgeries, patient reports of core biopsies are placed in this receiving area so that the pathologist has immediate access to these reports as fresh lumpectomy or mastectomy specimens are received from the operating rooms. The pathologist then uses these reports as a guide as to how to handle any given specimen. For example, patients who have had ADH or DCIS on a core biopsy have all of their surgical excision specimen sequentially processed for microscopy entirely, according to the mapping procedures that have been described for DCIS.[55] Simultaneously, upon receipt of specimens from the operating rooms, tissue is immediately banked for the breast tissue bank; this includes both normal tissue and tumor tissue. The technician who receives these tissues records the cold ischemic time that is recorded by the operating room circulating nurse.

The previously described detail for preanalytic handling of both core biopsies and surgical excisions requires teamwork. This process has been accomplished by virtue of the medical director meeting with operating room personnel as well as managers of the operating room and surgical suites. These processes are explained in detail and are presented as essential to compliance for accrediting agencies. The reality is that managers and personnel at all levels have no resistance to this change. They realize that it is in the best interest of the patient and, of course, is mandated compliance by accrediting agencies.

ANALYTIC FACTORS

The analytic process begins when the pathologist receives the five stained levels of a core biopsy or the slides from the case of a breast resection specimen.

All breast core biopsies have a documented second review by another pathologist. This includes all benign breast core biopsies that undergo a rapid second review by a second pathologist before signout. This is documented by the second reviewer, by initialing the backside of the surgical requisition, which is stored for 7 years. All new cases of atypia, including ADH or atypical lobular hyperplasia and above, receive a documented second review by a pathologist. Each pathologist has a consult book in which she or he places the diagnosis and hands this book off along with the slides to the second pathologist reviewer. If the second pathologist agrees, he or she initials the agree column. If there is disagreement, the case undergoes multiheaded microscope review.

As a part of the core biopsy signout, any concurrent fine-needle aspiration biopsy specimens of the same site in the breast or of an axillary lymph node are assigned to the same pathologist who interprets the core biopsy. This is performed for sake of completeness so that the pathologist knows the entire patient case and all the nuances of the entire case. The cytology report is signed out with a comment that annotates the core biopsy findings, and the core biopsy is signed out with annotation in the comment that discusses the results of the fine-needle aspiration biopsy.

All prior core biopsies of the patient are mandated for review when a patient has a breast resection, and the review is documented in the comment section of the surgical pathology report. Acknowledging that there are many entities of atypia in breast pathology that generate differences of opinion, it is prudent of a practice to attempt to minimize these differences and discuss difficult cases. This is performed at Magee-Women's Hospital of UPMC by use of a daily conference among pathologists that occurs around a multiheaded microscope that also has a flat screen display. Pathologists, residents, and fellows discuss cases that are difficult or where there are differences of opinion among pathologists. This daily conference, entitled "Pathology Slide Review for Patient Safety and Quality Assurance," receives Council on Medical Education (CME) credits for patient safety from the hospital CME office. Attendance is monitored by pathologists, who signed in on a sign in sheet and document the cases that are reviewed.

The microscopic examination of breast core biopsies and surgical excisions often requires the use of IHC. Immunohistochemical panels have been set up and approved by the group practice. These fundamentally revolve around prognostic and predictive factors (estrogen receptor/progesterone receptor [ER/PgR], *HER2*, Ki-67), determination of ductal versus lobular carcinoma, or discerning ADH versus atypical lobular hyperplasia (E-cadherin, P120 catenin), myoepithelial markers (p63, smooth muscle myosin–heavy chain), special types of breast carcinoma such as metaplastic carcinoma (cytokeratin-7 [CK7], CK5, CK14, CK17, p63, cell adhesion molecule [CAM] 5.1, AE1/AE3, vimentin), and searching for breast carcinoma in metastatic sites (ER, gross cystic disease fluid protein-15 [GCDFP-15], mammaglobin, CK7). All panels are available through the Co-Path laboratory information system, and when ordered, controls are ordered automatically and they appear on the patient's slide. Controls for patient slides for hormone receptors include normal breast tissue, ductal breast carcinoma, lobular breast carcinoma, normal exocervix, and normal endocervix. This gamut of tissues demonstrates the dynamic range of hormone expression that is expected at each tissue site. Hormone receptor controls are semiquantitated daily by a single pathologist in order to detect any analytical drift. *HER2* IHC is interpreted according to the ASCO/CAP guidelines, and all *HER2* 2+ cases are sent to fluorescence in situ hybridization (FISH), where they are examined by a pathologist.

All *HER2* cases are imaged using the VIAS imaging system (Ventana, Tucson, AZ) and reviewed microscopically by the pathologist. All *HER2* 3+ cases are mandated for review and documented signoff by a second pathologist. Negative controls and *HER2* 3+ controls are present on each patient slide. All predictive/prognostic markers are performed using U.S. Food and Drug Administration (FDA) 510K cleared kits. The concordance between *HER2* IHC and FISH has been greater than 95% for 3 consecutive years at Magee-Women's Hospital of UPMC, using *HER2* antibody 4B5 for IHC and the Vysis FISH probes.

Surgical pathology reports for breast resection specimens are mandated to have synoptic reporting for in situ and invasive carcinomas. The synoptic fields are comprehensive and based on recommendations of CAP and ADASP guidelines, and synoptic fields are searchable for research purposes.

POSTANALYTIC FACTORS

The core biopsy reports, when released, have a comment that attest to the fact the radiologist will issue an addendum report to go to the ordering clinician once the radiologist reviews the pathologist's report for concordance with radiographic findings: "IMPORTANT INFORMATION REGARDING COMMUNICATION OF BREAST BIOPSY RESULTS: Please be aware that an important component of percutaneous breast biopsy includes correlation of this biopsy report with the radiology report in order to ensure radiologic-pathologic concordance of the lesion in question for proper patient management."

This is a "Rad-Path" correlation. If the radiologist feels uncomfortable that the morphologic findings reported by pathology are not consistent with the radiographic findings, she or he has the discretion to call the patient back for further procedures.

The majority of breast cancer cases at our institution are reviewed by the Breast Tumor Board, which occurs weekly. These cases are documented and are part of the accreditation process by the American College of Surgeons and the American Cancer Society. These reviews are considered to be a peer review quality activity and all slides are reviewed by the pathologist responsible for the tumor board that week. Paperwork accompanies these reviews, and the reviews are documented by our quality assurance clerk.

All operating room consultations that are generated in the department undergo peer review for accuracy and completeness. In addition, all amended/corrected reports that are generated in the department undergo detailed review by the medical director. There are quarterly peer review meetings for both pathologists and pathologists' assistants for recredentialing purposes. The results of the previously mentioned activities, including peer review of operating room consults and amended/corrected reports, are reviewed by a quality assurance committee. These findings are reported to the hospital credentialing office for recredentialing purposes. Pathologists' assistants are also reviewed in precisely the same manner with respect to their activities, which include the preanalytic and analytic (gross handling of specimens).

The medical director receives quarterly metrics reports from a quality assurance clerk who specifically documents the percent of breast cancer cases that are ER+/PgR+, ER+/PgR–, ER–/PgR+, and ER–/PgR–, as well as the percent of *HER2* 3+ cases, percent of *HER2* 2+ cases, and percent of *HER2* 2+ cases that are FISH positive. Quarterly review of these predictive/prognostic markers metrics is vital to ensure detection of potential undesirable assay analytic drift.

Finally, another postanalytic activity is the review of outside consults for patients seen at our institution. All surgeons who perform breast surgery at our institution are very strongly encouraged to engage in this practice, and this practice has been well received and robust. All patients who are seen at our institution for breast surgery have their outside biopsy reviewed by our pathology department. This activity was made easy after demonstrating to the clinical team the potential for variation in diagnostic interpretation in breast pathology. In a period of 1 year, our department monitored the outside diagnoses compared with internal diagnoses in surgical resection outcomes. Of the cases reviewed, 7.5% of all the cases demonstrated a diagnostic discrepancy; 3.5% of these (50% of the discrepancies) demonstrated diagnostic interpretation variation that had a significant impact on patient care. When reviewing outside consultations on patients who are to have surgery at our institution, if a diagnostic discrepancy is discovered, the surgeon is notified immediately by telephone and this is documented in the surgical pathology report. The immediate notification is to ensure that patients will not undergo unnecessary or harmful surgery.

The Magee Women's Hospital of UPMC sponsors three fellows in breast pathology who function in the environment described previously. The fellows communicate results to clinicians, review slides and present tumor boards weekly, view all outside patient consults, attend the daily working diagnostic patient safety conference, and conduct quality assurance activities with attending pathologists. The fellows are fully integrated into the breast health care team.

SUMMARY

Many of the issues that affect quality patient care and safety in breast pathology have been enumerated and discussed here. An example of executing implementation of the Masood[27] and Perkins and coworkers[35] suggestions had been presented. These are not all of the answers, and all of the issues have not yet been fully addressed. One of the major issues currently confronting pathologists is the direct marketing to oncologists of molecular tests that have not been properly studied for their clinical usefulness, clinical effectiveness, clinical utility, cost benefit, or patient safety. The benefits and harms of these tests remain unknown.[56] New challenges such as this will continue to affect patients, and how pathologists respond to such challenges will determine whether patients will be treated with unbiased, evidence-based medicine or with market-driven corporate-based tests.

REFERENCES

1. Tabar L, Fagerberg CJG, Gad A, et al. Reduction in mortality from breast cancer after mass screening with mammography. Lancet 1985;1:829-832.
2. Duffy SW, Smith RA, Gabe R, et al. Screening for breast cancer. Surg Oncol Clin North Am 2005;14:671-697.
3. Dershaw DD, Morris EA, Liberman L, Abramson AF. Non-diagnostic stereotaxic core breast biopsy: results of rebiopsy. Radiology 1996;198:313-315.
4. Masood S. Cytomorphology of the Breast. Chicago: American Society of Clinical Pathology Press; 1996; pp. 1–50.
5. Masood S, Frykberg E, McLellan GL, et al. Cytologic differentiation between proliferative and nonproliferative breast disease in mammographically guided fine needle aspirates. Diagn Cytopathol 1991;7:581-590.
6. Fisher B, Dignam J, Wolmark N, et al. Lumpectomy and radiation therapy for the treatment of intraductal breast cancer: findings from the National Surgical Adjuvant Breast and Bowel Project B-17. J Clin Oncol 1998;16:441-452.
7. Giuliano AE, Jones RC, Brennan M, Statman R. Sentinel lymphadenectomy in breast cancer. J Clin Oncol 1997;15:2345-2350.
8. Breast cancer and hormone replacement therapy: collaborative reanalysis of data from 51 epidemiological studies of 52,705 women with breast cancer and 108,411 women without breast cancer. Collaborative Group on Hormonal Factors in Breast Cancer. Lancet 1997;350:1047-1059.
9. Recht A, Edge SB, Solin LJ, et al. Postmastectomy radiotherapy: guidelines of the American Society of Clinical Oncology. J Clin Oncol 2001;19:1539-1569.
10. Early Breast Cancer Trialists' Collaboratorive Group. Effects of radiotherapy and chemotherapy in node-positive premenopausal women with breast cancer. N Engl J Med 1997;337:956-962.
11. Ingle JN. Current status of adjuvant endocrine therapy for breast cancer. Clin Cancer Res 2001;7:S4392-S4396.
12. Narod SA, Brunet JS, Ghadirian P, et al. Tamoxifen and the risk of contralateral breast cancer in BRCA1 and BRCA2 mutation carriers: a case-control study. Hereditary Breast Clinical Study Group. Lancet 2000;356:1876-1881.
13. Ganz PA, Rowland JH, Meyerowitz BE, Desmond KA. Impact of different adjuvant therapy strategies on quality of life in breast cancer survivors. Recent Results Cancer Res 1998;152:396-411.
14. Boone CW, Kelloff G. Biomarkers of premalignant breast disease and their use as surrogate endpoints in clinical trials of chemopreventive agents. Breast J 1995;1:228-235.
15. Fabian C, Kimler B, Brady D, et al. A phase II breast cancer chemoprevention trial of oral DFMO: breast tissue, imaging and serum and urine biomarkers. Clin Cancer Res 2002;8:3105-3117.
16. Singletary SE, Hansen NM, Klimberg VS, Simmons RM. Managing the cancer patient at a comprehensive breast-care center. Contemp Surg 2000;56:518-528.
17. Pinder SE, Murray S, Ellis IO, et al. The importance of the histologic grade of invasive breast carcinoma and response to chemotherapy. Cancer 1998;83:1529-1539.
18. Masood S. Prognostic factors in breast cancer: use of cytologic preparations. Diagn Cytopathol 1995;13:388-395.
19. Masood S, Bui M. Assessment of Her-2/neu overexpression in primary breast cancers and then metastatic lesions: An immunohistochemical study. Ann Clin Lab Sci 2000;30:259-265.
20. Yoshida B, Solkoloff M, Welch D, Rinker-Schaeffer C. Metastasis-suppressor genes: a review and perspective on an emerging field. J Natl Cancer Inst 2000;92:1717-1730.
21. Mauro MJ, O'Dwyer M, Heinrich MC, et al. STI571: a paradigm of new agents for cancer therapeutics. J Clin Oncol 2002;20:325-334.
22. Runsak JM, Kisabeth RM, Herbert FP, et al. Pharmacogenomics: a clinician's primer on emerging technologies for improved patient care. Mayo Clin Proc 2001;76:299-309.
23. Slamon DJ, Leyland-Jones B, Shak S, et al. Use of chemotherapy plus a monoclonal antibody against HER2 for metastatic breast cancer that overexpresses HER2. N Engl J Med 2001;344:783-792.
24. Slonim DK. Transcriptional profiling in cancer: the path to clinical pharmacogenomics. Pharmacogenomics 2001;2:123-136.
25. Hess JL. The advent of targeted therapeutics and implications for pathologists. Am J Clin Pathol 2002;117:355-357.
26. Cobleigh MA, Vogel CL, Tripathy D, et al. Multinational study of the efficacy and safety of humanized anti-HER2 monoclonal antibody in women who have HAER2-overexpressing metastatic breast cancer that has progressed after chemotherapy for metastatic disease. J Clin Oncol 1999;17:2639-2648.
27. Masood S. Raising the bar: a plea for standardization and quality improvement in the practice of breast pathology. Breast J 2006;12:409-412.
28. Masood S. The expanding role of pathologists in the diagnosis and management of breast cancer: Worldwide Excellence in Breast Pathology Program. Breast J 2003;9(Suppl 2):S94-S97.
29. Henson DE, Oberman HA, Hutter RVP, et al. Practice protocol for the examination of specimens removed from patients with cancer of the breast. Publication of the Cancer Committee, College of American Pathologists. Arch Pathol Lab Med 1997;121:27-33.
30. Fechner RE, Kempson RL, Livolsi VA, et al. Recommendations for the reporting of breast carcinoma. Association of Directors of Anatomic and Surgical Pathology. Am J Clin Pathol 1995;104:614-619.
31. Hammond ME, Hayes DF, Dowsett M, et al. American Society of Clinical Oncology/College of American Pathologists guideline recommendations for immunohistochemical testing of estrogen and progesterone receptors in breast cancer. Arch Pathol Lab Med 2010;134:907-922.
32. Wolf C, Hammond EH, Schwartz HN, et al. American Society of Clinical Oncology/College of American Pathologists guideline recommendations for human epidermal growth factor receptor 2 testing in breast cancer. Arch Pathol Lab Med 2007;131:18-43.
33. Wilkinson NW, Shahryarinejad A, Winston JS, et al. Concordance with breast cancer pathology reporting practice guidelines. J Am Coll Surg 2003;196:38-43.
34. Rosai J. Borderline epithelial lesions of the breast. Am J Surg Pathol 1991;15:209-221.
35. Perkins C, Balma D, Garcia R. Why current breast pathology practices must be evaluated. A Susan G. Komen for the Care White Paper, June 2006. Breast J 2007;13:443-447.
36. Rosen PP. Breast Pathology. 3rd ed. Philadelphia: Lippincott Williams & Wilkins; 2009; p. 250.
37. Schnitt SJ, Connolly JL, Tavassoli FA, et al. Interobserver reproducibility in the diagnosis of ductal proliferative breast lesions using standardized criteria. Am J Surg Pathol 1992;16:1133-1143.
38. Saul S. Prone to error: earliest steps to find cancer. New York Times, July 19, 2010; p. A1.
39. Masood S. Is it time to retire the term of "in situ carcinoma" and use the term of "borderline breast disease"? Breast J 2010;16:571-572.
40. Ellis OI, Schnitt SJ, Sastre-Garau X, et al. Invasive breast carcinoma. In Tavasolli FA, Devillee P, eds. Tumors of Breast and Female Genital Organs. Lyon, France: IARC Press; 2003; pp. 60-62.

TABLE 6-1	This Chart Helps the Physician Who Is Submitting a Breast Biopsy to Convey the Relevant Clinical Information to the Pathologist
Laterality: Right Left	Location: o'clock
Position/zone from nipple:	Type: Mass Calcifications Density
BIRADS:	Size:

BIRADS, Breast Imaging Reporting and Data System.

overlap with other chapters, and the reader is directed to those chapters for in-depth discussion of the topic. Finally, some tips for developing standard operating procedures in the gross room are presented that are intended to help the readers to either adopt or modify these guidelines for their own specific needs.

KEY DIAGNOSTIC POINTS

Handling and Processing of Breast Core Needle Biopsies

- Ideally, use a laboratory information system that allows for printing tissue cassettes instead of hand-written blocks.
- Work with the radiology department to establish methods to capture required clinical information.
- Develop mechanisms to clearly identify the cores more likely to contain the lesion of interest, such as calcifications, for thorough pathologic evaluation.
- Use printed instructions on the cassette for the histotechnologist performing microtomy, including the number of desired histologic sections or levels.
- Do not submit more than five cores per cassette.
- Try to embed all the cores and fragments in one plane in the paraffin block.
- Define levels and steps clearly. For example, three to five sections need to be cut at a 25-μm interval.
- The practice to exhaust the block upfront is not advised, because immunostains are often used in diagnostic evaluation.
- For core needle biopsies for calcifications, a specimen radiograph must be made available to the pathologist to make sure the tissue sections adequately represent the calcifications or any associated lesion.
- In cases in which calcifications either are not seen in routine histologic sections or do not match the specimen radiograph, all paraffin blocks should be x-rayed and then the tissue should be cut away to look for calcifications. Whether all the sections should be evaluated by H&E or some saved for possible immunostains should be left to the discretion of the pathologist.
- The guidelines for tissue sectioning should take into account the thickness of the tissue cores, that is, the lower the gauge, the thicker are the cores and more levels may be needed for adequate tissue evaluation.
- All efforts should be made to accomplish these tasks in the most time- and cost-efficient method.

TABLE 6-2	A Sample Template to Capture the Required Time Points for Breast Samples, which Can Be Potentially Used to Assess Predictive Biomarkers

Collection time and date:	Fixation start date and time:	Fixation end date and time:

PERCUTANEOUS CORE NEEDLE BIOPSIES

The majority of these biopsies are now done with the aid of imaging modalities, such as mammography, ultrasound, or magnetic resonance imaging (MRI; see Chapter 8), and most come to the pathology suite from radiology or a breast surgeon.[6,7] The pathology report on these samples requires correlation with findings on imaging studies that triggered the biopsy in addition to the clinical presentation and clinical breast examination. The physician who performed the biopsy then performs the final correlation.[8]

Stereotactic Needle Biopsies

The biopsies triggered by an abnormal mammogram are typically done by a radiologist and are mostly reserved for nonpalpable lesions or calcifications.[9] The most important initial step is to get all the necessary information about the clinical examination and imaging studies so that the pathologist can document the information required to perform the radiologic-pathologic correlation. We have found it useful to aid our physicians in providing us with useful clinical information. A strategy depicted later can be used as is or modified as necessary to help in this first step.

A sticker or preprinted area on the specimen requisition can help guide the submitting physician to provide relevant clinical information; this is often helpful for best compliance (see Table 6-1).

The radiologists almost always x-ray the cores to make sure the calcifications are present in the removed tissue (Figure 6-1).

A variety of methods are used to segregate the involved cores for the pathologist to ensure focused examination. The cores may be placed in a separate specimen container, which is labeled as "cores with calcifications," or they may be placed in a tissue cassette, which is itself placed in the specimen container. Some institutions use Petri dish–like containers with several compartments and may place the cores with calcifications in the central section (Figure 6-2). In this case, the tissue cassettes containing the targeted cores should be clearly identified in the gross description of the specimen. A variety of protocols are used in pathology laboratories regarding sectioning of these blocks. No specific protocol can be recommended here; however, these basic principles should be kept in mind. First, the tissue should be embedded in a fashion that all the cores lay separately and in a single plane. Second, enough

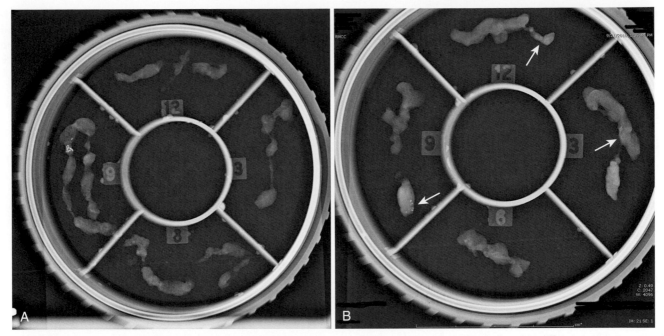

FIGURE 6-1 Specimen radiograph after a core needle biopsy procedure. The cores are separated and placed in different compartments of a Petri dish–like specimen container, which can undergo close examination in pathology. **A,** The 9 o'clock compartment contains one core with a cluster of calcifications. **B,** One core each in the 12, 3, and 9 o'clock compartments contain small clusters of calcifications, which have been marked by the radiologist *(arrows)*.

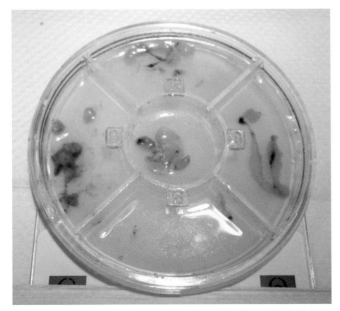

FIGURE 6-2 Stereotactic core needle biopsies. One of the methods of submitting core needle biopsies with calcifications is depicted. An accompanying radiograph (like the one shown in Figure 6-1) directs the attention of the pathologist to the cores containing the calcifications.

hematoxylin and eosin (H&E) levels should be cut to ensure that the pathologist can identify the lesion, that is, calcifications or a mass at the time of microscopic evaluation. Third, the pathologist should be liberal in examining additional sections, after reviewing the routine sections and the accompanying radiograph or digital image on the computer, to ensure adequate histologic examination of the imaging abnormality.

Ultrasound- and Magnetic Resonance Imaging–guided Biopsies

Breast ultrasound is the most common way to further characterize the nature of density or mass identified on mammogram. Ultrasound-guided biopsies are much easier to perform and are currently the method of choice to sample both the solid and the complex cystic lesions. The methods described previously for obtaining clinical information and handling of needle biopsies also apply to ultrasound-guided core needle biopsies. Conversely, MRI-guided biopsies are relatively difficult and more time consuming to perform and are reserved for lesions seen only on the MRI and cannot be located by the second-look, focused ultrasound of the area.

Handling and Documentation Requirements

Percutaneous minimally invasive biopsies have become the standard of practice in evaluation of breast lesions and have helped reduce the number of open biopsies for initial diagnosis, thus, potentially saving additional surgery and anesthesia for such patients. Because these samples are placed immediately in the surgical or radiology suites, tissue preservation is near ideal and tumor is directly exposed to the fixative for rapid fixation. CAP and ASCO, in their recent recommendations, have suggested using such core biopsies as the preferred type of samples to assess hormone receptors and Her2 in breast cancer cases.[5] However, the issue of sampling errors, because the amount of tumor may be limited in such cores, needs to be kept in mind, particularly in case of negative hormone receptor results. With the new guidelines, these samples also need documentation of the collection time and duration of minimum and total fixation times. Ten percent neutral phosphate-buffered formalin is the fixative of choice. Use of any other fixative is the responsibility of the laboratory director to properly validate.

In most cases, such as ultrasound-guided core biopsies, the specimen can be placed in the fixative right away, and within 15 to 20 minutes for stereotactic biopsies, which require x-ray of the cores to verify the presence of calcifications. Again, simple templates can be used for these and all other breast specimens to document the required times (see Table 6-2).

The documentation of this information requires a combined effort from the pathology personnel and staff in other departments or locations. A brief discussion and ways to accomplish these goals are provided later in the chapter.

Tissue Processing of Core Needle Biopsies

A quick turnaround time is desirable for breast biopsies owing to anxiety associated with abnormal breast imaging requiring biopsy. The use of appropriate tissue processors and processing protocols can keep the processing time to the minimum. The modern microwave-assisted tissue processors have the ability to process needle cores, including those with substantial amounts of fat, in less than 3 hours. These advances, when coupled with efficient work flow in histology, can help laboratories achieve the desired turnaround times.[10] However, it is the choice of individual laboratories to make the decisions that best serve their clients and patients. Tissue processors enhanced with heat need to be validated against processing in the traditional manner without heat for predictive and prognostic markers according to ASCO/CAP guidelines.

Microtomy of Core Needle Biopsies

In most anatomic pathology laboratories, the standard operating procedure provides guidelines for tissue sectioning and sampling. Often, these procedures outline the number of tissue blocks to be submitted for each type of specimen, appropriate for the clinical indication of the biopsy. Most of the current anatomic pathology information systems/softwares offer the capability to generate an appropriate number of tissue cassettes for each specimen at the time of case accession. It is often possible to create tissue codes in the software that will generate a standard number of prelabeled tissue cassettes. In laboratories that use bar-coding technology, the information for the histotechnologists can be added to the bar code, including instructions about the specifics of embedding and microtomy. Therefore, it is desirable that the decision about the number of tissue sections or levels of H&E sections to be prepared is made at the time of gross examination and tissue submission.

Minimally invasive core needle biopsies can provide information similar to that of an open excisional biopsy. All the necessary information that helps the breast surgeon in planning a definite surgery should be available in the pathology report for core needle biopsies. Therefore, it is critical that any atypical lesion that necessitates surgical excision and all cancers are reliably identified in the core biopsies. The false-negative rate in the core biopsies is relatively low, but it can be attributed to the level of tissue sectioning required to obtain the relevant information. This topic was addressed by Renshaw and coworkers in a series of publications in 2000 to 2002,[11,12] which helped the pathologists understand the critical decision-making points in reading core biopsies. In their studies, the histology laboratory was instructed to make eight slides from each tissue block, cutting through the entire tissue. Between two and five consecutive sections were placed on each of the eight slides. The tissue was trimmed approximately 50 to 75 μm between each of the slides to process the tissue block to exhaustion. On review of over 3000 core needle biopsies using this microtomy protocol, they found that five sections of breast core biopsy specimens were necessary to identify all atypical lesions, including atypical ductal hyperplasia (ADH).[13] In their report, 95 cases of ADH had follow-up surgical excision. Of these cases, only 43% were identified in the first slide, 17% on the second slide, 23% on the third slide, and 8% each on the fourth and fifth slides. In a related study with the similar guidelines for microtomy, they found that, in a small subset used for comparison purposes, the majority of core biopsies with the diagnosis of low- or intermediate-grade ductal carcinoma in situ (DCIS) had cancer in the follow-up excision.[14] They also suggested that the use of larger-gauge needles can potentially remove the entire lesion initially diagnosed as ADH, leading to no residual disease in the excisional specimen. The same is true for a small focus of low-grade DCIS. In subsequent studies, they validated the use of this method of microtomy for rare lesions, such as mucinous lesions and lobular neoplasia.

In a relatively recent publication, Cornea and colleagues[15] tried to establish the number of histologic sections of MRI-guided core needle biopsies of breast that were necessary to detect disease. Their laboratory had been preparing four levels for routine examination of such biopsies. In this series of 505 MRI-guided biopsies, the lesions were classified as those either necessitating surgical excision or not requiring subsequent open excision. All cases of papilloma, radial scar, ADH, DCIS, and invasive cancer were included in the first category, whereas other lesions, such as fibroadenoma, fibrocystic changes, and lobular neoplasia, were left in the second group. The authors found that they could make a complete and accurate diagnosis of all the lesions in 482 of the 505 (95.4%) specimens from the first slide alone. In 4.6% of all cases, the additional levels were helpful in further defining the characteristics of the lesion. Information obtained from subsequent levels did not make any difference in patient care. Therefore, they suggested that for MRI-guided core needle biopsies, one

TABLE 6-3	ASCO/CAP 2010 Summary of Guideline Recommendations for Optimal Tissue Handling Requirements: ER and PgR Testing by IHC in Breast Cancer Patients

Time from tissue acquisition to fixation should be as short as possible.

Samples for ER and PgR testing are fixed in 10% NPBF for 6 to 72 hours.

Large, preferably multiple, core biopsies of tumor are preferred for testing if they are representative of the tumor (grade and type) at resection.

Resection samples should be sliced at 5-mm intervals after appropriate gross inspection and margins designation and placed in sufficient volume of NPBF to allow adequate tissue penetration.

If tumor comes from a remote location, it should be bisected through the tumor on removal and sent to the laboratory immersed in a sufficient volume of NPBF.

Cold ischemia time, fixative type, and time the sample was placed in NPBF must be recorded.

As in the ASCO/CAP *HER2* guideline, storage of slides for more than 6 weeks before analysis is not recommended.

Time tissue is removed from patient, time tissue is placed in fixative, duration of fixation, and fixative type must be recorded and noted on the accession slip or in the report.

Specimen should be rejected and testing repeated on a separate sample if the sample has prolonged cold ischemia time or fixation duration, less than 6 hours or more than 72 hours and is negative on testing in the absence of internal control elements.

ASCO, American Society of Clinical Oncology; CAP, College of American Pathologists; ER, estrogen receptor; IHC, immunohistochemistry; NPBF, neutral phosphate-buffered formalin; PgR, progesterone receptor.

H&E-stained section is sufficient for routine evaluation. This significant degree of difference in obtaining diagnostic information on the first H&E slide (i.e., 43% vs. 95%) is difficult to explain but it can have tremendous impact on workload for both the histology laboratory and the pathologists. Additional studies addressing this important issue are needed to provide better guidance to practicing pathologists.

It is ultimately the responsibility of the medical director to establish procedures and guidelines for her or his histology laboratory. Several factors play a role in creating these standard operating procedures. Some of these should be kept in mind including pre-analytic variables, such as the quality and experience of the radiologists performing these biopsies, gauge of the needle, and number of tissue cores submitted. The main aspects for histology include the number of tissue cores or fragments in each cassette, embedding method, and clear definition of steps and levels of histologic sections. Finally, the pathologists interpreting the slides need to incorporate all the relevant clinical information to provide a pathology report, which addresses the clinical concerns such that the radiologist is able to perform the final radiologic-pathologic correlation. A summary of recommendations is provided in Table 6-3.

KEY DIAGNOSTIC POINTS

ASCO/CAP Elements to Be Included in Accession Slip for ER and PgR IHC Assays

- Patient identification information
- Physician Identification
- Date of procedure
- Clinical indication for biopsy
- Specimen site and type of specimen
- Collection time
- Time sample placed in fixative
- Type of fixative
- Fixation duration

ASCO, American Society of Clinical Oncology; CAP, College of American Pathologists; ER, estrogen receptor; IHC, immunohistochemistry; PgR, progesterone receptor.

KEY DIAGNOSTIC POINTS

Reporting Elements for ER and PgR IHC Assays

- Patient identification information.[*]
- Physician identification.[*]
- Date of service.[*]
- Specimen site and type.[*]
- Specimen identification (case and block number).[*]
- Fixative.
- Cold ischemia time (time between removal and fixation).
- Duration of fixation.
- Staining method used.
- Primary antibody and vendor.
- Assay details and other reagents/vendors.
- References supporting validation of assay (note: most commonly, these will be published studies performed by others that the testing laboratory is emulating).
- Status of FDA approval.
- Controls (high protein expression, low-level protein expression, negative protein expression, internal elements or from normal breast tissue included with sample).
- Adequacy of sample for evaluation.
- Results[*]

ER, estrogen receptor; IHC, immunohistochemistry; PgR, progesterone receptor.
*Patient and specimen demographics.

WIRE-GUIDED EXCISIONS/ LUMPECTOMIES

In order to aid the surgeon, nonpalpable lesions are often localized by the radiologist using a needle or guidewire through the center of the radiologic abnormality. In some cases, in which the nonpalpable lesion has some areas of

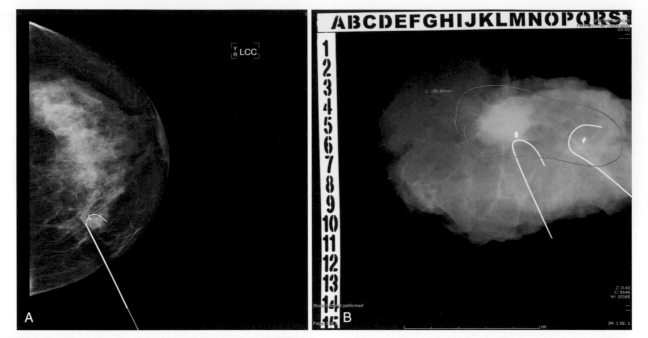

FIGURE 6-3   Needle localization of breast lesions. **A,** A digital mammogram in a patient with previously diagnosed invasive breast cancer. The presence of a metallic clip helps the radiologist place the needle with the guidewire. **B,** An example of bracketing type of needle localization. The placement of two guidewires allows the surgeon to remove two lesions in one specimen.

concern that extend beyond the main lesion or if two or more lesions are located in the same quadrant and are close enough to be removed by one incision, two wires are placed to mark the greatest extent or separation between the lesions; this is referred to as *bracketing*. In most cases, a needle biopsy has been done and a clip is present to aid the radiologist in placing the guidewires (Figure 6-3).

Some surgeons prefer to use intraoperative ultrasound as an aid during lumpectomy, although this does not generate any images for correlation for the pathologist. In rare instances, the area of mammographic or ultrasound abnormality is too small or difficult to see in two dimensions to accurately target for a needle biopsy and is localized for a diagnostic excisional biopsy. The term *lumpectomy* is used for excision of a palpable mass. Wire-guided excisions for nonpalpable lesions and lumpectomy are the main types of breast-conserving surgeries. In combination with radiation therapy, this approach is offered to the majority of patients with breast cancer. Breast-conserving surgery with radiation therapy is considered equivalent to mastectomy for local control of breast cancer.[16–19] For this reason, these specimens account for the majority of cancer surgery specimens that are processed in the pathology laboratory.

Radiologic-Pathologic Correlation

The first step in handling wire-guided excisions is to obtain the specimen x-ray or digital image.[20–23] A variety of options exists to accomplish this step and involves close communication among the surgeon, operating room staff, radiologist, gross room staff, and pathologist. In most cases, the specimen is placed on a radiopaque grid in the operating room or the radiology suite after it has been transported there. A specimen radiograph is obtained (Figure 6-4).

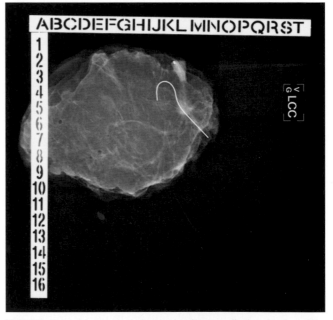

FIGURE 6-4   Specimen radiograph after needle localization. The specimen removed by the surgeon is placed on a grid and a faxitron is performed. The image can be sent to the pathology suite as either a film or a digital image. Note a spiculated mass that has been localized by the wire at the L-5 coordinates. This helps the pathologist mark the area of interest during tissue sampling.

If an analog machine is used, the image is developed on a film. The radiologist reviews the specimen radiograph and may need to compare it with the patient's preoperative mammogram and images taken at the time of wire placement. Then the surgeon is notified to make sure the intended radiographic abnormality has been adequately excised. The specimen radiograph is marked and sent to the pathology suite along with the specimen for handling. At this time, the pathologist or his or her assistant marks the specimen at the corresponding grid marks for the lesion. Alternate ways include using a faxitron machine in either the operating room or the gross room, obtaining the image and transmitting it to the radiologist, who makes the necessary communication. At certain institutions, this task is done in the pathology suite, where the surgeon brings the specimen to the gross room. The next steps are done together with the surgeon, the radiologist, and the pathologist. In this situation, a second round of images is often performed after the specimen has been inked and sliced. These images help direct the sampling as well as possible selection of tissue for intraoperative margin evaluation (see more details later). The choice for selecting the best method rests with the individual institution. Often, the location and proximity or lack thereof between operating room, radiology, and pathology suite play a key role in deciding the most cost- and time-efficient way of accomplishing this step.

Inking Protocol for the Surgical Margins

The orientation of surgical specimen has been required as a quality measure by the American Society of Breast Surgeons. A simple approach of "s for s" and "l for l," that is, short suture for superior and long suture for lateral, had been adopted by the surgeons across the world.[24] It makes sense to use a standardized method in the gross room for breast specimens as well. For some time, a limited number of colored inks or dyes were available to mark the surgical margins. However, six pigment-based tissue-staining systems have been available in addition to India ink. At our institutions, a standardized scheme has been in place for several years. It uses seven inks. We have reserved the red ink to first mark the area of mammographic abnormality after reviewing the specimen radiograph with the help of a breast radiologist. Once this is accomplished, the breast specimen is inked on its six surfaces in the following manner (Table 6-4).

The outer surface should be either dried using paper towels or immersed in 100% ethanol, which helps with drying the surface covered with fat. Whenever possible, the breast specimens should be inked fresh, before formalin fixation. The use of cotton-tipped applicators is preferable. Another option is to use a sponge to brush the specimen surfaces. One should not use a brush because it will push ink into crevices on the surface of the specimen, which do not represent the true margins. One should not dip the whole specimen in an ink container because it increases the likelihood of contaminating or carrying over tissue material from previous specimens. After applying the inks, the surface should be sprayed with a mordant solution, such as 5% acetic acid in water or any commercially available solution to make the ink adhere to the tissue. Then wash the entire specimen in flowing water to get rid of unattached ink, and dry using paper towels before cutting. These last

TABLE 6-4	A Scheme Using Six Dyes to Mark the Margins of Oriented Lumpectomy Specimens
Superior	Purple
Inferior	Green
Anterior	Orange
Posterior	Black
Medial	Blue
Lateral	Yellow

two steps are very helpful in making sure that the inks do not overflow onto unintended margins or be carried with the knife into the freshly cut surfaces. However, recently, some concerns have been raised about the accuracy of inking the surgical margins after the specimen has been compressed and distorted during the process of obtaining specimen radiograph.[25] There are no systematic data to correlate the incidence of residual tumor in second surgery after a positive margin and local recurrence. Recently, a sterile kit has become available for the surgeons to ink the surgical margins immediately after removing the specimen from the breast and before specimen radiography, potentially decreasing the effects of distortion. It remains to be seen whether this step will improve the orientation and thus outcome in terms of local recurrence.[26]

A method developed and optimized in our laboratory allows sectioning of fatty breast tissue into thin slices immediately without lengthy formalin fixation.[27] This involves cooling the specimen (after it has been inked and its surface dried) rapidly by direct immersion in an isopentane bath at –65°C for 5 to 60 seconds (based on size of the specimen). The outer surface of tissue quickly turns pale and firm while the center of the specimen remains soft. The specimen should be carefully observed during the immersion process to prevent overcooling. After the immersion, the tissue can be immediately sectioned easily at 3- to 5-mm intervals, thawed at room temperature, and fixed in 10% formalin (Figure 6-5).

The specimen should then be weighed (recorded in grams) and measured in millimeters (or centimeters) in the three planes (i.e., anterior-posterior, superior-inferior, and medial-lateral). It is recommended that the phrase "in the maximum dimension in each of the three planes" should be used. This helps avoid confusion in cases in which the lesion, such as DCIS, is reported to involve the two opposing margins but the maximum dimensions of the tumor do not match the specimen dimensions (e.g., a DCIS involving superior and inferior margin is estimated to be 20 mm in size but the specimen dimensions in the superior-inferior plane is 25 mm).

Lumpectomies and wire-guided excisions for nonpalpable lesions, associated with a sentinel lymph node mapping protocol, have raised concerns about exposure to radiation to personnel handling such specimens. Although the initial studies of sentinel lymph node

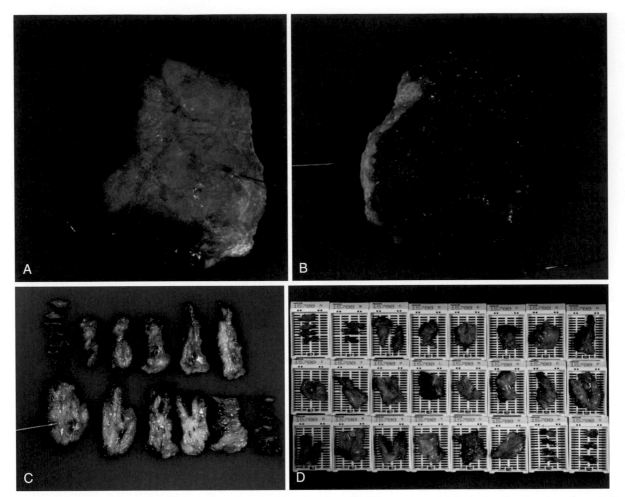

FIGURE 6-7 Submission of the entire specimen for non-palpable lesion. **A** and **B,** The specimen is inked using the six colors; the anterior surface is inked orange and the posterior surface is inked black. The entire specimen is serially sectioned into thin slices **(C)** and entirely submitted for histologic examination **(D).** This is easily accomplished in 24 cassettes by putting an ideal amount of tissue in each cassette to accomplish adequate fixation and processing. X-Ray of tissue cassette at this point can further aid in selecting those cassettes with the area of abnormality and additional hematoxylin and eosin (H&E) sections, if desired.

Most of the DCIS are detected by mammography and sometimes by other techniques, such as MRI, and not by clinical examination. For some years, the CAP has recommended using a tumor summary for reporting cases with DCIS without invasive cancer. The recently published update in 2009 has provided more details about the gross examination of such specimens, specifically focusing on a standardized method for tissue sampling in order to accurately estimate the extent of DCIS after microscopic examination.[2] Some of the details for examining specimens with the preoperative diagnosis of DCIS have been provided previously. In order to follow these recommendations, a standardized method for multicolor inking of surgical margin, correlation with specimen radiograph, and then images of sliced tissue are important sequential steps. One of the main emphases in the gross examination is uniform sectioning at 3- to 5-mm intervals. The method described previously can help in obtaining reliably consistent thickness in slicing fatty breast specimens. A diagram with details regarding the areas that are submitted with a detailed cassette summary is required to meet the recommendations. There are at least two ways to accomplish this

goal. One of the frequently used methods is to use the radiograph of the sliced breast specimen to mark the cassette summary.[33,34] However, for certain laboratories, access to an image or faxitron may be limited or cumbersome. The other method is to use a hand-drawn schema of the number of slices of the specimen and marking this with orientation and the cassette number in addition to a relatively detailed summary of cassettes (Figure 6-8).

In both these methods, the pathologist examining the slides can identify the number of slices involved with DCIS and calculate the extent of DCIS.

RE-EXCISION SPECIMENS

The re-excision specimen may be a biopsy cavity margin sampling or complete excisions. The indications for re-excision include microscopically positive margin on the original excision, invasive tumor with extensive intraductal component with close (<2-mm) margins, abnormal calcifications still present at the margin of the original excision, unoriented or poorly oriented initial lumpectomy, and additional margin clearance

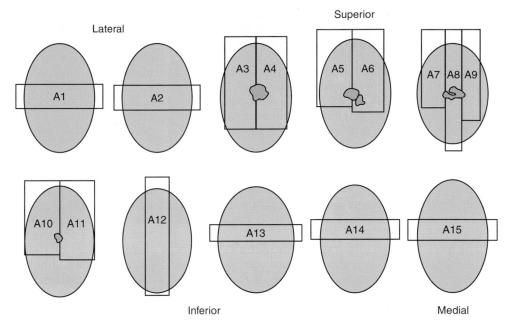

Lateral

Superior

Inferior

Medial

FIGURE 6-8 A scheme to supplement the summary of sections. This computer-generated template or a hand-drawn depiction of an oriented specimen, with location of the lesion and scheme of tissue submission can be a very useful aid to the pathologist performing the histologic examination and can also help in estimating the extent of nonpalpable lesions.

for MammoSite radiation. For a small shaved margin, the new margin should be inked and en face submission is appropriate. For larger re-excisions, the new margin should be inked and the specimen should be serially sectioned perpendicular to the inked surface. If small enough, usually approximately 3 cm or less, the entire specimen should be submitted. If the specimen is fatty and no residual tumor or induration is noted, either alternate slices or directed sampling may be considered. In general, the gross assessment and frozen section of residual margins is difficult owing to postsurgical changes associated with the initial excision and cannot be relied upon entirely for directed sampling.[35,36]

MASTECTOMIES

About one third of the patients with breast cancer either opt for or are offered a mastectomy as their definite surgical treatment for breast cancer. A few patients with known breast cancer gene mutations may choose prophylactic mastectomy. The goal of gross examination of mastectomies is to ensure documentation of margins, skin, or nipple involvement, and often, multifocal and/or multicentric disease.

A modified radical mastectomy is easy to orient, and after the standard procedure of obtaining the weight, the dimensions of the breast in three planes and the skin and nipple-areola complex, the margins can be inked. At our institution, we use this protocol (Table 6-5).

The purpose of differential inking is mainly to keep the orientation during the time of gross examination and sectioning. If one needs to go back to the specimen to submit additional sections, the different inks help maintain the orientation of the specimen. However, modified radical mastectomies have become relatively uncommon. Often, the patients undergo a simple mastectomy with a sentinel lymph node sampling. Such specimens can be challenging to orient, particularly the skin-sparing mastectomies. Therefore, it is critical that

TABLE 6-5	The Surgical Margins of the Mastectomy May Be Inked Using This Simple Scheme to Aid in Initial and Second-Look Sectioning
Lateral half	Blue
Medial half	Orange
Posterior/deep	Black

the surgeon provides orientation of the specimen to the pathologist, and use of long and short sutures, as employed for lumpectomies, are very helpful in simple mastectomy specimens as well.

Mastectomy for breast cancer is almost always preceded by a core needle or excisional biopsy, and therefore, correlation with the previous pathology report or imaging studies is a useful adjunct in both the orientation and the examination of the specimen. The important pieces of information that need to be captured in the external examination include the appearance of nipple, areola, and skin, making note of any scars or ulcers, and the presence of pectoralis fascia or muscle, axillary lymph nodes, and any palpable lesions in the breast.

The detailed examination of mastectomies has been traditionally done by placing the specimen on the cutting board with the skin surface down. The orientation is maintained by viewing the specimen as if one is standing behind the patient. The whole specimen should be sliced at approximately 5-mm intervals from the pectoralis fascia or muscle all the way to the dermis, leaving the skin intact to hold the specimen together. Once the lesional area is identified, first attention should be paid to accurate and detailed characteristics of the tumor as described previously for lumpectomy specimens. In addition, the distance of the tumor to the deep margin, skin, and nipple should be recorded. Careful attention should

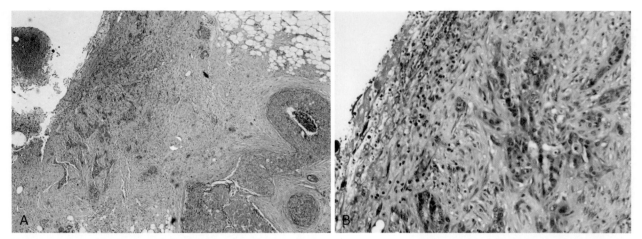

FIGURE 6-10 Ductal carcinoma in situ (DCIS) entrapped in the biopsy bed. **A,** A low-power view shows a focus of high-grade DCIS close to the biopsy cavity. Note irregular small nests of tumor cells close to the biopsy cavity. **B,** The entrapment of DCIS in tissue reaction mimics invasive cancer.

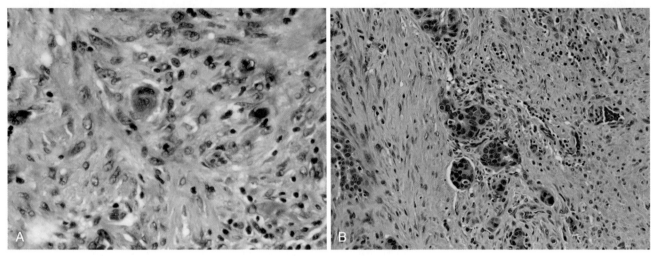

FIGURE 6-11 Seeding of the biopsy needle tract by tumor cells. **A** and **B,** DCIS can be dislodged by the needle used in the biopsy procedure and track along the granulation tissue. In such cases, the absence of invasive carcinoma elsewhere is indicative that the changes around the biopsy site are artifactual.

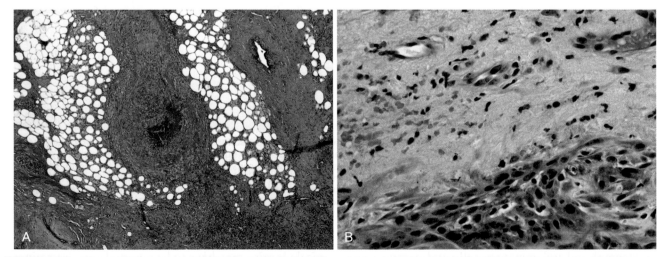

FIGURE 6-12 Changes in the stroma and blood vessels. **A,** A medium-sized vessel entrapped in the biopsy tract with organizing thrombus. **B,** A close view of capillaries with epithelioid endothelial cells and marked reactive stromal proliferation.

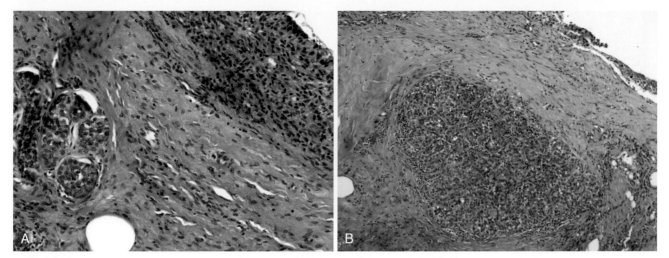

FIGURE 6-13 Lobular neoplasia hidden in the biopsy site changes. **A,** A focus of atypical lobular hyperplasia (ALH) identified close to the biopsy cavity. **B,** An intense chronic inflammatory response in the wall of biopsy cavity has masked a lobular unit involved by ALH.

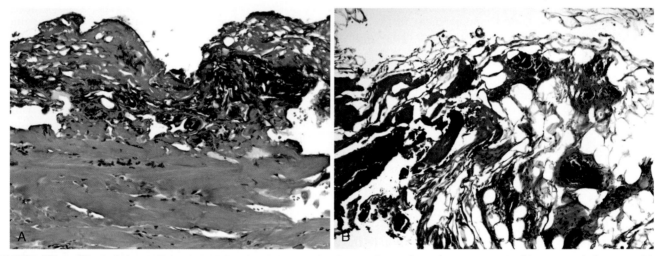

FIGURE 6-14 Effects of electrocautery on tissue preservation. **A,** The degree of tissue burn due to cautery in this case precludes recognition of the nature of underlying cell type. **B,** In this example, only the architecture of the tissue suggests normal breast tissue, although the cellular detail is not preserved enough to be certain.

activity and feedback to avoid excessive use of electrocautery, to a degree that it affects patient care.

In some cases, a combination of these changes and processing of breast tissue with less than adequate formalin fixation can create spaces that simulate lymphatic vessels. Sometimes, a retraction artifact around tumor nests during the dehydration process appears as if the tumor cells are in a vascular space (Figure 6-15).

All these changes and artifacts can pose difficulty and create challenges in interpretation of such cases. In general, the knowledge that a needle biopsy was done or a needle localization procedure was difficult is the most important first step in exercising caution during interpretation. Correlation with gross description and summary of submitted sections helps identify the tissue sections taken from a grossly identified biopsy site or wire track, and one can ask the question, Can these changes be artifactual? The distinction between epithelioid endothelial cells versus epithelial cells or tubules can be made using CD31 and cytokeratin immunostains.

When it comes to interpreting vascular or lymphatic invasion, the traditional criteria should be followed (i.e., location of the space in appropriate vascular bundle, tumor emboli attached to the vessel wall and, ideally, at least partially covered by endothelial cells). For cases in which there is a suspicion of "halo" artifact mimicking a lymphatic space, verification by immunostains, such as CD31 or D2-40 can be very helpful. The clinical significance of such displacements, in both breast and lymph nodes, in terms of long-term adverse effects is not established. There is a suggestion that these false emboli often do not survive unlike true vascular invasion and transport by the tumor, although no definite opinions exist at the present time.[45,46]

AXILLARY LYMPH NODES

Most of the chapter thus far has described aspects of gross examination, which are important and often time consuming, but the most important prognostic

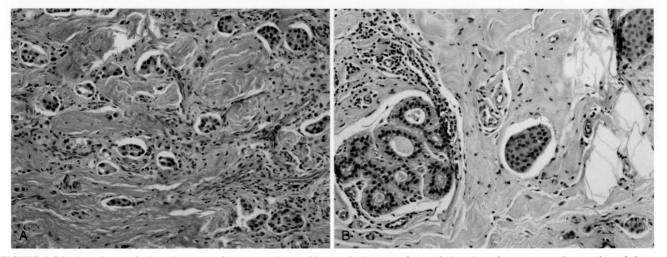

FIGURE 6-15 Pseudovascular invasion secondary to reaction to biopsy. **A,** An area of granulation tissue has entrapped a number of clusters of invasive tumor cells with a surrounding halo, which mimics lymphatic invasion. **B,** In comparison, here one sees true lymphatic invasion. The focus is located near normal epithelial compartment and adjacent to a capillary and a venule.

information in breast cancer management in the current practice is the number and status of axillary lymph nodes. Because sentinel lymph node biopsy has become the standard of care for all breast cancers, the rate of axillary lymph node dissection has steadily declined. A detailed discussion of various aspects of examination of sentinel lymph nodes is provided in Chapter 7. The procedure for obtaining the sentinel node is in Chapter 8. The procedures described later are limited to axillary lymph node dissection.

In the previous editions of the tumor-node-metastasis (TNM) staging system, the pathologic staging of the lymph nodes for breast cancer took into account not only the number and size of the involved lymph nodes but also the location of a positive node at different levels of the axilla divided according to the location of the pectoralis minor muscle. This is no longer true and, in the current practice, there is no specific reason to have exact orientation of axillary lymph nodes to perform the gross examination. Similarly, the issue of identifying internal mammary lymph nodes or the "Rotter" node is not considered relevant. Therefore, it is straightforward to perform the gross examination and isolation of axillary nodes. Usually, a careful manual dissection of relatively unfixed axillary fat permits identification of all the lymph nodes.[47] The identification of a vein can aid in identifying most of the nodes, which tend to be aligned close to the vessel. Some of the smaller nodes, typically those measuring 3 mm or less, can be difficult to separate from firm portions of adipose tissue. Therefore, it is advised that the word "possible" be used in the gross description because the exact number of nodes is determined by histologic confirmation of nodal tissue in the sections. As far as the larger nodes are concerned, these are often easy to recognize with the exception of fatty nodes. Such nodes often have central fatty infiltration and only a rim of lymphoid tissue under the capsule is present. A combination of fat and fibrous tissue in such nodes can lead to misinterpretation of grossly positive node for metastasis. A good observer should not have difficulty in identifying such pitfalls. In general, a combination of gentle pressure using the tip of the index finger together with the use of a surgical blade to splay apart the axillary fat helps in separating the nodes from surrounding adipose tissue.[48]

There is no consensus on methods of submission of lymph nodes isolated during the gross examination. A few principles, which are common to most of the lymph node dissections used elsewhere in the body, also apply to axillary nodes. Lymph nodes grossly positive for metastatic disease should be counted and measured carefully. A representative section from each of the positive nodes is sufficient for histologic examination. One of the important aspects of examination of such nodes, which can potentially show extranodal tumor extension, is to select the best section to demonstrate this important feature.[49,50] The submission of grossly negative nodes requires more work.[51] In general, the lymph nodes larger than 5 mm should be bisected or serially sectioned at 2-mm intervals and submitted entirely for examination; ideally, one node should be submitted per cassette. For lymph nodes measuring less than 5 mm, it is best to bisect and submit the entire node. In general, axillary nodes tend to be smaller than 10 mm and submitting only one node per cassette may lead to increased cost and time of tissue processing, embedding, and microtomy. Multiple small and intact nodes can be submitted in each cassette. In addition, bisected nodes can be differentially inked and then submitted with two to three nodes in one cassette. It is important to clearly dictate the summary of cassettes for lymph node submission, so it is clear at the time of histologic examination to obtain an accurate count of examined lymph nodes, because it is required for completing CAP-required tumor summaries. Finally, the highest lymph should be submitted separately, if it has been identified as such by the surgeon.

Over the years, the therapeutic value of axillary node clearing has been questioned. Therefore, we have observed that the amount of axillary adipose tissue removed as a part of axillary clearing has decreased in size, thus leading to the probability of identifying fewer numbers of axillary nodes. This raises the question of how many nodes need to be examined from the axillary dissection for an adequate nodal staging? This debate takes into account the risk of subsequent arm lymphedema associated with aggressive axillary clearing versus the benefit of accurate lymph node status. An additional complicating factor is the use of a minimum number of lymph nodes identified and reported as a measure of standard of surgical technique and has been used by some third-party payers to deny payments to surgeons. This has been the case with colon cancer surgery, but it is yet to be seen in axillary node dissection for breast cancer. Irrespective of these issues, every effort should be made to isolate as many nodes from axillary dissection as possible. At least a minimum of 10 nodes should be identified and verified at the time of histologic evaluation, because it has been shown that fewer than 10 nodes may understage the patient and adversely affect survival.[52] Therefore, the use of fat-clearing agents should be considered and applied as necessary. In the past, Bouin's and Carnoy's solutions have been used, but in the current practice, the use of such harmful chemicals is best avoided. Several relatively safe fat-clearing agents are commercially available for use and should be a part of all surgical pathology suites that deal with lymph node dissection specimens.

EXAMINATION OF BREAST SPECIMENS AFTER NEOADJUVANT THERAPY

Preoperative therapy in breast cancers has been used successfully for some time. It provides an in vivo test for effectiveness of therapies, which are usually used after primary cancer surgery. The main advantage of neoadjuvant therapy is obtaining reliable information of response or lack thereof to a particular treatment specific to that individual. The degree of response is used in the clinical setting to better predict the long-term outcome, often measured in terms of disease-free and overall survival. There remains controversy about the use of neoadjuvant versus adjuvant therapy and overall survival advantage among responders. However, there is more consistent evidence that a complete pathologic response (pCR), defined as no residual invasive or metastatic cancer in the lymph nodes, is a good prognostic factor. In addition, an assessment of response provides a short-term prognostic end point unlike disease-free or overall survival, making it an attractive measurable end point in the clinical trials setting.[53–55] Therefore, a systematic examination and documentation of residual disease after neoadjuvant therapy has become an important aspect of breast pathology.

Several studies have compared the pathologic response with clinical outcomes.[56] However, the criteria for defining and reporting pathologic response have not been standardized. Despite these shortcomings, there is a direct relationship between response and outcome. The definition of pCR is the same in all studies (i.e., no residual invasive cancer in breast).[57] The American Joint Commission on Cancer (AJCC) task

force has recommended that the definition of pCR is the absence of invasive cancer in the breast and axillary nodes.[58] The presence of noninvasive cancer is important in selection of patients for local therapy; it is not a determinant of survival. Most systems do not take into account response in the lymph nodes; however, studies that do consider response in lymph node as a part of the definition all require absence of residual metastatic tumor in the lymph nodes as pCR. For these reasons, the AJCC task force recommends pathologic tumor size after neoadjuvant therapy to be the largest contiguous tumor focus, with a suffix to alert the clinician when multiple scattered tumor foci are observed. This method of residual tumor size correlates with survival.[59] The definition and criteria for partial response remain markedly variable in different systems.

Taken together, several features need to be kept in mind when examining breast specimens from patients who have received neoadjuvant therapy. It is advised that the pathologist adopts a published system for measuring and reporting residual disease. This helps in developing gross examination protocols for such specimens. Some of the prerequisites for examination of specimens after neoadjuvant therapy include location and size of the lesion before treatment; specific history of type and duration of neoadjuvant therapy; pretreatment status of skin, nipple, chest wall, and axillary lymph nodes; and finally, the impression of clinical examination and relevant imaging studies that have specifically evaluated the response to treatment.

The main focus of the gross examination in this setting is identification of the residual tumor mass. In the majority of cases, pCR is not achieved and it is relatively easy to locate the tumor bed and the gross description follows the same principles as described previously for both breast-conserving surgery and mastectomy. However, the residual tumor looks and feels different from an untreated breast cancer. The desmoplastic stroma, which accompanies an untreated tumor, is often modified as a result of treatment, making it difficult to get a good feel of the tumor. Residual tumor is often softer and more rubbery than a typical untreated cancer. In most cases, the tumor regresses in a patchy fashion and may give an appearance of tan, fleshy nodules embedded in a soft, fibrotic stroma. The appearance of residual DCIS is also altered and high-grade DCIS may not appear as ropy structures with punctate cheesy material in the lumen, as is often the case with untreated high-grade DCIS with comedonecrosis. Once the residual tumor is identified, a complete description and its relationship to previous biopsy site and all the margins should be recorded.

In about 15% of cases, there is clinical complete response, and imaging studies show no residual tumor. Such cases make it quite difficult to identify the tumor bed. Correlation with findings from pretreatment biopsy, in terms of location and the most recent imaging study, helps identify the clip left at the time of pretreatment core biopsy. A careful inspection in a well-lighted grossing station, sometimes aided by a magnifying lens and gentle palpation, is a useful basic tool to locate the tumor bed. After that, a detailed description with measurements and distance from all the margins should follow. In case of mastectomy, the relationship of the tumor bed with nipple, skin, and skin margins is important to document. The examination of lymph nodes after neoadjuvant therapy follows similar principles. The only difference is in the lymph nodes, which were positive before the treatment. The pathologic response in the nodes is more variable; however, a rubbery and pale appearance or sometimes an obvious scar should be noted and described because this is not a common finding in untreated nodes.[60,61]

Unfortunately, there are no agreed upon guidelines for tissue sampling after neoadjuvant therapy. The goal of microscopic examination is to make sure a pCR is not missed.[62] For cases in which there is gross residual tumor, one block per centimeter is reasonable initial sampling. Attention should be paid to submit all the margins that fall within 1 cm so that they can be verified in histologic sections. If no tumor is found in a case for which the gross examination suggested residual disease, it is better to submit the residual grossly identified abnormal tissue for tumors up to 5 cm. One of the systems used at M.D. Anderson Cancer Center (called *residual cancer burden*) recommends at least five sections per the longest tumor dimension.[63] In cases in which a pCR is suspected at the time of gross examination, at least two sections per centimeter of the largest specimen dimension is a good start. If no residual tumor is found in these sections, the only reliable way to document pCR is to submit and examine the entire suspected tumor bed. The lymph nodes should be submitted completely, following the methods described previously. These general guidelines can be modified based on the system that the pathology department may adopt or develop to assess and report breast specimens after neoadjuvant therapy.

CHALLENGES IN EVALUATING SPECIMENS AFTER NEOADJUVANT THERAPY

The medications used in the neoadjuvant setting are often the same as those prescribed for adjuvant therapy. The main target of these drugs can be specific but their effect often alters a variety of processes and pathways involved in tumorigenesis. Several of these effects can then lead to morphologic changes in tumor cells and their environment that can pose challenges in histologic evaluation of breast specimens after therapy.[64] These histologic changes are often not specific to treatment type. In nonresponding tumors, there is often minimal change compared with the pretreatment sample (Figure 6-16).

Conversely, in tumors with some clinical response, the main effects are on either tumor size or cellularity and sometimes a combination of these two effects. In general, most of the therapeutic agents affect some aspects of cell cycle and some may induce apoptosis. Therefore, the main damage appears to be tumor cell shrinkage with loss of cytoplasm, followed by disintegration of the nuclear apparatus (Figure 6-17).

These changes are easy to recognize and do not cause any diagnostic problems. The viable cells can show cell

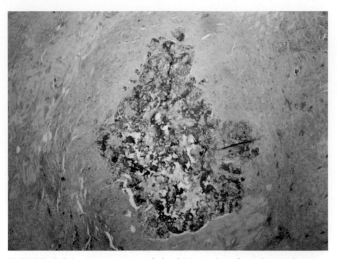

FIGURE 6-16 Appearance of the biopsy site after chemotherapy. In most cases, there is no significant change in the histologic features of the biopsy site, even after 4 to 6 months of neoadjuvant chemotherapy, as seen in this case.

enlargement and vacuolation of nucleus and cytoplasm. One of the challenges is the change in benign ductal epithelium, which can mimic in situ carcinoma. The key is to recognize a relatively uniform appearance in benign epithelium in terms of nuclear enlargement and prominent nucleolus and some cytoplasmic vacuolation (Figure 6-18).

Conversely, the degree of atypia in DCIS is uniform and other cytologic changes are more marked because most therapeutic agents target rapidly dividing cells (Figure 6-19). There are concurrent changes in the stroma. This is often more cellular and inflamed and may show abnormal vascular patterns.[65] In some cases, the tumor cells necrosis is followed by a highly collagenous stroma. Some of the entrapped vessels may shrink and endothelial cells can mimic epithelial cells (Figure 6-20).

The other area of difficulty is shrunken individual tumor cells in a cellular reactive stroma. These cells can be missed at scanning magnification. It is important to look at relatively high power in areas, which show altered stroma or some inflammation. In certain cases, immunostaining for cytokeratin can be very useful. In particular, lobular carcinomas after treatment may be quite difficult to recognize. Finally, the tumor grading may not be reliable after neoadjuvant therapy. The histologic grade of the tumor after neoadjuvant therapy has not been shown to be of significant clinical value and need not be reported. Further detailed discussion of the pathology of neoadjuvant treatment is found in Chapter 28.

EXAMINATION OF BREAST PROSTHESES (IMPLANTS)

Most of the medical and surgical devices removed during the surgery are submitted to the pathology department for either identification or recording pertinent information and storage. Therefore, each pathology department should have policies and procedures in

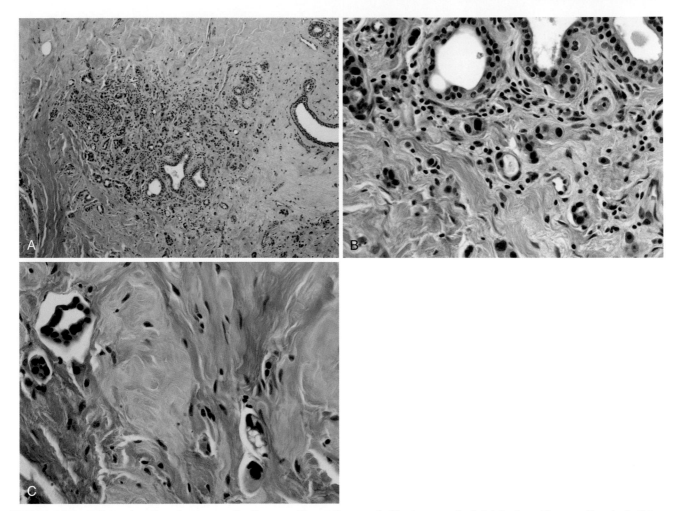

FIGURE 6-17   Cellular alterations in tumor cells after neoadjuvant therapy. **A,** The tumor cells shrink in size with some fibrosis. In this example, the residual tumor cells are intermixed with a focus of sclerosing adenosis. **B,** High-power view shows single and small clusters of tumor cells between benign tubules. **C,** Tumor cells may shrink in size while maintaining glandular architecture and thus create a pseudovascular space *(top left)* or enlarge with vacuolated cytoplasm and degenerative, hyperchromatic nucleus *(bottom right).*

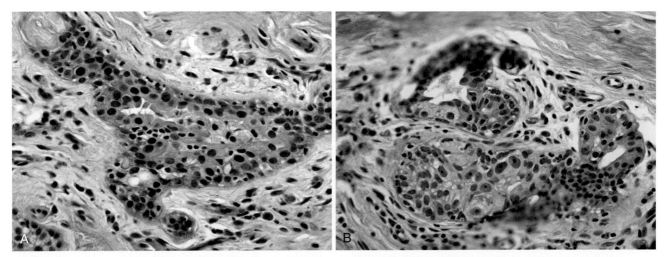

FIGURE 6-18   Effects of neoadjuvant therapy on normal epithelial cells. **A** and **B,** The alterations in the normal ductal epithelial cells are variable. There is nuclear enlargement and prominent nucleolus in most cells. In addition to changes described in the text, an edematous and inflamed stroma supports a benign ductal space with reactive changes over DCIS.

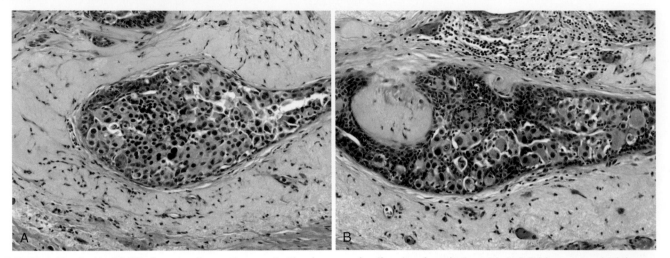

FIGURE 6-19 Residual DCIS after neoadjuvant therapy. **A,** The degree and uniformity of cytologic atypia in DCIS is more marked than normal reactive epithelium in this setting. The presence of mitotic figures and fibrotic and cellular periductal stroma are also helpful clues to the presence of residual DCIS. **B,** The diagnosis of pagetoid spread of DCIS after neoadjuvant treatment can be difficult. Note marked atypia in pagetoid cells, as compared with normal epithelium.

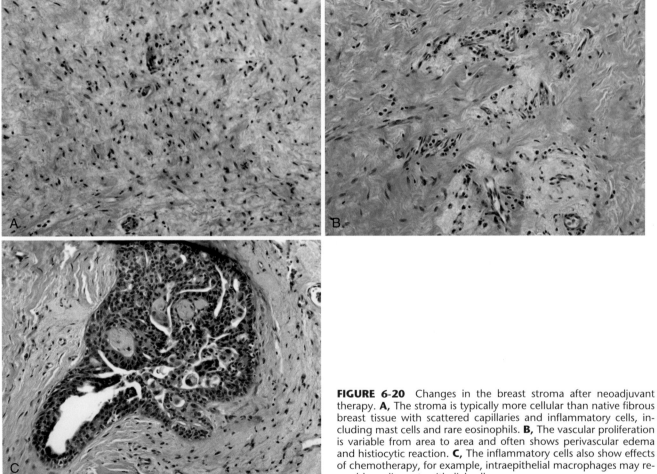

FIGURE 6-20 Changes in the breast stroma after neoadjuvant therapy. **A,** The stroma is typically more cellular than native fibrous breast tissue with scattered capillaries and inflammatory cells, including mast cells and rare eosinophils. **B,** The vascular proliferation is variable from area to area and often shows perivascular edema and histiocytic reaction. **C,** The inflammatory cells also show effects of chemotherapy, for example, intraepithelial macrophages may resemble malignant epithelial cells.

place to deal with these specimens for either potential medicolegal issues or possible recall or evaluation of removed prosthesis in the future. All such devices are biohazardous material and it is best to treat and keep them in accordance with the institution's and other agencies' regulations. In general, it is a good idea that the surgeon explains this to the patient and documents this discussion in the operative note. After examination, breast implants should be kept separately and stored in a secure place and retained in consultation with the

TABLE 6-6	A Template to Dictate Gross Examination of Breast Prostheses
Laterality	Right or Left
Type	Silicone or Saline
Shape	Round or Teardrop
Contents	Clear or Cloudy or Dark
Shell	Smooth or Textured (fine vs. coarse)
Surface	Dry or Oily or Sticky
Intact	Yes or No (describe the defect)
Manufacturer	If known
Imprinted Volume (mL)	
Other imprinted data	
Capsule	Absent or Present (brief description)
Implant retained for	5 years

risk management department. A breast implant without any attached tissue can be stored without fixative, but if there is any tissue or capsule with the implant, buffered formalin should be present in the container. All of the specifics about handling of breast implants should be a part of a separate procedure. It is suggested that the containers with breast implants are specifically labeled as such with clear instructions for retention. It is suggested that a bright-colored sticker is placed with the date before which it cannot be discarded. As a good practice, breast implants and other similar specimens are stored with access limited to only a few laboratory personnel. Some patients may request the return of implants to them. Similarly, the manufacturer may also request their return. A disposition form must be appropriately filled out with the description of the material that leaves the pathology department, ideally with a photo identification of the person who receives the breast implants. The containers should be labeled with the biohazard sign, and it should be explained to the person that biohazard risks are associated with the specimen.

The examination of breast implants should capture some specific details about the implant, and use of a simple template can assist the person recording this information not to forget any key elements (Table 6-6).

The important features to include in gross description are patient identification; laterality; weight and dimensions of the implant; type of implant; type of shell or encasing and its appearance; any numbers or other inscriptions; the color, appearance, and characteristics of contents; and most importantly, whether the prosthesis is intact. Any area of rupture should be measured and its extent clearly documented. It is a good idea to take photographs of all the implants with a front and back view and close-up views of inscribed information and site of rupture. If any tissue or capsule is attached to the implant, it should be described as any other surgical specimen. Attention should be paid to areas of nodule masses, calcifications, hemorrhage, and excessive fibrous tissue. At least one representative section from each of the different-appearing areas and any attached breast tissue should be submitted for histologic examination (Figure 6-21).

INTRAOPERATIVE EXAMINATION OF BREAST SPECIMENS

The role of intraoperative examination of breast and lymph node specimens is an integral part of the practice of breast pathology.[66] Over the years, the clinical management of breast disease, particularly the detection and options to either obtain or remove breast lesions, has transformed. At one time, intraoperative evaluation with frozen sections was heavily used for a number of indications in management of patients with breast disease, including initial diagnosis, diagnosis confirmation, extent of the primary tumor, evaluation of surgical margins, and assessment of lymph nodes, with reliable results.[67–69] However, several laboratories have seen a decline in frozen sections of breast.[70]

The main shift has been intraoperative evaluation from the primary lesion to assessment of margins and sentinel lymph nodes. The reason for this shift is advances in imaging and minimally invasive biopsy technology, leading to fairly accurate assessment of tumor size and extent using mammography, ultrasound, and sometimes MRI of the breast. In most institutions, the patient has already been diagnosed with a core needle biopsy or fine-needle aspiration. Another important aspect leading to minimal reliance on intraoperative frozen sections for initial diagnosis is detection of nonpalpable breast cancers, including small invasive cancers and most cases of DCIS. However, there is a small probability of false-negative and false-positive diagnosis of malignancy in frozen section evaluation of nonpalpable lesions in breast. In addition, there is a higher deferral rate of up to 3% in these circumstances, making frozen section for initial diagnosis not as attractive. Thus, the main indications for intraoperative evaluation of breast specimens are assessment of surgical margins and sentinel lymph nodes.

The majority of patients with breast cancer undergo breast-conserving surgery. The goal of the breast surgeon is to get clear margins in one surgical procedure, whenever possible.[71] Therefore, it is reasonable to request intraoperative assessment of the resection margins. In cases with a palpable mass, a careful gross examination after the specimen has been adequately inked and thinly sliced should allow the pathologist to reliably assess the margins. A combination of close inspection and gentle palpation helps demarcate the extent of the tumor. The margins can then be measured and reported to the surgeon. If any margin appears to be close (i.e., <5 mm), a frozen section may be considered. However, one must remember that it is difficult to obtain good sections of fat around the tumor and a reliance on frozen section on the slide alone can lead to an erroneous interpretation of margin (i.e., closer than the actual distance). It is reasonable to discuss the findings of the gross examination with the surgeon before proceeding with frozen

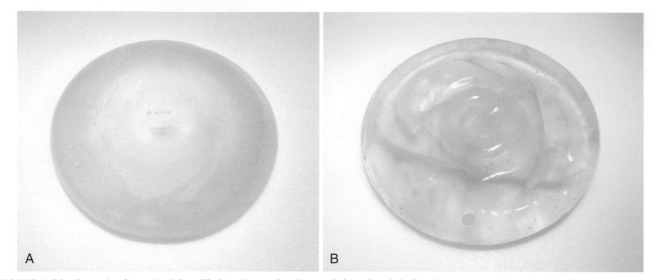

FIGURE 6-21 Breast implants. **A,** Saline-filled implants often have a light-colored shell and can vary in distention based on the volume of injected saline. The gross description of implants should include any inscriptions on the shell, such as the manufacturer's name and volume. **B,** Silicone implants tend to have a deeper yellow, often smooth shell. These prefilled implants should be evenly distended, unlike the one shown here. This implant is flaccid and contains inclusions, consistent with rupture.

sections. In most cases, a surgeon is comfortable with such an assessment and, if possible, may decide to take extra tissue for a close margin. Certain locations, such as anterior margin in a centrally located tumor, tumors close to medial edge of breast, and in some cases, tumors close to inframammary crease, may not leave much tissue to remove with good cosmetic results. In such cases, an accurate assessment of close margins can be of significant value to the surgeon and the patient. During the process of frozen section, the faced frozen tissue block can be very helpful to see the relationship with the tumor, which appears white or gray-white against bright yellow adipose tissue and the inked surface. The advantage of a good frozen section is that it allows measurements of margins in millimeters rather than a qualitative assessment as positive or negative.

The other method of intraoperative assessment of resection margin is touch imprint cytology.[72,73] Once an oriented specimen is received, it is weighed and measured in three planes. Then a glass slide is applied to each of the five or six surfaces, depending on whether there is any attached skin, and the slide is then air-dried. A simple and quick stain, such as Diff-quik or toluidine blue, is used to stain the imprinted slides. For surfaces measuring more than 5 cm, two imprints are prepared for that surface. The slides are screened to look for malignant cells. This method yields either no epithelial cells or rare clusters of benign epithelial and nonepithelial cells when the margin is negative versus atypical or malignant epithelial cells for positive margin. This method has been successfully used by several laboratories and, on average, takes about 10 minutes per specimen. In an initial study of 114 consecutive cases, Cox and associates[74] reported a sensitivity of 100% and a specificity of 96.6%. Klimberg and coworkers[75] studied 428 samples by this method and reported sensitivity, specificity, and positive (PPV) and negative (NPV) predictive values of almost 100%. D'Halluin and colleagues[76] evaluated the use of imprint cytology for margin assessment in 400

procedures and reported a sensitivity of 88.6% and a specificity of 92.2%, when they compared cytology with final surgical margin status of the case on permanent sections. They reported a PPV of 73.6% and an NPV of 97%. Conversely, this method has not enjoyed as much success in other laboratories. Saarela and associates[77] in their series of 55 cases reported the sensitivity to be very low, 7.5%. Similarly, Valdes and coworkers[78] studied a series of cases with invasive lobular carcinoma and found imprint cytology to be less than 10% sensitive with a PPV of 50%. Cox and colleagues[79] in a follow-up study of 701 cases found a very low recurrence rate of 2.7% with a median follow-up of 3.5 years in patients whose margins were evaluated by touch imprints during the surgical procedure. The advantages of touch imprint cytology for margin assessment for breast specimens are that it is safe, rapid, and in experienced hands, a relatively reliable method. The disadvantages are that it shows tremendous variability in sensitivity among different laboratories and may result in missing positive margins in low-grade malignancies.

The purpose of intraoperative resection margin assessment is to achieve breast conservation and to avoid a second surgery. Weber and associates[80] compared the benefits of specimen radiography versus frozen section in assessing surgical margins. In their study of 115 lesions, frozen section assessment of surgical margin rendered 27.5% margin-negative versus 14.3% by specimen radiography only, when these intraoperative results were used to re-excise the margins or to proceed to mastectomy during the first surgery. M.D. Anderson Cancer Center has reported their experience with use of intact and sliced specimen radiographs in conjunction with careful gross examination and frozen section of close margins. In a series of 264 patients with stages 0 to III breast cancer, Cabioglu and coworkers[81] reported that 92 patients had either a positive or a close margin on permanent sections of the main lumpectomy margin (i.e., 35% rate of positive margin, with no additional margin resection). However, with use of intraoperative margin assessment, approximately 25% of this population was rendered margin-negative. They verified this approach by reporting the 5-year local recurrence-free rate of 99% for invasive carcinoma and 100% for DCIS in this cohort, which underwent breast-conserving surgery with local radiation. In a subsequent study, Chagpar and colleagues[82] studied 109 cases of DCIS with intraoperative evaluation of resection margin. This assessment lead to positive (<1-mm) or close (<5-mm) margins in 59 patients, 43 of which were confirmed to have positive margins on permanent section diagnosis of the main lumpectomy specimen. Of the 59 patients, 44 had re-excision of the margin during the surgery and 31 were rendered margin-negative owing to intraoperative assessment. This significantly reduced the rate of a second procedure. These studies demonstrate the benefit of intraoperative margin assessment. There are some reports that the use of touch imprint can be successful in assessment of margin assessment during a second surgery to obtain clear margins.[35,36] However, it is important to exercise caution in interpreting either touch imprints or frozen section because the changes after the initial surgery can mimic malignancy.

Another indication for frozen section of breast specimens is assessment of skin margins in skin-sparing mastectomies. In addition, a frozen section may be used to rule out DCIS or invasive cancer in cases of nipple-sparing mastectomy. Usually, a section from the subareolar area is submitted for frozen section evaluation. In both of these situations, the tissue has minimal fat and it is relatively easy to obtain optimal sections for histologic evaluation. However, in such cases, the frozen section evaluation is to rule out malignancy (i.e., DCIS or invasive cancer), particularly in nipple-sparing mastectomy. Certain benign lesions, such as radial sclerosing lesions, intraductal papillomas, sclerosing adenosis, and subareolar sclerosing duct hyperplasia, can mimic either in situ or invasive carcinoma. Similarly, a small invasive lobular or tubular carcinoma may be difficult to diagnose. The differential diagnoses of these cases are discussed in detail in the respective chapters on these topics. Suffice it to say here that frozen section artifact can markedly enhance the complexity in evaluation of such lesions during intraoperative consultation.

STANDARD OPERATING PROCEDURES FOR GROSS EXAMINATION OF BREAST SPECIMENS

Several aspects should be kept in mind when creating a protocol for examination of breast specimens. One of the challenges in the current practice of breast pathology is to keep up with the new guidelines and the increasing volume of all types of breast specimens. In order to comply with these requirements, a greater degree of cooperation from other areas of the hospital, outpatient surgery centers, doctor offices, and radiology suites is needed.

An integral part of developing protocols for examination of breast specimens is the initial and continuous education of both the gross room and the other staff in the hospital and outpatient surgery centers. For example, the requirement to document the time of collection of a breast specimen to be used for assessment of predictive biomarkers is beyond the scope of the pathology staff. Because it is not possible to predict what types of breast specimen may contain malignancy, the only way to consistently acquire the collection time is to mandate this for all types of breast specimens, with rare exceptions such as re-excision margins, post-treatment excisions, or mastectomies. The most successful approach to this issue is to educate the staff in doctor's offices, radiology suites, outpatient surgery centers, and hospital operating rooms. Once these staff members understand the importance of documenting collection time, the probability of a high level of compliance is high. In this regard, it is important to advise the medical staff as well as relevant hospital committees, such as patient care quality committee or cancer committee, about the requirements for such documentation. One of the helpful activities is to collect compliance data and share them with the managers and supervisors for additional education and feedback to their staff. An effort like that at our institution has led to over 99% compliance in obtaining collection time for all breast specimens. The cold ischemic time (i.e., the interval between the time the tissue is removed from the patient and the time the tumor is exposed to formalin, and the total formalin fixation duration, which is now established at < 1 hr and 72 hr, respectively) requires education and training of the pathology staff. The standard operating procedure should establish specific cutoffs and processing start times to ensure adequate fixation of all breast specimens. Care should be taken for cases done on the last working day, especially before long weekends and holidays. A close communication between the surgeon and the pathologist or their assisting staff is necessary to accomplish this task.

As discussed previously, it is best to capture the microtomy guidelines on the tissue cassette. This is often easily accomplished using a laboratory information system that generates prelabeled cassettes at the time of accession of the case and each specimen. For example, many laboratories perform reflex immunostains for sentinel nodes, which are negative on intraoperative frozen section examination or touch imprint. The tissue cassettes for sentinel nodes can be prelabeled to cut extra sections for cytokeratin immunostain, thus saving time. In another situation in which a protocol can help reduce errors is not to assign consecutive accession numbers to same specimen types by site (e.g., two breast cases should not be accessioned or grossed consecutively) whenever possible. Another way to help reduce this type of error or troubleshooting possible case mix-up is to keep an exact count of each breast core or pieces in each tissue cassette. It has been suggested that the breast cores are inked differentially to reduce the chances of specimen mix-up. These simple steps can become very useful in case there is a concern of possible tissue mix-up or tissue contamination.[83]

TABLE 6-7	**Template for Gross Examination of Breast Surgical Specimen**
Site: Left breast.	
Procedure: Wire-guided excision.	
Fixative type/time: 10% NPBF; collected at 1235; fixation started at 1305.	
Dimensions/weight: 56-mm (AP) × 72-mm (SI) × 34-mm (ML), 72 g.	
Inking scheme: Ant—orange; Post—black; Med—blue; Lat—yellow; Sup—purple; Inf—green.	
Main findings: Poorly defined, irregular, tumor mass with gray-white rough-cut surface, firm to palpation with a central biopsy cavity. Tumor measures 21 × 15 × 9 mm. Located 2 mm from the inferior margin, 4 mm from the anterior, 6 mm from the lateral, and more than 10 mm from rest of the margins.	
Additional findings: Scattered small cysts. No skin or muscle.	
Summary of sections: A1—shaved medial margin; A2-4—tumor with inferior, anterior and lateral margins; A5—tumor with biopsy cavity; A6—tumor with surrounding breast tissue; A7-10—random sections including superior and deep margins.	

AP, anteroposterior; Ant, anterior; Inf, inferior; Lat, lateral; Med, medial; ML, mediolateral; NBPF, neutral phosphate-buffered formalin; Post, posterior; SI, superoinferior; Sup, superior.

The use of templates for dictating gross description is strongly encouraged (Table 6-7). Such templates should be developed by close communication between the residents, the fellows, the pathology assistants, and the pathologists with interest in breast pathology and should be a part of the gross room tissue dissection manual. Often, a review by a breast surgeon and a medical oncologist can help in adjusting the contents of such a template. The aim in developing such templates is to capture all the required information in a succinct form without omitting any pertinent positive or negative finding. At the same time, the template should keep some flexibility and should be reevaluated periodically to improve it, based on use and feedback from the physicians, who read the reports and explain them to patients.

Finally, protocols should take into consideration special issues for tissue procurement for either tissue banking or ancillary studies. Most tumor banks require submission of tumor and normal tissue to be saved as frozen tissue within 30 minutes of removal from the patient. A recently available gene-profiling test also requires collection of fresh tumor sample. The pathology suite should have specific written protocols and kits available to accomplish these tasks. As the field of theranostics evolves, new molecular and genetic tests will likely add to the complexity of tissue procurement.

SUMMARY

The grossing of breast specimens is the vital beginning of the diagnostic process. It is imperative that the pathologist, not only the pathologist assistant, see the gross specimen in the fresh state and guide the processing based on patient history and disease process. The guidelines offered here are just that—guidelines. Every patient specimen is unique, but the same goal of attainment of diagnostic accuracy for patient management is essential.

REFERENCES

1. Immediate management of mammographically detected breast lesions. Association of Directors of Anatomic and Surgical Pathology. Am J Surg Pathol 1993;17:850-851.
2. Lester SC, Bose S, Chen YY, et al. Protocol for the examination of specimens from patients with ductal carcinoma in situ of the breast. Arch Pathol Lab Med 2009;133:15-25.
3. Allred DC, Carlson RW, Berry DA, et al. NCCN Task Force Report: estrogen receptor and progesterone receptor testing in breast cancer by immunohistochemistry. J Natl Compr Canc Netw 2009;7(Suppl 6):S1-S21; quiz S2-S3.
4. Hammond ME, Hayes DF, Dowsett M, et al. American Society of Clinical Oncology/College of American Pathologists guideline recommendations for immunohistochemical testing of estrogen and progesterone receptors in breast cancer. Arch Pathol Lab Med 2010;134:907-922.
5. Hammond ME, Hayes DF, Dowsett M, et al. American Society of Clinical Oncology/College of American Pathologists guideline recommendations for immunohistochemical testing of estrogen and progesterone receptors in breast cancer. J Clin Oncol 2010;28:2784-2795.
6. American College of Radiology. *Breast Imaging Reporting and Data System (BI-RADS)*. 4th ed. Reston, VA: American College of Radiology; 2003; pp. 3-5.
7. Liberman L. Impact of image-guided core biopsy on the clinical management of breast disease. In Rosen PP, Hoda SA, eds. Breast Pathology: Diagnosis by Needle Core Biopsy. New York: Lippincott Williams & Wilkins; 2006; pp. 314-324.
8. Elvecrog EL, Lechner MC, Nelson MT. Nonpalpable breast lesions: correlation of stereotaxic large-core needle biopsy and surgical biopsy results. Radiology 1993;188:453-455.
9. Gershon-Cohen J, Colcher AE. An evaluation of the roentgen diagnosis of early carcinoma of the breast. JAMA 1937;108:867-871.
10. Morales AR, Essenfeld H, Essenfeld E, et al. Continuous-specimen-flow, high-throughput, 1-hour tissue processing. A system for rapid diagnostic tissue preparation. Arch Pathol Lab Med 2002;126:583-590.
11. Renshaw AA. Can mucinous lesions of the breast be reliably diagnosed by core needle biopsy? Am J Clin Pathol 2002;118:82-84.
12. Renshaw AA, Cartagena N, Derhagopian RP, et al. Lobular neoplasia in breast core needle biopsy specimens is not associated with an increased risk of ductal carcinoma in situ or invasive carcinoma. Am J Clin Pathol 2002;117:797-799.
13. Renshaw AA. Adequate histologic sampling of breast core needle biopsies. Arch Pathol Lab Med 2001;125:1055-1057.
14. Renshaw AA, Cartagena N, Schenkman RH, et al. Atypical ductal hyperplasia in breast core needle biopsies. Correlation of size of the lesion, complete removal of the lesion, and the incidence of carcinoma in follow-up biopsies. Am J Clin Pathol 2001;116:92-96.
15. Cornea V, Jaffer S, Bleiweiss IJ, et al. Adequate histologic sampling of breast magnetic resonance imaging-guided core needle biopsy. Arch Pathol Lab Med 2009;133:1961-1964.
16. Fisher B, Montague E, Redmond C, et al. Comparison of radical mastectomy with alternative treatments for primary breast cancer. A first report of results from a prospective randomized clinical trial. Cancer 1977;39(6 Suppl):2827-2839.
17. Epstein AH, Connolly JL, Gelman R, et al. The predictors of distant relapse following conservative surgery and radiotherapy for early breast cancer are similar to those following mastectomy. Int J Radiat Oncol Biol Phys 1989;17:755-760.
18. Gage I, Schnitt SJ, Nixon AJ, et al. Pathologic margin involvement and the risk of recurrence in patients treated with breast-conserving therapy. Cancer 1996;78:1921-1928.

19. Schnitt SJ, Abner A, Gelman R, et al. The relationship between microscopic margins of resection and the risk of local recurrence in patients with breast cancer treated with breast-conserving surgery and radiation therapy. Cancer 1994;74:1746-1751.

20. Koehl RH, Snyder RE, Hutter RV. The use of specimen roentgenography to detect small carcinomas not found by routine pathologic examination. CA Cancer J Clin 1971;21:2-10.

21. Snyder RE, Rosen P. Radiography of breast specimens. Cancer 1971;28:1608-1611.

22. Bauermeister DE, Hall MH. Specimen radiography—a mandatory adjunct to mammography. Am J Clin Pathol 1973;59:782-789.

23. Philip J, Harris WG, Rustage JH. Radiography of breast biopsy specimens. Br J Surg 1982;69:126-127.

24. Brenin DR. Management of the papable breast mass. In Harris JR, Harris ME, Morrow M, et al, eds. Diseases of the Breast. 3rd ed. Philadelphia: Lippincott Williams & Wilkins; 2004; pp. 33-46.

25. Molina MA, Snell S, Franceschi D, et al. Breast specimen orientation. Ann Surg Oncol 2009;16:285-288.

26. Singh M, Singh G, Hogan KT, et al. The effect of intraoperative specimen inking on lumpectomy re-excision rates. World J Surg Oncol 2010;8:1-4.

27. Miller B, Brownell MD. A cooling method to improve sectioning of fatty breast specimens. Lab Med 2008;39:467-469.

28. Giuliano AE, Kirgan DM, Guenther JM, et al. Lymphatic mapping and sentinel lymphadenectomy for breast cancer. Ann Surg 1994;220:391-398; discussion 398-401.

29. Treseler PA, Tauchi PS. Pathologic analysis of the sentinel lymph node. Surg Clin North Am 2000;80:1695-1719.

30. Schnitt SJ, Connolly JL. Processing and evaluation of breast excision specimens. A clinically oriented approach. Am J Clin Pathol 1992;98:125-137.

31. Schnitt SJ, Wang HH. Histologic sampling of grossly benign breast biopsies. How much is enough? Am J Surg Pathol 1989;13:505-512.

32. Owings DV, Hann L, Schnitt SJ. How thoroughly should needle localization breast biopsies be sampled for microscopic examination? A prospective mammographic/pathologic correlative study. Am J Surg Pathol 1990;14:578-583.

33. Dadmanesh F, Fan X, Dastane A, et al. Comparative analysis of size estimation by mapping and counting number of blocks with ductal carcinoma in situ in breast excision specimens. Arch Pathol Lab Med 2009;133:26-30.

34. Grin A, Horne G, Ennis M, et al. Measuring extent of ductal carcinoma in situ in breast excision specimens: a comparison of 4 methods. Arch Pathol Lab Med 2009;133:31-37.

35. Sauter ER, Hoffman JP, Ottery FD, et al. Is frozen section analysis of reexcision lumpectomy margins worthwhile? Margin analysis in breast reexcisions. Cancer 1994;73:2607-2612.

36. Valdes EK, Boolbol SK, Cohen JM, et al. Intra-operative touch preparation cytology; does it have a role in re-excision lumpectomy? Ann Surg Oncol 2007;14:1045-1050.

37. Douglas-Jones AG, Verghese A. Diagnostic difficulty arising from displaced epithelium after core biopsy in intracystic papillary lesions of the breast. J Clin Pathol 2002;55:780-783.

38. Nagi C, Bleiweiss I, Jaffer S. Epithelial displacement in breast lesions: a papillary phenomenon. Arch Pathol Lab Med 2005;129:1465-1469.

39. Youngson BJ, Cranor M, Rosen PP. Epithelial displacement in surgical breast specimens following needling procedures. Am J Surg Pathol 1994;18:896-903.

40. Youngson BJ, Liberman L, Rosen PP. Displacement of carcinomatous epithelium in surgical breast specimens following stereotaxic core biopsy. Am J Clin Pathol 1995;103:598-602.

41. Hoorntje LE, Schipper ME, Kaya A, et al. Tumour cell displacement after 14G breast biopsy. Eur J Surg Oncol 2004;30:520-525.

42. Carter BA, Jensen RA, Simpson JF, et al. Benign transport of breast epithelium into axillary lymph nodes after biopsy. Am J Clin Pathol 2000;113:259-265.

43. Gobbi H, Tse G, Page DL, et al. Reactive spindle cell nodules of the breast after core biopsy or fine-needle aspiration. Am J Clin Pathol 2000;113:288-294.

44. Rosen PP. Electrocautery instruments have been used routinely for the excision of tissue from the urinary bladder, prostate gland, and other sites for many years. Ann Surg 1986;204:612-613.

45. Diaz NM, Mayes JR, Vrcel V. Breast epithelial cells in dermal angiolymphatic spaces: a manifestation of benign mechanical transport. Hum Pathol 2005;36:310-313.

46. Diaz NM, Vrcel V, Centeno BA, et al. Modes of benign mechanical transport of breast epithelial cells to axillary lymph nodes. Adv Anat Pathol 2005;12:7-9.

47. Hartveit F, Samsonsen G, Tangen M, et al. Routine histological investigation of the axillary nodes in breast cancer. Clin Oncol 1982;8:121-126.

48. Durkin K, Haagensen CD. An improved technique for the study of lymph nodes in surgical specimens. Ann Surg 1980;191:419-429.

49. Fisher ER, Gregorio RM, Redmond C, et al. Pathologic findings from the national surgical adjuvant breast project (protocol no. 4). III. The significance of extranodal extension of axillary metastases. Am J Clin Pathol 1976;65:439-444.

50. Altinyollar H, Berberoglu U, Gulben K, et al. The correlation of extranodal invasion with other prognostic parameters in lymph node positive breast cancer. J Surg Oncol 2007;95:567-571.

51. Niemann TH, Yilmaz AG, Marsh WL Jr, et al. A half a node or a whole node: a comparison of methods for submitting lymph nodes. Am J Clin Pathol 1998;109:571-576.

52. Salama JK, Heimann R, Lin F, et al. Does the number of lymph nodes examined in patients with lymph node-negative breast carcinoma have prognostic significance? Cancer 2005;103:664-671.

53. Jones RL, Lakhani SR, Ring AE, et al. Pathological complete response and residual DCIS following neoadjuvant chemotherapy for breast carcinoma. Br J Cancer 2006;94:358-362.

54. Jones RL, Smith IE. Neoadjuvant treatment for early-stage breast cancer: opportunities to assess tumour response. Lancet Oncol 2006;7:869-874.

55. Mazouni C, Peintinger F, Wan-Kau S, et al. Residual ductal carcinoma in situ in patients with complete eradication of invasive breast cancer after neoadjuvant chemotherapy does not adversely affect patient outcome. J Clin Oncol 2007;25:2650-2655.

56. Connolly JL, Schnitt SJ. Evaluation of breast biopsy specimens in patients considered for treatment by conservative surgery and radiation therapy for early breast cancer. Pathol Annu 1988;23:1-23.

57. Pu RT, Schott AF, Sturtz DE, et al. Pathologic features of breast cancer associated with complete response to neoadjuvant chemotherapy: importance of tumor necrosis. Am J Surg Pathol 2005;29:354-358.

58. Kaufmann M, Hortobagyi GN, Goldhirsch A, et al. Recommendations from an international expert panel on the use of neoadjuvant (primary) systemic treatment of operable breast cancer: an update. J Clin Oncol 2006;24:1940-1949.

59. Carey LA, Metzger R, Dees EC, et al. American Joint Committee on Cancer tumor-node-metastasis stage after neoadjuvant chemotherapy and breast cancer outcome. J Natl Cancer Inst 2005;97:1137-1142.

60. Donnelly J, Parham DM, Hickish T, et al. Axillary lymph node scarring and the association with tumour response following neoadjuvant chemoendocrine therapy for breast cancer. Breast 2001;10:61-66.

61. Newman LA, Pernick NL, Adsay V, et al. Histopathologic evidence of tumor regression in the axillary lymph nodes of patients treated with preoperative chemotherapy correlates with breast cancer outcome. Ann Surg Oncol 2003;10:734-739.

62. Rajan R, Poniecka A, Smith TL, et al. Change in tumor cellularity of breast carcinoma after neoadjuvant chemotherapy as a variable in the pathologic assessment of response. Cancer 2004;100:1365-1373.

63. Symmans WF, Peintinger F, Hatzis C, et al. Measurement of residual breast cancer burden to predict survival after neoadjuvant chemotherapy. J Clin Oncol 2007;25:4414-4422.

64. Sharkey FE, Addington SL, Fowler LJ, et al. Effects of preoperative chemotherapy on the morphology of resectable breast carcinoma. Mod Pathol 1996;9:893-900.

65. Mohsin SK, Weiss HL, Chang J. Histological changes associated with Herceptin therapy in breast cancer [abstract]. Mod Pathol 2004;17(Suppl 1):43A.

66. Bianchi S, Palli D, Ciatto S, et al. Accuracy and reliability of frozen section diagnosis in a series of 672 nonpalpable breast lesions. Am J Clin Pathol 1995;103:199-205.

67. Ferreiro JA, Gisvold JJ, Bostwick DG. Accuracy of frozen-section diagnosis of mammographically directed breast biopsies. Results of 1,490 consecutive cases. Am J Surg Pathol 1995;19: 1267-1271.

68. Niemann TH, Lucas JG, Marsh WL Jr. To freeze or not to freeze. A comparison of methods for the handling of breast biopsies with no palpable abnormality. Am J Clin Pathol 1996;106:225-228.

69. Speights VO Jr. Evaluation of frozen sections in grossly benign breast biopsies. Mod Pathol 1994;7:762-765.

70. Laucirica R. Intraoperative assessment of the breast: guidelines and potential pitfalls. Arch Pathol Lab Med 2005;129: 1565-1574.

71. DiBiase SJ, Komarnicky LT, Schwartz GF, et al. The number of positive margins influences the outcome of women treated with breast preservation for early stage breast carcinoma. Cancer 1998;82:2212-2220.

72. Blair SL, Wang-Rodriguez J, Cortes-Mateos MJ, et al. Enhanced touch preps improve the ease of interpretation of intraoperative breast cancer margins. Am Surg 2007;73:973-976.

73. Creager AJ, Shaw JA, Young PR, et al. Intraoperative evaluation of lumpectomy margins by imprint cytology with histologic correlation: a community hospital experience. Arch Pathol Lab Med 2002;126:846-848.

74. Cox CE, Ku NN, Reintgen DS, et al. Touch preparation cytology of breast lumpectomy margins with histologic correlation. Arch Surg 1991;126:490-493.

75. Klimberg VS, Westbrook KC, Korourian S. Use of touch preps for diagnosis and evaluation of surgical margins in breast cancer. Ann Surg Oncol 1998;5:220-226.

76. D'Halluin F, Tas P, Rouquette S, et al. Intra-operative touch preparation cytology following lumpectomy for breast cancer: a series of 400 procedures. Breast 2009;18:248-253.

77. Saarela AO, Paloneva TK, Rissanen TJ, et al. Determinants of positive histologic margins and residual tumor after lumpectomy for early breast cancer: a prospective study with special reference to touch preparation cytology. J Surg Oncol 1997;66:248-253.

78. Valdes EK, Boolbol SK, Ali I, et al. Intraoperative touch preparation cytology for margin assessment in breast-conservation surgery: does it work for lobular carcinoma? Ann Surg Oncol 2007;14:2940-2945.

79. Cox CE, Pendas S, Ku NN, et al. Local recurrence of breast cancer after cytological evaluation of lumpectomy margins. Am Surg 1998;64:533-537; discussion 537-538.

80. Weber S, Storm FK, Stitt J, et al. The role of frozen section analysis of margins during breast conservation surgery. Cancer J Sci Am 1997;3:273-277.

81. Cabioglu N, Hunt KK, Sahin AA, et al. Role for intraoperative margin assessment in patients undergoing breast-conserving surgery. Ann Surg Oncol 2007;14:1458-1471.

82. Chagpar A, Yen T, Sahin A, et al. Intraoperative margin assessment reduces reexcision rates in patients with ductal carcinoma in situ treated with breast-conserving surgery. Am J Surg 2003;186:371-377.

83. Renshaw AA, Kish R, Gould EW. The value of inking breast cores to reduce specimen mix-up. Am J Clin Pathol 2007;127:271-272.

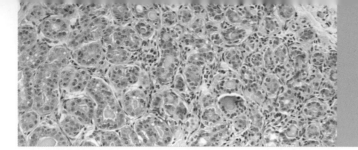

7

Sentinel Lymph Node Biopsy

Sunil Badve

INTRODUCTION

Systematic screening of women by mammography and clinical examination has resulted in early diagnosis of breast cancer and a 25% to 30% decrease in mortality.[1] Early breast cancer can be cured with locoregional treatment alone in some cases. However, subclinical metastases do occur, and in a significant percentage of women treated with an apparently curative locoregional therapy, distant metastases ultimately develop.[2,3] Trying to determine which women with clinically early breast cancer have metastases is an important issue in the management of patients with breast cancer. It is possible that these women might benefit from aggressive systemic therapy given at the time of diagnosis. One approach to stratify early breast cancer patients to various risk groups is to analyze the primary tumor for nuclear or histologic grade, kinetics of cell growth and division, hormone receptor expression, markers of invasive or metastatic capability, or angiogenesis. However, these prognostic markers used singly or in combinations have failed to achieve the same prognostic value as examination of the axillary lymph nodes (ALNs).[4] The probability of recurrence is higher for women with histologically positive ALNs and increases with each additional lymph node (Figure 7-1).[5,6] Although axillary lymph node dissection (ALND) provides prognostic information, it has minimal, if any, therapeutic value, particularly in patients with negative lymph nodes. ALND is also responsible for most of the morbidities associated with breast cancer surgery. Sentinel lymph node biopsy (SLNB) was devised as an alternative procedure to ALND. It is a minimally invasive procedure that accurately evaluates the status of the axilla and can obtain the same prognostic information derived from ALND with significantly less morbidity.

In 1977, the concept of a sentinel node was originally described by Cabanas[7] for penile cancer and is based on

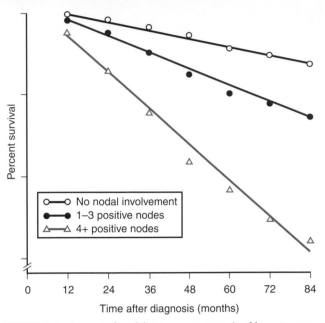

FIGURE 7-1 Impact of nodal status on prognosis of breast cancer. Note that the prognosis worsens as the number of involved lymph nodes increases.

the proposed concept of orderly progression of tumor cells within the lymphatic system. Cabanas proposed that the lymph nodes that first receive the drainage from a tumor (termed *sentinel lymph nodes [SLN]*) could be removed by limited surgery and examined to determine whether more extensive lymphadenectomy should be performed. This model was later applied to melanoma[8] and then to breast cancer,[9] first to prove the hypothesis and then to ask the question whether the technique can be applied to staging breast cancer. Incidentally, Kett and coworkers[10] reported that the first regional lymph node, "the Sorgius node" could be identified in breast cancer using direct mammolymphography. They infused contrast material, "lipoidol ultra fluide," into a lymphatic vessel that had been visualized by intradermal injection of patent blue violet into the areola. However, because this technique was labor intensive and time consuming, it did not get acceptance into clinical practice. More recent modifications of the technique such as dye-directed lymphatic mapping, isotope-based radiolocalization, and the combination of vital dye and isotope techniques have been critical steps that have led to the current practice of SLNB.[9,11,12] Although commonly used, the performance of SLNB requires significant experience as illustrated by the original study by Giuliano and colleagues[11] in which SLNB was performed in addition to complete ALND to verify the accuracy of the SLNB. In this study of 174 patients, the initial success rate for identifying the sentinel node was 58.6% with an accuracy of 94.3%. However, in the latter half of the study, this increased to 78% and 100%, respectively. Since the original studies,[11–15] several studies have examined and validated the SLN hypothesis in breast cancer. Currently, there is level 1 evidence that documents that SLNB is as accurate as ALND for staging breast cancer.[16] If the SLN is negative, it is predicted

that the rest of the ALNs will also be negative. Conversely, if SLN is positive, the rest of the ALNs might also contain metastatic tumor deposits. This made the SLN an extremely valuable piece of tissue requiring critical analysis. Thin slicing of the SLN and examination of multiple levels has become the standard practice for analysis of the specimens.

CLINICAL PARAMETERS AND FEASIBILITY ISSUES

The current body of literature shows that SLNB is suitable for virtually all clinically node-negative T1-2 invasive breast cancers[17]; however, patients with SLNB performed for ductal carcinoma in situ (DCIS), T3-4 tumors including inflammatory breast cancer, and after neoadjuvant therapy for histologically positive nodes are not included in the quality assessment measures by the American Society of Breast Surgeons.[16] Nuances associated with these specific settings are detailed later.

Age

The SLNB has been performed in individuals of all ages ranging from 20 to 90 years. However, the identification of the SLN has been significantly less successful in older patients.[18–20] The radioactive count within a node tends to be inversely proportional to age.[21] In this patient population, the combination of colored dye and radioactive material has led to significant improvement in the results.[22,23] It has also been reported that permitting a greater amount of time between injection and dissection may improve the success rate. It should also be remembered that ALND has a greater morbidity in the elderly[19,24] and that this patient population is less likely to have received chemotherapy than younger individuals. In a retrospective study of 194 cases of positive SLN with ALND, Turner and associates[25] did not find any association between clinical or patient parameters with SLN positivity.

Gender

Central core biopsy has been performed in men and women with equal success. Although the size of the studies has been relatively small,[26–28] the accuracy of identification of SLN has been reported to be approximately 95% with 100% accuracy for prediction of axillary status. However, it has been noted that this higher rate possibly reflects the late presentation of breast cancer in men.[27]

Body Habitus

SLNB is more challenging in obese patients.[20] The failure rate has been directly correlated with increased main body mass index (BMI). In a study of 1356 patients, it was found that, for an increase in one unit of BMI (or an increase in 1 yr of age), the odds of successful SLNB decrease by 0.05.[21]

Pregnancy and Lactation

Very limited data are available on the safety and utility of SLNB in the setting of pregnancy and lactation.[29] The American Society of Clinical Oncology (ASCO) 2005 guidelines do not recommend the procedure in these settings.[30] However, in a recent study, Gentilini and coworkers[31] demonstrated 100% accuracy in a series of 12 pregnant patients.

Prior Breast or Axillary Surgery

The performance of a needle core biopsy does not affect the accuracy of SLNB. Prior breast reduction surgery, surgical implants, extensive injuries, burns, previous reconstructive surgery to the breast or to the axilla, and congenital lymphatic problems could all theoretically affect the feasibility of SLNB; however, this has not been found to be a major issue.[30] More recently, Yararbas and colleagues[32] analyzed a series of 156 patients with prior excision biopsy. They were able to identify SLNs in approximately 95% of the patients. The common problems identified in this series were failure of SLN visualization, dilated lymphatics, and misleading radioactive accumulations. The use of combination techniques may lead to significant improvement in the identification rates and predictive ability of the SLNB in these situations. SLNB after axillary surgery has not been studied in detail. In a series of 32 cases, a high failure rate (25% vs. 5%) was noted in patients who had prior axillary surgery.[33] There are limited data with regard to application of SLNB to recurrent disease, especially of prior SLNB.[34]

Location of the Sentinel Node

The SLN is typically one of the level I or II lymph nodes in the ipsilateral axilla.[18] However, in certain circumstances, a contralateral ALN or internal mediastinal lymph node may be highlighted by the blue dye/radioactive material. This is particularly common in cases in which the tumor is located in the medial aspect of the breast.[35,36] The surgical management of these cases is controversial. More often than not, internal mammary node sampling is not performed at the time of breast surgery. This is, in part, because resection of the internal mammary nodes does not offer a survival advantage over conventional surgery, and untreated internal mammary lymph nodes are rarely a source of local recurrence in patients with early-stage breast cancer.[35,37,38]

Most studies of SLNB have excluded patients with clinically positive nodes in the axilla. It must be noted that approximately 25% of clinically positive ALNs do not have metastatic disease.[39] When SLNB is carried out in the setting of suspicious/palpable lymph nodes, these nodes should be excised and treated like SLNs.[30] An option to consider in these cases is ultrasound examination of the nodes with directed biopsy. Published reports suggest that up to 40% to 50% of node-positive patients can be identified by this method, with up to 90% sensitivity for patients with four or more positive nodes.[40,41] However, this technique has limited sensitivity (25%) for the detection of micrometastasis.[41]

Prior Chemotherapy

SLNB in patients with locally advanced breast cancer may be performed before or after neoadjuvant chemotherapy. The Guidelines of the ASCO Expert Panel[30] (2005) state that there are insufficient data to recommend SLNB or to suggest an appropriate time for SLNB for patients receiving preoperative systemic chemotherapy. Some authors regard downstaging of clinically positive ALNs as a contraindication for SLNB. Concerns with regard to altered patterns of lymphatic drainage, multiple obscured and undetected sources of lymphatic drainage, and possible nonuniform cytotoxic response within the axillary metastasis giving rise to false-negative SLNB results have been expressed. Several studies have documented an unexpectedly high false-negative rate of up to 15% when SLNBs are performed after neoadjuvant chemotherapy.[42–44] A more recent study by Schwartz and associates[45] showed that SLNs could be reliably used to predict ALN status in a series of 79 patients. They also noted that neoadjuvant chemotherapy frequently converted patients with N1-2 lymph node status to N0 status. Suffice to say that the issue is controversial and definitive data for management of patients with neoadjuvant chemotherapy are still not available.[17]

Prophylactic Mastectomy

SLNB may be performed in association with prophylactic mastectomy procedures because of the risk of occult carcinoma.[46] In a series of 245 unilateral prophylactic mastectomies, Cox and coworkers[47] identified occult carcinoma in 14 patients (5.7%); 2 of these patients had involvement of the sentinel node (0.8%). Similarly, in the review of 436 prophylactic mastectomies performed at M.D. Anderson Cancer Center, carcinoma was identified in 2 of the 108 patients who underwent SLNB.[48] King and colleagues[49] found the incidence of occult carcinoma in 8% of their 163 prophylactic mastectomies; 2 of these patients had positive SLNs. Incidentally, among the 130 women who did not have an occult primary tumor in the prophylactic mastectomies, metastatic carcinoma was identified in 1 patient. This was believed to arise from the contralateral breast, which had an AJCC (American Joint Committee on Cancer[50]) stage IIIC carcinoma. More recently, Nasser and associates[51] reviewed 99 patients undergoing prophylactic mastectomy and identified SLN metastasis in 2 patients; both of whom had inflammatory carcinoma in the contralateral side. Based on these studies, it appears that the incidence of SLN metastasis in the prophylactic mastectomy is approximately 1%, with patients with inflammatory carcinoma being at higher risk.

Tumor Characteristics

TUMOR TYPE

The vast majority of SLNBs have been performed for invasive ductal carcinoma; however, the procedure appears to also be efficient for other types of breast cancer. It should be noted that, in some studies, a slightly decreased sensitivity has been observed for invasive lobular carcinoma.[52] However, Grube and coworkers[53] have shown a 97% identification rate with an accuracy of 100% in a series of 105 consecutive patients with lobular carcinoma. Inflammatory carcinoma is a contraindication for SLNB.

DUCTAL CARCINOMA IN SITU AND MICROINVASIVE CARCINOMA

SLNBs have also been performed in patients with DCIS, with or without microinvasion. Micrometastases have been identified in a small percentage of these cases; however, the relevance of this finding is uncertain. In a recent meta-analysis, Ansari and colleagues[54] analyzed 22 published reports and found an incidence of 7.4% for patients with preoperative diagnosis of DCIS. However, this rate was only 3.7% when cases lacking an incidentally identified invasive component ("pure" DCIS) were analyzed. It is not known whether this includes cases with iatrogenic displacement and transport of tumor cells to the lymph nodes (discussed later). In T1mic patients, the rates of SLN involvement have been reported to range from 10% to 33%.[55,56]

TUMOR SIZE

In older literature, SLNB was not recommended for large (T3) tumors, because it was believed the altered lymphatic pattern due to the tumor may interfere with the correct identification of SLN. Multifocal and multicentric diseases have long been regarded as relative contraindications for SLNB; however, this viewpoint has been challenged. Recent studies show that these concerns might be overstated. A multi-institutional study of 130 patients with multicentric disease showed acceptable sensitivity and accuracy.[57] Tumor size and multicentricity are not absolute contraindications for SLNB. Periareolar injection of the dye has been shown to successfully identify SLNs in these situations.[58]

PREDICTORS OF SENTINEL NODE METASTASIS

A number of studies have looked at ways of preoperatively predicting the likelihood of identifying a positive SLN. However, many of these have been small single-institution studies that lacked adequate sample size and discriminative power. More recently, Bevilacqua and associates[59] (Figure 7-2) analyzed a series of 3786 patients to identify important parameters and integrate the findings into a simplified tool. The tool developed, a nomogram, was further validated in a series of 1545 independent cases. The nomogram is based on the following factors: age, tumor location, multifocality, tumor size, tumor type, lymphovascular involvement, nuclear grade, and estrogen receptor (ER) and progesterone receptor (PgR) expression. The overall frequency of SLN involvement in this study was 33%, with the vast majority of cases identified by intraoperative frozen section. Additional metastases were identified using serial sections in 6% and immunohistochemistry (IHC) in 4% of cases. In larger studies, the frequency of nodal involvement is about 10% in T1mic, 9% to 13% in T1a, 13% to 19% in T1b, 26% to 29% in T1c, 39% to 50% in T2 tumors less than 3 cm, 48% to 59% in T2 tumors greater than 3 cm, and 71% to 81% in T3 tumors.[59–67] The incidence of SLN positivity is slightly higher for ER+/PgR+ tumors than for ER–/PgR– tumors.[59,68–70] Also, a slight decrease in frequency for (axillary) SLN involvement is noted in tumors located in the upper inner quadrant; this may, in part, be due to drainage to nonaxillary sites.[59] It must be noted that this Memorial Sloan-Kettering Cancer Center (MSKCC) nomogram had an area under the receiver operating characteristic (ROC) curve (AUC) of 0.754, indicating that it was less than perfect. These data indicate that prediction of positivity of SLNB is difficult and that, in most cases, the risk of axillary metastasis is sufficiently high enough to warrant SLNB for all breast cancers.

PATHOLOGIC EVALUATION

The SLNB can be performed as an office procedure under local anesthesia to allow better planning of subsequent surgery. More commonly, it is performed during surgery to the primary tumor and accessed intraoperatively using frozen sections or postoperatively after fixation and paraffin embedding. There are no standardized protocols for handling of the SLN; this has resulted in marked differences in the handling and processing of nodes, number of sections examined, cutting intervals, and the use of IHC for detection of isolated tumor cells (ITCs). A survey of 240 European laboratories identified close to 123 somewhat different histologic protocols.[71]

Gross Evaluation

The amount of radioactive material used in the SLNB procedure is one tenth of that used for a bone scan. Because of the short half-life and limited penetration of technetium, health risks to those handling SLNs are negligible, although appropriate care should be taken.[72]

The basic principle underlying the gross examination of the SLN is similar to the evaluation of other specimens. The node should be dissected away from the adjoining fat, and thinly (<2 mm) sliced; both cut surfaces should be closely examined for the presence of metastatic carcinoma, and the entire lymph node should be submitted for histologic examination. A survey conducted on behalf of the European Working Group for Breast Screening Pathology (EWGBSP)[71] identified marked variations in the practice of 382 respondents, with less than 3% of the laboratories examining the entire SLN in a single piece. Lymph nodes tend to be bean-shaped with short and long axes. Cutting parallel to the long axis produces a fewer number of slices than slicing along the short axis and has been recommended.[30,73] An important point to remember is that opposing surfaces of the slices need to be examined, so care should be taken when putting the sliced node

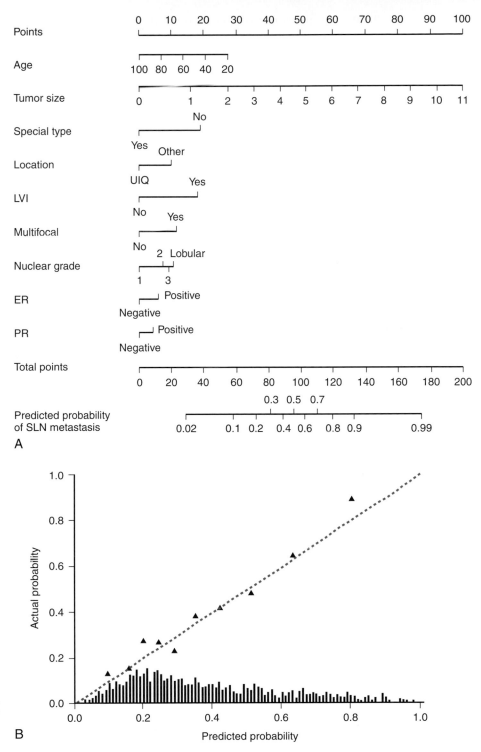

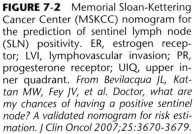

FIGURE 7-2 Memorial Sloan-Kettering Cancer Center (MSKCC) nomogram for the prediction of sentinel lymph node (SLN) positivity. ER, estrogen receptor; LVI, lymphovascular invasion; PR, progesterone receptor; UIQ, upper inner quadrant. *From Bevilacqua JL, Kattan MW, Fey JV, et al. Doctor, what are my chances of having a positive sentinel node? A validated nomogram for risk estimation. J Clin Oncol 2007;25:3670-3679.*

in the cassettes for processing and embedding.[73] It should be noted that some of the older recommendations (Association of Directors of Anatomic and Surgical Pathology [ADASP],[74] 2001) involved slicing the lymph node at 3- to 4-mm intervals; this is no longer considered acceptable because a number of micrometastasis would be missed using this protocol. An alternative approach is slicing the lymph nodes very thin (~1 mm); the advantage of this approach is that it decreases the need for examining multiple levels from

the paraffin block. We have very successfully used this approach at our institution without significant loss of sensitivity and specificity.

Histologic Evaluation

Although the general principles remain identical, a number of protocols have been used in the examination of SLNs. In the 2004 EWGBSP study,[71] 60% of the centers carried out intraoperative assessment of the nodes, although it is likely that intraoperative evaluation is much more frequent today.

Intraoperative Evaluation

Intraoperative evaluation can be performed using imprint cytology and frozen sections.

IMPRINT CYTOLOGY

Advocates of imprint cytology believe that the preparation of frozen sections is wasteful because samples are trimmed in the microtome in order to obtain a surface suitable for sectioning.[75] This is particularly so for fatty lymph nodes, which are difficult to section. Initial studies reported a high sensitivity and sensitivity for the technique. However, these results have not been substantiated in the larger, recent studies. The success rate of imprint cytology is high, although it tends to vary according to the institutions and the staining methods used. Respectively, the sensitivity and specificity for Diff-Quik stain has been reported to be 53% and 99%,[76] whereas that for the Papanicolaou stain is 91% and 99%.[77] Hematoxylin and eosin (H&E) staining achieved a sensitivity of 94% and a specificity of 99%.[78] H&E staining has the added advantage of increasing the ease with which the surgical pathologist can interpret the findings of the touch preparation. A meta-analysis performed by Tew and coworkers[79] reported 63% sensitivity for imprint cytology with significantly lower sensitivity for micrometastasis compared with macrometastasis (22% vs. 81%). In a more recent study, Lorand and colleagues[80] analyzed the utility of intraoperative imprint cytology in a series of 355 procedures and an observed total sensitivity was 36%; 15% of patients with nodal metastasis were not detected. The technique was also less effective for detection of micrometastases. False negativity due to poor-quality imprints can be a significant issue with fatty lymph nodes. In such situations, some workers prefer to use a scraping method rather than touch imprints to prepare the cytology preparation. Sensitivity is significantly lower for the oldest patients, small (T1a-b) tumors, and lobular subtype.[80]

FROZEN SECTION

Intraoperative frozen section for evaluation of SLNs has become routine at most institutions. However, there are no specific guidelines as to whether the entire lymph node (all the slices) should be examined by this method; some institutions examine only a single slice of the node; this could significantly increase the false-negative rate. The number of sections examined from the frozen section block is also variable, with most places examining two to three levels. This is in contrast to some protocols in which the entire block is sectioned to generate hundreds of sections, resulting in no tissue left for permanent sectioning.[81]

The false-negative rate for frozen section is typically less than 10%. It is estimated that, for every 100 patients who have intraoperative SLN evaluation, 16% to 17% will have positive lymph nodes and 8% to 9% will have false-negative results.[30] Technical difficulties such as fatty lymph nodes and incomplete sections contribute significantly to the false-negative results. Suspicious findings should be reported as not diagnostic for tumor and deferred for permanent sections.[30]

The advantages and disadvantages of intraoperative assessment of SLNs are discussed later under "Critical Issues."

Permanent Sections

The standard approach for examination of permanent sections involves performance of multilevel assessment; this increases the likelihood of finding metastases.[75,82] This ranges from evaluation of 2 to 5 levels to up to 100 levels separated by 40-μm intervals. In a 2004 survey performed by Cserni and associates,[71] the most common practice was assessing three levels; however, this was performed by only 26% of institutions. More importantly, the distance between the levels is not standardized and ranges from 10 to 500 μm. The 2005 ASCO guidelines recommend taking step-sections at 200- to 500-μm intervals into the block.[30] This is recommended to enhance the detection of micrometastasis by allowing evaluation of more of the subcapsular sinus, the location in which micrometastases are most often found.

Role of Immunostains

Immunohistochemical stains are commonly performed to increase the likelihood of detection of micrometastasis. A number of different broad-spectrum or low-molecular-weight cytokeratin (CK) antibodies including AE1/AE3, MNF116, CAM5.2, CK19 have been used for this purpose.[83,84] The routine use of immunohistochemical staining for the assessment of SLNs is not without controversy and is not uniformly recommended by professional organizations. The major reason for the controversy, apart from the increased cost, is that these methods detect scattered ITCs. The significance and practical relevance of these single cells is poorly understood, and in many countries, nodes containing ITCs are considered negative for malignancy (see the discussions on AJCC and other staging systems).

IHC is more commonly performed for evaluation of nodes from a patient with lobular carcinoma. In this regard, it is important to note the recent modification in the AJCC staging system[50] in which "more than 200 nonconfluent or nearly confluent cells in the single histologic cross-section of a lymph node" (such as seen in lobular carcinoma [Figures 7-3 to 7-5]) can be classified as micrometastasis.[50]

Molecular Methods

Molecular methods designed for both intraoperative and paraffin sections have been used to analyze SLNs for the presence of micrometastasis. Intraoperative reverse-transcriptase polymerase chain reaction (RT-PCR) analysis has been performed using commercially available assays such as GeneSearch breast lymph node (BLN)

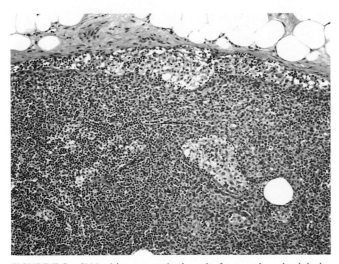

FIGURE 7-3 SLN with metastatic deposits from an invasive lobular carcinoma of breast cancer. Note the diffuse pattern of infiltration.

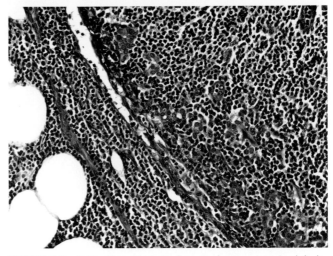

FIGURE 7-5 SLN with metastatic deposits from an invasive lobular carcinoma of breast cancer. Note that reactive endothelial cells can mimic some of the morphologic features of carcinoma.

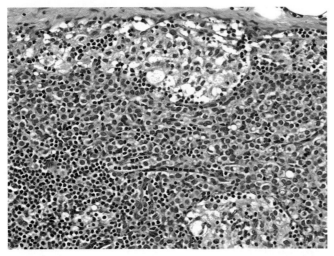

FIGURE 7-4 SLN with metastatic deposits from an invasive lobular carcinoma of breast cancer. The cytologic features of the tumor cells can be difficult to differentiate from lymphocytes even at high magnification.

assay (Veridex) and the one-step nucleic acid assay. These assays involve extracted RNA from part of or the entire lymph node; these processes significantly impede complete histologic analysis of excised SLN and, therefore, are not generally recommended for routine use. These assays have been compared in a number of studies with traditional frozen sections.[85–87] The studies have failed to demonstrate a quantum benefit in terms of time to result or sensitivity when compared with the gold standard (permanent paraffin section). It seems unlikely that any of the current methods of intraoperative molecular assessment will increase the efficacy of breast cancer surgery or lead to net cost saving.[41] The BLN assay is no longer commercially available.

RT-PCR on paraffin blocks has been able to identify epithelial markers in a significant number of lymph nodes with a negative result by both histology and IHC (AJCC, N0(mol+)). This is not surprising given that RT-PCR is capable of identifying single cells. The prognostic or staging significance of such RT-PCR assay results remains unclear (AJCC). It should be noted that the data from the long-term follow-up for a multicenter clinical trial using molecular detection methods have recently been published.[88] In this study, molecular analysis upstaged 13% (52 of 394) node-negative patients. At mean follow-up of 7 years, these patients had a significantly lower distant recurrence-free survival compared with node-negative polymerase chain reaction (PCR) negative patients (80% vs. 91%; $P < .04$). Patients with N0(mol+) disease are 3.4 times more likely to experience relapse than PCR-negative patients (odds ratio 3.4; $P = .001$). However, molecular staging failed to correctly predict most of the N0 patients with recurrences and was not a statistically significant independent predictor of distant recurrence. One of the caveats of this trial was that patients were not randomized and did not receive standardized adjuvant chemotherapy.

AMERICAN JOINT COMMISSION ON CANCER STAGING OF SENTINEL LYMPH NODES

The AJCC staging system[50] recognizes three categories of lymph node involvement: macrometastasis (>2 mm) (Figure 7-6), micrometastasis (Figure 7-7) (<2 mm but > 0.2 mm), and ITC (<0.2 mm).[50] The upper limit of this cutoff is based on the 1971 study by Huvos and coworkers,[89] which showed that the prognosis of patients with tumor deposits smaller than 2 mm was similar to that of node-negative patients. A recent analysis of the Surveillance Epidemiology and End Results (SEER) database revealed that the prognosis of T1 tumors with nodal deposits less than 2 mm (micrometastasis) was associated with only a 1% decrease in survival at 5 and 10 years of follow-up when compared with patients with no nodal disease.[90]

The greater than 0.2 mm criterion is arbitrary but has been tested in one retrospective study of occult metastasis.[91] Using these definitions, a 2-mm metastasis

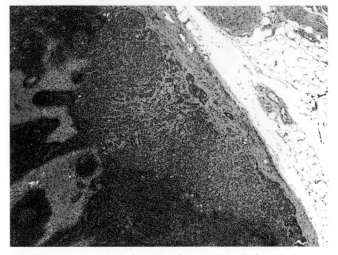

FIGURE 7-6 Lymph node with a large (>2-mm) deposit (macrometastasis) of invasive ductal carcinoma. Note that the tumor involves the subcapsular sinus as well as the nodal parenchyma.

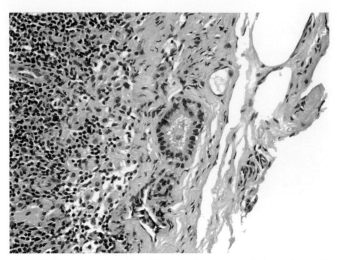

FIGURE 7-8 Lymph node with capsular metastasis from the well-differentiated invasive ductal carcinoma. Note the well-differentiated nature of the tumor; this might raise concerns of epithelial inclusions.

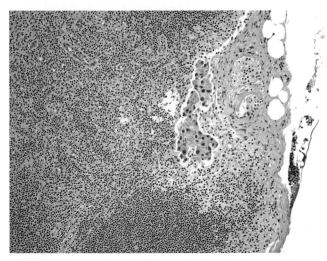

FIGURE 7-7 Lymph node with small (<2-mm) deposits (micrometastasis) of invasive ductal carcinoma. In this case, the tumor predominantly involves the subcapsular sinus with focal involvement of nodal parenchyma.

contains approximately 1 million tumor cells whereas up to a 0.2-mm metastasis contains approximately 1000 tumor cells. It is recognized that the practical applications of the definitions are difficult, particularly for lobular carcinoma. Hence, the current AJCC staging guidelines have provided some additional guidance. When more than 200 nonconfluent or nearly confluent tumor cells are present in a single histologic cross section of the lymph node, there is a high probability that more than 1000 cells are present in the node; the cumulative volume of these cells exceeds the volume of an ITC and the node should be classified as containing a micrometastasis. Cases with borderline or indeterminate findings, such as at the end of the spectrums, are classified into the lower stage category.

Another point that requires clarification pertains to measuring the size of the tumor deposit. When multiple tumor deposits are present in a lymph node with the ITC or micrometastasis, the size of only the largest contiguous tumor deposit is used to classify the node. As in the case of multicentric tumors, the size of different metastatic deposits within the same node is not added up. When a tumor deposit has induced a fibrous (desmoplastic) stromal reaction, the combined contiguous dimension of tumor cells and fibrous tissue determines the size of the metastasis. This is regardless of whether the deposit is confined to the lymph node, extends outside the node (extranodal or extracapsular extension) (Figure 7-8), or is totally present outside the lymph node and invading adipose tissue.

CONTROVERSIAL ISSUES WITH REGARD TO HISTOLOGIC ASSESSMENT

The occurrence of ITCs in the blood has been described as early as 1896.[92] Because the formation of a metastatic deposit is a complex process, only a very small percentage of circulating tumor cells survive to initiate metastasis.[93,94] This raises the issue of how to distinguish isolated (disseminated or circulating) tumor cells from micrometastasis. Hermanek and colleagues[94] defined ITCs as single cells or small clusters that do not show invasion or penetration of a vessel or lymph sinuses (extravasation). These clusters are also not associated with stromal reaction or tumor cell proliferation. This interpretation continues in the International Union Against Cancer (UICC) staging system.[95] In contrast, the AJCC definitions rely entirely on the size of tumor cell clusters. The EWGBSP does not consider lesions purely outside the lymph node (e.g., in afferent lymphatic channels or perinodal fat) as evidence of nodal involvement (Figures 7-9 and 7-10).[96] More importantly, tumor cell clusters, if located within the parenchyma of the lymph node (not in vessels or sinuses), irrespective of their size, are considered as micrometastasis. The size criteria to distinguish ITCs from micrometastasis (0.2 mm and 2 mm, respectively) are used only when tumor cell clusters are identified within vessels and sinuses. EWGBSP

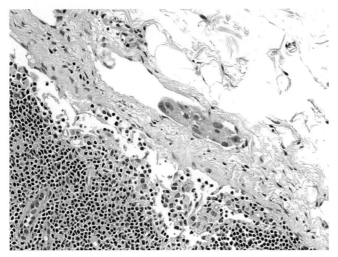

FIGURE 7-9 Micrometastasis or isolated tumor cells? Deposits of invasive ductal carcinoma in capsular afferent sinus of the SLN. Please see discussion with regards to differences in the International Union Against Cancer (UICC) and the American Joint Committee on Cancer (AJCC) staging systems.

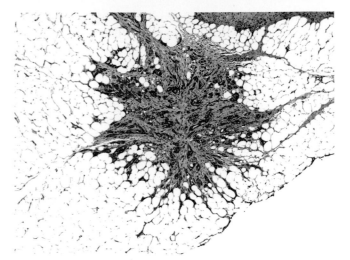

FIGURE 7-11 Ductal carcinoma of the breast involving the adipose tissue in proximity to an SLN.

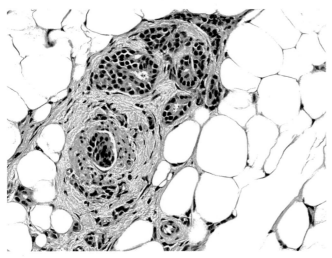

FIGURE 7-10 Micrometastasis or isolated tumor cells? Metastatic ductal carcinoma in the afferent vessel of the sentinel lymph node. Please see discussion with regards to differences in the UICC and the AJCC staging systems.

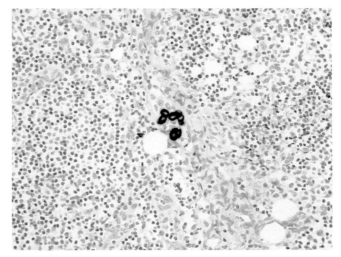

FIGURE 7-12 Isolated tumor cells in the parenchyma of the SLN.

HISTOLOGIC PITFALLS

False-Negative Sentinel Node Biopsy

In addition to the parameters discussed at the beginning of this chapter, one of the principal determinants of the efficacy of SLNB is the experience of the surgeons performing the biopsy, with rates ranging from 65% to 98% according to the surgeon's experience.[98] In review of their experience of the first 500 cases, Cox and colleagues[99] found that one half of their false-negative cases occurred within the first six cases of each surgeon. They also found that, to correctly identify the SLN, surgeons required an average of 23 cases to achieve 90% success and 53 cases to achieve 95% success. The American Society of Breast Surgeons[17,30] recommends that surgeons (1) take a formal course on the technique, with didactic and hands-on training components; (2) have an experienced mentor; (3) keep track of individual results, including the proportion of successful mappings, false-negative rate, and complication rates; and (4) maintain follow-up on all patients over time.

definitions permit cell clusters arranged in a discontinuous manner (separated by more than a distance of a few cells) but dispersed homogeneously (evenly) in the definable part of lymph node to be considered as a single focus for measurement of the size of the tumor cell cluster. These variations in the definition led to 24% discordance in a series of 517 cases reviewed by Cserni and associates.[96] In a comparative study using these two definitions, van Deurzen and coworkers[97] reported that the EWGBSP definition might be better suited for managing high-risk patients. To reiterate, the AJCC definition is based entirely on size of tumor cell clusters (Figures 7-11 and 7-12; see also Figures 7-9 and 7-10) and does not require mitotic activity, stromal reaction, or any other qualifiers. Necrotic and/or nonviable cells, by themselves, are not considered evidence of metastatic disease.

Apart from surgical expertise, variations in the mapping techniques contribute significantly to the efficacy of SLNB.[100] Some workers prefer deep peritumoral injections[101,102]; others prefer subcutaneous injections[12] over the area of the tumor; and still others inject the marker in the region of the areola closest to the tumor.[103] Although the blue dye and the radioisotope techniques are both good, some studies suggest that a combination of the two leads to greater sensitivity for identifying SLNs.[102,104]

The International (Ludwig) Cancer Group[105] retrospectively examined ALNs from 921 patients using deeper sections and IHC and found metastases in 9% of cases. It has also been demonstrated that SLNs are more likely to harbor micrometastases than non-SLNs. Examination of SLNs that were reported as negative by H&E examination detected micrometastases in 15% to 30% of the same cases by IHC.[84,106] Lack of meticulous search for micrometastases in SLNs by using IHC could have contributed significantly to the low negative predictive value in the present study. Even after using IHC, a small percentage of cases are associated with false-negative SLNs; these are attributed to skip metastases. In a multicenter trial conducted by the University of Vermont,[107,108] the incidence of false-negative SLNs even after performing IHC was 1.4% (3 of 214 cases).

Pseudosentinel Node

On rare occasions, an area highlighted in an SLN does not contain any lymphoid tissue. More commonly, the identified node may not be a "true" SLN but may represent altered lymphatic drainage secondary to blockage of the main SLN by metastatic tumor. In order to avoid this possibility, the ASCO guidelines[30] recommend that SLNB should not be performed in cases with clinically positive lymph nodes.

It should also be emphasized that the presence of tumor cells within perinodal lymphatics or adipose tissue should be regarded as evidence of nodal involvement. In the AJCC staging system, this is regarded as nodal involvement. Subjective interpretation of the guidelines can result in misclassification of nodes as ITCs or micrometastasis.[97]

Lastly, tumor cells with unusual morphology can be missed on routine examination. Altered morphology is particularly characteristic after neoadjuvant chemotherapy, where the cells often take on a foamy appearance and can be mistaken for macrophages (Figures 7-13 to 7-17).

False-Positive Sentinel Lymph Nodes

In general, false-positive SLNs are extremely rare. The most common cause of concern is identification of plump endothelial cells (Figure 7-18) on frozen section. The linear distribution of these cells as well as the presence of rare red blood cells provides clues to the identification of these cells. In addition, these cells are located in the cortical region of the lymph node and are rarely, if ever, present in the subcapsular sinuses. They are almost never associated with a stromal reaction. Epithelial inclusions (Figures 7-19 to 7-24) within

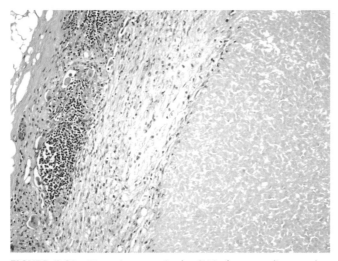

FIGURE 7-13 Necrotic tumor in the SLN after neoadjuvant chemotherapy.

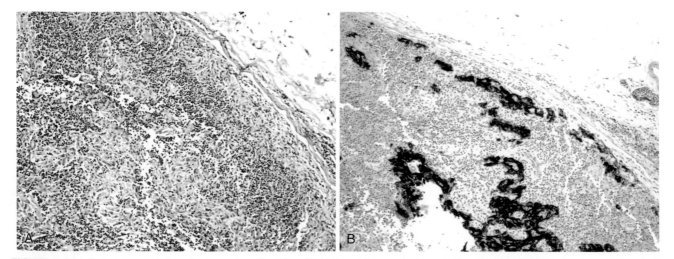

FIGURE 7-14 **A,** Invasive ductal carcinoma in lymph node with histiocytoid morphology. **B,** Keratin immunostain of same tumor as in **A.**

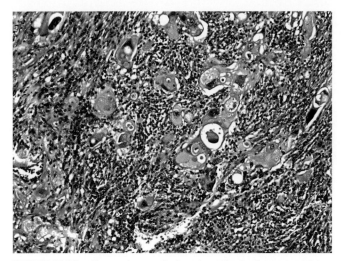

FIGURE 7-15 Chemotherapy-induced cytologic changes and nuclear atypia in metastatic carcinoma.

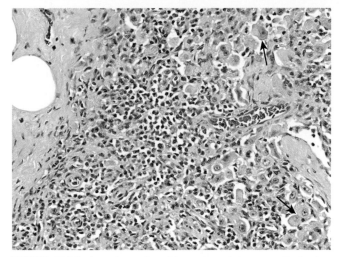

FIGURE 7-16 Lymph node with scattered tumor cells having foamy cytoplasm mimicking macrophages.

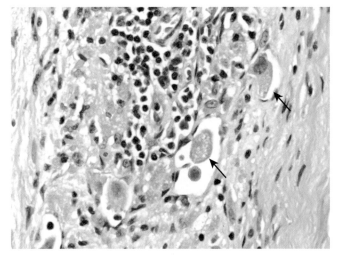

FIGURE 7-17 Lymph node with scattered tumor cells having foamy cytoplasm mimicking macrophages.

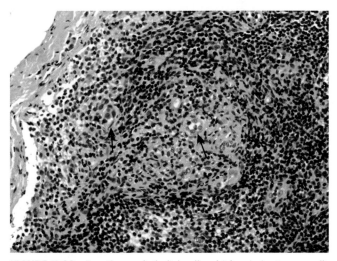

FIGURE 7-18 Reactive endothelial cells which mimics tumor cells of ductal carcinoma.

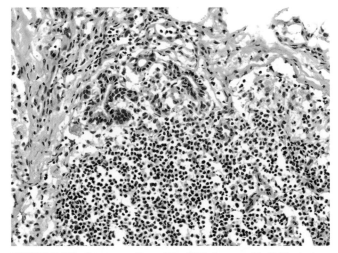

FIGURE 7-19 Frozen section of the SLN shows epithelial inclusion.

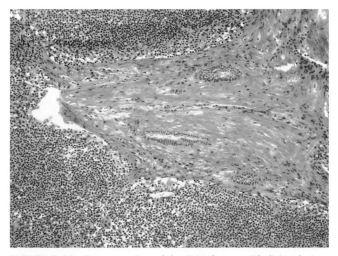

FIGURE 7-20 Frozen section of the SLN shows epithelial inclusion.

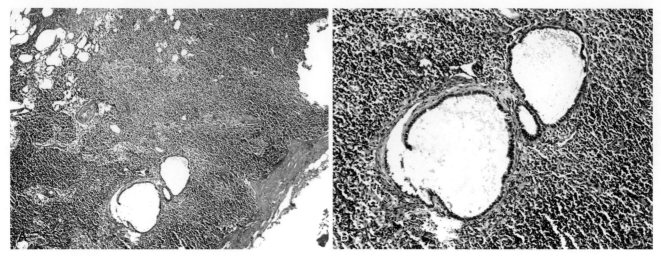

FIGURE 7-21 Frozen section of the SLN shows epithelial inclusion cyst at low **(A)** and high **(B)** magnifications.

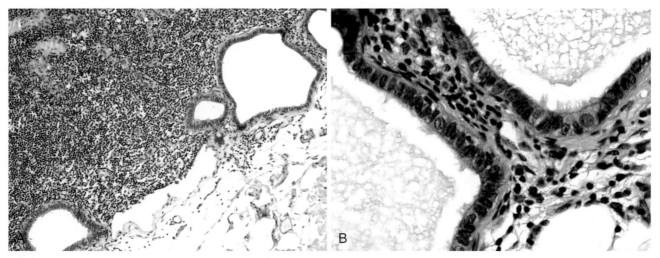

FIGURE 7-22 **A,** Cystic epithelial inclusion in a lymph node. **B,** Note the presence of cilia in the image taken at high magnification.

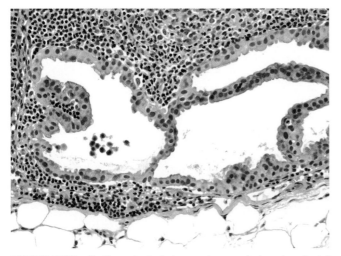

FIGURE 7-23 Cystic metastasis from a low-grade invasive ductal carcinoma mimicking epithelial inclusion.

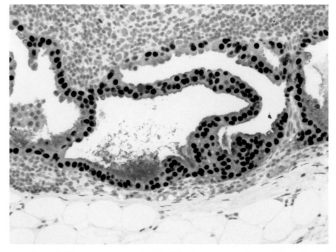

FIGURE 7-24 Cystic metastatic from a low-grade invasive ductal carcinoma mimicking epithelial inclusion. Note the strong ER expression within the tumor cells. Stain for p63 did not identify myoepithelial cells.

the lymph node are rare but well described.[109–114] These are commonly cystic and not dissimilar to those seen in the pelvic lymph nodes. Even more rarely, they can take a papillary architecture and can be confused with a well-differentiated carcinoma. The comparison of the morphology of these inclusions with the primary tumor offers a simple way to validate the interpretation. In the rare cases, molecular markers such as ER, p53, and p63 may be employed to aid the distinction. Much more common than epithelial inclusions are nests of nevus cells (Figures 7-25 and 7-26), typically located in the capsule of the lymph node. The nevus cells may contain melanin; however, it is not always apparent on an H&E and is sometimes better seen on the negative control of the CK immunostain. Once the possibility of nevus is raised, diagnosis is seldom a problem; however, in difficult cases, IHC stains for keratins and melanoma markers such as S100 may be used for confirmation.

The use of IHC has resulted in misinterpretation in some cases. Artifacts due to staining of mast cells (Figure 7-27) or blobs of DAB (3,3'-diaminobenzidine) have been misinterpreted as evidence of nodal positivity. These are typically not in the same plane and lack cellular outlines. Keratin expression in macrophages (Figure 7-28) (due to phagocytosed debris) or dendritic cells (Figure 7-29) can be a cause of false positivity. The interstitial distribution of the cells and the presence of dendritic processes provide clues to the correct diagnosis. The presence of necrotic debris is a much more common cause of overinterpretation of IHC. Nonviable cells should not be considered as evidence of nodal metastasis.

Benign Transport

Diagnostic procedures such as needle core biopsies have been shown to cause seeding of tumor cells in the needle track. Similar processes could lead to displacement of tumor cells from the tumor bed and enter into lymphatic channels (Figure 7-30). In some cases, this could lead to detection of tumor cells within the sinusoids of the SLN. Early reports by Youngson and associates[115,116] were confirmed by Carter and coworkers,[117] who

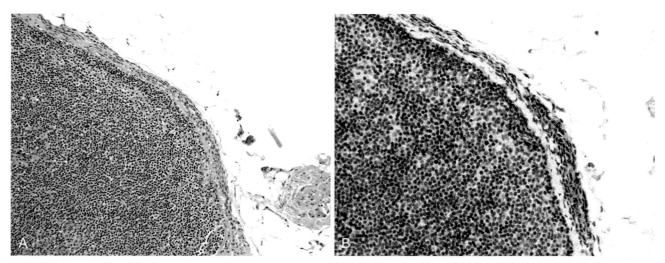

FIGURE 7-25   A, SLN of the breast cancer with capsular nevus. **B,** Note these nevus cells are highlighted by immunostain with melan A.

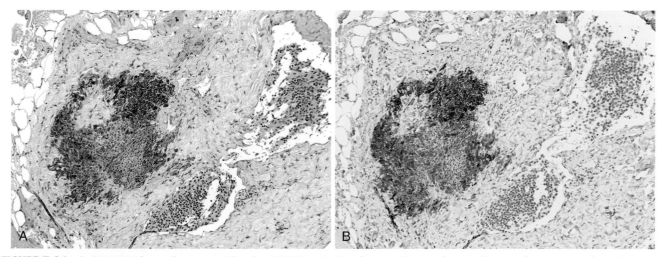

FIGURE 7-26   A, Pigmented capsular nevus within the SLN. **B,** Note that the prominent melanin in the capsular nevus can be mistaken for cytokeratin expression on immunostain.

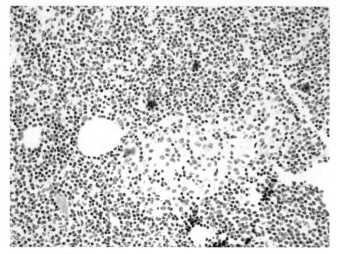

FIGURE 7-27 Reactivity within a mast cell can be falsely interpreted as metastasis.

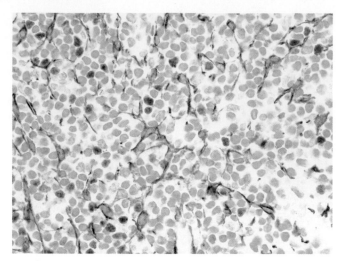

FIGURE 7-29 Cytokeratin (cell adhesion molecule [CAM] 5.2) staining of the lymph node highlighting interdigitating dendritic cells.

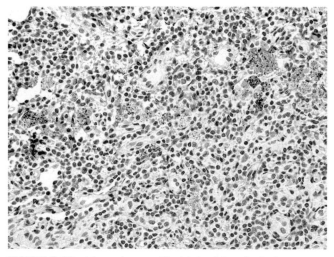

FIGURE 7-28 Macrophages with debris giving rise to immunoreactivity with cytokeratin.

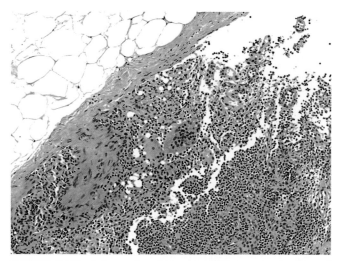

FIGURE 7-30 Subcapsular sinus containing macrophages and giant cells. These can be associated with scattered keratin-positive cells.

introduced the term "benign transport." Bleiweiss and colleagues[118,119] have further documented iatrogenic displacement and transport of benign cells, usually originating from a papilloma, within the sinuses of SLNs. The morphology of these cells was shown to be clearly distinct from those of the tumor cells. This highlights an important caveat in the interpretation of IHC stains of SLNs. These cases should be carefully evaluated before a diagnosis of benign transport is made.

PREDICTORS OF NONSENTINEL LYMPH NODE INVOLVEMENT

A recent review of 97,000 patients in the National Cancer Database[120] indicates that ALND is not routinely necessary in all patients with involved SLNs. A randomized clinical trial[121] has shown that patients with negative SLNs had the same outcomes at 10 years whether or not they underwent ALND. Thus, patients having SLNB may or may not undergo

conventional ALND. The presence of SLN involvement is the strongest predictor of non-SLN involvement. Non-SLN metastasis is detected in 30% to 50% of patients with positive SLNs.[25,122] It is important to identify parameters within the SLN that might be used to predict the presence of additional lymph node involvement. Numerous studies have identified several individual parameters that are important. These include (1) patient age; (2) tumor parameters such as type, size, grade, presence of lymphatic invasion, and hormone receptor status; and (3) lymph node parameters such as number of involved lymph nodes, size of the metastatic deposit, and extracapsular spread. The number of positive SLNs has been consistently associated with non-SLN involvement, even in clinical trials.[123] In order to synthesize the information obtained from individual predictors, nomograms based on composite analysis of these parameters have been developed and validated; these are detailed later.

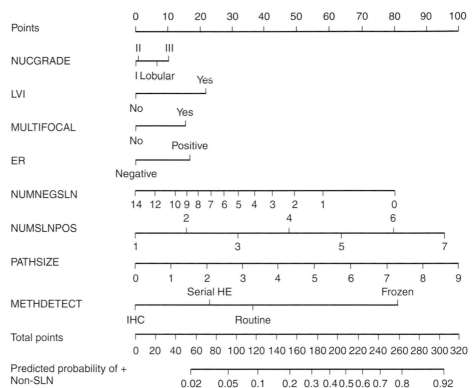

FIGURE 7-31 MSKCC nomogram predictors of non-SLN positivity. ER, estrogen receptor; HE, hematoxylin/eosin; IHC, immunohistochemistry; LVI, lymphovascular invasion; NUMNEGSLN, number of negative sentinel lymph nodes; NUMSLNPOS, number of positive sentinel lymph nodes. PATHSIZE, pathologic size.

Memorial Sloan-Kettering Cancer Center Nomogram (Figure 7-31)

In 2003, Van Zee and associates[124] from MSKCC (http://www.mskcc.org/mskcc/html/15938.cfm) published the first nomogram. They used multivariate logistic regression to identify parameters associated with non-SLN involvement in a series of 702 patients treated at MSKCC. The following parameters are included: pathologic tumor size, tumor type, nuclear grade, lymphovascular invasion (LVI), multifocality, ER status, method of detection of the positive SLN, and the number of metastatic and nonmetastatic SLNs. They obtained a "good" AUC for prediction of non-SLN metastasis. The method was demonstrated to be reliable and practical.

The MSKCC nomogram does not take into account factors such as patient age, size of SLN metastasis, and the presence of extracapsular extension. In spite of these limitations, the MSKCC nomogram is the most commonly used and validated nomogram for the prediction of non-SLN involvement.

Tenon Nomogram

In 2005, Barranger and coworkers[125] found that the SLN was the only positive node in 52 of 71 patients (73.2%) who underwent ALND. The risk of having non-SLN positivity was 0% in patients with pT1a/b tumors, 17% in pT1c tumors, and 67% in tumors larger than 20 mm. A significant correlation was observed between positive non-SLNs and tumor size, tumor histology, macrometastasis, number of SLNs involved, the proportion of involved SLNs, and the size of SLN metastasis. On the basis of these parameters, an axillary scoring system

based on three variables was developed: the ratio of positive SLNs to the number of nodes removed, the presence of macrometastasis, and the histologic primary tumor size. Using this scoring system, a score of less than 3.5 indicated a probability of non-SLN negativity to be 97.3%. In the Barranger and coworkers' study,[125] size of SLN metastasis was a strong predictor of non-SLN involvement; 14% of patients with SLN micrometastasis had non-SLN metastasis compared with 40% with macrometastasis.

The limitations of the Tenon nomogram include the relatively low AUC obtained in the validation studies. It also does not take into account the presence of lymphovascular invasion and extracapsular extension.

The Cambridge Model

Pal and colleagues[126] described a formula that included three factors: tumor grade, overall metastatic tumor size, and the proportion of involved SLNs to uninvolved lymph nodes. The AUC with the Cambridge model was 0.84, suggesting it as a superior discriminating power when compared with the MSKCC nomogram; in their study, it had a value of 0.69.

The limitations of this model include the fact that it does not take into account the size of the primary tumor or tumor type.

The Stanford Online Calculator

Kohrt and associates[127] evaluated 13 parameters for correction of non-SLNs and found that three of these (tumor size, lymphovascular invasion, and size of metastasis) were significant in multivariate analysis. An online calculator was developed using these parameters. The overall diagnostic accuracy for prediction of non-SLN involvement was found to be 77%.

M.D. Anderson Nomogram

In 2008, Jeruss and coworkers[128] identified 18 parameters that could affect the rate of non-SLN involvement in women who had positive SLNs after neoadjuvant chemotherapy. Five of these factors that were significant on multivariate analysis were used to develop the nomogram. These factors are pathologic tumor size, initial lymph node status, multicentricity, method of detection, and lymphovascular invasion. The data were validated in an independent cohort from the University of Michigan.

Others

A number of other nomograms have been described in the literature but they have not been widely used. Hwang and colleagues[129] developed a model based on the retrospective analysis of 131 patients, whereas the Saidi and associates' score[130] is based on the analysis of 116 patients. Degnim and coworkers[131] developed a new model from the analysis of 574 patients and found it to be better than the MSKCC nomogram. Viale and colleagues[132] developed a model based on the analysis of 1228 patients but found that even the patients with the best predictive features still had up to a 13% risk of non-SLN involvement. Houvenaeghel and associates,[133] based on the analysis of 909 patients with micrometastasis and ALND, developed a micrometastasis nomogram to predict non-SLN involvement. In a similar study, Kumar and coworkers[134] examined the MSKCC experience of micrometastasis in SLNs and found that different methods of assessment did not make a significant difference.

A nomogram for the prediction of involvement of more than four non-SLN has also been reported.[135]

Limitations of Nomograms

Although a number of nomograms are available, their success in prediction of non-SLN involvement is variable and institution dependent (Table 7-1).[136–147a] This is, in part, due to variations in institutional practices with regard to methods used for identifying SLNs, use of intraoperative frozen sections, and methods used for analysis and reporting. The subjectivity in reporting of the parameters used such as tumor grade and angiolymphatic invasion is well documented. The accuracy of the predictions made by a nomogram may depend on the number of cases with micrometastasis in the series.[138,148,149] The AUC results were obtained and ranged from 0.58 to 0.86 in these studies, with studies having more than 200 patients showing an AUC value of approximately 0.72. The predictive value of nomograms is affected by neoadjuvant chemotherapy.[142] Another important issue is at what cutoff point is ALND omitted. Poirier and colleagues[150] indicate that a value of less than 10% could be used as a cutoff point. In summary, nomograms are less than perfect and their use does not replace detailed discussion of the risks and benefits of ALND.[17]

CRITICAL ISSUES

Advantages and Disadvantages of a Sentinel Lymph Node Assessment

ALND is the best predictor of survival for patients with invasive breast cancer; as the number of lymph node metastases increases, survival decreases.[5,6] The

TABLE 7-1	Studies Evaluating Nomograms for the Prediction of Nonsentinel Lymph Node Metastases							
			AUC Value					
Author	Year	No. of Patients	MSKCC	Tenon	Cambridge	Stanford	Mayo	Degnim
Van Zee et al[124]	2003	373	0.78					
Smidt et al[144]	2005	222	0.77					
Degnim et al[131]	2005	462	0.72					0.77
Lambert et al[145]	2006	200	0.71					
Alran et al[148]	2007	588	0.724					
Bevilacqua et al[59]	2007	1545	0.75					
Zgajnar et al[146]	2007	276	0.72					
*Evrensel et al[147]	2008	233	0.73					
Coutant et al[149]	2009	561	0.78	0.81	0.73	0.72	0.74	
Poirier et al[150]	2008	209	0.687					
Scow et al[147a]	2009	464	0.74			0.72	0.77	
Gur et al[136]	2009	607	0.7006	0.5825	0.711	0.7306		

*Patients received neoadjuvant chemotherapy.
AUC, area under the curve; MSKCC, Memorial Sloan-Kettering Cancer Center.

predictive value of ALND increases with the thoroughness of the procedure. A total ALND consists of removal of all the nodes in the axilla (i.e., removal of levels I, II, and III nodes). Anything less than total ALND is associated with some staging inaccuracy.[100] When compared with total ALND, dissection of only level I nodes results in a staging error rate of 2% to 3% and blind (nonanatomic) sampling has an error rate of 14% to 45%.[151] Total ALND is seldom performed nowadays because it is associated with a marked increase in postoperative morbidity and complications. SLNB is an alternative procedure for staging the axilla. It is associated with a significant risk of morbidity and complications such as long-term lymphedema, shoulder stiffness, pain, and parasthesia.[17,152–156]

Trojani and associates[157,158] examined the lymph nodes of 150 patients with node-negative breast cancers with serial sectioning and IHC. Microscopic foci of metastasis were identified in 14% of patients. Conversion rates ranging from 10% to 50% have been reported when the protocol for histologic assessment of lymph node changed from a single section to multiple levels and use of IHC stains.[100,159–161] These studies highlight the upstaging patients by using more detailed analyses of the SLN. The clinical impact of finding micrometastasis (<2 mm) is as yet not very clear. An analysis of the SEER database showed that micrometastasis was associated with a decreased overall survival at 10 years of 1%, 6%, and 2% for T1, T2, and T3 tumors, respectively, compared with patients with no nodal metastasis.[90] In contrast, Millis and coworkers[162] and Nasser and colleagues[91] reexamined additional sections from lymph nodes of 447 and 159 patients, respectively, 10 years after primary surgery and did not find a prognostic impact for micrometastasis. More recently, Andersson and associates[163] performed a prospective analysis of 3369 patients with breast cancer and demonstrated a worse prognosis for patients with micrometastasis than for patients with node-negative disease.

The National Surgical Adjuvant Breast and Bowel Project (NSABP) B04 study has shown that complete ALND results in better outcomes than radiotherapy to the axilla.[3,164] The purpose of intraoperative evaluation is to decrease the need for a second procedure to perform ALND. Intraoperative assessment using either imprint cytology or frozen section techniques requires significant amounts of resources that may not be available at all sites. Intraoperative assessment, particularly of fatty lymph nodes, can lead to false negativity. Fritzsche and coworkers[75] reported a comparative analysis of the incidence of SLN positivity in patients with and without intraoperative assessment. They found the incidence of nodal positivity significantly lower in patients undergoing intraoperative assessment using frozen sections; suggesting that, owing to loss of tissue during the frozen section procedure, this could contribute to false-negative assessment of the SLN. In most centers today, even a single focus of tumor identified at frozen section results in completion ALND. In a majority of these cases, particularly for women with T1 tumors, these additional ALNs are negative for tumor. This, in some opinions, results in unnecessary ALND and mitigating advantages of SLNB. Questions are being raised as to whether intraoperative assessment of SLN could be safely avoided in a subgroup of patients.[41]

The major advantage of intraoperative SLNB assessment is that it prevents a second surgical procedure, which increases the hospital stay.[165] The recall rates for completion ALND have been shown to be approximately 10%.[41] It should be noted that patients who have positive margins (at the primary tumor site) do not receive significant benefit from intraoperative assessment of SLNs. Interestingly, preliminary results of the After Mapping of the Axilla: Radiotherapy or Surgery? (AMAROS) trial suggest radiotherapy could be a substitute for completion ALND in patients with low-volume nodal disease.[166,167] The combined analysis of Z10 and Z11 trials (see later) suggests morbidity.[168] With respect to staging and complications, there was no clear detriment for patients with positive SLN who underwent a second procedure for completion ALND.

It is still controversial as to whether patients with positive SLNs require complete ALND. Depending on institutional practices, these patients may or may not undergo further ALND.

Number of Sentinel Lymph Nodes to Be Removed

The number of SLNs biopsied varies significantly in different studies. It is recommended that surgeons intraoperatively excise all nodes with radioactive counts more than 10% of the "hottest" node.[169,170] Wong and colleagues[171] analyzed the impact of removal of multiple SLNs as opposed to a single SLNB. In their study of 146 patients, the false-negative rate was 14.3% when a single SLN was removed. This is compared with 4.3% when multiple nodes were removed. Zervos and associates[172] showed that removal of the first two lymph nodes identified axillary status in 98% of cases. In another study, 98% accuracy was obtained by removal of three lymph nodes.[173] However, in 4% of cases in this study, a positive SLN was detected in four to eight additional sites. In a study involving 3882 patients undergoing SLNB, these guidelines resulted in a number of nodes removed, ranging from 1 to 18. Although it must be noted that more than four nodes were removed in less than 10% of cases and surgeons with lesser experience removed more nodes.[174] The number of nodes removed was inversely related to the experience of the surgeons. A number of studies have shown that removal of more than four SLNs may be superfluous and does not improve the accuracy.[58,172,173,175,176] However, some studies have shown that 1.5% to 10.3% of metastases were detected after the fourth node.[171,174,177,178] Dabbs and Johnson,[179] in a study of 662 patients, found that, in all the patients where the first sign of metastasis was in a fourth or higher lymph node, the micrometastasis was found by IHC alone. Although it is controversial as to how many lymph nodes are sufficient for accurate staging of the axilla,[58,173,175,178] some have proposed that the procedure should be terminated after the identification of three nodes.[176] Some authors state that there is no upper limit for the number of central lymph nodes that are at risk for metastasis and that all "blue and hot" lymph nodes should be removed.[173,177] This recommendation should be tempered with the increased risk of complications, such as lymphedema, that the patients can develop.

Extranodal Invasion

The presence of tumor outside the lymph node is a prognostic parameter in breast cancer.[180,181] It has also been shown to be associated with increased likelihood of non-SLN involvement.[181–185] Extranodal invasion is often further classified into minimal (if < 1 mm beyond the capsule) or prominent (if > 1 mm). Documentation of extranodal fat involvement is easier on the capsular surface of the lymph node but is often difficult in the hilar region. Prominent extranodal invasion is often used by radiation oncologists to guide therapy, although there is no hard evidence that this makes a difference to the outcomes.[180]

Sentinel Lymph Node Positivity and Plastic Reconstruction

The presence of metastatic deposits in more than three ALNs is often used as an indication for radiotherapy. If more than one SLN is positive intraoperatively, the surgical team may reconsider whether to perform a one-stage reconstruction of the breast because radiation therapy significantly affects the cosmetic results. In such situations, reconstruction is performed after completion of radiation therapy.

Sentinel Node Biopsy in Major Clinical Trials

MILAN TRIAL

Veronesi and coworkers[121] randomized 516 patients with less than 2 cm tumors to receive either SLNB plus axillary dissection (AD arm) or SLNB and ALND only if the SLN is positive (SN arm). There were 23 breast cancer-related events in the SN arm and 26 in the AD arm. The overall survival at 10 years of follow-up was slightly (but not significantly) greater in the SN arm. They concluded that ALND should not be performed in breast cancer patients without first examining the SLN.

AXILLARY LYMPHATIC MAPPING AGAINST NODAL AXILLARY CLEARANCE (ALMANAC) TRIAL

Mansel and colleagues[186] conducted a multicenter randomized trial to compare quality of life outcomes between patients with clinically node-negative invasive breast cancer who received SLNB and patients who received standard axillary treatment. From November 1999 to October 2003, 1031 patients were randomly assigned to undergo SLNB (n = 515) or standard axillary surgery (n = 516). Patients with SLN metastases

proceeded to delayed axillary clearance or received axillary radiotherapy (depending on the protocol at the treating institution). The relative risks of any lymphedema and sensory loss for the SLNB group compared with the standard axillary treatment group at 12 months was significantly lower in the SLNB group (absolute rates: 11% vs. 31%). The overall patient-recorded quality of life and arm functioning scores were statistically significantly better in the SLNB group throughout. These benefits were seen with no increase in anxiety levels in the SLNB group ($P > .05$).

NATIONAL SURGICAL ADJUVANT BREAST AND BOWEL PROJECT B 32

The NSABP B 32 (Figure 7-32) randomized clinical trial investigated the role of axilla resection after SLN resection in patients with clinically node-negative breast cancer.[187–189] A total of 5611 women with clinically negative ALNs underwent SLNB. Patients with positive SLNs underwent full ALN whereas patients with negative SLNs were randomized to receiving either no further surgery (n = 2011) or ALND (n = 1975). After an average follow-up of 95 months, there was no difference in overall survival or disease-free survival in women who received ALND versus those who did not.[187] Rates for local and regional recurrence were similar in both groups; however, in patients receiving full ALND, there was significantly more arm morbidity including more deficits in shoulder abduction, arm swelling, arm numbness, and arm tingling compared with patients not having ALND.[190] This study is seen as a validation of the common practice of not completing ALND in women with low-risk early breast cancer.

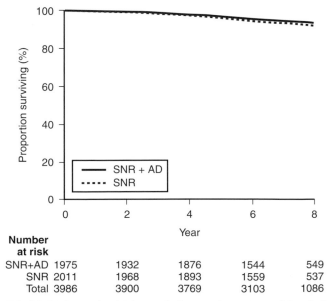

Number at risk					
SNR+AD	1975	1932	1876	1544	549
SNR	2011	1968	1893	1559	537
Total	3986	3900	3769	3103	1086

FIGURE 7-32 Kaplan-Meier survival curves from National Surgical Adjuvant Breast and Bowel Project (NSABP-32) clinical trial. AD, axillary dissection; SNR, sentinel node resection. *From Krag DN, Anderson SJ, Julian TB, et al. Sentinel-lymph-node resection compared with conventional axillary-lymph-node dissection in clinically node-negative patients with breast cancer: overall survival findings from the NSABP B-32 randomised phase 3 trial. Lancet Oncol 2010;11:927-933.*

AMERICAN COLLEGE OF SURGEONS ONCOLOGY GROUP Z0010 TRIAL

The American College of Surgeons Oncology Group (ACOSOG) Z0010 trial evaluated the prognostic significance of metastasis detected in bone marrow by IHC and in SLNs detected by H&E stain.[191] The study enrolled 5210 patients with stage I or II disease and clinically negative axilla. Patients underwent breast conservation surgery with SLN dissection and iliac crest bone marrow aspiration. If the SLN was negative by traditional H&E, it was then centrally assessed for micrometastasis with IHC. Overall, SLNs were positive in 24% of patients. Another 10% of patients had lymph nodes that were negative by H&E but were found to be positive by IHC. In multivariate analysis, there was no difference in outcomes (local recurrence, distant recurrence, disease-free survival, or overall survival) in patients who tested negative by both (H&E and IHC) stains or were positive by IHC. Thus, micrometastasis detected in SLN by IHC did not correlate with survival. In addition, there was no correlation within micrometastasis in SLN and micrometastasis in bone marrow. This study calls in question the practice of routinely performing IHC stains for all SLNs.

AMERICAN COLLEGE OF SURGEONS ONCOLOGY GROUP Z0011 TRIAL

The ACOSOG Z0011 was a prospect of a randomized trial comparing ALN resection versus no further surgery in women with SLN-positive early breast cancer. The trial enrolled approximately 900 patients and did not show significant differences in the two arms with respect to overall survival, disease-free survival, or locoregional recurrence. This trial, because of logistic issues, was underpowered to detect a survival difference and the data need to be interpreted with care in part because patients received traditional tangent radiation. It showed that omitting ALND after the identification of positive SLNs resulted in residual axillary disease in 27% of patients, but the risk of axillary recurrence was less than 1% and there was no effect on survival.[192] The decision to omit complete ALND should arise from a balanced discussion between the surgeon and the patient.[17]

THE AFTER MAPPING OF THE AXILLA: RADIOTHERAPY OR SURGERY? TRIAL

The randomized EORTC 10981-22023 AMAROS trial is investigating whether breast cancer patients with a tumor-positive SLNB are best treated with an ALND or axillary radiotherapy (ART). The trial will enroll 4767 patients and is currently ongoing. Interim analysis of the first 2000 patients showed that the SLN identification rate was 97%.[167] The SLNB results of 65% of the patients ($n = 1220$) were negative and the patients underwent no further axillary treatment. The SLNB results were positive in 34% of the patients ($n = 647$), including macrometastases ($n = 409$, 63%), micrometastases ($n = 161$, 25%), and ITCs ($n = 77$, 12%). The rates of nodal involvement in patients undergoing an ALND for SLN macrometastases was 41% but was similar (18%) for patients with SLN micrometastases or ITCs. The interim analysis also showed that the absence of knowledge regarding the extent of nodal involvement in the ART arm did not appear to have a major impact on the administration of adjuvant therapy.[166]

SUMMARY

The examination of ALNs is a vitally important aspect of breast pathology. The preponderance of evidence indicates that the SLN is key to properly staging breast cancer patients. Optimal protocol for SLN examination includes sectioning along the short axis at 2-mm intervals to maximize the area of lymph node examined. The current AJCC guidelines for SLN examination, although sometimes controversial, are in a state of chronic change based on our knowledge of tumor biology.

REFERENCES

1. Kerlikowske K, Grady D, Rubin SM, et al. Efficacy of screening mammography. A meta-analysis. JAMA 1995;273:149-154.
2. Tabar L, Fagerberg G, Day NE, et al. Breast cancer treatment and natural history: new insights from results of screening. Lancet 1992;339:412-414.
3. Fisher B. Biological and clinical considerations regarding the use of surgery and chemotherapy in the treatment of primary breast cancer. Cancer 1977;40(1 Suppl):574-587.
4. Hortobagyi GN. Treatment of breast cancer. N Engl J Med 1998;339:974-984.
5. Moore MP, Kinne DW. Axillary lymphadenectomy: a diagnostic and therapeutic procedure. J Surg Oncol 1997;66:2-6.
6. Wilking N, Rutqvist LE, Carstensen J, et al. Prognostic significance of axillary nodal status in primary breast cancer in relation to the number of resected nodes. Stockholm Breast Cancer Study Group. Acta Oncol 1992;31:29-35.
7. Cabanas RM. An approach for the treatment of penile carcinoma. Cancer 1977;39:456-466.
8. Morton DL, Wen DR, Wong JH, et al. Technical details of intraoperative lymphatic mapping for early stage melanoma. Arch Surg 1992;127:392-399.
9. Alex JC, Krag DN. Gamma-probe guided localization of lymph nodes. Surg Oncol 1993;2:137-143.
10. Kett K, Varga G, Lukacs L. Direct lymphography of the breast. Lymphology 1970;3:2-12.
11. Giuliano AE, Kirgan DM, Guenther JM, Morton DL. Lymphatic mapping and sentinel lymphadenectomy for breast cancer. Ann Surg 1994;220:391-398; discussion 398-401.
12. Veronesi U, Paganelli G, Galimberti V, et al. Sentinel-node biopsy to avoid axillary dissection in breast cancer with clinically negative lymph-nodes. Lancet 1997;349:1864-1867.
13. Albertini JJ, Lyman GH, Cox C, et al. Lymphatic mapping and sentinel node biopsy in the patient with breast cancer. JAMA 1996;276:1818-1822.
14. Giuliano AE, Jones RC, Brennan M, Statman R. Sentinel lymphadenectomy in breast cancer. J Clin Oncol 1997;15:2345-2350.
15. Krag DN, Weaver DL, Alex JC, Fairbank JT. Surgical resection and radiolocalization of the sentinel lymph node in breast cancer using a gamma probe. Surg Oncol 1993;2:335-339; discussion 340.
16. The American Society of Breast Surgeons. Quality measures for sentinel node biopsy in breast cancer. 2010 [12/29/2010]. Available at http://breastsurgeons.org/statements/QM/Sentinel_Lymph_Node_Biopsy_For_Breast_Cancer11042010.pdf.
17. The American Society of Breast Surgeons. Guidelines for performing sentinel lymph node biopsy in breast cancer. 2010 [12/29/2010]. Available at http://breastsurgeons.org/statements/2010-Nov-05_Guidelines_on_Performing_SLN.pdf.
18. Krag DN, Anderson SJ, Julian TB, et al. Technical outcomes of sentinel-lymph-node resection and conventional axillary-lymph-node dissection in patients with clinically node-negative breast cancer: results from the NSABP B-32 randomised phase III trial. Lancet Oncol 2007;8:881-888.

19. McMahon LE, Gray RJ, Pockaj BA. Is breast cancer sentinel lymph node mapping valuable for patients in their seventies and beyond? Am J Surg 2005;190:366-370.

20. Posther KE, McCall LM, Blumencranz PW, et al. Sentinel node skills verification and surgeon performance: data from a multicenter clinical trial for early-stage breast cancer. Ann Surg 2005;242:593-599; discussion 599-602.

21. Cox CE, Dupont E, Whitehead GF, et al. Age and body mass index may increase the chance of failure in sentinel lymph node biopsy for women with breast cancer. Breast J 2002;8:88-91.

22. Cody HS 3rd, Fey J, Akhurst T, et al. Complementarity of blue dye and isotope in sentinel node localization for breast cancer: univariate and multivariate analysis of 966 procedures. Ann Surg Oncol 2001;8:13-19.

23. Motomura K, Inaji H, Komoike Y, et al. Combination technique is superior to dye alone in identification of the sentinel node in breast cancer patients. J Surg Oncol 2001;76:95-99.

24. DiFronzo LA, Hansen NM, Stern SL, et al. Does sentinel lymphadenectomy improve staging and alter therapy in elderly women with breast cancer? Ann Surg Oncol 2000;7:406-410.

25. Turner RR, Chu KU, Qi K, et al. Pathologic features associated with nonsentinel lymph node metastases in patients with metastatic breast carcinoma in a sentinel lymph node. Cancer 2000;89:574-581.

26. Gentilini O, Chagas E, Zurrida S, et al. Sentinel lymph node biopsy in male patients with early breast cancer. Oncologist 2007;12:512-515.

27. Rusby JE, Smith BL, Dominguez FJ, Golshan M. Sentinel lymph node biopsy in men with breast cancer: a report of 31 consecutive procedures and review of the literature. Clin Breast Cancer 2006;7:406-410.

28. Boughey JC, Bedrosian I, Meric-Bernstam F, et al. Comparative analysis of sentinel lymph node operation in male and female breast cancer patients. J Am Coll Surg 2006;203:475-480.

29. Pandit-Taskar N, Dauer LT, Montgomery L, et al. Organ and fetal absorbed dose estimates from 99mTc-sulfur colloid lymphoscintigraphy and sentinel node localization in breast cancer patients. J Nucl Med 2006;47:1202-1208.

30. Lyman GH, Giuliano AE, Somerfield MR, et al. American Society of Clinical Oncology guideline recommendations for sentinel lymph node biopsy in early-stage breast cancer. J Clin Oncol 2005;23:7703-7720.

31. Gentilini O, Cremonesi M, Toesca A, et al. Sentinel lymph node biopsy in pregnant patients with breast cancer. Eur J Nucl Med Mol Imaging 2010;37:78-83.

32. Yararbas U, Argon AM, Yeniay L, Kapkac M. Problematic aspects of sentinel lymph node biopsy and its relation to previous excisional biopsy in breast cancer. Clin Nucl Med 2009;34:854-858.

33. Port ER, Fey J, Gemignani ML, et al. Reoperative sentinel lymph node biopsy: a new option for patients with primary or locally recurrent breast carcinoma. J Am Coll Surg 2002;195:167-172.

34. Port ER, Garcia-Etienne CA, Park J, et al. Reoperative sentinel lymph node biopsy: a new frontier in the management of ipsilateral breast tumor recurrence. Ann Surg Oncol 2007;14:2209-2214.

35. Dupont EL, Salud CJ, Peltz ES, et al. Clinical relevance of internal mammary node mapping as a guide to radiation therapy. Am J Surg 2001;182:321-324.

36. Klauber-DeMore N, Bevilacqua JL, Van Zee KJ, et al. Comprehensive review of the management of internal mammary lymph node metastases in breast cancer. J Am Coll Surg 2001;193:547-555.

37. Veronesi U, Marubini E, Mariani L, et al. The dissection of internal mammary nodes does not improve the survival of breast cancer patients. 30-year results of a randomised trial. Eur J Cancer 1999;35:1320-1325.

38. Mansel RE, Goyal A, Newcombe RG. Internal mammary node drainage and its role in sentinel lymph node biopsy: the initial ALMANAC experience. Clin Breast Cancer 2004;5:279-284; discussion 285-286.

39. Fisher B, Wolmark N, Bauer M, et al. The accuracy of clinical nodal staging and of limited axillary dissection as a determinant of histologic nodal status in carcinoma of the breast. Surg Gynecol Obstet 1981;152:765-772.

40. Britton PD, Goud A, Godward S, et al. Use of ultrasound-guided axillary node core biopsy in staging of early breast cancer. Eur Radiol 2009;19:561-569.

41. Benson JR, Wishart GC. Is intra-operative nodal assessment essential in a modern breast practice? Eur J Surg Oncol 2010;36:1162-1164.

42. Gimbergues P, Abrial C, Durando X, et al. Sentinel lymph node biopsy after neoadjuvant chemotherapy is accurate in breast cancer patients with a clinically negative axillary nodal status at presentation. Ann Surg Oncol 2008;15:1316-1321.

43. Lee S, Kim EY, Kang SH, et al. Sentinel node identification rate, but not accuracy, is significantly decreased after pre-operative chemotherapy in axillary node-positive breast cancer patients. Breast Cancer Res Treat 2007;102:283-288.

44. Mamounas EP, Brown A, Anderson S, et al. Sentinel node biopsy after neoadjuvant chemotherapy in breast cancer: results from National Surgical Adjuvant Breast and Bowel Project Protocol B-27. J Clin Oncol 2005;23:2694-2702.

45. Schwartz GF, Tannebaum JE, Jernigan AM, Palazzo JP. Axillary sentinel lymph node biopsy after neoadjuvant chemotherapy for carcinoma of the breast. Cancer 2010;116:1243-1251.

46. Dupont EL, Kuhn MA, McCann C, et al. The role of sentinel lymph node biopsy in women undergoing prophylactic mastectomy. Am J Surg 2000;180:274-277.

47. Cox CE, White L, Stowell N, et al. Clinical considerations in breast cancer sentinel lymph node mapping: a Moffitt review. Breast Cancer 2004;11:225-232; discussion 264-266.

48. Boughey JC, Khakpour N, Meric-Bernstam F, et al. Selective use of sentinel lymph node surgery during prophylactic mastectomy. Cancer 2006;107:1440-1447.

49. King TA, Ganaraj A, Fey JV, et al. Cytokeratin-positive cells in sentinel lymph nodes in breast cancer are not random events: experience in patients undergoing prophylactic mastectomy. Cancer 2004;101:926-933.

50. Edge SB, Byrd DR, Compton CC, et al, eds. AJCC Cancer Staging Manual. 7th ed. New York: Springer; 2010; pp. 352-362.

51. Nasser SM, Smith SG, Chagpar AB. The role of sentinel node biopsy in women undergoing prophylactic mastectomy. J Surg Res 2010;164:188-192.

52. Ilum L, Bak M, Olsen KE, et al. Sentinel node localization in breast cancer patients using intradermal dye injection. Acta Oncol 2000;39:423-428.

53. Grube BJ, Hansen NM, Ye X, Giuliano AE. Tumor characteristics predictive of sentinel node metastases in 105 consecutive patients with invasive lobular carcinoma. Am J Surg 2002;184:372-376.

54. Ansari B, Ogston SA, Purdie CA, et al. Meta-analysis of sentinel node biopsy in ductal carcinoma in situ of the breast. Br J Surg 2008;95:547-554.

55. Dauway EL, Giuliano R, Pendas S, et al. Lymphatic mapping: a technique providing accurate staging for breast cancer. Breast Cancer 1999;6:145-154.

56. Zavotsky J, Hansen N, Brennan MB, et al. Lymph node metastasis from ductal carcinoma in situ with microinvasion. Cancer 1999;85:2439-2443.

57. Knauer M, Konstantiniuk P, Haid A, et al. Multicentric breast cancer: a new indication for sentinel node biopsy—a multiinstitutional validation study. J Clin Oncol 2006;24:3374-3380.

58. Schrenk P, Wayand W. Sentinel-node biopsy in axillary lymphnode staging for patients with multicentric breast cancer. Lancet 2001;357:122.

59. Bevilacqua JL, Kattan MW, Fey JV, et al. Doctor, what are my chances of having a positive sentinel node? A validated nomogram for risk estimation. J Clin Oncol 2007;25:3670-3679.

60. Fehr MK, Köchli OR, Helfenstein U, et al. Multivariate analysis of clinico-pathologic predictors of axillary lymph node metastasis in invasive breast carcinoma [in German]. Geburtshilfe Frauenheilkd 1995;55:182-188.

61. Maibenco DC, Weiss LK, Pawlish KS, Severson RK. Axillary lymph node metastases associated with small invasive breast carcinomas. Cancer 1999;85:1530-1536.

62. Mustafa IA, Cole B, Wanebo HJ, et al. The impact of histopathology on nodal metastases in minimal breast cancer. Arch Surg 1997;132:384-390; discussion 390-391.

63. Olivotto IA, Jackson JS, Mates D, et al. Prediction of axillary lymph node involvement of women with invasive breast carcinoma: a multivariate analysis. Cancer 1998;83:948-955.

64. Port ER, Tan LK, Borgen PI, Van Zee KJ. Incidence of axillary lymph node metastases in T1a and T1b breast carcinoma. Ann Surg Oncol 1998;5:23-27.

65. Rivadeneira DE, Simmons RM, Christos PJ, et al. Predictive factors associated with axillary lymph node metastases in T1a and T1b breast carcinomas: analysis in more than 900 patients. J Am Coll Surg 2000;191:1-6; discussion 6-8.

66. Voogd AC, Coebergh JW, Repelaer van Driel OJ, et al. The risk of nodal metastases in breast cancer patients with clinically negative lymph nodes: a population-based analysis. Breast Cancer Res Treat 2000;62:63-69.

67. Giuliano AE, Barth AM, Spivack B, et al. Incidence and predictors of axillary metastasis in T1 carcinoma of the breast. J Am Coll Surg 1996;183:185-189.

68. Gann PH, Colilla SA, Gapstur SM, et al. Factors associated with axillary lymph node metastasis from breast carcinoma: descriptive and predictive analyses. Cancer 1999;86:1511-1519.

69. Ravdin PM, De Laurentiis M, Vendely T, Clark GM. Prediction of axillary lymph node status in breast cancer patients by use of prognostic indicators. J Natl Cancer Inst 1994;86:1771-1775.

70. Viale G, Zurrida S, Maiorano E, et al. Predicting the status of axillary sentinel lymph nodes in 4351 patients with invasive breast carcinoma treated in a single institution. Cancer 2005;103:492-500.

71. Cserni G, Amendoeira I, Apostolikas N, et al. Discrepancies in current practice of pathological evaluation of sentinel lymph nodes in breast cancer. Results of a questionnaire based survey by the European Working Group for Breast Screening Pathology. J Clin Pathol 2004;57:695-701.

72. Fitzgibbons PL, LiVolsi VA. Recommendations for handling radioactive specimens obtained by sentinel lymphadenectomy. Surgical Pathology Committee of the College of American Pathologists, and the Association of Directors of Anatomic and Surgical Pathology. Am J Surg Pathol 2000;24:1549-1551.

73. Weaver DL. Pathology evaluation of sentinel lymph nodes in breast cancer: protocol recommendations and rationale. Mod Pathol 2010;23(Suppl 2):S26-S32.

74. ADASP recommendations for processing and reporting lymph node specimens submitted for evaluation of metastatic disease. Am J Surg Pathol 2001;25:961-963.

75. Fritzsche FR, Reineke T, Morawietz L, et al. Pathological processing techniques and final diagnosis of breast cancer sentinel lymph nodes. Ann Surg Oncol 2010;17:2892-2898.

76. Cox C, Centeno B, Dickson D, et al. Accuracy of intraoperative imprint cytology for sentinel lymph node evaluation in the treatment of breast carcinoma. Cancer 2005;105:13-20.

77. Motomura K, Nagumo S, Komoike Y, et al. Intraoperative imprint cytology for the diagnosis of sentinel node metastases in breast cancer. Breast Cancer 2007;14:350-353.

78. Henry-Tillman RS, Korourian S, Rubio IT, et al. Intraoperative touch preparation for sentinel lymph node biopsy: a 4-year experience. Ann Surg Oncol 2002;9:333-339.

79. Tew K, Irwig L, Matthews A, et al. Meta-analysis of sentinel node imprint cytology in breast cancer. Br J Surg 2005;92:1068-1080.

80. Lorand S, Lavoue V, Tas P, et al. Intraoperative touch imprint cytology of axillary sentinel nodes for breast cancer: A series of 355 procedures. Breast 2011;20:119-123.

81. Viale G, Mastropasqua MG, Maiorano E, Mazzarol G. Pathologic examination of the axillary sentinel lymph nodes in patients with early-stage breast carcinoma: current and resolving controversies on the basis of the European Institute of Oncology experience. Virchows Arch 2006;448:241-247.

82. Groen RS, Oosterhuis AW, Boers JE. Pathologic examination of sentinel lymph nodes in breast cancer by a single haematoxylin-eosin slide versus serial sectioning and immunocytokeratin staining: clinical implications. Breast Cancer Res Treat 2007;105:1-5.

83. Dowlatshahi K, Fan M, Anderson JM, Bloom KJ. Occult metastases in sentinel nodes of 200 patients with operable breast cancer. Ann Surg Oncol 2001;8:675-681.

84. Dowlatshahi K, Fan M, Snider HC, Habib FA. Lymph node micrometastases from breast carcinoma: reviewing the dilemma. Cancer 1997;80:1188-1197.

85. Blumencranz P, Whitworth PW, Deck K, et al. Scientific Impact Recognition Award. Sentinel node staging for breast cancer: intraoperative molecular pathology overcomes conventional histologic sampling errors. Am J Surg 2007;194:426-432.

86. Mansel RE, Goyal A, Douglas-Jones A, et al. Detection of breast cancer metastasis in sentinel lymph nodes using intra-operative real time GeneSearch BLN Assay in the operating room: results of the Cardiff study. Breast Cancer Res Treat 2009;115:595-600.

87. Tsujimoto M, Nakabayashi K, Yoshidome K, et al. One-step nucleic acid amplification for intraoperative detection of lymph node metastasis in breast cancer patients. Clin Cancer Res 2007;13:4807-4816.

88. Verbanac KM, Min CJ, Mannie AE, et al. Long-term follow-up study of a prospective multicenter sentinel node trial: molecular detection of breast cancer sentinel node metastases. Ann Surg Oncol 2010;17(Suppl 3):368-377.

89. Huvos AG, Hutter RV, Berg JW. Significance of axillary macrometastases and micrometastases in mammary cancer. Ann Surg 1971;173:44-46.

90. Chen SL, Hoehne FM, Giuliano AE. The prognostic significance of micrometastases in breast cancer: a SEER population-based analysis. Ann Surg Oncol 2007;14:3378-3384.

91. Nasser IA, Lee AK, Bosari S, et al. Occult axillary lymph node metastases in "node-negative" breast carcinoma. Hum Pathol 1993;24:950-957.

92. Ashwort TR. A case of cancer in which cells similar to those in the tumors were seen in the blood after death. Aust Med J 1896;14:146. Cited by Abati A, Liotta LA. Looking forward in diagnostic pathology. Cancer 1996;78:1-3.

93. Abati A, Liotta LA. Looking forward in diagnostic pathology: the molecular superhighway. Cancer 1996;78:1-3.

94. Hermanek P, Hutter RV, Sobin LH, Wittekind C. Classification of isolated tumor cells and micrometastasis. International Union Against Cancer. Cancer 1999;86:2668-2673.

95. Breast tumors. Sobin LH, Gospodarowicz MK, Wittekind C, International Union Against Cancer. TNM Classification of Malignant Tumours. 7th ed. Chichester, West Sussex, UK, and Hoboken, NJ: Wiley-Blackwell; 2010; pp. 181-193.

96. Cserni G, Bianchi S, Vezzosi V, et al. Variations in sentinel node isolated tumour cells/micrometastasis and non-sentinel node involvement rates according to different interpretations of the TNM definitions. Eur J Cancer 2008;44:2185-2191.

97. van Deurzen CH, Cserni G, Bianchi S, et al. Nodal-stage classification in invasive lobular breast carcinoma: influence of different interpretations of the pTNM classification. J Clin Oncol 2010;28:999-1004.

98. Farshid G, Pradhan M, Kollias J, Gill PG. Computer simulations of lymph node metastasis for optimizing the pathologic examination of sentinel lymph nodes in patients with breast carcinoma. Cancer 2000;89:2527-2537.

99. Cox CE, Bass SS, Boulware D, et al. Implementation of new surgical technology: outcome measures for lymphatic mapping of breast carcinoma. Ann Surg Oncol 1999;6:553-561.

100. Giuliano AE, Dale PS, Turner RR, et al. Improved axillary staging of breast cancer with sentinel lymphadenectomy. Ann Surg 1995;222:394-399; discussion 399-401.

101. Krag D, Harlow S, Weaver D, Ashikaga T. Technique of sentinel node resection in melanoma and breast cancer: probe-guided surgery and lymphatic mapping. Eur J Surg Oncol 1998;24:89-93.

102. O'Hea BJ, Hill AD, El-Shirbiny AM, et al. Sentinel lymph node biopsy in breast cancer: initial experience at Memorial Sloan-Kettering Cancer Center. J Am Coll Surg 1998;186:423-427.

103. Borgstein PJ, Meijer S, Pijpers R. Intradermal blue dye to identify sentinel lymph-node in breast cancer. Lancet 1997;349:1668-1669.

104. Barnwell JM, Arredondo MA, Kollmorgen D, et al. Sentinel node biopsy in breast cancer. Ann Surg Oncol 1998;5:126-130.

105. Prognostic importance of occult axillary lymph node micrometastases from breast cancers. International (Ludwig) Breast Cancer Study Group. Lancet 1990;335:1565-1568.

106. Cserni G. Metastases in axillary sentinel lymph nodes in breast cancer as detected by intensive histopathological work up. J Clin Pathol 1999;52:922-924.

107. Weaver DL, Krag DN, Ashikaga T, et al. Pathologic analysis of sentinel and nonsentinel lymph nodes in breast carcinoma: a multicenter study. Cancer 2000;88:1099-1107.

108. Weaver DL. Sentinel lymph node biopsy in breast cancer: creating controversy and defining new standards. Adv Anat Pathol 2001;8:65-73.

109. Corben AD, Nehhozina T, Garg K, et al. Endosalpingiosis in axillary lymph nodes: a possible pitfall in the staging of patients with breast carcinoma. Am J Surg Pathol 2010;34:1211-1216.

110. Jaffer S, Lin R, Bleiweiss IJ, Nagi C. Intraductal carcinoma arising in intraductal papilloma in an axillary lymph node: review of the literature and proposed theories of evolution. Arch Pathol Lab Med 2008;132:1940-1942.

111. Kadowaki M, Nagashima T, Sakata H, et al. Ectopic breast tissue in axillary lymph node. Breast Cancer 2007;14:425-428.

112. Maiorano E, Mazzarol GM, Pruneri G, et al. Ectopic breast tissue as a possible cause of false-positive axillary sentinel lymph node biopsies. Am J Surg Pathol 2003;27:513-518.

113. Norton LE, Komenaka IK, Emerson RE, et al. Benign glandular inclusions a rare cause of a false positive sentinel node. J Surg Oncol 2007;95:593-596.

114. Ohsie SJ, Moatamed NA, Chang HR, Apple SK. Heterotopic breast tissue versus occult metastatic carcinoma in lymph node, a diagnostic dilemma. Ann Diagn Pathol 2010;14:260-263.

115. Youngson BJ, Cranor M, Rosen PP. Epithelial displacement in surgical breast specimens following needling procedures. Am J Surg Pathol 1994;18:896-903.

116. Youngson BJ, Liberman L, Rosen PP. Displacement of carcinomatous epithelium in surgical breast specimens following stereotaxic core biopsy. Am J Clin Pathol 1995;103:598-602.

117. Carter BA, Jensen RA, Simpson JF, Page DL. Benign transport of breast epithelium into axillary lymph nodes after biopsy. Am J Clin Pathol 2000;113:259-265.

118. Bleiweiss IJ, Nagi CS, Jaffer S. Axillary sentinel lymph nodes can be falsely positive due to iatrogenic displacement and transport of benign epithelial cells in patients with breast carcinoma. J Clin Oncol 2006;24:2013-2018.

119. Nagi C, Bleiweiss I, Jaffer S. Epithelial displacement in breast lesions: a papillary phenomenon. Arch Pathol Lab Med 2005;129:1465-1469.

120. Bilimoria KY, Bentrem DJ, Hansen NM, et al. Comparison of sentinel lymph node biopsy alone and completion axillary lymph node dissection for node-positive breast cancer. J Clin Oncol 2009;27:2946-2953.

121. Veronesi U, Viale G, Paganelli G, et al. Sentinel lymph node biopsy in breast cancer: ten-year results of a randomized controlled study. Ann Surg 2010;251:595-600.

122. Chu KU, Turner RR, Hansen NM, et al. Do all patients with sentinel node metastasis from breast carcinoma need complete axillary node dissection? Ann Surg 1999;229:536-541.

123. Goyal A, Douglas-Jones A, Newcombe RG, Mansel RE. Predictors of non-sentinel lymph node metastasis in breast cancer patients. Eur J Cancer 2004;40:1731-1737.

124. Van Zee KJ, Manasseh DM, Bevilacqua JL, et al. A nomogram for predicting the likelihood of additional nodal metastases in breast cancer patients with a positive sentinel lymph node biopsy. Ann Surg Oncol 2003;10:1140-1151.

125. Barranger E, Coutant C, Flahault A, et al. An axilla scoring system to predict non-sentinel lymph node status in breast cancer patients with sentinel lymph node involvement. Breast Cancer Res Treat 2005;91:113-119.

126. Pal A, Provenzano E, Duffy SW, et al. A model for predicting non-sentinel lymph node metastatic disease when the sentinel lymph node is positive. Br J Surg 2008;95:302-309.

127. Kohrt HE, Olshen RA, Bermas HR, et al. New models and online calculator for predicting non-sentinel lymph node status in sentinel lymph node positive breast cancer patients. BMC Cancer 2008;8:66.

128. Jeruss JS, Newman LA, Ayers GD, et al. Factors predicting additional disease in the axilla in patients with positive sentinel lymph nodes after neoadjuvant chemotherapy. Cancer 2008;112:2646-2654.

129. Hwang RF, Krishnamurthy S, Hunt KK, et al. Clinicopathologic factors predicting involvement of nonsentinel axillary nodes in women with breast cancer. Ann Surg Oncol 2003;10:248-254.

130. Saidi RF, Dudrick PS, Remine SG, Mittal VK. Nonsentinel lymph node status after positive sentinel lymph node biopsy in early breast cancer. Am Surg 2004;70:101-105; discussion 105.

131. Degnim AC, Reynolds C, Pantvaidya G, et al. Nonsentinel node metastasis in breast cancer patients: assessment of an existing and a new predictive nomogram. Am J Surg 2005;190:543-550.

132. Viale G, Maiorano E, Pruneri G, et al. Predicting the risk for additional axillary metastases in patients with breast carcinoma and positive sentinel lymph node biopsy. Ann Surg 2005;241:319-325.

133. Houvenaeghel G, Nos C, Giard S, et al. A nomogram predictive of non-sentinel lymph node involvement in breast cancer patients with a sentinel lymph node micrometastasis. Eur J Surg Oncol 2009;35:690-695.

134. Kumar S, Bramlage M, Jacks LM, et al. Minimal disease in the sentinel lymph node: how to best measure sentinel node micrometastases to predict risk of additional non-sentinel lymph node disease. Ann Surg Oncol 2010;17:2909-2919.

135. Katz A, Smith BL, Golshan M, et al. Nomogram for the prediction of having four or more involved nodes for sentinel lymph node-positive breast cancer. J Clin Oncol 2008;26:2093-2098.

136. Gur AS, Unal B, Johnson R, et al. Predictive probability of four different breast cancer nomograms for nonsentinel axillary lymph node metastasis in positive sentinel node biopsy. J Am Coll Surg 2009;208:229-235.

137. Gur AS, Unal B, Ozbek U, et al. Validation of breast cancer nomograms for predicting the non-sentinel lymph node metastases after a positive sentinel lymph node biopsy in a multi-center study. Eur J Surg Oncol 2010;36:30-35.

138. Jamal MH, Rayment JH, Meguerditchian A, et al. Impact of the sentinel node frozen section result on the probability of additional nodal metastases as predicted by the MSKCC nomogram in breast cancer. Jpn J Clin Oncol 2011;41:314-319.

139. Moghaddam Y, Falzon M, Fulford L, et al. Comparison of three mathematical models for predicting the risk of additional axillary nodal metastases after positive sentinel lymph node biopsy in early breast cancer. Br J Surg 2010;97:1646-1652.

140. Sanjuan A, Escaramis G, Vidal-Sicart S, et al. Predicting non-sentinel lymph node status in breast cancer patients with sentinel lymph node involvement: evaluation of two scoring systems. Breast J 2010;16:134-140.

141. Scow JS, Degnim AC, Hoskin TL, et al. Assessment of the performance of the Stanford Online Calculator for the prediction of nonsentinel lymph node metastasis in sentinel lymph node-positive breast cancer patients. Cancer 2009;115:4064-4070.

142. Unal B, Gur AS, Kayiran O, et al. Models for predicting non-sentinel lymph node positivity in sentinel node positive breast cancer: the importance of scoring system. Int J Clin Pract 2008;62:1785-1791.

143. D'Eredita G, Troilo VL, Giardina C, et al. Sentinel lymph node micrometastasis and risk of non-sentinel lymph node metastasis: validation of two breast cancer nomograms. Clin Breast Cancer 2010;10:445-451.

144. Smidt ML, Kuster DM, van der Wilt GJ, et al. Can the Memorial Sloan-Kettering Cancer Center nomogram predict the likelihood of nonsentinel lymph node metastases in breast cancer patients in the Netherlands? Ann Surg Oncol 2005;12:1066-1072.

145. Lambert LA, Ayers GD, Hwang RF, et al. Validation of a breast cancer nomogram for predicting nonsentinel lymph node metastases after a positive sentinel node biopsy. Ann Surg Oncol 2006;13:310-320.

146. Zgajnar J, Perhavec A, Hocevar M, et al. Low performance of the MSKCC nomogram in preoperatively ultrasonically negative axillary lymph node in breast cancer patients. J Surg Oncol 2007;96:547-553.

147. Evrensel T, Johnson R, Ahrendt G, et al. The predicted probability of having positive non-sentinel lymph nodes in patients who received neoadjuvant chemotherapy for large operable breast cancer. Int J Clin Pract 2008;62:1379-1382.

147a. Scow JS, Degnim AC, Hoskin TL, et al. Assessment of the performance of the Stanford Online Calculator for the prediction of nonsentinel lymph node metastasis in sentinel lymph node positive breast cancer patients. Cancer 2009;115:4064-4070.

148. Alran S, De Rycke Y, Fourchotte V, et al. Validation and limitations of use of a breast cancer nomogram predicting the likelihood of non-sentinel node involvement after positive sentinel node biopsy. Ann Surg Oncol 2007;14:2195-2201.

149. Coutant C, Olivier C, Lambaudie E, et al. Comparison of models to predict nonsentinel lymph node status in breast cancer patients with metastatic sentinel lymph nodes: a prospective multicenter study. J Clin Oncol 2009;27:2800-2808.

150. Poirier E, Sideris L, Dube P, et al. Analysis of clinical applicability of the breast cancer nomogram for positive sentinel lymph node: the canadian experience. Ann Surg Oncol 2008;15: 2562-2567.

151. Moffat FL Jr, Senofsky GM, Davis K, et al. Axillary node dissection for early breast cancer: some is good, but all is better. J Surg Oncol 1992;51:8-13.

152. Baron RH, Fey JV, Borgen PI, et al. Eighteen sensations after breast cancer surgery: a 5-year comparison of sentinel lymph node biopsy and axillary lymph node dissection. Ann Surg Oncol 2007;14:1653-1661.

153. Crane-Okada R, Wascher RA, Elashoff D, Giuliano AE. Long-term morbidity of sentinel node biopsy versus complete axillary dissection for unilateral breast cancer. Ann Surg Oncol 2008;15:1996-2005.

154. Goldberg JI, Wiechmann LI, Riedel ER, et al. Morbidity of sentinel node biopsy in breast cancer: the relationship between the number of excised lymph nodes and lymphedema. Ann Surg Oncol 2010;17:3278-3286.

155. Langer I, Guller U, Berclaz G, et al. Morbidity of sentinel lymph node biopsy (SLN) alone versus SLN and completion axillary lymph node dissection after breast cancer surgery: a prospective Swiss multicenter study on 659 patients. Ann Surg 2007;245:452-461.

156. Land SR, Kopec JA, Julian TB, et al. Patient-reported outcomes in sentinel node-negative adjuvant breast cancer patients receiving sentinel-node biopsy or axillary dissection: National Surgical Adjuvant Breast and Bowel Project phase III protocol B-32. J Clin Oncol 2010;28:3929-3936.

157. Trojani M, de Mascarel I, Bonichon F, et al. Micrometastases to axillary lymph nodes from carcinoma of breast: detection by immunohistochemistry and prognostic significance. Br J Cancer 1987;55:303-306.

158. Trojani M, de Mascarel I, Coindre JM, Bonichon F. Micrometastases to axillary lymph nodes from invasive lobular carcinoma of breast: detection by immunohistochemistry and prognostic significance. Br J Cancer 1987;56:838-839.

159. Carter BA, Page DL. Sentinel lymph node histopathology in breast cancer: minimal disease versus artifact. J Clin Oncol 2006;24:1978-1979.

160. Rutgers EJ. Sentinel node biopsy: interpretation and management of patients with immunohistochemistry-positive sentinel nodes and those with micrometastases. J Clin Oncol 2008;26:698-702.

161. Weaver DL, Le UP, Dupuis SL, et al. Metastasis detection in sentinel lymph nodes: comparison of a limited widely spaced (NSABP protocol B-32) and a comprehensive narrowly spaced paraffin block sectioning strategy. Am J Surg Pathol 2009;33:1583-1589.

162. Millis RR, Springall R, Lee AH, et al. Occult axillary lymph node metastases are of no prognostic significance in breast cancer. Br J Cancer 2002;86:396-401.

163. Andersson Y, Frisell J, Sylvan M, et al. Breast cancer survival in relation to the metastatic tumor burden in axillary lymph nodes. J Clin Oncol 2010;28:2868-2873.

164. Fisher B, Montague E, Redmond C, et al. Findings from NSABP Protocol No. B-04-comparison of radical mastectomy with alternative treatments for primary breast cancer. I. Radiation compliance and its relation to treatment outcome. Cancer 1980;46:1-13.

165. Goyal A, Newcombe RG, Chhabra A, Mansel RE. Morbidity in breast cancer patients with sentinel node metastases undergoing delayed axillary lymph node dissection (ALND) compared with immediate ALND. Ann Surg Oncol 2008;15:262-267.

166. Straver ME, Meijnen P, van Tienhoven G, et al. Role of axillary clearance after a tumor-positive sentinel node in the administration of adjuvant therapy in early breast cancer. J Clin Oncol 2010;28:731-737.

167. Straver ME, Meijnen P, van Tienhoven G, et al. Sentinel node identification rate and nodal involvement in the EORTC 10981-22023 AMAROS trial. Ann Surg Oncol 2010;17:1854-1861.

168. Olson JA Jr, McCall LM, Beitsch P, et al. Impact of immediate versus delayed axillary node dissection on surgical outcomes in breast cancer patients with positive sentinel nodes: results from American College of Surgeons Oncology Group Trials Z0010 and Z0011. J Clin Oncol 2008;26:3530-3535.

169. Cox CE, Pendas S, Cox JM, et al. Guidelines for sentinel node biopsy and lymphatic mapping of patients with breast cancer. Ann Surg 1998;227:645-651; discussion 651-653.

170. Martin RC 2nd, Edwards MJ, Wong SL, et al. Practical guidelines for optimal gamma probe detection of sentinel lymph nodes in breast cancer: results of a multi-institutional study. For the University of Louisville Breast Cancer Study Group. Surgery 2000;128:139-144.

171. Wong SL, Edwards MJ, Chao C, et al. Sentinel lymph node biopsy for breast cancer: impact of the number of sentinel nodes removed on the false-negative rate. J Am Coll Surg 2001;192:684-689; discussion 689-691.

172. Zervos EE, Badgwell BD, Abdessalam SF, et al. Selective analysis of the sentinel node in breast cancer. Am J Surg 2001;182: 372-376.

173. McCarter MD, Yeung H, Fey J, et al. The breast cancer patient with multiple sentinel nodes: when to stop? J Am Coll Surg 2001;192:692-697.

174. Chagpar AB, Carlson DJ, Laidley AL, et al. Factors influencing the number of sentinel lymph nodes identified in patients with breast cancer. Am J Surg 2007;194:860-864; discussion 864-865.

175. Low KS, Littlejohn DR. Optimal number of sentinel nodes after intradermal injection isotope and blue dye. Aust N Z J Surg 2006;76:472-475.

176. Zakaria S, Degnim AC, Kleer CG, et al. Sentinel lymph node biopsy for breast cancer: how many nodes are enough? J Surg Oncol 2007;96:554-559.

177. Chagpar AB, Scoggins CR, Martin RC 2nd, et al. Are 3 sentinel nodes sufficient? Arch Surg 2007;142:456-459; discussion 459-460.

178. Woznick A, Franco M, Bendick P, Benitez PR. Sentinel lymph node dissection for breast cancer: how many nodes are enough and which technique is optimal? Am J Surg 2006;191:330-333.

179. Dabbs DJ, Johnson R. The optimal number of sentinel lymph nodes for focused pathologic examination. Breast J 2004;10:186-189.

180. Leonard C, Corkill M, Tompkin J, et al. Are axillary recurrence and overall survival affected by axillary extranodal tumor extension in breast cancer? Implications for radiation therapy. J Clin Oncol 1995;13:47-53.

181. Bucci JA, Kennedy CW, Burn J, et al. Implications of extranodal spread in node positive breast cancer: a review of survival and local recurrence. Breast 2001;10:213-219.

182. Abdessalam SF, Zervos EE, Prasad M, et al. Predictors of positive axillary lymph nodes after sentinel lymph node biopsy in breast cancer. Am J Surg 2001;182:316-320.

183. Altinyollar H, Berberoglu U, Gulben K, Irkin F. The correlation of extranodal invasion with other prognostic parameters in lymph node positive breast cancer. J Surg Oncol 2007;95:567-571.

184. Palamba HW, Rombouts MC, Ruers TJ, et al. Extranodal extension of axillary metastasis of invasive breast carcinoma as a possible predictor for the total number of positive lymph nodes. Eur J Surg Oncol 2001;27:719-722.

185. Fujii T, Yanagita Y, Fujisawa T, et al. Implication of extracapsular invasion of sentinel lymph nodes in breast cancer: prediction of nonsentinel lymph node metastasis. World J Surg 2010;34:544-548.

186. Mansel RE, Fallowfield L, Kissin M, et al. Randomized multicenter trial of sentinel node biopsy versus standard axillary treatment in operable breast cancer: the ALMANAC Trial. J Natl Cancer Inst 2006;98:599-609.

187. Krag DN, Anderson SJ, Julian TB, et al. Sentinel-lymph-node resection compared with conventional axillary-lymph-node dissection in clinically node-negative patients with breast cancer: overall survival findings from the NSABP B-32 randomised phase 3 trial. Lancet Oncol 2010;11:927-933.

188. Krag DN, Anderson SJ, Julian TB, et al. Primary outcome results of NSABP B-32, a randomized phase III clinical trial to compare sentinel node resection (SNR) to conventional axillary dissection (AD) in clinically node-negative breast cancer patients. Lancet 2010;10:927-933.

189. Weaver DL, Ashikaga T, Krag DN, et al. Effect of occult metastases on survival in node-negative breast cancer. N Engl J Med 2011;364:412-421.

190. Ashikaga T, Krag DN, Land SR, et al. Morbidity results from the NSABP B-32 trial comparing sentinel lymph node dissection versus axillary dissection. J Surg Oncol 2010;102:111-118.

191. Cote R, Giuliano AE, Hawes D, et al. ACOSOG Z0010: A multicenter prognostic study of sentinel node (SN) and bone marrow (BM) micrometastases in women with clinical T1/T2 N0 M0 breast cancer [abstract CRA504]. J Clin Oncol 2010;28:7s.

192. Giuliano AE, McCall L, Beitsch P, et al. Locoregional recurrence after sentinel lymph node dissection with or without axillary dissection in patients with sentinel lymph node metastases: the American College of Surgeons Oncology Group Z0011 randomized trial. Ann Surg 2010;252:426-432; discussion 432-433.

8

Breast Imaging Modalities for Pathologists

Christiane M. Hakim • Marie A. Ganott • Amy Vogia • Jules H. Sumkin

INTRODUCTION

Just as there have been rapid changes in the world of breast pathology in recent years, the changes have been just as dramatic in the field of breast imaging. As the body of knowledge for breast cancer diagnosis and treatment expands, it is increasingly important for the various specialties involved in the care of breast cancer patients to understand what is happening in related fields so that effective communication can occur. The types of imaging tests and biopsy techniques available for breast cancer diagnosis and staging have undergone many changes in recent years. This chapter attempts to highlight the current diagnostic modalities and biopsy techniques available to the radiologist. Special attention is placed on the appropriate utilization of the various techniques and the imaging appearances of the various pathologic entities that the pathologist will see. It is important for the pathologist to understand the strengths and limitations of imaging and how imaging can complement pathology.

Mammography remains the most basic and important test in breast imaging. It has evolved from an analog technique to a digital one, but it is still typically the initial test that women will undergo in both the screening and the diagnostic environment. There are ongoing controversies involving what age to initiate screening mammography, when to stop it, and at what intervals it should be employed. Despite these controversies, all agree that some form of screening is important and improves survival by identifying cancer at an earlier and more treatable stage.[1] Mammography is performed as both a screening test (asymptomatic women) and a diagnostic test (symptomatic women). When an abnormality is identified, it will be further evaluated by special mammographic techniques and other imaging modalities. Usually, the first additional modality to be employed is ultrasound. Even though there is new evidence to suggest that, in certain instances, ultrasound may be a valuable screening test,[2] currently, its primary use is to complement mammography. For example, when a woman has a palpable lesion that has no mammographic correlate, other tools become warranted. Figure 8-1 demonstrates the image of a young woman with a palpable abnormality in her right breast. The mammogram is unimpressive; however, the ultrasound targeted to the area of interest demonstrates a densely shadowing lesion. Once a lesion is identified, the ultrasound can be used for guidance to perform a percutaneous biopsy. If a lesion is identified mammographically and is non-mass-like (e.g., calcifications), a biopsy could be performed with mammographic guidance (stereotactic biopsy). Figure 8-2 illustrates a patient with new indeterminate calcifications in her right breast. Special magnification views to further characterize the calcifications were performed, but they remained indeterminate by imaging criteria. Therefore, a mammography-guided stereotactic biopsy was performed. The diagnosis was ductal carcinoma in situ (DCIS), solid and cribriform, with moderate comedonecrosis.

Once a malignancy is defined by mammography and/or ultrasound, magnetic resonance imaging (MRI) may be performed to further define the extent of disease. In Figure 8-1, the MRI shows that the extent of the lobular cancer is considerably greater than expected by physical examination, mammography, and ultrasound. If the patient undergoes neoadjuvant chemotherapy, MRI is a way to follow tumor response.

On the day of surgery, wire localization will be performed for nonpalpable lesions to assist the surgeon in

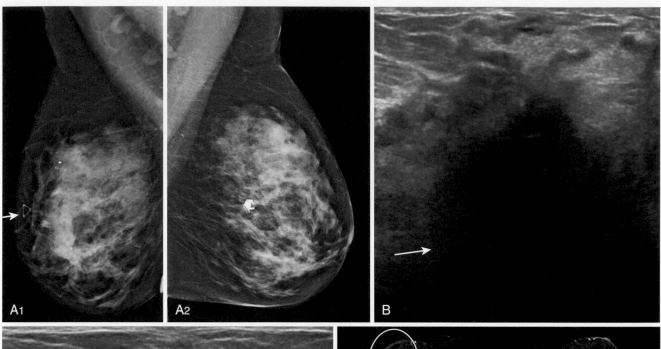

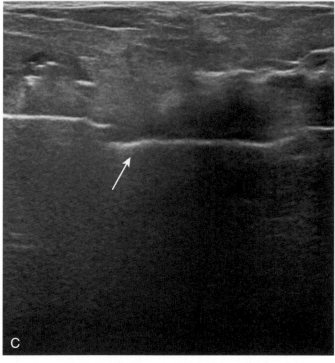

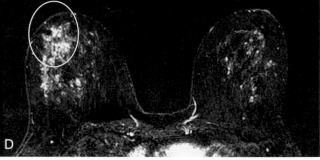

FIGURE 8-1 A1 and **A2,** Young woman with a palpable abnormality in her right breast. The mammogram is unimpressive. The triangular marker *(arrow* in A1) indicates the palpable finding. **B,** Ultrasound demonstrates a densely shadowing lesion *(arrow).* **C,** Ultrasound-guided core biopsy shows the linear bright echogenic core needle placed through the lesion for tissue sampling. *Arrow* demonstrates the trough of the core biopsy needle through the lesion. **D,** Magnetic resonance imaging (MRI) shows the multiple enhancing foci within the right breast. The extent of the lobular cancer within the right breast *(circled area)* is considerably greater than expected by physical examination, mammography, and ultrasound.

finding and excising the tumor. If the lesion is an invasive cancer and there is no known axillary nodal disease, a sentinel lymph node injection will be performed so that the sentinel lymph node can be removed.

Depending on physical examination, the size of the tumor, the histology, and the appearance of the axilla, a metastatic workup will ensue before the anticipated surgery. This typically consists of computed tomography (CT) or positron-emission tomography (PET)/CT of the chest, abdomen, and pelvis and a bone scan if a plain CT is performed. If the patient is going to receive cardiotoxic chemotherapy, she will typically undergo a multigated angiogram (MUGA) scan to ensure that left ventricular function is normal.

MAMMOGRAPHY

Mammography, developed in the 1930s, has experienced progressive refinements in image quality and reduction in radiation dose due to improvements in the equipment generating x-rays and the receptors to display images, resulting in high-resolution and high-contrast radiographic images of the breast.[3] Mammographic images are produced either digitally (digital mammography [DM]), and displayed on a high-resolution monitor, or directly, onto special mammography film (film screen [FS] mammography).

For most women, the start of the radiological workup begins with a mammogram. The American Cancer

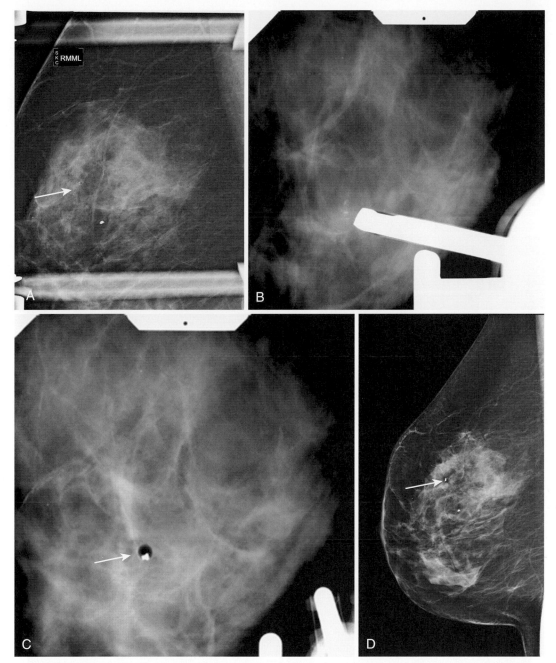

FIGURE 8-2 **A,** Indeterminate calcifications within the right breast *(arrow)*. RMML, right magnification mediolateral. **B,** Mammography-guided stereotactic-guided biopsy was performed. **C,** Air in the marker cavity surrounds the biopsy clip *(arrow)*. **D,** The clip marks the site of calcifications for future surgical intervention *(arrow)*.

Society guidelines for evaluation of average-risk individuals include annual mammograms beginning at age 40. Mammography screening ages can be altered if there is a history of breast cancer in a first-degree relative. Symptomatic women presenting with abnormalities, including a palpable lump, erythema, skin or nipple retraction, arm or breast swelling, and discoloration, will also begin with the standard mammographic views but will require additional mammographic views, ultrasound, or both.

To achieve a high-quality image, the skilled mammography technologist must include as much breast tissue as possible in the field of view and compress the breast firmly against the x-ray receptor plate, reducing the chance for motion blurring. The standard mammogram consists of a craniocaudal (CC) and a mediolateral oblique (MLO) view of each breast. The MLO view is used instead of a true lateral in order to include the axillary tail of the breast and as much of the axilla as possible. The CC image is viewed rotated with the lateral side up and with the CC label on the lateral aspect of the breast (Figure 8-3).

Owing to considerable variation in the mammographic appearance of women's breasts, the detection of malignancy may be challenging, and comparison with prior mammograms is often critical to accurate interpretation of the current examination. The interpreting

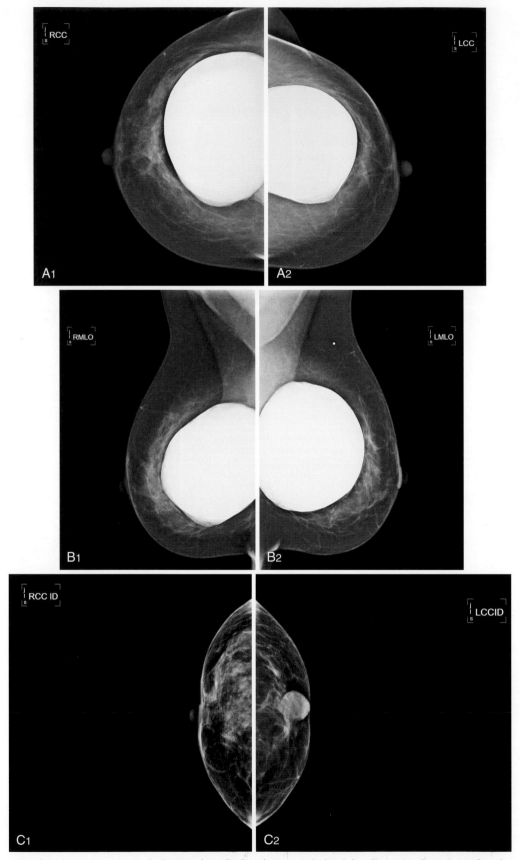

FIGURE 8-3 Routine digital mammogram including implant-displaced views. Subglandular silicone implants were placed over 20 years ago. Labels denoting views are placed in the upper outer quadrants. Craniocaudal (**A1** and **A2**) and mediolateral oblique (MLO; **B1** and **B2**) views with implants seen in view. Craniocaudal (**C1** and **C2**) and MLO (**D1-3**) views with the implants displaced. LCC, left craniocaudal; LCCID, left craniocaudal implant displaced; LMLO, left mediolateral oblique; LMLO ID, left mediolateral oblique implant displaced; RCC, right craniocaudal; RCCID, right craniocaudal implant displaced; RMLO, right mediolateral oblique; RMLO ID, right mediolateral oblique implant displaced.

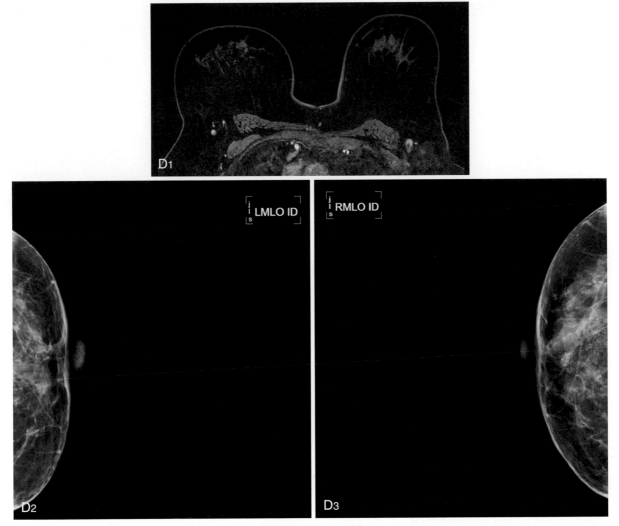

FIGURE 8-3, cont'd

radiologist must meet experience and education requirements mandated by the federal government in accordance with the MQSA (Mammography Quality and Standards Act).

The "density of breast tissue" refers to the amount of glandular tissue relative to the amount of fat and has been classified into four groups: These include fatty (<25% glandular tissue), scattered (25–50% glandular tissue), heterogeneously dense (50–75% glandular tissue), and extremely dense (>75%). The more glandular the breast tissue, the more likely a noncalcified lesion will be obscured by the dense tissue on one or both views.

Similar to computer-aided Papanicolaou (Pap) smear analysis, computer-aided detection (CAD) has been employed to aid radiologists in detecting abnormalities detected by mammography. The programs are designed to detect and highlight masses and calcifications with suspicious/indeterminate features. Some CAD programs attempt to assign a likelihood of malignancy by varying the size of the mark or providing a percentage depicting level of concern.[4–6] The sensitivity and specificity of the CAD algorithm may be adjusted with the

goal of assisting the radiologist to detect malignancy without unnecessarily increasing the false positives (Figure 8-4).[7,8]

Currently, facilities perform either full-field (whole breast) digital mammography (FFDM) or analog FS mammography. The diagnostic accuracy of digital and FS imaging was studied in the DMIST (Digital Mammographic Imaging Screening Trial) conducted by ACRIN (American College of Radiology Imaging Network).[9] The DMIST study concluded that, whereas both methods produce a mammogram of diagnostic quality, FFDM performed better for pre- and perimenopausal women younger than 50 and also for women of all ages with dense breast tissue (Figure 8-5).[9,10]

A distinct advantage of FFDM systems is the speed at which the images are obtained and the ability of the radiologist to manipulate the images at the workstation. Digital mammography tends to shorten the length of performing the examination with a decrease in the number of additional images needed to complete the evaluation but is more expensive than FS.[10,11]

The mammographic abnormalities that may be seen as a manifestation of malignancy are microcalcifications,

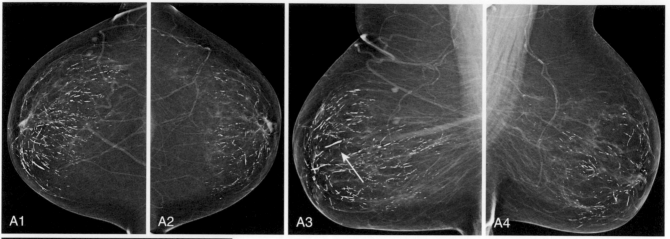

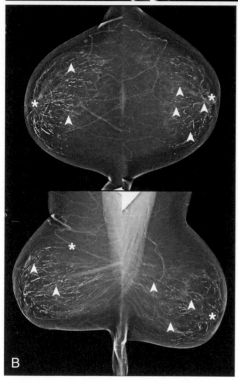

FIGURE 8-4   A1-A4, Diffuse bilateral benign secretory calcifications are present *(arrow on linear calcification* **[A3]***).* **B,** Computer-aided detection (CAD) images have numerous marks, all denoting benign stable findings *(arrowheads,* calcifications; *asterisks,* masses).

masses, architectural distortion, asymmetrical or developing densities, edema of the breast or skin, and axillary lymphadenopathy.

Microcalcifications can be associated with benign and malignant processes. Pleomorphism, linear shape and orientation, and clustered or segmental distribution of calcifications suggest malignancy, whereas a more diffuse distribution and rounded shape favor a benign etiology. Magnified views in the CC and MLO projection are performed to more accurately assess their morphology. Certain features of calcifications such as central lucency or meniscal layering are classic for benign disease, but often, the calcifications cannot be categorized as benign or malignant and are reported as "indeterminate." Stereotactic biopsy is recommended for suspicious calcifications, and usually for indeterminate calcifications, whereas 6-month

follow-up mammography is advised for those thought to be probably benign (Figure 8-6).

Masses are evaluated mammographically with spot compression or spot-magnified views to better visualize their margins. Smooth margins suggest a benign etiology, whereas irregular, microlobulated, ill-defined, or spiculated margins suggest malignancy. Large coarse calcifications in a well-defined mass are typical features of a fibroadenoma (Figure 8-7).

Carcinomas are rarely well defined but, frequently, are very dense for their size. Phyllodes tumors are well defined and often become quite large.

Architectural distortion is defined as disturbance of the normal architecture without an apparent mass. This appearance is most commonly the result of a surgical scar but can be due to a subtle invasive cancer, DCIS, radial scar, and other entities.

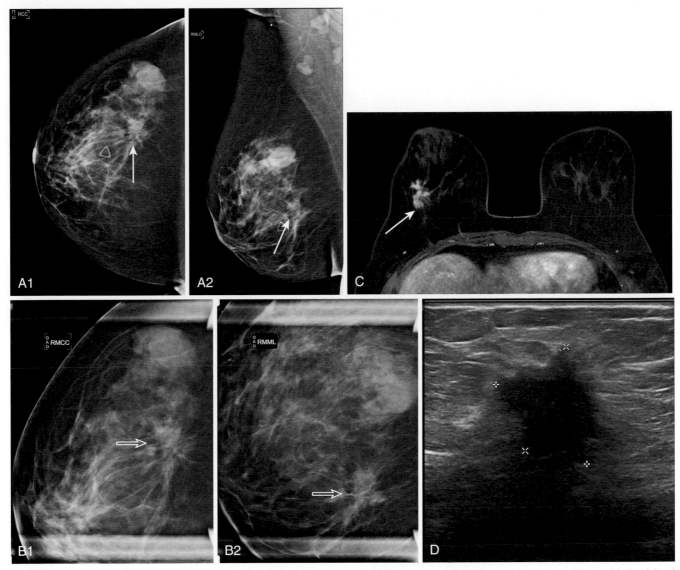

FIGURE 8-5 Craniocaudal (CC) and MLO routine images **(A1** and **A2)** and CC and MLO spot magnification views **(B1** and **B2)** of focal asymmetry (*solid arrows* in **A1** and **A2**) reveal a spiculated mass (*open arrows* in **B1** and **B2**). MRI **(C)** and ultrasound images **(D)** of the same lesion. RMCC, right magnification craniocaudal; RMML, right magnification mediolateral.

Magnified views will better demonstrate the distortion and may reveal a subtle mass. Biopsy should be performed unless the area is shown to correspond to a surgical scar (Figure 8-8).

Asymmetrical densities, also called *asymmetry* and *focal asymmetry,* are sometimes due to malignancy but more often represent areas of glandular tissue. These are evaluated by comparison with old studies, spot compression views, angled or rolled views, and ultrasound. Persistence on multiple views and change from prior study suggests a true mass, which will be evaluated with ultrasound (Figure 8-9).

Edema of the breast and skin can be due to radiation, mastitis, inflammatory carcinoma, or lymphatic obstruction. Lymphadenopathy may be visible on the mammogram if the axilla is visualized. Abnormally large dense nodes may be reactive, metastatic, or due to lymphoma.

Establishing the size of a lesion as well as the multiplicity of lesions is important in planning definitive therapy. Other modalities such as ultrasound and MRI can be helpful in evaluating the true extent of disease once a diagnosis of malignancy is made.

Mammography is important not only in the diagnosis of breast cancer but also in surveillance and assessment of neoadjuvant chemotherapy (Figure 8-10).

Ductography is performed to evaluate nipple discharge of clinical concern (i.e., bloody or clear to golden discharge from a single duct) in order to detect an intraductal pathology that is too subtle to be seen on mammography or ultrasound. A papilloma is often seen as a retroareolar lobulated filling defect whereas DCIS may appear as a narrowed, irregularly marginated duct. Ductography is performed by cannulating the discharging duct with a 30-gauge sialogram catheter and injecting the duct with a small amount of contrast material.

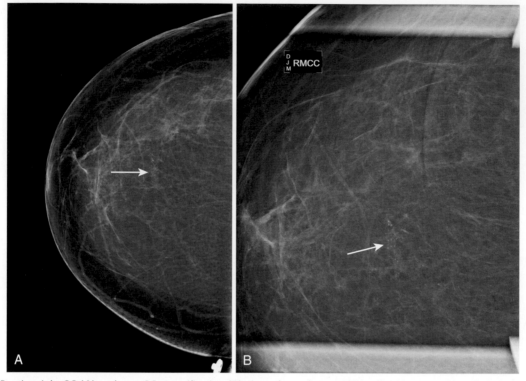

FIGURE 8-6   Routine right CC **(A)** and spot CC magnification **(B)** views show pleomorphic malignant-appearing calcifications *(arrows)*. Invasive ductal carcinoma and ductal carcinoma in situ (DCIS) with comedonecrosis, both nuclear grade 3, were shown on biopsy and confirmed at surgical excision.

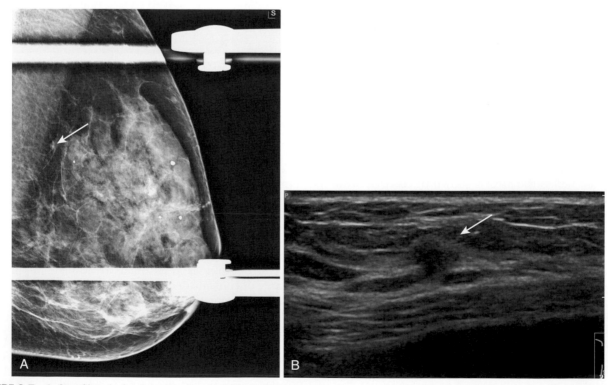

FIGURE 8-7   **A,** Spot film of a focal density demonstrates an 8-mm invasive ductal carcinoma *(arrow)*. **B,** Ultrasound of the same lesion shows a hypoechoic irregular mass *(arrow)*.

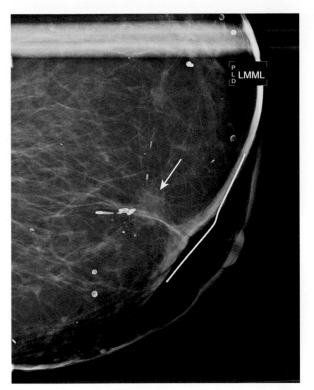

FIGURE 8-8 Spot film of architectural distortion *(arrow)* secondary to a previous lumpectomy. LMML, left magnification mediolateral.

Mammogram views are performed with the catheter in place. The contrast opacifies the duct so that an intraluminal lesion will be visible (Figure 8-11). In order to identify and cannulate the proper duct, the radiologist must be able to express the discharge.

KEY FEATURES

Mammography

- Screening for asymptomatic women, age of onset is controversial, 40 versus 50.
- Diagnostic mammogram for lesions found on screening.
- CAD programs for assisted interpretation.
- Digital (FFDM) performs better than analog (film based).
- Calcifications classified as benign, indeterminate, suspicious.

CAD, computer-aided detection; FFDM, full-field digital mammography.

ULTRASOUND

Breast ultrasound has become an important adjunct to mammography for the detection and diagnosis of breast cancer and for the evaluation of palpable breast masses. Ultrasound technology has advanced with improvements in image quality and resolution, expanding from its initial role in distinguishing cysts from solid masses to its current use in solid mass characterization and biopsy guidance. Ultrasound images are created by the reflection

of sound waves emanating from the ultrasound transducer from the interfaces in the tissue being insonated that return to the transducer and are converted into a gray scale image based on the distance of the reflected interfaces (echoes) from the transducer. The use of sound waves rather than x-rays allows this modality to be used freely in young patients and pregnant women.

In most patients older than 30 years, imaging will begin with mammography, and ultrasound will be used to evaluate a mass seen or suspected on the mammogram or to evaluate a palpable mass that cannot be visualized mammographically. In the case in which a well-defined mass is definitely present on the mammogram, sonography will usually enable the radiologist to determine whether or not it is fluid filled (a cyst or a seroma) or solid. In cases of uncertainty, ultrasound can be used to guide aspiration or biopsy of the lesion. If the lesion is solid, the shape, orientation, internal echogenicity, sound transmission features, vascularity, and margins of the lesion are evaluated to aid in determining the need for biopsy. The decision to biopsy versus follow with imaging surveillance will also be influenced by the risk status of the patient and the presence of other masses. If the abnormality on the mammogram cannot be seen on two orthogonal views, ultrasound will be used to help determine whether it is a true lesion or an area of glandular tissue appearing to be a lesion. If a true mass is present but hidden by glandular tissue on one or both orthogonal mammographic views, it can most often be found with sonography.

Sonographic features of simple cysts include well-defined margins, anechoic contents, and acoustic enhancement (increased sound transmission through the fluid compared with the surrounding tissue) (Figure 8-12). Simple cysts are rarely aspirated except for relief of patient symptoms, and the fluid obtained is often discarded rather than sent for cytologic evaluation. However, some cysts contain internal echoes and are aspirated or percutaneously biopsied to determine whether they are indeed *complicated cysts* or solid masses (Figure 8-13). The aspirate cytology of these complicated cysts does not always contain ductal epithelial cells, leading the pathologist to report the sample as suboptimal. A *complex cyst* is one that contains a mass or has complex internal architecture and will undergo biopsy of the noncystic portion, which may represent an intracystic papilloma or carcinoma (Figure 8-14).

Sonographic features of benign masses, originally reported by Stavros and coworkers,[12] include three or fewer gentle lobulations, orientation parallel to the chest wall, and a thin echogenic pseudocapsule, along with absence of any malignant features. Other features favoring a benign etiology are oval shape, circumscribed borders, and uniform hyperechogenicity (Figure 8-15). However, many benign-appearing masses undergo percutaneous or excisional biopsy because they are new or enlarging and cannot be unequivocally distinguished from well-circumscribed malignancies (Figure 8-16). A very large but well-defined mass is suspect for a phyllodes tumor (Figure 8-17).

If a mass has suspicious features on mammography, ultrasound will be performed to further characterize

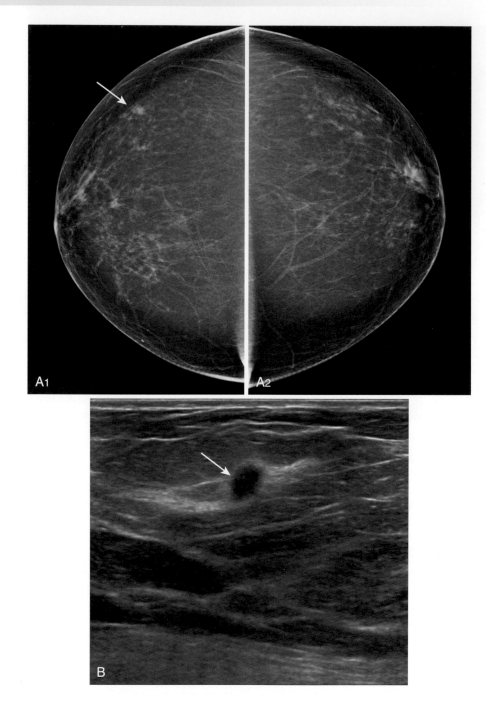

FIGURE 8-9 A1 and **A2,** Small nodule (*arrow* in **A1**) in the anterior right breast on CC view. **B,** Sonogram of a 6-mm invasive carcinoma *(arrow).*

it, to guide percutaneous needle biopsy, and to assess for additional disease in the breast and axilla. Sonographic features associated with invasive carcinoma are irregular shape, marked hypoechogenicity, ill-defined or angular margins, anteroposterior diameter greater than transverse diameter (taller than wide), and acoustic shadowing (greater attenuation of sound by the lesion compared with surrounding tissue, allowing less to pass through it)[13] (Figure 8-18). The appearance of a surgical scar can mimic malignancy, so careful correlation with the mammogram, physical examination, and history is essential (Figure 8-19).

Ultrasound is ideal for evaluation of suspected breast infection, because the patient's breast is often too tender and swollen to tolerate the compression required for mammography. If an abscess (Figure 8-20) is identified, it can be drained with ultrasound guidance, and if there is any question of the area representing a necrotic tumor, its wall can be sampled with ultrasound guidance for pathologic evaluation.

The axillary lymph nodes are well visualized sonographically in most patients, unless they are very deep in a large patient. Diffuse cortical thickening, rounded shape, loss or narrowing of the hilus, and eccentric bulging of the cortex of an axillary node are features that may be seen with reactive or metastatic lymphadenopathy (Figure 8-21).[14] The presence of multiple bilateral abnormally cortically prominent axillary nodes suggests a chronic inflammatory process such as rheumatoid arthritis or a lymphoproliferative disorder.

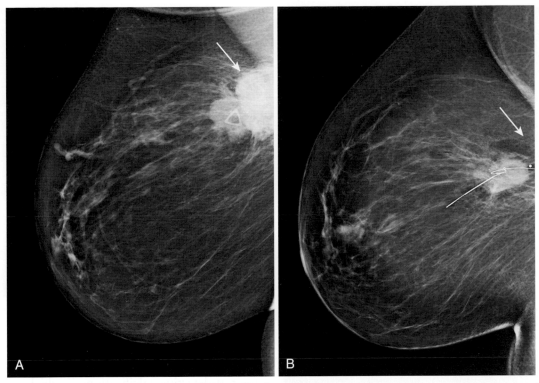

FIGURE 8-10   An oblique view, before **(A)** and after **(B)** 8 months of neoadjuvant chemotherapy *(arrows* mark the known carcinoma, shown to be smaller after neoadjuvant chemotherapy. This allowed for improved cosmesis after a smaller lumpectomy. The after film contains the localizing wire.

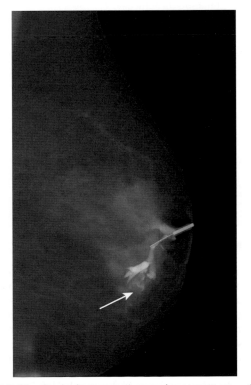

FIGURE 8-11   Single ductogram image shows contrast outlining a lobulated filling defect (papilloma; *arrow*).

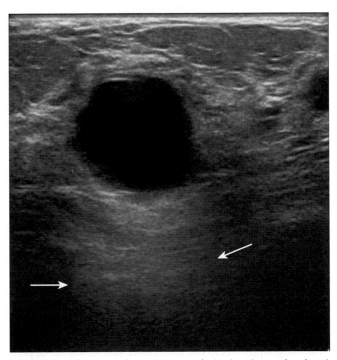

FIGURE 8-12   A simple cyst is anechoic (no internal echoes) because it is fluid filled and has no interfaces within, has smooth walls, and exhibits acoustic enhancement *(arrows)* owing to greater transmission of sound through fluid compared with adjacent tissue, where more sound is absorbed or reflected owing to the multiple interfaces in solid tissue.

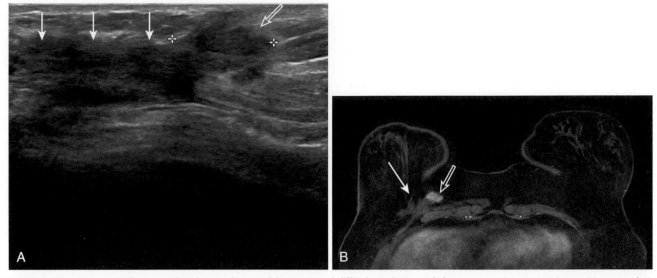

FIGURE 8-19 **A,** A surgical scar is often hypoechoic *(solid arrows)* and difficult to distinguish from a mass *(open arrow),* requiring correlation with the location of the lumpectomy site on mammography and physical examination. **B,** The hypoechoic mass merging with the scar was identified by its enhancement on MRI *(open arrow),* seen medial to the scar *(solid arrow).* Ultrasound-guided core biopsy revealed recurrent IDC.

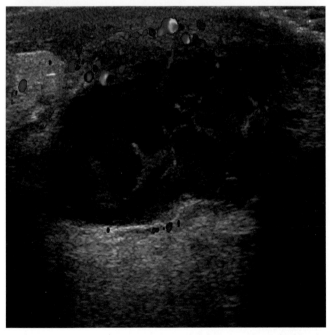

FIGURE 8-20 Sonography of this painful periareolar palpable abscess reveals a 3.5-cm mixed echogenicity lesion from which was aspirated creamy material, which grew *Staphlococcus aureus.*

To perform high-quality MRI of the breast, it is necessary to have hardware and software capable of scanning both breasts simultaneously and within the necessary time constraints of observing the inflow and egress of contrast material. In addition, the scanning protocol must suppress fat because much of the breast is composed of fatty tissue. Scanning parameters must have sufficient spatial resolution to depict the shape and margin so that accurate morphologic characterization is possible. To do this, magnets must have current software and should have a magnetic strength of at least 1.5 Tesla. Dedicated breast coils are critical.

A confounding factor to be considered with MRI is the presence of physiologic enhancement. The enhancement of the breast is subject to change based on the hormonal status during the menstrual cycle or during pregnancy and lactation.[31] At times, physiologic enhancement can mimic cancer. It is, therefore, recommended that, when MRI is completely elective, such as when it is performed for high-risk screening, it should be performed during the first week or so of the menstrual cycle. When a newly diagnosed breast cancer patient is scanned, it may not be possible to wait for the beginning of the cycle because treatment could be delayed. In addition, women who have had hysterectomy are problematic because the menstrual cycle is not apparent. Figures 8-24 and 8-25 demonstrate these points in two different clinical scenarios.

High-risk lesions such as **atypical ductal hyperplasia (ADH)** have a variable MRI appearance. The kinetic features are variable ranging from washout to progressive. Contrast enhancement is thought to be the result of increased microvessel density and/or capillary permeability. The morphology is typically non-mass-like; however, sometimes, these lesions can present as masses.[24,32,33] When ADH is diagnosed by MRI-guided biopsy, recent literature suggests an upgrade rate of approximately 30% to malignancy. This is considerably higher than the upgrade rate of approximately 19% for stereotactic biopsy. According to Liberman and colleagues,[32] this may be related to the fact that the women undergoing MRI are at a higher risk than those routinely undergoing mammography.[33,34] Figure 8-26 demonstrates one appearance of ADH. It is non-masslike with a predominantly plateau pattern enhancement. Similar to high-risk lesions, the kinetic pattern of DCIS is variable. The typical morphologic appearance of DCIS is described as non-masslike clumped linear or segmental enhancement. Occasionally, an enhancing ductal branching pattern or filling defects within

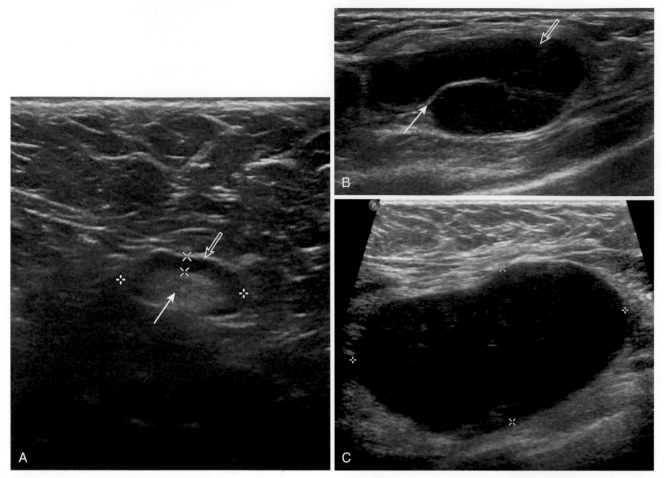

FIGURE 8-21   A, A normal lymph node has a thin cortex *(open arrow)* and a visible hilus *(solid arrow).* An abnormal lymph node has a thickened cortex *(open arrow* in **B**), which may compress the hilus *(solid arrow* in **B**) or render the hilus invisible **(C).** A grossly abnormal lymph node may lose the normal bean shape and smooth margin.

fluid-filled ducts can be identified (Figure 8-27). Similar to mammography and ultrasound, DCIS rarely may present as a mass on MRI. It is not currently possible to reliably predict whether there is a coexistent invasive component or the exact histologic type of DCIS based on the morphology or kinetic characteristics. The sensitivity of MRI for detecting DCIS is lower than for invasive breast cancer, with reported sensitivities ranging from 77% to 96%. The specificity is considered to be similar to that of invasive cancer. MRI is better at depicting high-grade DCIS than low-grade disease. It is better at demonstrating high-grade DCIS without necrosis than mammography because DCIS is most frequently detected when the mammogram demonstrates calcifications. Unfortunately, it is well known that microcalcifications identified mammographically are often nonspecific. Because MRI does not detect DCIS by imaging the calcium, it is difficult at times to make a direct correlation between the mammogram and the MRI; therefore, at present, MRI and mammography are complementary tests.[35–40] Figure 8-28 shows malignant calcifications on a mammogram and the MRI demonstrates malignant morphology typical of DCIS.

One of the most common uses of breast MRI is to evaluate for **extent of disease** in patients with biopsy-proven breast cancer. Liberman and associates,[41] in a study across multiple series, reported that up to 48% of women with breast cancer will have unsuspected additional cancer that was not expected from mammography. This could be either multifocal or multicentric disease. MRI has been reported to depict additional tumors that necessitated wider excision in 27% to 34% of patients.[41–43] Berg and coworkers[42] point out that this closely mirrors the 25% to 36% rate of local recurrence in patients treated without chemotherapy or radiation therapy.[44] MRI is relatively accurate at estimating tumor size but can overestimate and underestimate size on average by 15 mm in approximately 48% and 40%, respectively. Because the size variation between MRI and pathologic truth is relatively small, it is unlikely to have clinical implications.[24] Lobular cancer is especially difficult to evaluate because it is well known that mammography, physical examination, and ultrasound tend to underestimate the extent and size of the tumors.[42,45] Perhaps just as important, Lehman and colleagues[46] reported that approximately 3% of women will have an unsuspected cancer in the contralateral breast (Figure 8-29).

Despite the belief by most of the imaging community that breast MRI is a valuable staging tool, there are critics who believe that MRI may cause overestimation and overtreatment of breast cancer with no significant a specimen sonogram is necessary to confirm removal of the lesion.

NEW METHODS ON THE HORIZON

The future holds promise by virtue of enhancements of conventional imaging techniques and novel molecular imaging approaches. *Digital breast tomosynthesis (DBT)* or three-dimensional tomography is essentially FFDM (full-field digital mammography) with the ability to examine the breast with thin (1-mm) sections. By removing overlapping structures, DBT helps to differentiate true lesions from summation densities and also helps to delineate the margins of lesions, which may help to increase the specificity of mammography (e.g., the differentiation of benign from malignant lesions). To date, DBT has not been shown to increase the sensitivity of mammography for finding additional breast cancers, but it has been shown to decrease the recall rate in screening mammography by approximately 30% when used in combination with standard two dimensional mammography.[75,76] The DBT machine is essentially a modified mammography unit with a moving x-ray tube. Another related technology that does sectional imaging of the breast is *cone-beam CT*. Cone-beam CT creates high-resolution tomographic images of the breast using CT technology. Initial reports show high-quality images that may be

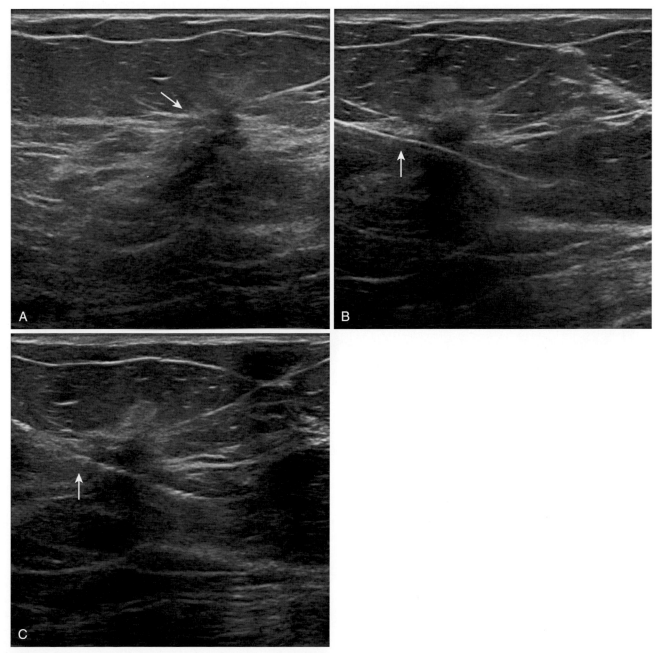

FIGURE 8-41 Ultrasound-guided needle localization. **A,** The carcinoma is sonographically visualized *(arrow)*. The needle *(arrow* in **B**) is passed through it then removed, leaving the wire *(arrow* in **C**) traversing the mass.

Continued

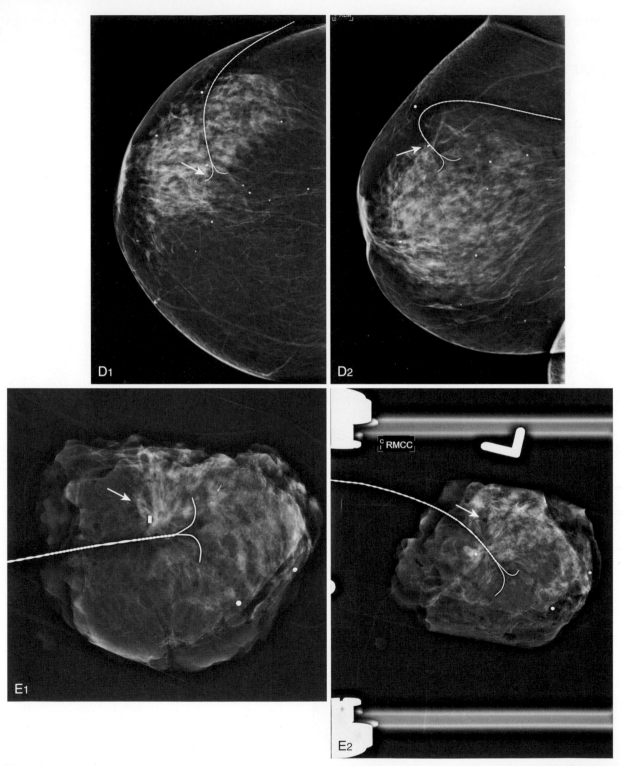

FIGURE 8-41, cont'd   D1 and **D2,** CC and mediolateral radiographs show the wire and clip *(arrows)* that had been placed at the time of biopsy. **E1** and **E2,** The mass is not well seen in the mammogram views but is visible as a spiculated lesion *(arrows)* on the two-view specimen radiograph.

viewed using contrast enhancement.[77] Women would likely prefer this test owing to its lack of compression, which is necessary with conventional mammography or DBT.

Another advancement of an existing technology is *elastography*. Using the underlying premise that malignant tissue is less compressible than benign tissue,

such as complex cysts, elastography uses ultrasound to measure the compressive force of tissue. This should theoretically increase the specificity of conventional ultrasound.[78]

Radiology begins to merge with pathology as we enter the realm of molecular imaging. One such technology is positron-emission mammography (PEM). PEM

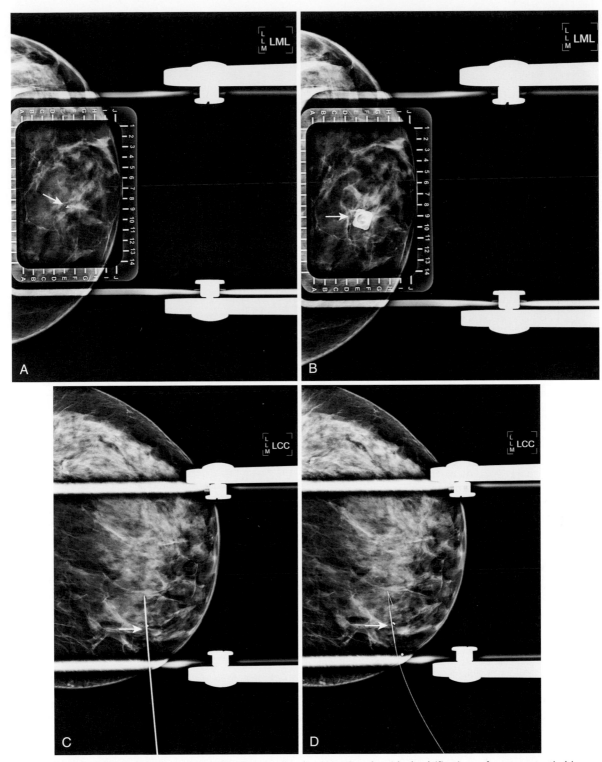

FIGURE 8-42 Mammography-guided needle localization. **A,** The clip *(arrow)* and residual calcifications after stereotactic biopsy revealed DCIS are located mammographically using the alphanumeric grid. **B,** The needle placement *(arrow),* with the hub seen en face, is confirmed. **C,** The orthogonal view shows the distance from the tip of the needle to the lesion *(arrow on the clip).* **D,** The needle is removed, leaving the wire in place *(arrow).*

uses PET agents, which are radiolabeled glucose molecules used to measure tumor metabolism. In the future, PET scans may be fused with cone-beam CT, which may be even more useful because the functional information provided by PET can be viewed with the anatomic imaging gleaned from CT.[64,79]

SUMMARY

This chapter presents the pathologist with the tools necessary to comprehend the critical information that the radiologist gathers and presents to the pathologist, so that there can be complete radiographic-pathologic

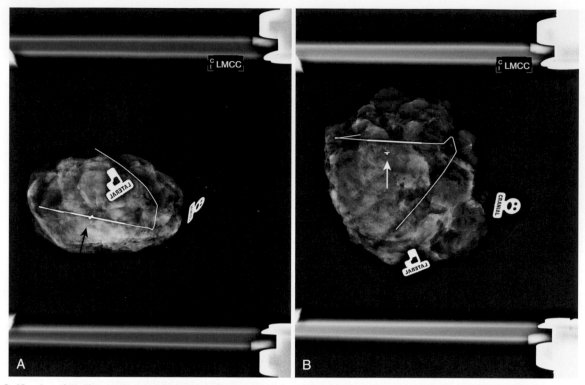

FIGURE 8-43 **A** and **B,** The specimen radiograph in two projections shows the wire, clip *(arrows),* and residual calcifications and their location relative to the margins of the specimen. Note the metallic markers placed on the specimen by the surgeon to help the radiologist and pathologist orient the specimen. LMCC, left magnification craniocaudal.

correlation of breast specimens to optimize patient care and patient safety. The future suggests closer ties between radiology and pathology, as imaging and molecular flow studies blur the boundaries for these two disciplines.

REFERENCES

1. Calonge N, Petitti DB, DeWitt TG, et al. Screening for breast cancer: US Preventive Services Task Force recommendation statement. Ann Intern Med 2009;151:I44.
2. Adams AM, Jong RA, Barr RG, et al. Reasons women at elevated risk of breast cancer refuse breast MR imaging screening: ACRIN 6666. Radiology 2010;254:79-87.
3. Bassett LW, Gold RH. The evolution of mammography. AJR Am J Roentgenol 1988;150:493-498.
4. Gromet M. Comparison of computer-aided detection to double reading of screening mammograms: review of 231,221 mammograms. AJR Am J Roentgenol 2008;190:854-859.
5. Destounis SV, DiNitto P, Logan-Young W, et al. Can computer-aided detection with double reading of screening mammograms help decrease the false-negative rate? Initial experience. Radiology 2004;232:578-584.
6. Zheng B, Lu A, Hardesty LA, et al. A method to improve visual similarity of breast masses for an interactive computer-aided diagnosis environment. Med Phys 2006;33:111-117.
7. Gur D, Stalder JS, Hardesty LA, et al. Computer-aided detection performance in mammographic examination of masses: Assessment. Radiology 2004;233:418-423.
8. The JS, Schilling KJ, Hoffmeister JW, et al. Detection of breast cancer with full-field digital mammography and computer-aided detection. AJR Am J Roentgenol 2009;192:337-340.
9. Pisano ED, Gatsonis CA, Yaffe MJ, et al. American College of Radiology Imaging Network digital mammographic imaging screening trial: objectives and methodology. Radiology 2005;236:404-412.
10. Pisano ED, Hendrick RE, Yaffe MJ, et al. DMIST Investigators Group. Diagnostic accuracy of digital versus film mammography: exploratory analysis of selected population subgroups in DMIST. Radiology 2008;246:376-383.
11. Hendrick RE, Pisano ED, Averbukh A, et al. Comparison of acquisition parameters and breast dose in digital mammography and screen-film mammography in the American College of Radiology imaging network digital mammographic imaging screening trial. AJR Am J Roentgenol 2010;194:362-369.
12. Stavros AT, Thickman D, Rapp CL, et al. Solid breast nodules: use of sonography to distinguish between benign and malignant lesions. Radiology 1995;196:123-134.
13. Raza S, Goldkamp AL, Chikarmane SA, Birdwell RA. US of breast masses categorized as BI-RADS 3, 4, and 5: pictorial review of factors influencing clinical management. Radiographics 2010;30:1199-1213.
14. Vassallo P, Wernecke K, Roos N, Peters PE. Differentiation of benign from malignant lymphadenopathy: the role of high-resolution US. Radiology 1992;183:215-220.
15. Mandelson MT, Osetreicher N, Porter PL. Breast density as a predictor of mammographic detection: comparison of interval and screen detected cancers. J Natl Cancer Inst 2000;92:1081-1087.
16. Porter G, Evans A, Cornford E, et al. Influence of mammographic parenchymal pattern in screening detected and interval invasive breast cancers on pathologic features, mammographic features, and patient survival. AJR Am J Roentgenol 2007;188:676-683.
17. Boyd NF, Guo H, Marin LJ, et al. Mammographic density and the risk and detection of breast cancer. N Engl J Med 2007;356:227-236.
18. Harvey JA, Bovberg VE. Quantitative assessment of breast density: relationship with breast cancer risk. Radiology 2004;230:29-41.
19. Nothacker M, Duda V, Hahn M, et al. Early detection of breast cancer: benefits and risks of supplemental breast ultrasound in asymptomatic women with mammographically dense breast tissue. A systematic review. BMC Cancer 2009;9:335.

20. Berg WA, Blume JD, Cormack JB, et al. Combined screening with ultrasound and mammography compared to mammography alone in women with elevated risk of breast cancer: results of the first-year screen in ACRIN 6666. JAMA 2008;299:2151-2163.
21. Soo M, Baker J, Rosen E. Sonographic detection and sonographically guided biopsy of breast calcification. AJR Am J Roentgenol 2003;180:941-948.
22. Kuhl CH. The current status of breast MR imaging part 1. Choice of technique, image interpretation, diagnostic accuracy, and transfer to clinical practice. Radiology 2007;244:356-378.
23. Schnall MD, Blume J, Bluemke DA, et al. Diagnostic architectural and dynamic features at breast MR imaging: multicenter study. Radiology 2006;238:42-52.
24. Baltzer PAT, Benndorf M, Dietzel M, et al. False-positive findings at contrast-enhanced breast MRI: a BI-RADS descriptor study. AJR Am J Roentgenol 2010;194:1658-1663.
25. Bazzocchi M, Zuiani C, Panizza P, et al. Contrast-enhanced breast MRI in patients with suspicious micro-calcifications on mammography: results of a multicenter trial. AJR Am J Roentgenol 2006;186:1723-1732.
26. Heywang-Köbrunner SH, Viehweg P, Heinig A, et al. Contrast-enhanced MRI of the breast: accuracy, value, controversies, solutions. Eur J Radiol 1997;24:94-108.
27. Szabo BK, Aspelin P, Kristoffersen Wiberg M, et al. Dynamic MR imaging of the breast. Acta Radiol 2003;44:379-386.
28. Schnall MD, Rosten S, Englander S, et al. A combined architectural and kinetic interpretation model for breast MR images. Acad Radiol 2001;8:591-597.
29. Kuhl CK, Schild HH, Morakkabati N. Dynamic bilateral contrast-enhanced MR imaging of the breast: trade off between spatial and temporal resolution. Radiology 2005;236:789-800.
30. Williams TC, DeMartini WB, Partridge SC, et al. Breast MR imaging: computer-aided evaluation program for discriminating benign from malignant lesions. Radiology 2007;244:94-104.
31. Ellis RL. Optimal timing of breast MRI examinations of premenopausal women who do not have a normal menstrual cycle. AJR Am J Roentgenol 2009;193:1738-1740.
32. Liberman L, Holland AE, Marjan D, et al. Underestimation of atypical ductal hyperplasia at MRI-guided 9-gauge vacuum-assisted breast biopsy. AJR Am J Roentgenol 2007;188:684-690.
33. Strigel RM, Eby PR, DeMartini WB, et al. Frequency, upgrade rates, and characteristics of high-risk lesions initially identified with breast MRI. AJR Am J Roentgenol 2010;195:792-798.
34. Jackman RJ, Birwell BL, Ikeda DM. Atypical ductal hyperplasia: can some lesions be defined as probably benign after stereotactic 11-gauge vacuum-assisted biopsy, eliminating the recommendation for surgical excision? Radiology 2002;224:548-554.
35. Kuhl CK, Schrading S, Bieling HB, et al. MRI for diagnosis of pure ductal carcinoma in situ: a prospective observational study. Lancet 2007;370:485-492.
36. Esserman LJ, Kumar AS, Herrera AF, et al. Magnetic resonance imaging captures the biology of ductal carcinoma in situ. J Clin Oncol 2006;24:4603-4610.
37. Orel SG, Mendonca MH, Reynolds C, et al. MR imaging of ductal carcinoma in situ. Radiology 1997;202:413-420.
38. Jansen SA, Newstead GM, Abe H, et al. Pure ductal carcinoma in situ: kinetic and morphologic MR characteristics compared with mammographic appearance and nuclear grade. Radiology 2007;245:684-691.
39. Raza S, Vallejo M, Chikarmane SA, et al. Pure ductal carcinoma in situ: a range of MRI features. AJR Am J Roentgenol 2008;191:689-699.
40. Kuhl CK. Science to practice: why do purely intraductal cancers enhance on breast MR images? Radiology 2009;253:281-284.
41. Liberman L, Morris EA, Dershaw DD, et al. MR imaging of the ipsilateral breast in women with percutaneously proven breast cancer. AJR Am J Roentgenol 2003;180:901-910.
42. Berg WA, Gutierrez L, Nessaiver MS, et al. Diagnostic accuracy of mammography, clinical examination, US and MR imaging in preoperative assessment of breast cancer. Radiology 2004;233:830-849.
43. Orel SG, Schnall MD, Powell CM, et al. Staging of suspected breast cancer: effect of MR imaging and MR-guided biopsy. Radiology 1995;196:115-122.
44. Fisher ER, Anderson S, Tan-Chiu E, et al. Fifteen-year prognostic discriminants for invasive breast carcinoma. Cancer 2001;91:1679-1687.
45. Hilleren DJ, Andersson IT, Lindholm K, et al. Invasive lobular carcinoma; mammographic findings in a 10-year experience. Radiology 1991;178:149-154.
46. Lehman CD, Gatsonis C, Kuhl CK, et al. MRI evaluation of the contralateral breast in women with recently diagnosed breast cancer. N Engl J Med 2007;356:1295-1303.
47. Turnbull L, Brown S, Harvey I, et al. Comparative effectiveness of MRI in breast cancer (COMICE) trial: a randomised controlled trial. Lancet 2010;375:563-571.
48. Katipamula R, Degnim AC, Hoskin T, et al. Trends in mastectomy rates at the Mayo Clinic Rochester: Effect of surgical year and preoperative magnetic resonance imaging. J Clin Oncol 2009;27:4082-4088.
49. Yuan Y, Chen XS, Liu SY, et al. Accuracy of MRI in prediction of pathologic complete remission in breast cancer after preoperative therapy: a meta-analysis. AJR Am J Roentgenol 2010;195:260-268.
50. Rosen EL, Blackwell KL, Baker JA, et al. Accuracy of MRI in the detection of residual breast cancer after neoadjuvant chemotherapy. AJR Am J Roentgenol 2003;181:1275-1282.
51. Kuhl CK. Current status of breast MR imaging part 2, clinical applications. Radiology 2007;244:672-692.
52. Kriege M, Brekelmans CTM, Boetes C, et al. Efficacy of MRI and mammography for breast-cancer screening in women with a familial or genetic predisposition. N Engl J Med 2004;351:427-437.
53. Smith RA, Saslow D, Sawyer KA, et al. American Cancer Society guidelines for breast cancer screening: update 2003. CA Cancer J Clin 2003;53:141-169.
54. Lee CH, Dershaw DD, Kopans D, et al. Breast cancer screening with imaging: recommendations from the Society of Breast Imaging and the ACR on the use of mammography, breast MRI, breast ultrasound, and other technologies for the detection of clinically occult breast cancer. J Am Coll Radiol 2010;7:18-27.
55. DeMartini WB, Eby PR, Peacock S, Lehman CD. Utility of targeted sonography for breast lesions that were suspicious on MRI. AJR Am J Roentgenol 2009;192:1128-1134.
56. Jardines L, Fowble B, Schultz D, et al. Factors associated with a positive re-excision after excisional biopsy for invasive breast cancer. Surgery 1995;118:803-809.
57. Gwin JL, Eisenberg BL, Hoffman JP, et al. Incidence of gross and microscopic carcinoma in specimens from patients with breast cancer after re-excision lumpectomy. Ann Surg 1993;218:729-734.
58. Solin LJ, Fowble B, Martz K, et al. Results of re-excisional biopsy of the primary tumor in preparation for definitive irradiation of patients with early stage breast cancer. Int J Radiat Oncol Biol Phys 1985;11:721-725.
59. Schnitt SJ, Connolly JL, Khettry U, et al. Pathologic findings on re-excision of the primary site in breast cancer patients considered for treatment by primary radiation therapy. Cancer 1987;59:675-681.
60. McCormick B, Kinne D, Petrek J, et al. Limited resection for breast cancer: a study of inked specimen margins before radiotherapy. Int J Radiat Oncol Biol Phys 1987;13:1667-1671.
61. Lee JM, Orel SG, Czerniecki BJ, et al. MRI before reexcision surgery in patients with breast cancer. AJR Am J Roentgenol 2004;182:473-480.
62. Brem RF, Floerke AC, Rapelyea JA, et al. Breast-specific gamma imaging as an adjunct imaging modality for the diagnosis of breast cancer. Radiology 2008;247:651-657.
63. Klaus AJ, Klingensmith III WC, Parker SH, et al. Comparative value of ^{99m}Tc-sestamibi scintimammography and sonography in the diagnostic workup of breast masses. AJR Am J Roentgenol 2000;174:1779-1783.
64. Rosen EL, Eubank WB, Mankoff DA. FDG PET, PET/CT, and breast cancer imaging. Radiographics 2007;27(Suppl 1):S215-S229.
65. Kim T, Guiliano AM, Lyman GH. Lymphatic mapping and sentinel lymph node biopsy in early-stage breast carcinoma. A meta analysis. Cancer 2006;106:4-16.

66. Philpotts LE, Hooley RJ, Lee CH. Comparison of automated versus vacuum assisted biopsy methods for sonographically guided core biopsy of the breast. AJR Am J Roentgenol 2003;180:347-351.

67. Semiz OA, Kaya H, Gulluoglu B, Aribal E. Comparison of sonographically guided vacuum-assisted and automated core-needle breast biopsy methods. Tani Girisim Radyol 2004;10:44-47.

68. Breuning W, Fontanarosa J, Tipton K, et al. Systematic review: comparative effectiveness of core needle and open surgical biopsy to diagnose breast lesions. Ann Intern Med 2010;152:238-246.

69. Cho N, Moon WK, Cha JH. Sonographically guided core biopsy of the breast: comparison of 14-gauge automated gun and 11-gauge directional vacuum-assisted biopsy methods. Korean J Radiol 2005;6:102-109.

70. O'Flynn EAM, Wilson ARM, Mitchell MJ. Image-guided breast biopsy: state of the art. Clin Radiol 2010;65:259-270.

71. Pisano ED, Fajardo LL, Caudry DJ, et al. Fine-needle aspiration biopsy of nonpalpable breast lesions in a multicenter clinical trial: results from the Radiologic Diagnostic Oncology Group V. Radiology 2001;219:785-792.

72. Oruwari JU, Chung MA, Koeliker S, et al. Axillary staging using ultrasound-guided fine needle aspiration biopsy in locally advanced breast cancer. Am J Surg 2002;184:307-309.

73. Koeliker SL, Chung MA, Maniero MB, et al. Axillary lymph nodes: US-guided fine-needle aspiration for initial staging of breast cancer—correlation with primary tumor size. Radiology 2008;246:81-89.

74. Hiroyuki A, Schmidt R, Kulkami K, et al. Axillary lymph nodes suspicious for breast cancer metastasis: sampling with US guided 14-gauge core-needle biopsy—clinical experience in 100 patients. Radiology 2009;250:41-49.

75. Hakim CH, Chough DM, Ganott MA, et al. Digital breast tomosynthesis in the diagnostic environment: a subjective side-by-side review. AJR Am J Roentgenol 2010;195:172-176.

76. Gur D, Abrams GS, Chough DM, et al. Digital breast tomosynthesis: observer performance study. AJR Am J Roentgenol 2009;193:586-591.

77. O'Connell A, Conover DL, Zhang Y, et al. Cone-beam CT for breast imaging: Radiation dose, breast coverage, and image quality. AJR Am J Roentgenol 2010;195:496-509.

78. Ginat DT, Destouis SV, Barr RG, et al. US elastography of breast and prostate lesions. Radiographics 2009;29:2007-2016.

79. MacDonald L, Edwards J, Lewellen T, et al. Clinical imaging characteristics of the positron emission mammography camera: PEM Flex Solo II. J Nucl Med 2009;50:1666-1675.

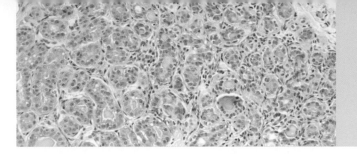

Predictive and Prognostic Marker Testing in Breast Pathology: Immunophenotypic Subclasses of Disease

D. Craig Allred • Rohit Bhargava • David J. Dabbs

INTRODUCTION

This chapter is divided into three main sections that include discussion of well-known prognostic/predictive markers, namely, steroid hormone receptors (estrogen and progesterone) and one of the most well studied oncogenes in breast cancer, HER2 (ERBB2). These two sections are followed by a brief discussion of other relevant single gene or gene products that are being increasing assessed in breast cancer. The discussion is mainly focused on analysis of these single gene/gene products within breast cancer tissue specimens. Other recently described multigene predictors are discussed in Chapter 20.

HORMONE RECEPTORS IN BREAST CARCINOMA

Estrogen receptor-alpha (ER-α) and progesterone receptor (PgR) are prognostic and predictive biomarkers that play a major role in determining the therapy of patients with invasive breast cancer (IBC). In this setting, the term *prognostic* refers to factors associated with the innate aggressiveness of untreated IBCs and, if adverse enough, usually results in the use of additional (i.e., adjuvant) therapies after surgery. *Predictive* refers to factors associated with the responsiveness of IBCs to specific types of adjuvant therapies. Many biomarkers have both prognostic and predictive significance to varying degrees. ER-α and PgR are weak prognostic factors but very strong predictive factors of response to endocrine therapies. It is currently mandatory to evaluate ER-α and PgR in all IBCs for the purpose of predicting therapeutic response. In current practice, immunohistochemistry (IHC) on formalin-fixed paraffin-embedded tissue (FFPET) samples is the primary method used to evaluate ER-α and PgR.

The American Society of Clinical Oncology (ASCO) and College of American Pathologists (CAP) recently jointly published guidelines for ER-α and PgR testing in breast cancer, recommending that specific IHC assays must be rigorously standardized and validated to be utilized in routine clinical practice (Table 9-1).[1] Adherence to these guidelines is now mandatory for laboratory accreditation by the CAP, which also provides many educational and support materials to facilitate compliance.

Estrogen Receptor-Alpha

ER-α is a nuclear transcription factor activated by the hormone estrogen to regulate the development, growth, and differentiation of normal breast tissue.[2–4] These pathways remain active to varying degrees in IBCs, including estrogen-stimulated growth of tumor epithelial cells expressing ER-α, which can be detrimental to patients.[3–5] ER-α expression has been evaluated in IBCs since the 1970s. Until the mid 1990s, it was primarily

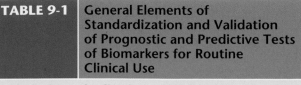

TABLE 9-1	General Elements of Standardization and Validation of Prognostic and Predictive Tests of Biomarkers for Routine Clinical Use

Technical Standardization and Validation—The Test is

Highly specific for the analyte.
Highly sensitive for the analyte.
Reproducible
- Confirmed by comprehensive ongoing quality assurance.
- Confirmed by comprehensive ongoing proficiency testing (true expertise).
Scored in a comprehensive and uniform manner.

Clinical Validation

The test identifies patients with significantly different risks of relapse, survival, and/or response to therapy.
Positive versus negative results (interpretation) are calibrated to values corresponding to optimal clinical outcome.
Clinical utility is demonstrated and confirmed in multiple comprehensive and well-designed studies (ideally, randomized clinical trials).
The test is used in clinical practice to determine therapy.

TABLE 9-2	Examples of Standardized Immunohistochemical Assays for Evaluating Estrogen Receptor-Alpha and Progesterone Receptor in Breast Cancers That Have Been Validated in a Comprehensive Manner

Reference	Primary Antibody	Definition of "Positive"
Estrogen Receptor		
Harvey, 1999[17]	6F11	Allred score ≥ 3 (1–10% weakly positive cells)
Cheang, 2006[27]	SP1	≥1%
Regan, 2006[31] Viale, 2007[15] Viale, 2008[33]	1D5	1–9% (low) and ≥ 10% (high)
Phillips, 2007[30]	ER.2.123 + 1D5 (cocktail)	Allred score ≥ 3
Dowsett, 2008[28]	6F11	H-score >1 (equivalent to ≥ 1%)
Progesterone Receptor		
Mohsin, 2004[29]	1294	Allred score ≥ 3
Regan, 2006[31] Viale, 2007[15] Viale, 2008[33]	1A6	1–9% (low) and ≥ 10% (high)
Phillips, 2007[30]	1294	Allred score ≥ 3

measured by biochemical ligand-binding assays (LBAs) on whole tissue extracts prepared from fresh-frozen tumor samples, which was costly and difficult. Many studies using LBAs in large randomized clinical trials demonstrated that ER-α was a weak prognostic factor but a very strong predictive factor for response to endocrine therapies such as tamoxifen.[5] Tamoxifen binds ER-α and inhibits the estrogen-stimulated growth of tumor cells, which significantly reduces cancer recurrences and prolongs survival in patients with ER-α–positive IBCs of all stages.[5–10] More recently, tamoxifen has also been shown to reduce subsequent breast cancer in patients with ER-α–positive ductal carcinoma in situ (DCIS)[11] and in patients who are cancer-free but at high risk for developing breast cancer.[12] The clinical response to newer types of endocrine therapies, such as the aromatase inhibitors, which suppress the production of estrogen, is also dependent on the status of ER-α, and only positive tumors benefit.[13–16]

Although the clinical utility of assessing ER-α was initially based almost entirely on studies using standardized LBAs, beginning in the early 1990s, laboratories around the world abandoned LBAs in favor of IHC, which is used for nearly all testing today. There are advantages to using IHC over LBAs, especially its ability to measure ER-α on routine FFPET samples, eliminating the need for fresh-frozen samples and the burdensome infrastructure required to provide it. Other advantages include lower cost, higher safety, and superior sensitivity and specificity (providing it is done correctly) because assessment of ER-α expression is restricted to tumor cells under direct microscopic visualization—independent of the numbers of tumor cells present or the presence of receptor-positive benign epithelium, which are problematic for LBAs. Several head-to-head comparisons have demonstrated that assessing ER-α by IHC can be equivalent to or better than LBAs in predicting response to

endocrine therapy,[1,17,18] which is comforting, because IHC replaced LBA before such proof was available.

IHC was approved in the 1990s by the CAP and ASCO for routine clinical testing of ER-α and PgR.[8] Despite these approvals, there were significant problems with the technical and clinical validation of IHC that persist today, resulting in inaccurate interpretations (i.e., positive vs. negative) in 20% or more of cases.[19–24] Most of the errors are false negatives, which is potentially catastrophic because the patients involved will usually not get the endocrine therapy that would greatly improve their outcome.

There are many causes and no easy solutions to the problem of inaccurate testing, although there are useful guidelines and recommendations intended to help avoid mistakes including, in particular, those more recently published by ASCO and CAP.[1,25,26] Surprisingly, there are relatively few IHC assays for ER-α or PgR that entirely satisfy all of these guidelines and recommendations, although a few come close[17,27–33] (Table 9-2). The strategy published by Harvey and colleagues[17] was among the first to be well validated (Figure 9-1). It is based on a highly specific and sensitive primary antibody to ER-α (mouse monoclonal 6F11), a quantitative and reproducible method of scoring results (the so-called Allred score [Figure 9-2]), and a definition of positive results calibrated to clinical outcome in several large studies, including randomized clinical trials. The latter

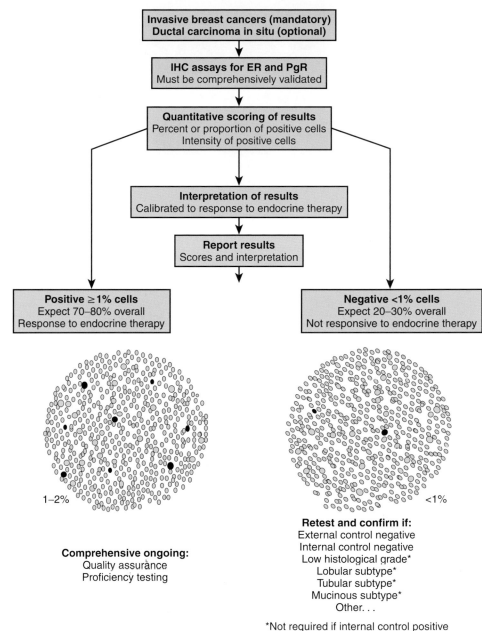

FIGURE 9-1 Overview of guideline recommendations for immunohistochemical testing of estrogen and progesterone receptors in breast cancer by the American Society of Clinical Oncology and College of American Pathologists.[1] ER, estrogen receptor; IHC, immunohistochemical; PgR, progesterone receptor.

involved patients with all stages of breast cancer treated with tamoxifen or aromatase inhibitors in adjuvant, neoadjuvant, and advanced disease settings.[11,17,18,34,35] It is extremely difficult to standardize and validate IHC assays for ER-α and PgR in a comprehensive manner, but any laboratory can utilize assays that have already been validated.

Studies evaluating ER-α by IHC in breast cancer collectively demonstrate that about 75% to 80% express ER-α, that it is almost entirely nuclear in location, and that there is tremendous variation of expression on a continuum ranging from 0% to nearly 100% positive cells (Figure 9-3).[36] More importantly, they show a direct correlation between the likelihood of clinical response to endocrine therapies and the level of ER-α expression.[17] Surprisingly, the gradient is skewed such that tumors expressing even very low levels show a

significant benefit far above that of entirely ER-α–negative tumors, which are essentially unresponsive. This evidence provides support for laboratories adopting 1% or greater positive-staining tumor cells as the definition of "ER-α–positive," which has now been validated in several other comprehensive studies and is endorsed by the ASCO/CAP guidelines.[1,14,15,17,27,29,30,33]

Two studies have reported an essentially bimodal (either entirely negative or strongly positive) distribution of ER-α assessed by IHC in IBCs, leading some to conclude that reporting results as simply positive or negative is sufficient,[37,38] but these assays do not reflect the quantitative continuum that is expected for a proper technically validated assay. There does appear to be a recent shift toward an increasing incidence of ER-positive IBCs, which may be partially due to earlier detection before additional genetic alterations are acquired

SCORING IMMUNOSTAINED SLIDES

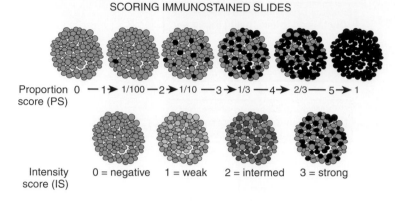

Proportion 0 — 1➤ 1/100 —2➤ 1/10 —3➤ 1/3 —4➤ 2/3 — 5➤ 1
score (PS)

Intensity   0 = negative   1 = weak   2 = intermed   3 = strong
score (IS)

Total score (TS) = PS + IS (range 0–8)

Modern pathol 11(2):155-168, 1998.

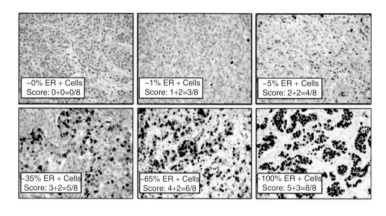

~0% ER + Cells
Score: 0+0=0/8

~1% ER + Cells
Score: 1+2=3/8

~5% ER + Cells
Score: 2+2=4/8

~35% ER + Cells
Score: 3+2=5/8

~65% ER + Cells
Score: 4+2=6/8

~100% ER + Cells
Score: 5+3=8/8

FIGURE 9-2 Diagram illustrating the Allred scoring method for quantifying IHC results for estrogen receptor (ER) and PgR in breast cancers. The score is assigned based on evaluating all tumor cells on the slide. The illustrations demonstrate the broad range of Allred scores observed in breast cancers. *From Allred DC, et al. Prognostic and predictive factors in breast cancer by immunohistochemical analysis. Mod Pathol 1998;11:155-168.*

Allred score	LBA (fmol/mg)	#Patients (%)
0	10	517 (26%)
2	50	67 (3%)
3	59	117 (6%)
4	67	190 (10%)
5	104	320 (16%)
6	141	370 (19%)
7	193	318 (16%)
8	282	83 (4%)

Near-linear correlation with LBA

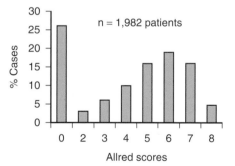

Wide distribution expression

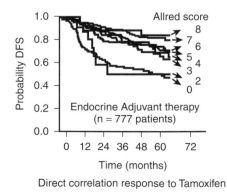

Direct correlation response to Tamoxifen

	DFS		OS		
	HR	p-val	HR	p-val	
No Rx	0.90	0.48	0.76	0.06	IHC:
(n = 688)	0.74	0.62	0.79	0.0001	LBA:
Chemo	1.01	0.96	0.97	0.86	IHC:
(n = 404)	0.97	0.86	0.82	0.23	LBA:
Chemo	0.56	0.008	0.50	0.004	IHC:
+Endo	0.51	0.01	0.58	0.05	LBA:
(n = 260)					
Endo	0.47	0.0008	0.35	0.0001	IHC:
(n = 517)	0.71	0.32	0.38	0.0003	LBA:

Multivariate analyses

FIGURE 9-3 Summary of ER results from a study by Harvey and colleagues. In this large retrospective study, there is a near-linear correlation between immunohistochemical (IHC) and ligand-binding-assay (LBA) ER results, a broad distribution of IHC ("Allred") scores, a skewed but direct correlation between Allred scores and improved disease-free survival (DFS) in patients treated with adjuvant hormonal therapy (primarily tamoxifen), and significantly stronger prediction of response to hormonal therapy associated with ER by IHC vs. LBA. HR, hazard ratio; OS, overall survival. *From Harvey JM, et al. Estrogen receptor status by immunohistochemistry is superior to the ligand-binding assay for predicting response to adjuvant endocrine therapy in breast cancer. J Clin Oncol 1999;17:1474-1481.*

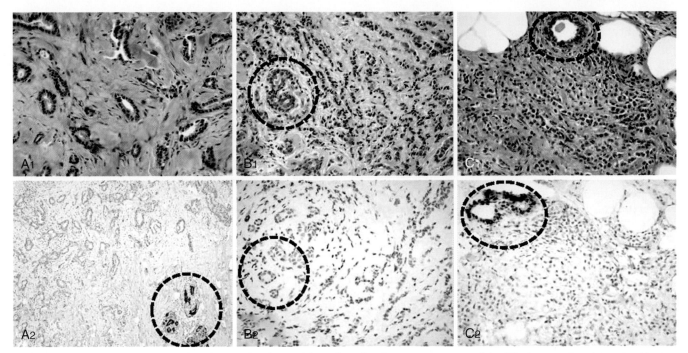

FIGURE 9-4 Representative examples of unusual and unanticipated results of estrogen receptor-alpha (ER-α) expression determined by immunohistochemistry in invasive breast cancers. **A1** and **A2**, Invasive tubular carcinoma, which is ER-α–negative but accurate and does not need to be confirmed because the normal internal control cells are ER-α–positive. **B1** and **B2**, Invasive lobular carcinoma that is apparently ER-α–negative but needs to be confirmed because normal internal control cells are also ER-α–negative. **C1** and **C2**, Invasive lobular carcinoma, which is ER-α–negative and does not need to be confirmed because the normal internal control cells are ER-α–positive.

TABLE 9-3	Approximate Average Percent Expression of Estrogen Receptor-Alpha in Common Types of Normal, Benign, and Malignant Categories of Breast Tissue														
	TDLU	CCH	ADH	ALH	DCIS	LCIS	IDC	ILC	ITC	IMUC	IMED	LUM A	LUM B	HER 2+	Basal
ER-α+	>90	>90	>90	>90	75	>90	75	>90	>90	>90	<10	>80	>90	<10	<5
ER-α+ cells	30	90	90	90	V	90	V	90	90	90	V	NA	NA	NA	NA

ADH, atypical ductal hyperplasia; ALH, atypical lobular hyperplasia; Basal, basal molecular subtype; CCH, columnar cell hyperplasia; DCIS, ductal carcinoma in situ; ER-α+, average % category expressing any ER-α; ER-α+ cells, average % cells within category expressing ER-α; IDC, invasive ductal carcinoma; ILC, invasive lobular carcinoma; IMED, invasive medullary carcinoma; IMUC, invasive mucinous carcinoma; ITC, invasive tubular carcinoma; LCIS, lobular carcinoma in situ; LUM A, luminal A molecular subtype; LUM B, luminal B molecular subtype; NA, not available; TDLU, normal terminal duct lobular unit; V, variable (ranging from 1–100%).

resulting in loss of expression.[39–41] However, many IHC assays today are also far too sensitive, obscuring any underlying continuum of expression.[42] This is unfortunate because accurate quantitative results provide patients and their physicians with more precise predictions of response to therapy, which can greatly influence therapeutic decisions. For example, clinical trials have demonstrated that postmenopausal patients with node-positive IBCs expressing high levels of ER-α may forego the rigors of adjuvant chemotherapy and experience equivalent benefit with endocrine therapy alone.[6]

The ASCO/CAP guidelines for IHC testing of ER-α and PgR in breast cancer were partly developed to help remedy an alarmingly high rate of inaccurate results, which was costing patients' lives.[21,43] They were conceptually modeled after the previously published guidelines for *HER2* testing by ASCO/CAP,[44] which have already shown an impact on improving quality.[45] Hopefully, the new guidelines for ER-α and PgR testing will also

be helpful. Figure 9-1 outlines the essential elements of the guidelines, which includes a recommendation to repeat and confirm negative results in unexpected situations. For example, an apparently negative IBC in a sample in which all the normal epithelial cells are also all negative should be repeated and confirmed because a significant proportion of normal cells are usually positive in most (>90%) samples. Similarly, apparently negative lobular, tubular, and mucinous IBCs should be repeated and confirmed because these special subtypes are also usually (>90%) positive—although this is not necessary if internal controls are positive (Figure 9-4). Table 9-3 provides a summary of average ER-α expression in a variety of benign and malignant categories of breast tissue,[5,46–49] which can be helpful in identifying potential problems if there is a significant departure from expected results. The recommendation to repeat suspicious negative results may help improve accuracy more than any other in the ASCO/CAP guidelines, although the new requirement for comprehensive ongoing quality assurance and proficiency testing for laboratory accreditation by the CAP should also make an important beneficial contribution.

Several strategies based on technologies other than IHC have been developed to assess multiple prognostic and predictive biomarkers simultaneously (see details in Chapter 10). For example, one promising strategy evaluates RNA expression of 21 genes that are important in breast cancer (including ER and PgR) by quantitative reverse transcriptase polymerase chain reaction (qRT-PCR) on FFPET samples, and it appears to be very powerful in predicting clinical outcome in several settings.[19,50-53] Another strategy uses microarray technology to determine an RNA expression profile of estrogen-induced genes in IBCs, which appears to be very powerful in predicting response to endocrine therapy.[54] Yet another is the expression ratio of the *HOXB13* and *IL17BR* genes determined by qRT-PCR, which also appears to be highly predictive of endocrine response.[55-57] Other examples could be discussed.[58]

Multifactorial molecular approaches offer strategies different from IHC for determining prognostic and predictive factors in IBCs, including responsiveness to endocrine therapy. This should not be too surprising in the sense that clinical outcomes in any setting are biologically very complex and measuring one or two gene products by IHC cannot account for this complexity, regardless of how accurately they are measured. However, it is also likely that IHC will remain the primary method of assessing ER and PgR in IBCs for some time, so doing it properly is very important. There are new immunofluorescence strategies that can simultaneously measure multiple proteins in a highly quantitative manner,[59-61] which may revitalize the usefulness of IHC-like methods for the in situ assessment of prognostic biomarkers, which has advantages over assays evaluating homogenates of tumor tissue.

Progesterone Receptor

PgR is also routinely assessed by IHC in IBCs. ER-α regulates the expression of PgR, so the presence of PgR usually indicates that the ER-α pathway is functionally intact.[2,5,62,63] PgR is activated by the hormone progesterone to help regulate several normal cellular functions, including proliferation that, like estrogen and ER-α, is detrimental to patients with breast cancer.[2,5,62,63] Most of the discussion regarding the historical assessment of ER-α in IBCs also applies to PgR. It was measured by standardized LBAs for nearly two decades and shown to be a weak prognostic factor but a relatively strong predictive factor for response to endocrine therapy. LBAs for PgR were replaced by IHC beginning in mid-1990s and IHC was eventually approved by the CAP and ASCO for routine clinical use, despite persistent shortcomings.[8,26,64]

Compared with ER-α, there are fewer studies in the medical literature standardizing and validating IHC assays for PgR.[15,18,29,33,35] Those available show that PgR is expressed in the nuclei of 60% to 70% of IBCs, that expression varies on a continuum ranging from 0% to nearly 100% positive cells, that there is a direct correlation between PgR levels and response to hormonal therapies, and that tumors with even very low levels of PgR-positive cells (≥1%) have a significant chance of responding.[29,35] Thus, the ASCO/CAP guidelines also recommend a cut point of 1% or greater IHC-positive cells to define PgR positive. PgR expression is also associated with reduced local recurrence in patients with DCIS treated with lumpectomy and radiation followed by endocrine therapy.[11]

The expression of PgR is highly correlated with ER-α, but the correlation is not perfect, resulting in four possible phenotypes of combined expression, each with significantly different rates of response to hormonal therapy, which would not be apparent measuring one or the other factor alone (Table 9-4). For example, in a comparison of patients with IBC treated with adjuvant tamoxifen, the relative risk of disease recurrence was 28% higher in patients with ER-α–positive/PgR-negative than ER-α–positive/PgR-positive tumors.[65,66] Distinguishing these significantly different outcomes is the primary reason that both ER-α and PgR are measured in routine clinical practice.

It appears that ER-α may also reside on the outer cell membrane in a subset of IBCs.[67-72] A majority of these tumors are negative for PgR, but positive for *HER2* and nuclear ER-α, and the latter is thought to be nonfunctional in many of these tumors, consistent with their PgR-negative status. However, membrane ER-α appears to be functional and promotes tumor cell proliferation in cooperation with overexpressed *HER2*.[67,68] To further complicate matters, there is also evidence that tamoxifen has a stimulatory or agonist effect on membrane ER-α, leading to the speculation that aromatase inhibitors may remain effective in this setting because they inhibit the upstream production of estrogen, which is the ligand for both nuclear and membrane ER-α. If these preliminary studies are confirmed, the quantitative

TABLE 9-4	Frequency and Relative Risk of Disease Recurrence in Breast Cancer Patients Receiving Adjuvant Hormonal Therapy Stratified by Estrogen Receptor-Alpha and Progesterone Receptor Status

ER-α/PgR Status	Frequency (% Cases)	RR* of Recurrence
Positive/positive	50	0.47
Positive/negative	25	0.75
Negative/positive	3	1.08
Negative/negative	22	1.0

*Comparisons made to ER-negative/PgR-negative patients with RR defined as 1.0. Overall *P* value < .0001.
ER-α, estrogen receptor-alpha; PgR, progesterone receptor; RR, relative risk.
Data from Bardou VJ, et al. Progesterone receptor status significantly improves outcome prediction over estrogen receptor status alone for adjuvant endocrine therapy in two large breast cancer databases. J Clin Oncol 2003;21:1973-1979.

assessment of PgR may take on added importance, especially in the ER-α/erbB2–positive subset of IBCs.[28,67,71]

Assessment of ER-α and PgR is mandatory in the routine care of all patients with IBC. Both are targets and/or indicators of response to highly effective endocrine therapies in many clinical settings, so accurate assessment is essential. Unfortunately, IHC results for ER-α and PgR are inaccurate (usually false negative) in up to 20% of patients. The recently published ASCO/CAP guidelines for evaluating ER-α and PgR by IHC make several recommendations to help improve accuracy.[1] It is the responsibility of every pathologist and laboratory performing these tests to ensure accurate test results, and compliance with the guideline will go a long way toward achieving this.

HER2 (ERBB2) ONCOGENE IN BREAST CARCINOMA

The ERBB2 (HER2) gene was originally called NEU because it was first derived from rat neuro/glioblastoma cell lines.[73] Coussens and coworkers[74] named it HER2 because its primary sequence was very similar to human epidermal growth factor receptor (EGFR or ERBB or ERBB1). Semba and colleagues[75] independently identified an ERBB-related but distinct gene which they named as ERBB2. DiFiore and associates[76] indicated that both NEU and HER2 were the same as ERBB2. Akiyama and coworkers[77] precipitated the ERBB2 gene product from adenocarcinoma cells and demonstrated it to be a 185-kD glycoprotein with tyrosine kinase activity. In 1987, 3 years after its discovery, the clinical significance of HER2 gene amplification was shown in breast cancer.[78] We now know that approximately 15% to 20% of breast cancers demonstrate HER2 gene amplification and/or protein overexpression.[79,80] In the absence of adjuvant systemic therapy, HER2-positive breast cancer patients have a worse prognosis, that is, a higher rate of recurrence and mortality, clearly demonstrating its prognostic significance. An even more important aspect of determining HER2 status is its role as a predictive factor. HER2 positivity is predictive of response to anthracycline- and taxane-based therapy, whereas the benefits derived from nonanthracyclines and nontaxane therapy may be inferior.[81–85] It is also important to note that HER2-positive tumors generally show relative resistance to all endocrine therapies; however, this effect may be more toward selective endocrine receptor modulators like tamoxifen and less likely toward estrogen depletion therapies like aromatase inhibitors.[86,87] Most importantly, the availability of HER2-targeted therapy brought this biomarker at the forefront of theranostic testing for breast cancer. Trastuzumab is a humanized monoclonal antibody to HER2 that was approved by the U.S. Food and Drug Administration (FDA) in 1998 for use in metastatic breast cancer. Trastuzumab improves response rates, time to progression, and survival when used alone or in combination with chemotherapy in treatment of metastatic breast cancer. Although approved for use in metastatic

cancer, several prospective, randomized clinical trials have shown significant therapeutic benefits from trastuzumab in early-stage breast cancers.[88–91] The same paradigm has also shifted to neoadjuvant chemotherapy using trastuzumab in HER2-positive tumors.

Immunohistochemistry for HER2

Given the enormous therapeutic benefit derived from trastuzumab in HER2-positive tumors, it is absolutely critical that an accurate determination of HER2 status be made in each case. Owing to its prognostic and predictive value, HER2 status should be determined on all newly diagnosed IBCs, which is now also recommended in the recently released CAP/ASCO guidelines.[46] These guidelines provide a detailed review of the literature and recommendations for optimal HER2 testing. The issues ensuring reliable HER2 testing by IHC can be divided in three categories: preanalytic, analytic, and postanalytic. All three issues are equally important and require a commitment to continuous quality improvement.

PREANALYTIC

Preanalytic mainly relates to time of fixation and type of fixative used. Because most studies with clinical outcome have been performed using FFPET, the current CAP/ASCO recommendation is to use 10% neutral buffered formalin and the tissue should be fixed for 6 to 48 hours. If an alternative fixative or fixation method is used, it has to be validated with standard fixation before it is implemented in clinical testing. Although the guidelines stress more regarding overfixation, we believe that underfixation seems to be the real problem with HER2 testing. The antigen can be retrieved by various methodologies and the enzymatic digestion times for in situ hybridization can be altered if the tissue is overfixed, but nothing can be done if the tissue is underfixed. Overfixation may become an issue with alcohol fixation, which can lead to antigen diffusion, but is generally not an issue with formalin fixation. We have validated tissue fixation times up to 96 hours for performing hormone receptors and HER2 testing on breast carcinoma at our institution. The effect of underfixation on biomarker testing has been nicely shown by Goldstein and colleagues,[92] using ER as an example. Using semiquantitative IHC, the authors demonstrated that, with 40 minutes of standard antigen retrieval, tissues fixed for less than 6 hours had very low "Q score" for ER and the "Q score" plateaued at 8 hours to 7 days. It should also be noted that CAP/ASCO guidelines for fixation times were addressed to resection specimens, but there is no reason to believe that these cannot be applied to needle core biopsies. As a matter of fact, the guidelines should remain the same irrespective of the size of the specimen. This is because tissue permeation (which is roughly 1 mm/hr) is not equal to fixation. It is true that formalin will permeate core biopsy samples faster and make it harder for sectioning, but actual fixation or chemical reaction of aldehyde cross-linking takes time and is independent of specimen size.

ANALYTIC

Analytic refers to the actual testing protocol including IHC equipment, reagents, competency of the staff performing IHC, use of appropriate controls, and finally, the type of antibody used. The last issue of the type of antibody used deserves special mention. The very first clinical trial assay for assessing the effect of trastuzumab on metastatic breast cancer used CB11 and 4D5 antibodies for determining *HER2* status. In these studies, only patients with 2+ or 3+ scores were eligible to receive trastuzumab. Retrospective analyses have revealed therapeutic benefit in cases with either 3+ score or *HER2* amplification by fluorescence in situ hybridization (FISH).[93] Only 24% of 2+ cases showed amplification by FISH. At the time of FDA approval of trastuzumab, a polyclonal antibody (HercepTest; Dako Corporation) was compared with the clinical trial assay antibody CB11 using the same scoring criteria. HercepTest received FDA approval based on its 79% concordance with CB11. A few additional studies showed that HercepTest had a slightly higher false-positive rate than other monoclonal antibodies (CB11, TAB250) when compared with FISH.[94–96] Later, it was recommended that laboratories performing *HER2* testing using HercepTest should strictly adhere to manufacturer's recommendation for appropriate staining. Even to this day, several different antibodies are being used, but all IHC 2+ cases are sent for reflex FISH testing, which in the majority of cases, resolves the clinical dilemma about *HER2* status. A more reliable rabbit monoclonal antibody 4B5 has become available, and it has a higher avidity. In a recent study, Powell and associates[97] showed that rabbit monoclonal 4B5 demonstrates sharper membrane staining with less cytoplasmic and stromal background staining than CB11. The major advantage of 4B5 was its excellent interlaboratory reproducibility (kappa of 1.0).

POSTANALYTIC

Postanalytic involves interpretation criteria, reporting methods, and quality assurance measures including competency of the interpreting pathologist. Although less often mentioned, the suboptimal interpretation of *HER2* IHC score is one of the major factors responsible for discordance between IHC and FISH. The literature regarding *HER2* IHC testing would suggest that 2+ score is the most problematic[98–100]; however, we believe that the 3+ score, which is often misinterpreted, has the most grave clinical consequences. Nowadays, most laboratories would do FISH for *HER2* gene copy number assessment when the IHC score is 2+ but would skip *HER2* FISH testing for 0, 1+, or 3+ scores.[101–103] There are ample data that *HER2* FISH has excellent correlation with response to trastuzumab treatment.[104,105] Therefore, a 2+ *HER2* IHC score coupled with a *HER2* FISH has no adverse clinical consequences. In contrast, a false-positive *HER2* IHC 3+ score would result in inappropriate (ineffective, expensive, and potentially harmful) therapy. We urge that the utmost care should be exercised in interpreting *HER2* IHC results, especially when the staining intensity is "strong 2+ or weak 3+." One may also argue using FISH alone as the diagnostic assay for *HER2*, but it should be realized that IHC is significantly less expensive than FISH, and moreover, IHC provides an opportunity to scan the tumor for any significant heterogeneity compared with FISH.

The CAP/ASCO guidelines recently modified the criteria by changing the number of positive cells for 3+ score from 10% to 30%.[46] Although the numeric change appears large, this will have negligible practical effect.

HER2 heterogeneity with respect to IHC is much more common in weakly positive cases where the score ranges from 1+ to 2+. The change in criteria is an attempt to reduce the number of 3+ false positives, because a small percentage of cells may show intense staining owing to edge artifacts. Moreover, scoring these cases (cases with 11–30% of strongly staining cells) as 2+ (which is now "called equivocal" per the guidelines) will result in additional confirmation by FISH if they are true positives. Image analysis systems could be further used to achieve consistency in interpretation. However, these instruments should be calibrated and undergo regular maintenance just like any other laboratory equipment. Apart from judging the *HER2* score, it is also important that it is effectively communicated to the treating physician. A standardized template could be used that states the time the tissue was fixed, the controls used, the antibody used, and the *HER2* IHC score with description of staining. An example of such a template is shown in Figure 9-5.

Furthermore, a quality assurance program should be in place for the laboratories that perform *HER2* testing. Quality control procedures for *HER2* IHC should include the laboratory statistics of percentage of positive cases and the percentage of IHC cases that are amplified by FISH. Periodic laboratory assessment of these correlations is essential for quality reporting. Rigorous adherence to quality, tissue fixation times, control tissues/cell lines, and improved interobserver interpretation agreement, or image-assisted analysis is preferable.[106–108] The CAP/ASCO guidelines recommend participation in a proficiency testing program specific to each method used.

KEY DIAGNOSTIC POINTS

HER2 *Immunohistochemistry*

- Owing to its predictive value, *HER2* is currently the most important theranostic test for breast cancer.

- Accurate assessment of *HER2* status is critical and the lessons learned from *HER2* testing will be applied for future biomarkers assessment.

- Tissues should be fixed in 10% NBF for at least 6 hours for accurate assessment.

- Choice of antibody may vary but must be mentioned in the report.

- Scoring criteria should be rigidly followed so that there are no 3+ false positives.

- All 2+ cases should go for reflex FISH testing.

- Continuous quality measures should be in place for any laboratory performing *HER2* testing.

FISH, fluorescence in situ hybridization; NBF, neutral buffered formalin.

HER2 IHC Template

HER2 IMMUNOHISTOCHEMISTRY: Using appropriate formalin fixed (6–48 hours) controls and tissue test block, ...antibody (clone, vendor information) is used to assess HER2 status and is interpreted as follows:

0 (NEGATIVE): No staining is observed or membranous staining is observed in less than 10% of the tumor cells.

1+ (NEGATIVE): A faint/barely perceptible staining is detected in more than 10% of the tumor cells. The cells are stained in part of their membrane.

2+ (EQUIVOCAL): A weak to moderate complete membrane staining is observed in more than 10% of the tumor cells OR strong complete membranous staining is observed in less than 30% of the tumor cells. HER2 FISH is being performed and will be subsequently reported.

3+ (POSITIVE): A strong complete membrane staining is observed in more than 30% of the tumor cells.

FIGURE 9-5 Template for reporting *HER2* protein expression by IHC. FISH, fluorescence in situ hybridization.

HER2 Fluorescence In Situ Hybridization

FISH is a molecular cytogenetic technique that uses fluorescent probes to detect specific DNA sequences on the chromosome. In case of *HER2* FISH, a *HER2* probe is used to identify *HER2* gene amplification. The probe could be a single-color *HER2* probe or a dual-color probe with one sequence labeled for the *HER2* gene and another for the chromosome 17 centromere (chromosome enumeration probe 17 [*CEP 17*]) on which the *HER2* gene resides. For a single-color probe, an absolute *HER2* gene copy number determines amplification, whereas for a dual-color probe, a ratio of *HER2* to *CEP17* is used to define amplification. DNA is a more robust molecule than protein, and therefore, *HER2* gene amplification studies could be performed on a wide variety of samples. However, owing to the significance of this test result and to avoid any variability, the CAP/ASCO guidelines recommend the similar preanalytic conditions as required for *HER2* IHC. In the available literature, *HER2* FISH has a better track record than *HER2* IHC in predicting response to trastuzumab. This may be due to several factors, including tissue fixation, criteria used to define positivity, wide number of antibodies used, and subjectivity in interpreting *HER2* IHC test result compared with FISH. However, after years of experience in both *HER2* IHC and FISH, the current CAP/ASCO guidelines demand 95% concordance (of negative and unequivocal positive results) between the two methods.[44] This seems like a high number, but theoretically, it is not unreasonable because *HER2* gene amplification almost always results in *HER2* protein overexpression. For many genes, there are alternative ways of protein overexpression, but *HER2* gene is unique in the sense that its gene amplification is very tight coupled with protein overexpression. In the past few years, it has also been realized that, just like IHC, a FISH assay may also give equivocal results. Until recently, *HER2* gene amplification was defined as *HER2/CEP17* ratio of 2 or higher, and lack of amplification was defined as a ratio less than 2. This was also the cutoff used for the clinical trial assay. Using the cutoff value of 2 makes sense, but it has been realized over

the years that there is variability in interpretation when the value is around 2.[109] Therefore, the recently released CAP/ASCO guidelines recommended that a ratio of 1.8 to 2.2 should be considered as equivocal for *HER2* gene amplification.[46] A ratio less than 1.8 is negative for amplification and a ratio greater than 2.2 is positive for amplification. If a laboratory is using a single-color probe to define gene amplification, a positive result is an average *HER2* gene copy number greater than 6, a negative result is an average *HER2* copy number less than 4, and an equivocal result is *HER2* gene copy number of 4 to 6.

Apart from its better prediction value than IHC, FISH is also very useful when the *HER2* IHC test result is equivocal (i.e., IHC score of 2+).[110] An IHC 2+ score is seen in up to 25% of all breast cancers.[111] It is now standard of care to FISH these 2+ cases to determine whether they show gene amplification. We reviewed FISH results on all 2+ IHC cases (186 cases) in 1 year at our institution and found that a majority (~80%) of these 2+ cases do not show amplification (i.e., *HER2/CEP 17* ratio < 1.8). An equal number of cases (10% in each category) demonstrated equivocal (ratio of 1.8–2.2) or true amplification (ratio > 2.2). However, it was extremely unusual (even in cases with ratio > 2.2) for IHC 2+ cases to show large *HER2* gene clusters, which is a characteristic of IHC 3+ cases (Figure 9-6). Although FISH is useful for clinical decision making in these cases, it appears that *HER2* IHC 2+ cases may be biologically different from the *HER2* IHC 3+ cases. Our review also showed that some of these *HER2* nonamplified, IHC 2+ cases contained more than three copies of *HER2* and *CEP 17*, indicative of polyploidy/aneuploidy for chromosome 17 as reported previously.[100,112] Whether the presence of ploidy predicts response to trastuzumab is currently not well known. In one study of 103 patients, polysomy was observed in 27% of patients; 6 responded to trastuzumab treatment. However, all 6 cases showed *HER2* overexpression (IHC 3+); 2 were FISH negative based on *HER2:CEP17* ratio due to chromosome 17 polysomy.[113] It appears that some of the polysomy/ploidy cases with *HER2* IHC 3+ expression likely represent co-amplification of *HER2* gene and chromosome 17 centromere.

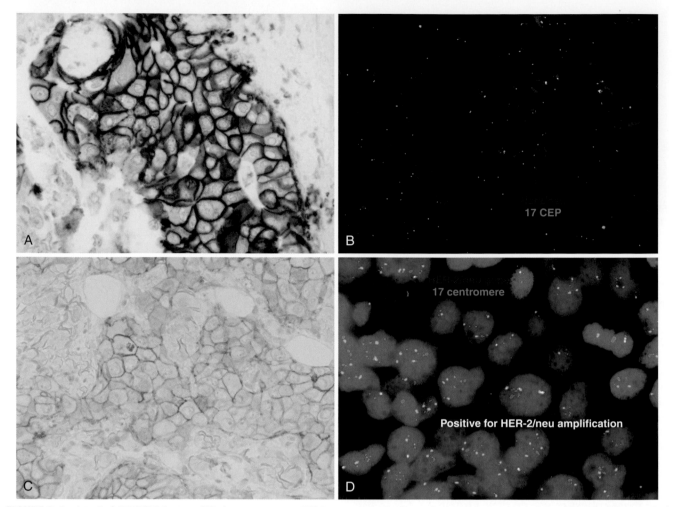

FIGURE 9-6 A typical *HER2* IHC 3+ case **(A)** shows numerous *HER2* gene copies (red) consistent with unequivocal amplification **(B)**. A typical *HER2* IHC 2+ case **(C)** with some increase in *HER2* gene copies **(D)**. CEP, chromosome enumeration probe.

Another caveat for *HER2* equivocal FISH result is whether FISH was performed on core biopsy or resection specimen. Recently, Striebel and coworkers[114] showed that evaluating *HER2* status by FISH on a larger tumor sample (resection specimen) affects patient management if the core biopsy shows an equivocal FISH result, indicating genetic heterogeneity in tumors showing low-level *HER2* gene copy numbers.

In spite of its usefulness, there are some limitations to FISH assay, mainly related to dark field fluorescence microscopy and lack of morphologic details (Table 9-5). In order to overcome some of these limitations, the chromogenic in situ hybridization (CISH) method has gained popularity. There are a range of studies comparing FISH and CISH showing average to 100% concordance.[115–118] CISH uses diaminobenzidine (DAB) as the chromogen and, therefore, results in brown signals. It is a method that combines the expertise of an IHC and cytogenetic laboratory. This may be the reason for the lack of wide acceptance for CISH, which we believe can improve with automation. Some pathologists also feel uncomfortable interpreting *HER2* CISH slides when there are between two and eight gene signals per nucleus because the signals may not be very discrete, especially when one is looking under a 40× objective using

bright-field microscopy. Silver in situ hybridization (SISH) has been developed specifically to overcome this problem. SISH uses an enzyme-linked probe to deposit silver ions from the solution to the target site, which provides a dense, punctate, high-resolution black stain that is readily distinguished from other commonly used stains. It appears that these innovative in situ hybridization assays will become more widely available and will be more acceptable to laboratories if these assays are automated and do not interfere with the current workflow. Because FISH slides are evaluated under 100× oil immersion lens, the amount of tumor analyzed is fairly limited. An added advantage of these other in situ hybridization assays would be to examine the tumor for heterogeneity with respect to *HER2* gene copy number.

Nonmorphologic Methods for *HER2* Assessment

Although Southern blot was the initial procedure used to show clinical usefulness of *HER2* gene in breast cancer, it is a very laborious procedure and is not favored in this day and age of faster and cheaper molecular assays. qRT-PCR for *HER2* mRNA measurement is

TABLE 9-5	Benefits and Limitations of Immunohistochemistry and In Situ Hybridization Assays		
	Immunohistochemistry	**FISH**	**CISH/SISH**
Availability of the test	Widely available.	Available at major laboratories.	Available at major laboratories.
Microscopy	Bright field.	Fluorescent.	Bright field.
Training for interpretation	No special training required.	Special training required.	Minimal training required.
Amount of tumor analyzed with ease	Large tumor area can be analyzed.	Generally, a small tumor area is analyzed.	Large tumor area can be analyzed.
Morphology	Morphology well preserved.	Morphology not well preserved.	Morphology well preserved.
Turnaround time	4–6 hr.	3 days.	2 days with CISH; 4–6 hr with SISH.
Average time for interpretation	<1 min.	20 min.	1–2 min.
Number of equivocal results	~25%.	<5%.	<5% (but limited experience).
Cost	Relatively inexpensive.	Expensive.	Intermediate.
Automation	Possible.	Possible.	Possible; available with SISH.

CISH, chromogenic (generally DAB as chromogen) in situ hybridization; FISH, fluorescence in situ hybridization; SISH, silver in situ hybridization.

KEY DIAGNOSTIC POINTS

HER2 *Fluorescence In Situ Hybridization*

- All IHC 2+ cases should go for reflex FISH testing.
- The preanalytic variables are similar to IHC testing.
- FISH interpretation also has an equivocal category (*HER2:CEP17* ratio of 1.8–2.2 or average *HER2* gene copy number between 4 and 6).
- Alternate in situ hybridization assays, especially SISH may become more widely available and acceptable.
- Continuous quality measures should be in place for any laboratory performing *HER2* FISH testing.

FISH, fluorescence in situ hybridization; IHC, immunohistochemical; SISH, silver in situ hybridization.

---

an attractive technique because it is more quantitative than IHC. mRNA measurement using expression microarrays is also possible. Both these techniques are being currently utilized in multigene expression assays for prognostic and predictive purposes in breast cancer. Genomic Health Inc. (GHI; Redwood City, CA) recently started reporting *ER, PR,* and *HER2* expression levels as a separate report to onco*type* DX test, and Agendia BV (Amsterdam, The Netherlands) offers the same with TargetPrint assay. A recent corporate study from GHI suggests excellent concordance between *HER2* FISH and *HER2* qRT-PCR onco*type* DX test. However, a quality assurance study at our institution (data currently in press) suggests otherwise. Although we have found excellent concordance on IHC/FISH-negative cases, the onco*type* DX *HER2* assay fails to identify a substantial number of unequivocally *HER2*-positive cases.

It should be noted that we have recently reported our results of a multi-institutional study on HER2 immunohistochemistry/FISH concordance with GHI qRT-pCR results and found excellent percent negative agreement but sub-optimal percent positive agreement (article in press; see also http://www.asco.org/ascov2/Meetings/Abstract?&vmview=abst_detail_view&confID=102&abstractID=82476). Specifically, GHI qRT-PCR assay failed to identify more than 50% of unequivocally positive HER2 cases, and failed to identify 100% of Her2 FISH equivocal cases. The results were consistent for the three participating institutions. Our analysis pointed towards dilution of tumor mRNA with non-tumoral tissues as one of the prominent explanations for sub-optimal positive agreement. In the breast, the contamination of invasive tumor mRNA can result from admixed and surrounding in-situ carcinoma, normal ductal breast tissue, fibro-adipose tissue, lymphocytic infiltrate, necrosis, benign cellular proliferations, or even biopsy cavities. In these situations, qRT-PCR assay, a non-morphologic technique, may give a false negative result for a gene not expressed by normal tissues such as *HER2*. This contamination from non-invasive tissue also has the potential to impact hormone receptors, proliferation genes and quantitative RT-PCR results and together these can impact the overall recurrence score which according to published literature is heavily affected by tumor hormone receptor content, *HER2* status, and proliferation.

A critical review of these cases suggests either sub-optimal microdissection or no microdissection at all on the tissue sections, resulting in a false-negative *HER2* qRT-PCR assay. Most breast cancers generally contain an admixture of non-neoplastic tissue (lymphocytes, fibrous breast stroma, adipose breast tissue, normal breast tissue, necrosis, benign cellular proliferations, or even biopsy cavities) either admixed within invasive tumor or in the immediate vicinity. Therefore, most cases will have some degree of contamination with non-neoplastic tissue that can proportionately reduce

HER2 mRNA levels, resulting in an equivocal or negative result by qRT-PCR on an unequivocally positive case. This is a well-known drawback of nonmorphologic techniques utilized for assessment of individual gene or gene product in tumor tissue.[119–121] Although a careful microdissection of invasive tumor under a stereomicroscope may be helpful, this drawback could be completely overcome only by performing laser-capture microdissection.[122–125] Therefore, caution is advised to currently accept these nonmorphologic assays for treatment purposes in lieu of FDA-approved IHC and FISH assays.

Other HER2 Assays

HER2 dimerization assays such as HERmark (monogram biosciences, South San Francisco, CA) based on VeraTag technology, has been described to provide a continuous quantitative measure of total HER2 protein and HER2 homodimers as a potential to stratify patients more accurately for HER2-targeted therapy. The test uses a dual-antibody format, whereby a fluorescent tag on one analyte-specific antibody is cleaved when in close proximity to a second antibody containing a photoactivated molecule. The fluorescent tags are then quantified using capillary electrophoresis.[126,127] HER2 protein quantification is then normalized to the tumor area. This method again brings into question some of the same issues that occur with nonmorphologic assays. Because the amount of measured protein is normalized to the tumor area, it is very difficult not to include the intermixed non-neoplastic stroma and sometimes in situ carcinoma with different HER2 expression level while determining the area, which can potentially alter the quantification.

HER2 receptor can be activated owing to autophosphorylation, and therefore, phosphorylated HER2 antibodies have been utilized by some investigators to assess its usefulness.[128] Although a few studies have shown a worse outcome for HER2-positive patients with phosphorylated receptor compared with HER2-positive patients without phosphorylated receptors,[129] the available antibodies lack specificity for accurate determination. Moreover, it is currently unknown whether phosphorylated HER2 receptor is a better predictor of response to trastuzumab.

Enzyme-linked immunosorbent assay (ELISA) on primary invasive tumor cytosol suffers from the same drawbacks as nonmorphologic assays and is generally not recommended/performed within the United States. In contrast, ELISA to detect extracellular domain (ECD) of HER2 protein in circulation is a more popular test. A number of studies have shown an association between serum HER2 protein levels and disease recurrence, metastasis, or shorter survival.[130–132] However, the assay is still not widely used for primary tumor HER2 status assessment because a high cutoff value of 37 μg/L gives a high 95% specificity but significantly affects the sensitivity.[133] HER2 ECD determination via ELISA is more often used for monitoring of patients with HER2-positive disease undergoing anti–HER2-targeted therapy.[134]

HER2 Status, Tumor Morphology, and Prognostic/Predictive Factors

HER2-positive tumors are mostly Nottingham grade 2 or 3 (i.e., Nottingham score 6–9).[135] The majority of the HER2-positive tumors are of ductal type (i.e., E-cadherin positive).[136] Among lobular tumors, HER2 amplification/overexpression is mainly seen in pleomorphic type tumors[137] demonstrating some degree of apocrine differentiation. Some studies suggest HER2 overexpression in 50% of pleomorphic lobular carcinomas,[138] but if strict criteria are applied, unequivocal amplification (ratio > 2.2)/overexpression is seen in not more than 25% of these cases.[139,140] The majority of classic lobular carcinomas are negative for HER2. We recently reviewed data at our institution and identified unequivocal HER2 positivity in approximately 5% of classic lobular carcinoma cases.[141] The morphoimmunohistologic factors that correlated with HER2 positivity included histiocytoid (which some consider part of apocrine differentiation) morphology and reduced PgR (not ER) expression.

The literature also suggests an inverse correlation between HER2 and hormone receptors.[87,135] Although ER or PgR expression is decreased in HER2-positive tumors, a substantial proportion of them still express hormone receptors. If a detailed semiquantitative evaluation is performed, approximately 15% of all breast cancers are HER2 positive. Of these, one third (5%) are completely negative for ER, one third (5%) are weak to moderately positive for ER, and the remaining one third (5%) are strongly positive for ER.[142] Therefore, of all HER2-positive tumors, two thirds are still ER positive using standard cutoffs according to ASCO/CAP guidelines. However, even in ER-positive tumors, many are PR-negative or the PR expression level is significantly reduced. These findings suggest that, despite ER positivity,

---

KEY DIAGNOSTIC POINTS

HER2 Status and Clinical-Pathologic Factors

- Most HER2-positive tumors are of ductal type and Nottingham grade 2 or 3.

- Many HER2-positive tumors demonstrate apocrine differentiation.

- Regional lymph node metastases are common in HER2-positive tumors.

- HER2 overexpression correlates inversely more with PgR than with ER.

- Proliferation rate for HER2-positive tumors is intermediate between ER+/HER2– tumors and triple-negative tumors.

- Brain metastases with HER2-positive tumors are more common in the trastuzumab era.

- HER2 status generally remains unchanged after therapy and in metastatic tumors.

ER, estrogen receptor; PgR, progesterone receptor.

the ER pathway may be dysfunctional in many *HER2*-positive tumors.

As far as special morphologic subtypes of breast carcinomas are concerned, *HER2* is generally negative in tubular,[143] mucinous (except on rare occasions),[144] and medullary carcinomas.[145] In contrast, *HER2* overexpression appears to be quite common with apocrine tumors.[139] This association deserves special mention. Although pure apocrine carcinomas are very rare; some degree of apocrine differentiation in breast carcinoma is fairly common and seen in approximately 15% of all cancers. If one specifically examines all breast cancers with apocrine differentiation, the association with *HER2* is rather weak or not at all present. In our study of 205 consecutive breast carcinoma cases, apocrine differentiation was seen in 26 cases.[142] Of these 26 cases, 35% were ER–/HER2–, 27% were ER–/HER2+, 23% were ER+/HER2–, and 15% were ER+/HER2+.[142] There is no association between *HER2* and apocrine differentiation when one looks at them in this manner because the majority of breast cancers are actually *HER2* negative and ER positive. However, when we examined our data in the reverse manner, apocrine differentiation was identified in 87% of ER–/HER2+ tumors, in 28% of ER–/HER2– tumors, in 22% of ER+/HER2+ tumors, and in only 4% of ER+/HER2– tumors.

The proliferation rate in *HER2*-positive tumors is generally variable. They are generally more proliferative than ER+/HER2–, but less proliferative than triple-negative tumors. The average proliferation index as determined by Ki-67 is approximately 25% to 50%. Another important aspect of *HER2*-positive disease is the frequent presence of regional lymph node metastases in these tumors. Distant metastases are also more common in *HER2*-positive tumors than in *HER2* negative, hormone receptor–positive disease. Prior to the availability of trastuzumab, the site of distant metastases mainly included lung and liver.[146] However, in the trastuzumab era, brain metastases have become more frequent because trastuzumab cannot cross the blood-brain barrier.[147] This unmasking of brain metastases is the major cause of death in *HER2*-positive tumors nowadays. It is hoped that the dual *(HER1* and *HER2)* tyrosine kinase inhibitor lapatinib would be more effective in the treatment of brain metastases.[148]

HER2 Status after Therapy and Metastatic Disease

A number of studies suggest that *HER2* expression does not change with therapy or at metastatic site.[149–152] However, a few studies have suggested otherwise.[153] We believe most of the discordance is either due to true heterogeneity of *HER2* expression within the primary tumor, which is not uncommon with large tumors (Figure 9-7), or to testing/scoring method in equivocal cases or cases that are near the equivocal range.[154] Owing to heterogeneity issues, it is important to determine *HER2* status in metastatic tumors because it may significantly affect treatment decisions. The ASCO/CAP guidelines recommend retesting for *HER2* and hormone receptors for all patients with recurrences.

HER2 Status and Response to Therapy

The *HER2*-positive tumors are clearly sensitive to *HER2*-targeted therapy (trastuzumab) and studies have shown that combination chemotherapy along with trastuzumab is even more effective than trastuzumab alone.[155] Trastuzumab-containing chemotherapy is now used in metastatic, adjuvant, and even neoadjuvant setting. However, some *HER2*-positive tumors are more sensitive to trastuzumab therapy than others. In the neoadjuvant setting, we have found that pathologic complete response and percentage tumor volume reduction are inversely related to tumor hormone receptor content as semiquantitatively measured by IHC.[156] This relative resistance to trastuzumab therapy may be due to activation of other growth factor receptors such as insulin-like growth factor-1 receptor (IGF-1R) in ER-positive tumors.[157–159] Several other studies have also described biomarkers that may predict resistance to trastuzumab therapy, such as loss of *PTEN* tumor suppressor gene and activation of *PI3K* pathway,[160–162] and overexpression of vascular endothelial growth factor.[163] In contrast, *CMYC* and *TOP2A* have been linked to responsiveness to trastuzumab therapy.[164,165]

In summary, *HER2* is a vitally important prognostic and predictive marker in a subset of breast carcinomas. Even in this era of multigene expression assays, accurate assessment of *HER2* status is of vital importance owing to the availability of highly effective targeted therapy. Every laboratory performing *HER2* assay must possess the expertise of providing highly accurate results because both over- and underassessment have grave clinical consequences.

OTHER RELEVANT PROGNOSTIC/PREDICTIVE MARKERS

p53

p53 is a tumor suppressor gene, commonly mutated in several human cancers. In routine diagnostic surgical pathology, mutation status is assessed based on its expression by IHC. In some tumor types, such as bladder carcinomas, it has been shown that diffuse strong p53 expression by IHC correlate with *P53* mutation by molecular techniques.[166,167] The commonly used antibody clone DO7 recognizes both the wild-type and the mutant p53 proteins. However, because the mutant protein has a longer half-life than the wild-type protein, the mutant protein is more diffusely and intensely stained on IHC. Therefore, weak or patchy staining with p53 antibodies should be considered as a negative result. Some of the confusion regarding p53 staining in breast and other cancers stems from the interpretation. In any event, p53 staining has been associated with poor prognosis in breast carcinoma. With our continued improved understanding of breast carcinoma, we now know that a large majority of

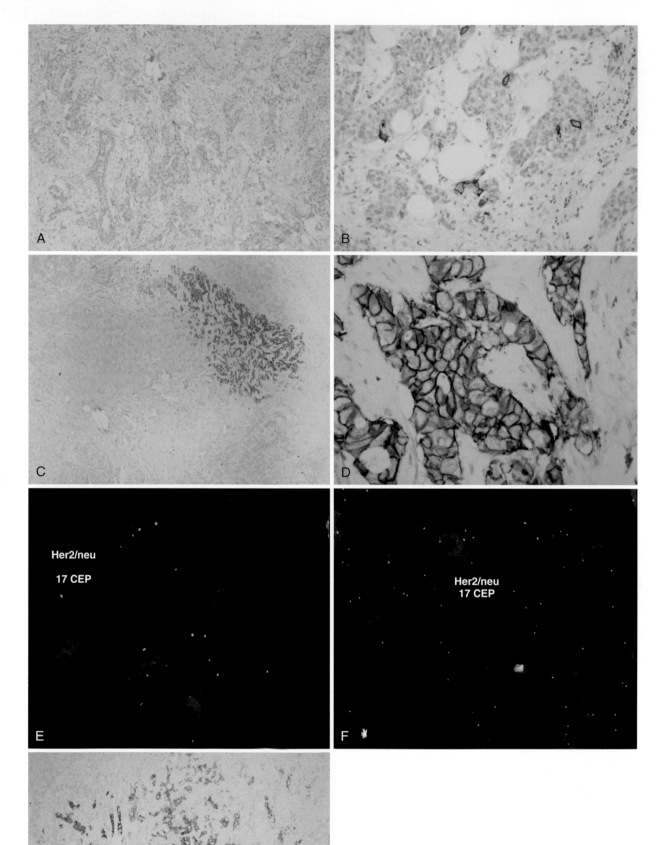

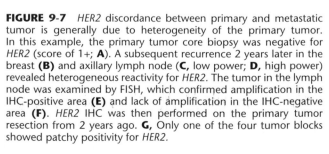

FIGURE 9-7 *HER2* discordance between primary and metastatic tumor is generally due to heterogeneity of the primary tumor. In this example, the primary tumor core biopsy was negative for *HER2* (score of 1+; **A**). A subsequent recurrence 2 years later in the breast (**B**) and axillary lymph node (**C**, low power; **D**, high power) revealed heterogeneous reactivity for *HER2*. The tumor in the lymph node was examined by FISH, which confirmed amplification in the IHC-positive area (**E**) and lack of amplification in the IHC-negative area (**F**). *HER2* IHC was then performed on the primary tumor resection from 2 years ago. **G**, Only one of the four tumor blocks showed patchy positivity for *HER2*.

tumors that demonstrate strong p53 immunoreactivity or show *P53* mutations belong to the basal-like subtype.[168] The clinical usefulness of p53 mutation analysis or diffuse strong immunoreactivity in nonbasal tumors has not been well studied. However, a recent study showed that *P53* gene abnormalities, as defined by sequencing, were associated with worse prognosis and that *P53* mutations/deletions were particularly prognostic in node-negative, ER-positive patients.[169] However, the present data are insufficient to recommend use of p53 measurements for management of patients with breast cancer as per the 2007 ASCO tumor guidelines for breast cancer.[170]

Ki-67

Numerous studies have been published regarding proliferation activity of breast carcinomas, many of which date back to the pre-expression profiling era. Investigators have used either flow cytometry to determine S-phase fraction or immunohistochemistry to study expression of proliferating cell nuclear antigen (PCNA) or Ki-67.[171,172] There has been good correlation between different methodologies. Many studies analyzing Ki-67 labeling index (LI) have shown high LI to be a poor prognostic factor in breast cancer.[173,174] However, different cutoff points have been used to define high-proliferation index. In addition, different techniques have been used to determine the LI. Owing to these factors, it is somewhat difficult to compare these studies and likely explain the reluctance to universally accept Ki-67 LI as a prognostic marker in breast cancer. Colozza and colleagues[175] performed a thorough review of 132 articles including 159,516 patients regarding the prognostic and predictive value of Ki-67 and other proliferation markers (cyclin D, cyclin E, p27, p21, TK, and topoisomerase II-alpha). The authors appropriately pointed out that all studies concerning these markers are level IV or III evidence at best (level I or II evidence is required for use in clinical practice) and demonstrated the difficulty in interpreting the literature owing to lack of standardization of assay reagents, procedures, and scoring. Therefore, the authors recommended not using these markers in routine clinical practice, a view also endorsed by the 2007 ASCO tumor guidelines for breast cancer.[170]

The scoring of Ki-67 LI is also compounded by the lack of consensus as to which area of the tumor should be counted—should it be the entire tumor section, the advancing edge of the tumor, or within the field of highest proliferative activity? Depending on where one chooses to count (regardless of the manual or image analysis method), variability in Ki-67 will be expected. In spite of the previous argument, it is interesting to note that the very first gene expression profiling study not only revealed "molecular portraits" but also identified genes responsible for the biologic differences between the tumor types.[176,177] One of the largest distinct gene clusters identified by expression profiling was of the proliferation genes and included both PCNA and Ki-67.

Subsequently, a few studies have primarily focused on the issue of Ki-67 LI and its correlation to all the molecular classes. We examined the Ki-67 LI using image analysis in approximately 200 consecutive breast carcinomas

divided into molecular class using IHC criteria.[142] It was interesting to note that the average Ki-67 LI was highest in triple-negative tumors and most tumors showed an index above 50%. The ER–/HER2+ tumors were a distant second, followed by hormone receptor–positive tumors. Although the mean Ki-67 LI was low in hormone receptor–positive tumors, not all tumors had low Ki-67 LI and showed a wide range. This difference in proliferation activity coupled with quantitative difference in ER/PgR expression has been exploited in the development of a commercial assay (onco*type*Dx) for predicting breast cancer prognosis and treatment.[54] Cheang and associates[178] have also used Ki-67 proliferation index (cutoff of 14%) to distinguish between luminal A and luminal B tumors.

Although not the most robust prognostic or predictive marker, Ki-67 LI is an additional piece of information that may be used in clinical decision making, provided the physician understands the limitations of the test and the test result.

Epidermal Growth Factor Receptor

The EGFR *(EGFR, HER-1, c-erbB-1)* is one of the four transmembrane growth factor receptor proteins that share similarities in structure and function. Using a criterion similar to assessing *HER2* IHC expression, EGFR overexpression in breast carcinoma is seen in fewer than 10% of all tumors.[179] The best correlation of EGFR increased gene copy number is with 3+ IHC score. Breast tumors that show EGFR expression/overexpression are generally negative for steroid hormone receptors. With our current understanding of breast carcinoma molecular classification, EGFR expression would be predominantly seen in basal-like breast carcinomas. Therefore, it has been proposed to use EGFR along with cytokeratin 5/6 (CK5/6) in identifying basal-like carcinomas.[180,181] It seems that EGFR does have a diagnostic use in breast pathology.

As far as prognostic and predictive value is concerned, the role of EGFR IHC is unknown. As per our understanding from lung carcinoma studies, the tumors that are responsive to small molecule tyrosine kinase inhibitors demonstrate mutations in exon 19 and 21 of EGFR. Such mutations have not been identified in breast carcinomas.[179,182] In colon carcinoma, use of an EGFR inhibitor (cetuximab) was initially based on EGFR expression. However, subsequent studies have found no correlation between EGFR expression and response to cetuximab. Whether cetuximab therapy would have a role in breast cancer (especially basal-like) remains to be seen.[183,184] Until further clinical trial and additional studies, the role of EGFR is limited to diagnostic use only.

Urokinase Plasminogen Activator and Plasminogen Activator Inhibitor-1

Urokinase plasminogen activator (uPA)/plasminogen activator inhibitor-1 (PAI-1) are part of the plasminogen-activating system, which includes the receptor for uPA and other inhibitors (PAI-2 and PAI-3). This system has been shown experimentally to be associated with invasion, angiogenesis, and metastasis.[185] Low levels of both markers are associated with a sufficiently low risk of recurrence (especially in hormone receptor–positive women who will receive adjuvant endocrine therapy) that chemotherapy will only contribute minimal additional benefit. Furthermore, cytoxan, and 5-fluorouracil–based adjuvant chemotherapy provides substantial benefit, compared with observation alone, in patients with high risk of recurrence as determined by high levels of uPA and PAI-1. Although any technique (IHC, qRT-PCR, ELISA) could be used to determine levels of uPA and PAI-1, the outcome is best correlated with ELISA.[186–188] Unfortunately, IHC results do not reliably predict outcomes, and the prognostic value of ELISA using smaller tissue specimens, such as tissue collected by core biopsy, has not been validated.[189] It appears that the clinical utility of this test is limited, because the availability of 300 mg of fresh or frozen breast tumor would be a significant impediment in this era of mammographically or magnetic resonance imaging (MRI)-detected cancers.

Insulin-like Growth Factor Receptor-1

IGF-1R is an integral part of the insulin-like growth factor (IGF) system that plays an important role in neoplastic processes.[190] The IGF family includes the two ligands (IGF-1 and IGF-2), two cell surface receptors (IGF-1R and IGF-2R), and a family of six Insulin-like growth factor-1–binding proteins (IGFBPs) that regulates the free IGF levels. Of the entire IGF system, IGF-1R appears to be the most critical molecule that can be analyzed in tumor samples. Moreover, with the advent of IGF-1R–targeted therapies, it may be useful to analyze IGF-1R expression levels in the tumor tissue. Studies evaluating tissue expression of IGF-1R have shown IGF-1R expression in a significant number of breast carcinomas.[191–194] In our own study of IGF-1R expression in normal breast tissue, proliferative breast lesions, and breast carcinomas, we found that even normal breast ducts and lobules also express membranous IGF-1R to a moderate degree.[157] Defining over-, normal, and underexpression in comparison with normal breast tissue, IGF-1R overexpression was predominantly seen in ER-positive tumors. The tumor group that consistently showed reduced expression was the ERBB2 group *(ER–/PR–/HER2+)*. The expression was somewhat heterogeneous in the triple-negative group. IGF-1R expression was not predictive of pathologic complete response or tumor volume reduction in ER-negative tumors, but reduced IGF-1R was associated with pathologic complete response and significant tumor volume reduction in ER-positive tumors.[157] Therefore, it appears that therapies targeting IGF-1R will be useful in a majority of ER-positive and a subset of triple-negative tumors that express IGF-1R.

BCL2

BCL2 is an antiapoptotic gene that is expressed in approximately 75% of breast carcinomas and its expression level correlates with ER expression.[195–198] Recently, an additional role for *BCL2* in breast tumor prognostication has been described. Abdel-Fateh and coworkers proposed a modified grading system by combining mitotic index and *BCL2* reactivity that can be applied to both ER-positive and ER-negative tumors and would be helpful in eliminating or reducing the number of tumors classified as Nottingham grade 2, in which clinical decision making is often difficult.[199] The investigators divided the tumors into low risk and high risk based on mitotic activity score (M1 = low if < 10 mitoses; M2 = medium if 10–18 mitoses; and M3 = high if > 18 mitoses per 10 high-power fields with field diameter 0.56 mm) and *BCL2* reactivity (used a cutoff of 10%). The low-risk tumors were described as M1/BCL2 ± and M2/BCL2+ and the high-risk tumors included M2-3/BCL2– and M3/BCL2+. The results showed that 87% of Nottingham grade 2 tumors (a clinically ambiguous category) were reclassified as either good (M1-2/BCL2+; 74%) or poor (M2-3/BCL2–; 13%) prognosis and only 13% (69/531) of Nottingham grade 2 tumors were allocated to an intermediate prognosis (M1/BCL2–). In a further subset analysis of ER-positive patients treated with hormonal therapy alone, cases with M2-3/BCL2– and M3/BCL2+ showed a 2.5- to 4.0-fold increase in risk of death, recurrence, and distant metastasis after 10 years, compared with patients with M1-2/BCL2+ and M1/BCL2– phenotypes. These findings suggest that ER+/*HER2*– tumors can be classified as luminal A (good-prognosis tumors) if they are Nottingham grade 1 or 2 and positive for *BCL2*, and all other ER+/*HER2*– tumors could be considered as luminal B (poor-prognosis tumors).

FOXA1

FOXA1 is a forkhead family transcription factor that segregates with genes that characterize the luminal subtypes in DNA microarray analyses.[200] Using genome-wide analysis, Laganiere and colleagues[201] identified 153 promoters bound by ER-α in the breast cancer cell line MCF-7 in the presence of estradiol. One of the promoters identified was for FOXA1, whose expression correlated with expression of ER-α. These authors further found that ablation of FOXA1 expression in MCF-7 cells suppressed ER-α binding to the prototypic TFF1 promoter (which contains a FOXA1-binding site), hindered the induction of TFF1 expression by estradiol, and prevented hormone-induced reentry into the cell cycle. The practical utility of FOXA1 was assessed by Badve and associates[200] where they showed positive correlation between FOXA1 expression and ER/PgR expression by IHC. Another immunohistochemical study by Thorat and coworkers[202] demonstrated a positive correlation between FOXA1 expression and ER-α ($P < .0001$), PgR ($P < .0001$), and luminal subtype ($P < .0001$); and a negative correlation with basal subtype ($P < .0001$), and proliferation markers and high histologic grade ($P = .0327$). Although FOXA1 was a significant predictor of overall survival in univariate analysis in this study, only nodal status and ER expression were significant predictors of overall survival on multivariate analyses. FOXA1 has also been proposed as a clinical/immunohistochemical marker to identify luminal A molecular subtype,[203] but data are currently limited on this subject.

GATA3

GATA-binding protein 3 (GATA3) is a transcriptional activator highly expressed by the luminal epithelial cells in the breast. It is involved in growth and differentiation. Gene expression profiling has shown that GATA3 is highly expressed in the luminal A subtype of breast cancer.[168,204] In an immunohistochemical study of 139 breast cancers, Mehra and colleagues[205] showed that low GATA3 expression was associated with higher histologic grade ($P < .001$), positive nodes ($P = .002$), larger tumor size ($P = .03$), negative ER and PgR ($P < .001$ for both), and HER2-neu overexpression ($P = .03$). Patients whose tumors expressed low GATA3 had significantly shorter overall and disease-free survival when compared with those whose tumors had high GATA3 levels. In a much larger series of 3119 breast cancer cases, Voduc and associates[206] showed somewhat similar findings; however, they also clarified some of the issues. In their study, GATA3 was almost exclusively expressed in ER-positive patients and was also associated with lower tumor grade, older age at diagnosis, and the absence of HER2 overexpression. GATA3 was a marker of good prognosis and predicted for superior breast cancer-specific survival, relapse-free survival, and overall survival in univariate analysis.[206] However, in multivariate models including patient age, tumor size, histologic grade, nodal status, ER status, and HER2 status, GATA3 was not independently prognostic for these same outcomes. Furthermore, in the subgroups of ER-positive patients treated with or without tamoxifen, GATA3 was again nonprognostic for all outcomes.[206]

Both FOXA1 and GATA3 are molecular markers that are highly associated with ER expression, but they do not seem to have prognostic value independent of ER. Additional clinical validation studies are required before their use can be recommended in routine practice.

Several other prognostic/predictive markers published in the literature (nm23, cathepsin D, microvascular density, PS2, p-glycoprotein, fibroblast growth factor, transforming growth factor-beta, androgen receptor, matrix metalloproteinase) are not discussed here owing to their current limited clinical utility.

SUMMARY

IHC is a critical tool for pathologists in evaluating and validating biomarkers in breast pathology. As more and more targeted therapy is applied in breast cancer patients, pathologists will be under pressure to analyze additional biomarkers. We also predict that pathologists will have to reconcile not only with morphology and IHC but also with additional multigene expression assays that clinicians are going to use in the future.

REFERENCES

1. Hammond ME, et al. American Society of Clinical Oncology/College of American Pathologists guideline recommendations for immunohistochemical testing of estrogen and progesterone receptors in breast cancer. J Clin Oncol 2010;28:2784-2795.
2. Clarke RB. Steroid receptors and proliferation in the human breast. Steroids 2003;68:789-794.
3. Fuqua SAW, Schiff S. The biology of estrogen receptors. In: Harris JR, et al, eds. Diseases of the Breast. Philadelphia: Lippincott Williams & Wilkins; 2004:585-602.
4. Keen JC, Davidson NE. The biology of breast carcinoma. Cancer 2003;97(Suppl 3):825-833.
5. Elledge RM, Allred DC. Clinical aspects of estrogen and progesterone receptors. In Harris JR, et al, eds. Diseases of the Breast. Philadelphia: Lippincott Williams & Wilkins; 2004:602-617.
6. Albain K, et al. Concurrent (CAFT) versus sequential (CAF-T) chemohormonal therapy (cyclophosphamide, doxorubicin, 5-fluorouracil, tamoxifen) versus T alone for postmenopausal, node-positive, estrogen (ER) and/or progestorn (PR-recpetor-positive breast cancer: mature outcomes and new biological correlates on phase III Intergroup Trial 0100 (SWOG-8814) [abstract 37]. Breast Cancer Res Treat 2004;88(Suppl 1):A37.
7. Dahabreh IJ, et al. Trastuzumab in the adjuvant treatment of early-stage breast cancer: a systematic review and meta-analysis of randomized controlled trials. Oncologist 2008;13:620-630.
8. Fitzgibbons PL, et al. Prognostic factors in breast cancer. College of American Pathologists Consensus Statement 1999. Arch Pathol Lab Med 2000;124:966-978.
9. Prat A, Baselga J. The role of hormonal therapy in the management of hormonal-receptor-positive breast cancer with co-expression of HER2. Nat Clin Pract Oncol 2008;5:531-542.
10. Early Breast Cancer Trialists' Collaborative Group (EBCTCG). Effects of chemotherapy and hormonal therapy for early breast cancer on recurrence and 15-year survival: an overview of the randomised trials. Lancet 2005;365:1687-1717.
11. Allred DC, et al. Adjuvant tamoxifen reduces subsequent breast cancer in women with hormone receptor-positive DCIS: a study based on NSABP protocol B-24. 2011.
12. Fisher B, et al. Tamoxifen for the prevention of breast cancer: current status of the National Surgical Adjuvant Breast and Bowel Project P-1 Study. J Natl Cancer Inst 2005;97:1652-1662.
13. Buzdar A, Vergote I, Sainsbury R. The impact of hormone receptor status on the clinical efficacy of the new-generation aromatase inhibitors: a review of data from first-line metastatic disease trials in postmenopausal women. Breast J 2004;10:211-217.
14. Dowsett M, et al. Retrospective analysis of time to recurrence in the ATAC trial according to hormone receptor status: an hypothesis-generating study. J Clin Oncol 2005;23:30.
15. Viale G, et al. Prognostic and predictive value of centrally reviewed expression of estrogen and progesterone receptors in a randomized trial comparing letrozole and tamoxifen adjuvant therapy for postmenopausal early breast cancer: BIG 1-98. J Clin Oncol 2007;25:3846-3852.
16. Goss PE, et al. Efficacy of letrozole extended adjuvant therapy according to estrogen receptor and progesterone receptor status of the primary tumor: National Cancer Institute of Canada Clinical Trials Group MA.17. J Clin Oncol 2007;25:2006-2011.
17. Harvey JM, et al. Estrogen receptor status by immunohistochemistry is superior to the ligand-binding assay for predicting response to adjuvant endocrine therapy in breast cancer. J Clin Oncol 1999;17:1474-1481.
18. Elledge RM, et al. Estrogen receptor (ER) and progesterone receptor (PgR) by ligand-binding assay compared with ER, PgR, and pS2 by immunohistochemistry in predicting response to tamoxifen in metastatic breast cancer: a Southwest Oncology Group Study. Int J Cancer 2000;89:111-117.
19. Allred DC. Problems and solutions in the evaluation of hormone receptors in breast cancer. J Clin Oncol 2008;26:2433-2435.
20. Gown AM. Current issues in ER and HER2 testing by IHC in breast cancer. Mod Pathol 2008;21(Suppl 2):S8-S15.
21. Hede K. Breast cancer testing scandal shines spotlight on black box of clinical laboratory testing. J Natl Cancer Inst 2008;100:836-837; 844.
22. Rhodes A, et al. Immunohistochemical demonstration of oestrogen and progesterone receptors: correlation of standards achieved on in house tumours with that achieved on external quality assessment material in over 150 laboratories from 26 countries. J Clin Pathol 2000;53:292-301.
23. Rhodes A, et al. Reliability of immunohistochemical demonstration of oestrogen receptors in routine practice: interlaboratory variance in the sensitivity of detection and evaluation of scoring systems. J Clin Pathol 2000;53:125-130.

24. Rhodes AR, et al. Study of interlaboratory reliability and reproducibility of estrogen and progesterone receptor assays in Europe. Am J Clin Pathol 2001;115:44-58.

25. Hayes DF, et al. Tumor marker utility grading system: a framework to evaluate clinical utility of tumor markers. J Natl Cancer Inst 1996;88:1456-1466.

26. Bast RC, et al. Update of recommendations for the use of tumor markers in breast and colorectal cancer: clinical practice guidelines for the American Society of Clinical Oncology. J Clin Oncol 2001;19:1865-1878.

27. Cheang MC, et al. Immunohistochemical detection using the new rabbit monoclonal antibody SP1 of estrogen receptor in breast cancer is superior to mouse monoclonal antibody 1D5 in predicting survival. J Clin Oncol 2006;24:5637-5644.

28. Dowsett M, et al. Relationship between quantitative estrogen and progesterone receptor expression and human epidermal growth factor receptor 2 (HER-2) status with recurrence in the Arimidex, Tamoxifen, Alone or in Combination trial. J Clin Oncol 2008;26:1059-1065.

29. Mohsin SK, et al. Progesterone receptor by immunohistochemistry and clinical outcome in breast cancer: a validation study. Mod Pathol 2004;7:1545-1554.

30. Phillips T, et al. Development of standard estrogen and progesterone receptor immunohistochemical assays for selection of patients for antihormonal therapy. Appl Immunohistochem Mol Morphol 2007;15:325-331.

31. Regan MM, et al. Re-evaluating adjuvant breast cancer trials: assessing hormone receptor status by immunohistochemical versus extraction assays. J Natl Cancer Inst 2006;98:1571-1581.

32. Dowsett M, et al. International Web-based consultation on priorities for translational breast cancer research. Breast Cancer Res 2007;9:R81.

33. Viale G, et al. Chemoendocrine compared with endocrine adjuvant therapies for node-negative breast cancer: predictive value of centrally reviewed expression of estrogen and progesterone receptors—International Breast Cancer Study Group. J Clin Oncol 2008;26:1404-1410.

34. Ellis MJ, et al. Outcome prediction for estrogen receptor-positive breast cancer based on postneoadjuvant endocrine therapy tumor characteristics. J Natl Cancer Inst 2008;100:1380-1388.

35. Love RR, et al. Oophorectomy and tamoxifen adjuvant therapy in premenopausal Vietnamese and Chinese women with operable breast cancer. J Clin Oncol 2002;20:2559-2566.

36. Allred DC, Brown P, Medina D. The origins of estrogen receptor alpha-positive and estrogen receptor alpha-negative human breast cancer. Breast Cancer Res 2004;6:240-245.

37. Collins LC, Botero ML, Schnitt SJ. Bimodal frequency distribution of estrogen receptor immunohistochemical staining results in breast cancer: an analysis of 825 cases. Am J Clin Pathol 2005;123:16-20.

38. Nadji M, et al. Immunohistochemistry of estrogen and progesterone receptors reconsidered: experience with 5,993 breast cancers. Am J Clin Pathol 2005;123:21-27.

39. Allred DC, et al. Ductal carcinoma in situ and the emergence of diversity during breast cancer evolution. Clin Cancer Res 2008;14:370-378.

40. Magne N, et al. Different clinical impact of estradiol receptor determination according to the analytical method: a study on 1940 breast cancer patients over a period of 16 consecutive years. Breast Cancer Res Treat 2006;95:179-184.

41. Ries LAG, Eisner MP, Kosary CL. SEER Cancer Statistics Review 1975-2000. Vol. Bethesda, MD: National Cancer Institute; 2003. Available at http://seer.cancer.gov/csr/1975_2000.

42. Allred DC, Mohsin SK. ER expression is not bimodal in breast cancer. Am J Clin Pathol 2005;124:474-475; author reply 475-476.

43. Allred DC. Commentary: hormone receptor testing in breast cancer: a distress signal from Canada. Oncologist 2008;13:1134-1136.

44. Wolff AC, Hammond ME, Schwartz JN, et al. American Society of Clinical Oncology/College of American Pathologists guideline recommendations for human epidermal growth factor receptor 2 testing in breast cancer. J Clin Oncol 2007;25:118-145.

45. Middleton LP, et al. Implementation of American Society of Clinical Oncology/College of American Pathologists *HER2* Guideline Recommendations in a tertiary care facility increases *HER2* immunohistochemistry and fluorescence in situ hybridization concordance and decreases the number of inconclusive cases. Arch Pathol Lab Med 2009;133:775-780.

46. Allred DC. Biological features of human premalignant breast disease and the progression to cancer. In Harris JR, et al, eds. Diseases of the Breast. New York: Lippincott Williams & Wilkins; 2009:323-334.

47. Arpino G, et al. Infiltrating lobular carcinoma of the breast: tumor characteristics and clinical outcome. Breast Cancer Res 2004;6:R149-R156.

48. Diab SG, et al. Tumor characteristics and clinical outcome of tubular and mucinous breast carcinomas. J Clin Oncol 1999;17:1442-1448.

49. Carey LA, et al. Race, breast cancer subtypes, and survival in the Carolina Breast Cancer Study. JAMA 2006;295:2492-2502.

50. Albain KS, et al. Prognostic and predictive value of the 21-gene recurrence score assay in postmenopausal women with node-positive, oestrogen-receptor-positive breast cancer on chemotherapy: a retrospective analysis of a randomised trial. Lancet Oncol 2010;11:55-65.

51. Badve S, et al. Estrogen- and progesterone-receptor status in ECOG 2197: comparison of immunohistochemistry by local and central laboratories and quantitative reverse polymerase chain reaction by central laboratory. J Clin Oncol 2008;26:2473-2481.

52. Paik S, Shak S, Tang G, et al. A multigene assay to predict recurrence of tamoxifen-treated, node-negative breast cancer. N Engl J Med 2004;351:2817-2826.

53. Paik S, et al. Gene expression and benefit of chemotherapy in women with node-negative, estrogen receptor-positive breast cancer. J Clin Oncol 2006;24:3726-3734.

54. Oh DS, et al. Estrogen-regulated genes predict survival in hormone receptor-positive breast cancers. J Clin Oncol 2006;24:1656-1664.

55. Goetz MP, et al. A two-gene expression ratio of homeobox 13 and interleukin-17B receptor for prediction of recurrence and survival in women receiving adjuvant tamoxifen. Clin Cancer Res 2006;12:2080-2087.

56. Ma XJ, et al. The HOXB13:IL17BR expression index is a prognostic factor in early-stage breast cancer. J Clin Oncol 2006;24:4611-4619.

57. Ma XJ, et al. A two-gene expression ratio predicts clinical outcome in breast cancer patients treated with tamoxifen. Cancer Cell 2004;5:607-616.

58. Loi S, et al. Definition of clinically distinct molecular subtypes in estrogen receptor-positive breast carcinomas through genomic grade. J Clin Oncol 2007;25:1239-1246.

59. Chung GG, et al. Quantitative analysis of estrogen receptor heterogeneity in breast cancer. Lab Invest 2007;87:662-669.

60. Rojo MG, Bueno G, Slodkowska J. Review of imaging solutions for integrated quantitative immunohistochemistry in the pathology daily practice. Folia Histochem Cytobiol 2009;47:349-354.

61. Tholouli E, et al. Quantum dots light up pathology. J Pathol 2008;6:275-285.

62. Anderson E. Progesterone receptors—animal models and cell signaling in breast cancer: the role of oestrogen and progesterone receptors in human mammary development and tumorigenesis. Breast Cancer Res 2002;4:197-201.

63. Jacobsen BM, et al. Expression profiling of human breast cancers and gene regulation by progesterone receptors. J Mammary Gland Biol Neoplasia 2003;8:257-268.

64. Carlson RW, et al. NCCN Breast Cancer Practice Guidelines Panel. Cancer Control 2001;8(6 Suppl 2):54-61.

65. Bardou VJ, et al. Progesterone receptor status significantly improves outcome prediction over estrogen receptor status alone for adjuvant endocrine therapy in two large breast cancer databases. J Clin Oncol 2003;21:1973-1979.

66. Cui X, et al. Biology of progesterone receptor loss in breast cancer and its implications for endocrine therapy. J Clin Oncol 2005;23:7721-7735.

67. Schiff R, et al. Cross-talk between estrogen receptor and growth factor pathways as a molecular target for overcoming endocrine resistance. Clin Cancer Res 2004;10:31S-36S.

68. Kampa M, Pelekanou V, Castanas E. Membrane-initiated steroid action in breast and prostate cancer. Steroids 2008;73:953-960.

69. Levin ER, Pietras RJ. Estrogen receptors outside the nucleus in breast cancer. Breast Cancer Res Treat 2008;108:351-361.

70. Silva CM, Shupnik MA. Integration of steroid and growth factor pathways in breast cancer: focus on signal transducers and activators of transcription and their potential role in resistance. Mol Endocrinol 2007;21:1499-1512.

71. Song RX. Membrane-initiated steroid signaling action of estrogen and breast cancer. Semin Reprod Med 2007;25:187-197.

72. Song RX, Santen RJ. Membrane initiated estrogen signaling in breast cancer. Biol Reprod 2006;75:9-16.

73. Schechter AL, Stern DF, Vaidyanathan L, et al. The neu oncogene: an erb-B-related gene encoding a 185,000-Mr tumour antigen. Nature 1984;312:513-516.

74. Coussens L, Yang-Feng TL, Liao YC, et al. Tyrosine kinase receptor with extensive homology to EGF receptor shares chromosomal location with neu oncogene. Science 1985;230:1132-1139.

75. Semba K, Kamata N, Toyoshima K, Yamamoto T. A v-erbB-related protooncogene, c-erbB-2, is distinct from the c-erbB-1/epidermal growth factor-receptor gene and is amplified in a human salivary gland adenocarcinoma. Proc Natl Acad Sci U S A 1985;82:6497-6501.

76. Di Fiore PP, Pierce JH, Kraus MH, et al. erbB-2 is a potent oncogene when overexpressed in NIH/3T3 cells. Science 1987;237:178-182.

77. Akiyama T, Sudo C, Ogawara H, et al. The product of the human c-erbB-2 gene: a 185-kilodalton glycoprotein with tyrosine kinase activity. Science 1986;232:1644-1646.

78. Slamon DJ, Clark GM, Wong SG, et al. Human breast cancer: correlation of relapse and survival with amplification of the HER-2/neu oncogene. Science 1987;235:177-182.

79. Owens MA, Horten BC, Da Silva MM. HER2 amplification ratios by fluorescence in situ hybridization and correlation with immunohistochemistry in a cohort of 6556 breast cancer tissues. Clin Breast Cancer 2004;5:63-69.

80. Yaziji H, Goldstein LC, Barry TS, et al. HER-2 testing in breast cancer using parallel tissue-based methods. JAMA 2004;291:1972-1977.

81. Hayes DF, Thor AD, Dressler LG, et al. HER2 and response to paclitaxel in node-positive breast cancer. N Engl J Med 2007;357:1496-1506.

82. Konecny GE, Thomssen C, Luck HJ, et al. Her-2/neu gene amplification and response to paclitaxel in patients with metastatic breast cancer. J Natl Cancer Inst 2004;96:1141-1151.

83. Menard S, Valagussa P, Pilotti S, et al. Response to cyclophosphamide, methotrexate, and fluorouracil in lymph node-positive breast cancer according to HER2 overexpression and other tumor biologic variables. J Clin Oncol 2001;19:329-335.

84. Pritchard KI, Shepherd LE, O'Malley FP, et al. HER2 and responsiveness of breast cancer to adjuvant chemotherapy. N Engl J Med 2006;354:2103-2111.

85. Thor AD, Berry DA, Budman DR, et al. erbB-2, p53, and efficacy of adjuvant therapy in lymph node-positive breast cancer. J Natl Cancer Inst 1998;90:1346-1360.

86. Ellis MJ, Coop A, Singh B, et al. Letrozole is more effective neoadjuvant endocrine therapy than tamoxifen for ErbB-1- and/or ErbB-2-positive, estrogen receptor-positive primary breast cancer: evidence from a phase III randomized trial. J Clin Oncol 2001;19:3808-3816.

87. Konecny G, Pauletti G, Pegram M, et al. Quantitative association between HER-2/neu and steroid hormone receptors in hormone receptor-positive primary breast cancer. J Natl Cancer Inst 2003;95:142-153.

88. Joensuu H, Kellokumpu-Lehtinen PL, et al. Adjuvant docetaxel or vinorelbine with or without trastuzumab for breast cancer. N Engl J Med 2006;354:809-820.

89. Piccart-Gebhart MJ, Procter M, Leyland-Jones B, et al. Trastuzumab after adjuvant chemotherapy in HER2-positive breast cancer. N Engl J Med 2005;353:1659-1672.

90. Romond EH, Perez EA, Bryant J, et al. Trastuzumab plus adjuvant chemotherapy for operable HER2-positive breast cancer. N Engl J Med 2005;353:1673-1684.

91. Smith I, Procter M, Gelber RD, et al. 2-year follow-up of trastuzumab after adjuvant chemotherapy in HER2-positive breast cancer: a randomised controlled trial. Lancet 2007;369:29-36.

92. Goldstein NS, Ferkowicz M, Odish E, et al. Minimum formalin fixation time for consistent estrogen receptor immunohistochemical staining of invasive breast carcinoma. Am J Clin Pathol 2003;120:86-92.

93. Slamon DJ, Leyland-Jones B, Shak S, et al. Use of chemotherapy plus a monoclonal antibody against HER2 for metastatic breast cancer that overexpresses HER2. N Engl J Med 2001;344:783-792.

94. Egervari K, Szollosi Z, Nemes Z. Immunohistochemical antibodies in breast cancer HER2 diagnostics. A comparative immunohistochemical and fluorescence in situ hybridization study. Tumour Biol 2008;29:18-27.

95. Gouvea AP, Milanezi F, Olson SJ, et al. Selecting antibodies to detect HER2 overexpression by immunohistochemistry in invasive mammary carcinomas. Appl Immunohistochem Mol Morphol 2006;14:103-108.

96. Roche PC, Ingle JN. Increased HER2 with U.S. Food and Drug Administration-approved antibody. J Clin Oncol 1999;17:434.

97. Powell WC, Hicks DG, Prescott N, et al. A new rabbit monoclonal antibody (4B5) for the immunohistochemical (IHC) determination of the HER2 status in breast cancer: comparison with CB11, fluorescence in situ hybridization (FISH), and interlaboratory reproducibility. Appl Immunohistochem Mol Morphol 2007;15:94-102.

98. Acs G, Wang L, Raghunath PN, et al. Role of different immunostaining patterns in HercepTest interpretation and criteria for gene amplification as determined by fluorescence in situ hybridization. Appl Immunohistochem Mol Morphol 2003;11:222-229.

99. Bhargava R, Naeem R, Marconi S, et al. Tyrosine kinase activation in breast carcinoma with correlation to HER-2/neu gene amplification and receptor overexpression. Hum Pathol 2001;32:1344-1350.

100. Perez EA, Roche PC, Jenkins RB, et al. HER2 testing in patients with breast cancer: poor correlation between weak positivity by immunohistochemistry and gene amplification by fluorescence in situ hybridization. Mayo Clin Proc 2002;77:148-154.

101. Garcia-Caballero T, Menendez MD, Vazquez-Boquete A, et al. HER2 status determination in breast carcinomas. A practical approach. Histol Histopathol 2006;21:227-236.

102. Tsuda H, Akiyama F, Terasaki H, et al. Detection of HER-2/neu (c-erb B-2) DNA amplification in primary breast carcinoma. Interobserver reproducibility and correlation with immunohistochemical HER-2 overexpression. Cancer 2001;92:2965-2974.

103. Tubbs RR, Pettay JD, Roche PC, et al. Discrepancies in clinical laboratory testing of eligibility for trastuzumab therapy: apparent immunohistochemical false-positives do not get the message. J Clin Oncol 2001;19:2714-2721.

104. Chorn N. Accurate identification of HER2-positive patients is essential for superior outcomes with trastuzumab therapy. Oncol Nurs Forum 2006;33:265-272.

105. Mass RD, Press MF, Anderson S, et al. Evaluation of clinical outcomes according to HER2 detection by fluorescence in situ hybridization in women with metastatic breast cancer treated with trastuzumab. Clin Breast Cancer 2005;6:240-246.

106. Clinical laboratory assays for HER-2/neu amplification and overexpression: quality assurance, standardization, and proficiency testing. Arch Pathol Lab Med 2002;126:803-808.

107. Rhodes A, Borthwick D, Sykes R, et al. The use of cell line standards to reduce HER-2/neu assay variation in multiple European cancer centers and the potential of automated image analysis to provide for more accurate cut points for predicting clinical response to trastuzumab. Am J Clin Pathol 2004;122:51-60.

108. Zarbo RJ, Hammond ME. Conference summary, Strategic Science symposium. Her-2/neu testing of breast cancer patients in clinical practice. Arch Pathol Lab Med 2003;127:549-553.

109. Persons DL, Tubbs RR, Cooley LD, et al. HER-2 fluorescence in situ hybridization: results from the survey program of the College of American Pathologists. Arch Pathol Lab Med 2006;130:325-331.

110. Chivukula M, Bhargava R, Brufsky A, et al. Clinical importance of *HER2* immunohistologic heterogeneous expression in core-needle biopsies vs resection specimens for equivocal (immunohistochemical score 2+) cases. Mod Pathol 2008;21:363-368.
111. Lal P, Salazar PA, Hudis CA, et al. *HER-2* testing in breast cancer using immunohistochemical analysis and fluorescence in situ hybridization: a single-institution experience of 2,279 cases and comparison of dual-color and single-color scoring. Am J Clin Pathol 2004;121:631-636.
112. Bose S, Mohammed M, Shintaku P, Rao PN. Her-2/neu gene amplification in low to moderately expressing breast cancers: possible role of chromosome 17/*Her-2/neu* polysomy. Breast J 2001;7:337-344.
113. Hofmann M, Stoss O, Gaiser T, et al. Central *HER2* IHC and FISH analysis in a trastuzumab (Herceptin) phase II monotherapy study: assessment of test sensitivity and impact of chromosome 17 polysomy. J Clin Pathol 2008;61:89-94.
114. Striebel JM, Bhargava R, Horbinski C, et al. The equivocally amplified *HER2* FISH result on breast core biopsy: indications for further sampling do affect patient management. Am J Clin Pathol 2008;129:383-390.
115. Bhargava R, Lal P, Chen B. Chromogenic in situ hybridization for the detection of *HER-2/neu* gene amplification in breast cancer with an emphasis on tumors with borderline and low-level amplification: does it measure up to fluorescence in situ hybridization? Am J Clin Pathol 2005;123:237-243.
116. Gupta D, Middleton LP, Whitaker MJ, Abrams J. Comparison of fluorescence and chromogenic in situ hybridization for detection of *HER-2/neu* oncogene in breast cancer. Am J Clin Pathol 2003;119:381-387.
117. Isola J, Tanner M, Forsyth A, et al. Interlaboratory comparison of *HER-2* oncogene amplification as detected by chromogenic and fluorescence in situ hybridization. Clin Cancer Res 2004;10:4793-4798.
118. Tanner M, Gancberg D, Di Leo A, et al. Chromogenic in situ hybridization: a practical alternative for fluorescence in situ hybridization to detect *HER-2/neu* oncogene amplification in archival breast cancer samples. Am J Pathol 2000;157:1467-1472.
119. Aubele M, Mattis A, Zitzelsberger H, et al. Intratumoral heterogeneity in breast carcinoma revealed by laser-microdissection and comparative genomic hybridization. Cancer Genet Cytogenet 1999;110:94-102.
120. Bohm M, Wieland I, Schutze K, Rubben H, Microbeam MOMe NT. Non-contact laser microdissection of membrane-mounted native tissue. Am J Pathol 1997;151:63-67.
121. Gjerdrum LM, Lielpetere I, Rasmussen LM, et al. Laser-assisted microdissection of membrane-mounted paraffin sections for polymerase chain reaction analysis: identification of cell populations using immunohistochemistry and in situ hybridization. J Mol Diagn 2001;3:105-110.
122. Emmert-Buck MR, Bonner RF, Smith PD, et al. Laser capture microdissection. Science 1996;274:998-1001.
123. Fend F, Emmert-Buck MR, Chuaqui R, et al. Immuno-LCM: laser capture microdissection of immunostained frozen sections for mRNA analysis. Am J Pathol 1999;154:61-66.
124. Lahr G. RT-PCR from archival single cells is a suitable method to analyze specific gene expression. Lab Invest 2000;80:1477-1479.
125. Schutze K, Lahr G. Identification of expressed genes by laser-mediated manipulation of single cells. Nat Biotechnol 1998;16:737-742.
126. Larson JS, Goodman LJ, Tan Y, et al. Analytical validation of a Highly Quantitative, Sensitive, Accurate, and Reproducible Assay (HERmark) for the measurement of *HER2* total protein and *HER2* homodimers in FFPE breast cancer tumor specimens. Pathol Res Int 2010:814176.
127. Shi Y, Huang W, Tan Y, et al. A novel proximity assay for the detection of proteins and protein complexes: quantitation of *HER1* and *HER2* total protein expression and homodimerization in formalin-fixed, paraffin-embedded cell lines and breast cancer tissue. Diagn Mol Pathol 2009;18:11-21.
128. DiGiovanna MP, Stern DF. Activation state-specific monoclonal antibody detects tyrosine phosphorylated p185neu/erbB-2 in a subset of human breast tumors overexpressing this receptor. Cancer Res 1995;55:1946-1955.
129. Thor AD, Liu S, Edgerton S, et al. Activation (tyrosine phosphorylation) of ErbB-2 (*HER-2/neu*): a study of incidence and correlation with outcome in breast cancer. J Clin Oncol 2000;18:3230-3239.
130. Fehm T, Maimonis P, Katalinic A, Jager WH. The prognostic significance of c-erbB-2 serum protein in metastatic breast cancer. Oncology 1998;55:33-38.
131. Isola JJ, Holli K, Oksa H, et al. Elevated erbB-2 oncoprotein levels in preoperative and follow-up serum samples define an aggressive disease course in patients with breast cancer. Cancer 1994;73:652-658.
132. Willsher PC, Beaver J, Pinder S, et al. Prognostic significance of serum c-erbB-2 protein in breast cancer patients. Breast Cancer Res Treat 1996;40:251-255.
133. Kong SY, Nam BH, Lee KS, et al. Predicting tissue *HER2* status using serum *HER2* levels in patients with metastatic breast cancer. Clin Chem 2006;52:1510-1515.
134. Esteva FJ, Cheli CD, Fritsche H, et al. Clinical utility of serum *HER2/neu* in monitoring and prediction of progression-free survival in metastatic breast cancer patients treated with trastuzumab-based therapies. Breast Cancer Res 2005;7:R436-R443.
135. Lal P, Tan LK, Chen B. Correlation of *HER-2* status with estrogen and progesterone receptors and histologic features in 3,655 invasive breast carcinomas. Am J Clin Pathol 2005;123:541-546.
136. Rosenthal SI, Depowski PL, Sheehan CE, Ross JS. Comparison of *HER-2/neu* oncogene amplification detected by fluorescence in situ hybridization in lobular and ductal breast cancer. Appl Immunohistochem Mol Morphol 2002;10:40-46.
137. Simpson PT, Reis-Filho JS, Lambros MB, et al. Molecular profiling pleomorphic lobular carcinomas of the breast: evidence for a common molecular genetic pathway with classic lobular carcinomas. J Pathol 2008;215:231-244.
138. Frolik D, Caduff R, Varga Z. Pleomorphic lobular carcinoma of the breast: its cell kinetics, expression of oncogenes and tumour suppressor genes compared with invasive ductal carcinomas and classical infiltrating lobular carcinomas. Histopathology 2001;39:503-513.
139. Varga Z, Zhao J, Ohlschlegel C, et al. Preferential *HER-2/neu* overexpression and/or amplification in aggressive histological subtypes of invasive breast cancer. Histopathology 2004;44:332-338.
140. Vargas AC, Lakhani SR, Simpson PT. Pleomorphic lobular carcinoma of the breast: molecular pathology and clinical impact. Future Oncol 2009;5:233-243.
141. Yu J, Dabbs DJ, Shuai Y, et al. Classical type invasive lobular carcinoma with *HER2* overexpression: clinical, histological and hormone receptor characteristics. Am J Clin Pathol 2011;136:88-97.
142. Bhargava R, Striebel J, Beriwal S, et al. Prevalence, morphologic features and proliferation indices of breast carcinoma molecular classes using immunohistochemical surrogate markers. Int J Clin Exp Pathol 2009;2:444-455.
143. Oakley GJ 3rd, Tubbs RR, Crowe J, et al. *HER-2* amplification in tubular carcinoma of the breast. Am J Clin Pathol 2006;126:55-58.
144. Lacroix-Triki M, Suarez PH, MacKay A, et al. Mucinous carcinoma of the breast is genomically distinct from invasive ductal carcinomas of no special type. J Pathol 2010;222:282-298.
145. Jacquemier J, Padovani L, Rabayrol L, et al. Typical medullary breast carcinomas have a basal/myoepithelial phenotype. J Pathol 2005;207:260-268.
146. Lin NU, Winer EP. Brain metastases: the *HER2* paradigm. Clin Cancer Res 2007;13:1648-1655.
147. Bendell JC, Domchek SM, Burstein HJ, et al. Central nervous system metastases in women who receive trastuzumab-based therapy for metastatic breast carcinoma. Cancer 2003;97:2972-2977.
148. Lin NU, Carey LA, Liu MC, et al. Phase II trial of lapatinib for brain metastases in patients with human epidermal growth factor receptor 2-positive breast cancer. J Clin Oncol 2008;26:1993-1999.
149. Simon R, Nocito A, Hubscher T, et al. Patterns of her-2/neu amplification and overexpression in primary and metastatic breast cancer. J Natl Cancer Inst 2001;93:1141-1146.

150. Symmans WF, Liu J, Knowles DM, Inghirami G. Breast cancer heterogeneity: evaluation of clonality in primary and metastatic lesions. Hum Pathol 1995;26:210-216.
151. Vincent-Salomon A, Jouve M, Genin P, et al. HER2 status in patients with breast carcinoma is not modified selectively by preoperative chemotherapy and is stable during the metastatic process. Cancer 2002;94:2169-2173.
152. Xu R, Perle MA, Inghirami G, et al. Amplification of Her-2/neu gene in Her-2/neu-overexpressing and -nonexpressing breast carcinomas and their synchronous benign, premalignant, and metastatic lesions detected by FISH in archival material. Mod Pathol 2002;15:116-124.
153. Lower EE, Glass E, Blau R, Harman S. HER-2/neu expression in primary and metastatic breast cancer. Breast Cancer Res Treat 2009;113:301-306.
154. Tapia C, Savic S, Wagner U, et al. HER2 gene status in primary breast cancers and matched distant metastases. Breast Cancer Res 2007;9:R31.
155. Hortobagyi GN. Overview of treatment results with trastuzumab (Herceptin) in metastatic breast cancer. Semin Oncol 2001;28:43-47.
156. Bhargava R, Dabbs DJ, Beriwal S, et al. Semiquantitative hormone receptor level influences response to trastuzumab-containing neoadjuvant chemotherapy in HER2-positive breast cancer. Mod Pathol 2011;24:367-374.
157. Bhargava R, Beriwal S, McManus K, Dabbs DJ. Insulin-like growth factor receptor-1 (IGF-1R) expression in normal breast, proliferative breast lesions, and breast carcinoma. Appl Immunohistochem Mol Morphol 2011;19:218-225.
158. Lu Y, Zi X, Zhao Y, et al. Insulin-like growth factor-1 receptor signaling and resistance to trastuzumab (Herceptin). J Natl Cancer Inst 2001;93:1852-1857.
159. Nahta R, Yuan LX, Zhang B, et al. Insulin-like growth factor-1 receptor/human epidermal growth factor receptor 2 heterodimerization contributes to trastuzumab resistance of breast cancer cells. Cancer Res 2005;65:11118-11128.
160. Berns K, Horlings HM, Hennessy BT, et al. A functional genetic approach identifies the PI3K pathway as a major determinant of trastuzumab resistance in breast cancer. Cancer Cell 2007;12:395-402.
161. Nagata Y, Lan KH, Zhou X, et al. PTEN activation contributes to tumor inhibition by trastuzumab, and loss of PTEN predicts trastuzumab resistance in patients. Cancer Cell 2004;6:117-127.
162. Pandolfi PP. Breast cancer—loss of PTEN predicts resistance to treatment. N Engl J Med 2004;351:2337-2338.
163. Pegram MD, Reese DM. Combined biological therapy of breast cancer using monoclonal antibodies directed against HER2/neu protein and vascular endothelial growth factor. Semin Oncol 2002;29:29-37.
164. Chang JC. HER2 inhibition: from discovery to clinical practice. Clin Cancer Res 2007;13:1-3.
165. Press MF, Sauter G, Buyse M, et al. Alteration of topoisomerase II-alpha gene in human breast cancer: association with responsiveness to anthracycline-based chemotherapy. J Clin Oncol 2011;29:859-867.
166. Gao JP, Uchida T, Wang C, et al. Relationship between p53 gene mutation and protein expression: clinical significance in transitional cell carcinoma of the bladder. Int J Oncol 2000;16:469-475.
167. Salinas-Sanchez AS, Atienzar-Tobarra M, Lorenzo-Romero JG, et al. Sensitivity and specificity of p53 protein detection by immunohistochemistry in patients with urothelial bladder carcinoma. Urol Int 2007;79:321-327.
168. Sorlie T, Tibshirani R, Parker J, et al. Repeated observation of breast tumor subtypes in independent gene expression data sets. Proc Natl Acad Sci U S A 2003;100:8418-8423.
169. Olivier M, Langerod A, Carrieri P, et al. The clinical value of somatic TP53 gene mutations in 1,794 patients with breast cancer. Clin Cancer Res 2006;12:1157-1167.
170. Harris L, Fritsche H, Mennel R, et al. American Society of Clinical Oncology 2007 update of recommendations for the use of tumor markers in breast cancer. J Clin Oncol 2007;25:5287-5312.
171. Caly M, Genin P, Ghuzlan AA, et al. Analysis of correlation between mitotic index, MIB1 score and S-phase fraction as proliferation markers in invasive breast carcinoma. Methodological aspects and prognostic value in a series of 257 cases. Anticancer Res 2004;24:3283-3288.
172. Gonzalez-Vela MC, Garijo MF, Fernandez F, Val-Bernal JF. MIB1 proliferation index in breast infiltrating carcinoma: comparison with other proliferative markers and association with new biological prognostic factors. Histol Histopathol 2001;16:399-406.
173. Molino A, Micciolo R, Turazza M, et al. Ki-67 immunostaining in 322 primary breast cancers: associations with clinical and pathological variables and prognosis. Int J Cancer 1997;74:433-437.
174. Nakagomi H, Miyake T, Hada M, et al. Prognostic and therapeutic implications of the MIB-1 labeling index in breast cancer. Breast Cancer 1998;5:255-259.
175. Colozza M, Azambuja E, Cardoso F, et al. Proliferative markers as prognostic and predictive tools in early breast cancer: where are we now? Ann Oncol 2005;16:1723-1739.
176. Perou CM, Jeffrey SS, van de Rijn M, et al. Distinctive gene expression patterns in human mammary epithelial cells and breast cancers. Proc Natl Acad Sci U S A 1999;96:9212-9217.
177. Perou CM, Sorlie T, Eisen MB, et al. Molecular portraits of human breast tumours. Nature 2000;406:747-752.
178. Cheang MC, Chia SK, Voduc D, et al. Ki67 index, HER2 status, and prognosis of patients with luminal B breast cancer. J Natl Cancer Inst 2009;101:736-750.
179. Bhargava R, Gerald WL, Li AR, et al. EGFR gene amplification in breast cancer: correlation with epidermal growth factor receptor mRNA and protein expression and HER-2 status and absence of EGFR-activating mutations. Mod Pathol 2005;18:1027-1033.
180. Cheang MC, Voduc D, Bajdik C, et al. Basal-like breast cancer defined by five biomarkers has superior prognostic value than triple-negative phenotype. Clin Cancer Res 2008;14:1368-1376.
181. Nielsen TO, Hsu FD, Jensen K, et al. Immunohistochemical and clinical characterization of the basal-like subtype of invasive breast carcinoma. Clin Cancer Res 2004;10:5367-5374.
182. Reis-Filho JS, Pinheiro C, Lambros MB, et al. EGFR amplification and lack of activating mutations in metaplastic breast carcinomas. J Pathol 2006;209:445-453.
183. Gholam D, Chebib A, Hauteville D, et al. Combined paclitaxel and cetuximab achieved a major response on the skin metastases of a patient with epidermal growth factor receptor-positive, estrogen receptor-negative, progesterone receptor-negative and human epidermal growth factor receptor-2-negative (triple-negative) breast cancer. Anticancer Drugs 2007;18:835-837.
184. Modi S, D'Andrea G, Norton L, et al. A phase I study of cetuximab/paclitaxel in patients with advanced-stage breast cancer. Clin Breast Cancer 2006;7:270-277.
185. Duffy MJ. Urokinase plasminogen activator and its inhibitor, PAI-1, as prognostic markers in breast cancer: from pilot to level 1 evidence studies. Clin Chem 2002;48:1194-1197.
186. Foekens JA, Schmitt M, van Putten WL, et al. Plasminogen activator inhibitor-1 and prognosis in primary breast cancer. J Clin Oncol 1994;12:1648-1658.
187. Look MP, van Putten WL, Duffy MJ, et al. Pooled analysis of prognostic impact of urokinase-type plasminogen activator and its inhibitor PAI-1 in 8377 breast cancer patients. J Natl Cancer Inst 2002;94:116-128.
188. Visscher DW, Sarkar F, LoRusso P, et al. Immunohistologic evaluation of invasion-associated proteases in breast carcinoma. Mod Pathol 1993;6:302-306.
189. Schmitt M, Sturmheit AS, Welk A, et al. Procedures for the quantitative protein determination of urokinase and its inhibitor, PAI-1, in human breast cancer tissue extracts by ELISA. Methods Mol Med 2006;120:245-265.
190. Grimberg A, Cohen P. Role of insulin-like growth factors and their binding proteins in growth control and carcinogenesis. J Cell Physiol 2000;183:1-9.
191. Belfiore A, Frasca F. IGF and insulin receptor signaling in breast cancer. J Mammary Gland Biol Neoplasia 2008;13:381-406.
192. Ouban A, Muraca P, Yeatman T, Coppola D. Expression and distribution of insulin-like growth factor-1 receptor in human carcinomas. Hum Pathol 2003;34:803-808.
193. Papa V, Gliozzo B, Clark GM, et al. Insulin-like growth factor-I receptors are overexpressed and predict a low risk in human breast cancer. Cancer Res 1993;53:3736-3740.
194. Railo MJ, von Smitten K, Pekonen F. The prognostic value of insulin-like growth factor-I in breast cancer patients. Results of a follow-up study on 126 patients. Eur J Cancer 1994;30A:307-311.

195. Castiglione F, Sarotto I, Fontana V, et al. Bcl2, p53 and clinical outcome in a series of 138 operable breast cancer patients. Anticancer Res 1999;19:4555-4563.

196. Ioachim EE, Malamou-Mitsi V, Kamina SA, et al. Immunohistochemical expression of Bcl-2 protein in breast lesions: correlation with Bax, p53, Rb, C-erbB-2, EGFR and proliferation indices. Anticancer Res 2000;20:4221-4225.

197. Kroger N, Milde-Langosch K, Riethdorf S, et al. Prognostic and predictive effects of immunohistochemical factors in high-risk primary breast cancer patients. Clin Cancer Res 2006;12: 159-168.

198. Leek RD, Kaklamanis L, Pezzella F, et al. bcl-2 in normal human breast and carcinoma, association with oestrogen receptor-positive, epidermal growth factor receptor-negative tumours and in situ cancer. Br J Cancer 1994;69:135-139.

199. Abdel-Fatah TM, Powe DG, Ball G, et al. Proposal for a modified grading system based on mitotic index and Bcl2 provides objective determination of clinical outcome for patients with breast cancer. J Pathol 2010;222:388-399.

200. Badve S, Turbin D, Thorat MA, et al. FOXA1 expression in breast cancer–correlation with luminal subtype A and survival. Clin Cancer Res 2007;13:4415-4421.

201. Laganiere J, Deblois G, Lefebvre C, et al. From the cover: location analysis of estrogen receptor alpha target promoters reveals that FOXA1 defines a domain of the estrogen response. Proc Natl Acad Sci U S A 2005;102:11651-11656.

202. Thorat MA, Marchio C, Morimiya A, et al. Forkhead box A1 expression in breast cancer is associated with luminal subtype and good prognosis. J Clin Pathol 2008;61:327-332.

203. Badve S, Nakshatri H. Oestrogen receptor-positive breast cancer: towards bridging histopathologic and molecular classifications. J Clin Pathol 2009;62:6-12.

204. Sorlie T. Molecular classification of breast tumors: toward improved diagnostics and treatments. Methods Mol Biol 2007;360:91-114.

205. Mehra R, Varambally S, Ding L, et al. Identification of GATA3 as a breast cancer prognostic marker by global gene expression meta-analysis. Cancer Res 2005;65:11259-11264.

206. Voduc D, Cheang M, Nielsen T. GATA-3 expression in breast cancer has a strong association with estrogen receptor but lacks independent prognostic value. Cancer Epidemiol Biomarkers Prev 2008;17:365-373.

Molecular-based Testing in Breast Disease for Therapeutic Decisions

Frederick L. Baehner* • Sunil Badve

INTRODUCTION

Breast carcinoma is a heterogeneous disease. Invasive duct carcinoma, not otherwise specified (NOS), is the largest histologic group, constituting 65% to 80% of mammary carcinomas, and within this cohort, patient outcome is extremely varied. Traditional clinical pathologic metrics have been shown to be prognostically useful for the determination of whether a carcinoma will recur; however, with the exception of the estrogen receptor (ER) for hormone therapy benefit[1] and *HER2* for trastuzumab benefit,[2] they largely have not been useful for the prediction of cytotoxic chemotherapy benefit.[3] Furthermore, these standard metrics suffer from problems of reproducibility; and thus, there is a significant need for more accurate and precise clinical instruments for recurrence risk assessment and prediction of hormone and chemotherapy benefit.[4] Rapid technologic advancements in molecular biology since the early 2000s have provided a strong foundation for the development of a new generation of prognostic and predictive multiple biomarker assays.

Just as Moore's law,[5] describing how the number of transistors that can be placed inexpensively on an integrated circuit doubles approximately every 2 years, a similar pace of innovation and technologic development in the biologic sciences has led to technologic improvements and new technologies permitting the study of hundreds to thousands of genes and their patterns of transcription, thus transforming the current understanding of breast carcinoma.[5] Since the year 2000, new technologies such as comparative genomic hybridization, gene expression arrays, and quantitative real-time polymerase chain reaction (qPCR) have led to a fundamental change in the understanding of breast cancer biology and culminated in the development of new prognostic and predictive assays for clinical treatment decision making for breast cancer physicians and patients. A first generation of diagnostic assays leverage these powerful technologies and provide personalized prognostic and predictive genomic information that is independent of information derived by traditional light microscopic evaluation of breast cancer.[6–8] These new multigene assays are currently used in clinical decision making, are part of treatment guidelines, and are now being used in a new generation of clinical trials that stratify patients for tailored treatments by gene expression risk profiles.[9]

This chapter first discusses key concepts for the development and validation of gene expression signatures, introduces the intrinsic subtype classifier, and then discusses in detail the development and validation of several commercially available gene expression assays for breast cancer.

GENOMIC TECHNOLOGIES

Gene expression is a term used to describe how active a particular gene is, for example, how many times it is transcribed ("expressed"), as messenger RNA (mRNA) to produce its encoded protein. A new generation of molecular biologic tools measures this activity by counting the number of mRNA molecules in a given cell type or tissue. Because the mRNA molecule is translated within the ribosome to produce a complete protein, counting mRNA transcripts in many cases provides an estimate of the number of corresponding proteins.[10,11] Unlike the subjective assessment of single markers of protein expression using immunohistochemistry, high-throughput technologies, such as DNA microarrays and

---

*F. L. Baehner is an employee of Genomic Health, Inc.

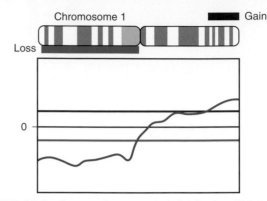

FIGURE 10-1   Comparative genomic hybridization. This is an example of the hybridization of reference DNA *(green)* and tumor DNA *(red)* to an interphase spread of cromosomes (ready for mitosis and frozen by adding colchicine to stop spindle apparatus). When the *blue line* is above the *red line,* this indicates amplification, and when it is below the *green line,* it indicates chromosomal deletion.

qPCR, allow for the precise quantitation of hundreds to thousands of gene transcriptions.[12] This expression profile provides a "portrait" of a tumor's global gene activity, which is called the *transcriptome.* The study of DNA is referred to as *genomics* and the study of mRNA is referred to as *functional genomics.* Improvements in genomic and functional genomics assessment technologies have provided the driving force for the new generation of genomic assays including comparative genomic hybridization (CGH), qPCR, gene expression microarrays, and next-generation high-throughput gene sequencing technologies.

Comparative Genomic Hybridization

METHODOLOGY

CGH provides an overview of DNA sequence copy number changes (losses, deletions, gains, amplifications) in a tumor specimen and maps these changes on normal chromosomes (Figure 10-1). CGH is a powerful method for molecular cytogenetic analysis of tumors. CGH is based on the in situ hybridization of differentially labeled total genomic tumor DNA (red) and normal reference DNA (green) to normal human metaphase chromosomes. It may be used with fixed or fresh tissue. and the fact that it works with fixed tissues explains its popularity. After hybridization and differential fluorescent staining of the bound DNAs, copy number variations among the different sequences in the tumor DNA are detected by measuring and comparing the tumor with normal fluorescence intensity ratio for each locus in the target metaphase chromosomes. Each chromosome is represented by a software package as an ideogram (see Figure 10-1). Areas of increased copy hybridization of tumor DNA are represented in red. Areas of decreased copy hybridization are represented in green.

CGH is excellent for low-resolution maps of genomic gains and losses. It is a poor method if a high-resolution map is required (sensitivity of ~50 kb).

CGH is particularly useful for analysis of DNA sequence copy number changes in common solid tumors in which high-quality metaphase preparations are often difficult to grow and in which complex karyotypes with numerous markers, double minutes, and homogeneously stained chromosomal regions are common. CGH detects only changes that are present in a substantial proportion of tumor cells (i.e., clonal aberrations). It does not reveal translocations, inversions, and other aberrations that do not change copy number. Gains or losses less than 50 kb will not be identified. At present, CGH is a research tool that complements previous methods for genetic analysis and may be used for the analysis of fixed paraffin-embedded tissues (FPETs).

ARRAY COMPARATIVE GENOMIC HYBRIDIZATION

Array-based comparative genomic hybridization (array-CGH or a-CGH) is a modification of standard chromosomal CGH using cloned fragments of DNA spotted onto glass slide arrays as the target of hybridization, rather than normal metaphase spreads. As in conventional CGH, differentially labeled tumor and normal reference DNA are hybridized to this array, and a normalized ratio of tumor to normal reference intensity is calculated for every clone. This application takes advantage of the mapping information and the cloned DNA fragments generated by the human genome project. The DNA, which is spotted onto glass slides to create CGH arrays, is prepared from bacterial artificial chromosomes (BACs), which contain approximately 100,000 base-pairs of cloned normal DNA derived from carefully mapped regions of the human genome. Current CGH arrays include BACs coding for 100 kb of DNA distributed on average every million base pairs (10% coverage, 1 megabase resolution). The next generation of CGH arrays currently being developed and validated contains approximately 30,000 BACs of 100 kb each, covering 100% of the genomic sequence. This may be used for the analysis of FPETs.

Expression Microarrays: "Expression Arrays"

FUNCTIONAL GENOMICS

Gene microarray analysis allows for the quantification of thousands of unique mRNA, obtained from fresh frozen tissue samples, on a single slide or chip. From an individual tumor, levels of mRNA can be detected, quantitated, and compared among multiple tumor samples. Typically RNA is converted to cDNA. This method is excellent for assessing correlations in gene expression, that is, expression patterns, obtained from thousands of genes that can be assessed on a single array.

cDNA microarrays are available commercially and are based on hybridization of nucleic acid strands but there are differences between platforms. An important distinction is the length of the probe. Probes are gene-specific and represent part of a gene. Microarrays may be classified as either cDNA arrays with probes up to a thousand base pairs (mer) or oligonucleotide arrays

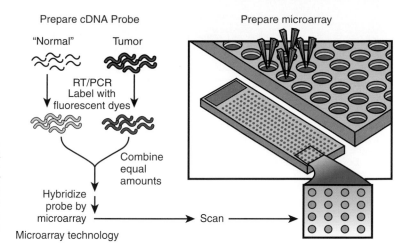

Prepare cDNA Probe

Prepare microarray

"Normal"   Tumor

RT/PCR
Label with
fluorescent dyes

Combine
equal
amounts

Hybridize
probe by
microarray

Scan

Microarray technology

FIGURE 10-2 Expression microarray methodology. **Left,** An example of the cDNA probe preparation process that often uses green fluorescence dyes for labeling of the reference cDNA and red fluorescene dyes for labeling of tumor cDNA and the hybridization process. **Right,** An example of the printing or "arraying" of thousands of copies of the probe at each site on an inert substrate (such as a glass slide or cartridge) in spatially specific locations. RT-PCR, reverse transcriptase polymerase chain reaction.

using short (25- to 30-mer) or long (60- to 70-mer) oligonucleotide probes. The probes can be either contact-spotted, ink-jet–deposited, or directly synthesized on the substrate. An array approximates the size of a glass microscope slide and it typically has thousands of individual genes represented on its surface, each gene represented multiple times (different segments of the gene at each site, respectively). Thousands of copies of the probe are printed or synthesized (*"arrayed"*) at each site on an inert substrate (such as a glass slide or cartridge) in spatially specific locations. However, in the DASL (cDNA-mediated annealing, selection, extension, and ligation technology; described later), random arrays are used.

TECHNICAL COMMENTS[13]

For the most part, DNA expression arrays require fresh frozen tissue, with the exception of a new assay, DASL (cDNA-mediated annealing, selection, extension, and ligation; Illumina) appears to be a promising exception (http://www.illumina.com/).[14] The sensitivities of the various platforms range from being able to detect from 1 to 10 copies per cell. They measure relative or absolute transcript concentrations of genes above the sensitivity level of the microarray (rendering approximately half of the transcriptome beyond reach of arrays). They have modest reproducibility (the best reported for Affymetrix, Agilent, and Codelink are 0.85).[15-17] Cross-platform correlations can be difficult owing to only moderate correlation coefficients.

METHODOLOGY

Typically, RNA is extracted from fresh frozen tissue and reverse transcribed into cDNA (Figure 10-2). Some newer assays are available for research purposes using FPETs. cDNA is labeled with a detectable fluorescent dye—the efficiency of this labeling step is crucial for assay precision and reproducibility. The cDNA is placed on the array and allowed to hybridize to the arrays. Individual molecules hybridize to complementary *gene-specific* probes on the array. Images are captured with the use of confocal laser scanning. The relative fluorescence intensity of each gene-specific probe is a measure

of the level of expression of the particular gene. The greater the degree of hybridization, the more intense the signal, implying a higher *relative* level of expression (more copies binding to the array).

Comparisons from different laboratories and across various types of microarray may differ significantly.[13] After collection, the data are normalized for comparison between the different assays. Normalization compensates for differences in labeling, hybridization, and detection methods. Normalization and filtering transformations must be carefully applied owing to effects on the results. The data are then filtered by objective criteria or statistical analyses to select expression levels that correlate with particular groups of samples. Different methods of statistical analysis applied to the same data set can produce different sets of significant genes.

Validation is important (confirmatory testing in a second series of patients/samples). Caution should be exercised in comparing data sets from different laboratories. Comparisons of published lists of genes can produce discordant results because they rarely take into account the differences in the methods of analysis of the data.[18,19]

QUANTITATIVE REAL-TIME POLYMERASE CHAIN REACTION

This method allows for the quantitation of mRNA transcripts from either fresh paraffin-embedded tissue or FPET. This technique is highly sensitive, specific, precise, and reproducible (Figure 10-3). It is generally considered to be the gold standard for measurement of gene expression.

Methodology

In brief, mRNA is extracted from fixed or fresh tissue, reverse transcribed to cDNA, and the specific target is amplified by polymerase chain reaction (PCR) using both a gene-specific probe and a pair of gene-specific primers. The probe has both a fluorescent reporter and a quencher attached to either end so there is no fluorescence signal when the probe is intact; however, when the specific primers and probe anneal to the specific target gene, due to the 5'-exonuclease activity of the Taq polymerase, the bound fluorescent-labeled probe is degraded

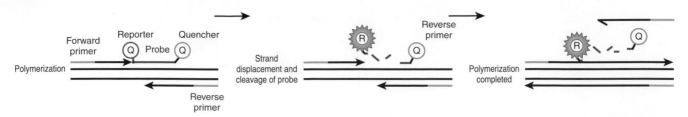

FIGURE 10-3 Quantitative real-time polymerase chain reaction (qPCR). The RNA is extracted, reverse transcribed, and mixed with two specific primers (generally within 100 base pairs of each other in the case of formalin-fixed tissue) and a fluorescently labeled probe specific for the same target. The probe has both a fluorescent reporter attached to one end and a quencher on the other—this quenches the fluorescent signal. **Left,** The primers and probe anneal to the specific target gene. **Middle,** Owing to the 5'-exonuclease activity of the Taq polymerase, the already-bound fluorescent-labeled probe is degraded while a new polymerase chain reaction (PCR) product is being synthesized. **Right,** This process releases the fluorescent tag from the quencher and generates a fluorescence signal that is directly proportional to the amount of PCR product in the tube. This signal can be quantitated and the amount of mRNA determined.

while the new PCR product is being synthesized. This process releases the fluorescent tag from the quencher and generates a fluorescence signal that is directly proportional to the amount of PCR product in the tube. It is highly sensitive, specific, precise, and reproducible. It is generally considered to be the gold standard for measurement of gene expression.

NEXT GENERATION SEQUENCING: SECOND-GENERATION SEQUENCING*

Owing to advances in sequencing approaches, the number of bases that can be sequenced for a given cost has increased 1 million–fold since 1990, more than doubling every year. Current advancements in gene sequencing technology, now in use in the research setting, involve high-throughput, massively parallel sequencing that allows for cost-efficient whole genome, whole exome and whole transcriptome sequencing. These methods, primarily using fresh tissues (although significant advancements are being made in FPETs) allow for detection of somatic cancer genome alterations including nucleotide substitutions, small insertions and deletions, copy number alterations, chromosomal rearrangements, and mRNA quantification.[20] These new methods generate huge sums of data and present a significant statistical and computational challenging: how to identify truly significant results from the noise. This technology is still in its infancy and since it is not used in diagnostic laboratories, it is not reviewed in this chapter. However, these evolving technologies will have a huge near-term impact on the practice of pathology, medicine, and the entire discipline of biology. Several excellent review articles are available.[20–22]

STATISTICAL METHODS OF ANALYSIS: SUPERVISED AND UNSUPERVISED APPROACHES

The "molecular portraits" give exquisite detail regarding the sum total of cellular processes, via global mRNA quantitation, inherent to the intrinsic subtypes of breast cancer. Using these new gene expression technologies generates massive amounts of genomic data and the use of statistical methodologies is requisite. Gene expression profiling defines, at the molecular level, the unique patterns of gene expression inherent to many kinds of tumors.

One of the common features of these studies has been the emergence, through *unsupervised*, hierarchical clustering analysis, of breast cancer subtypes with distinct gene expression patterns for each subtype. The differences in thousands of individual gene expression patterns among these subtypes likely reflect basic differences in the cell biology of the tumors; therefore, these molecular subtypes may be considered as separable diseases. The molecular differences between the tumor subtypes are often accompanied by differences in clinical features, such as statistically robust differences in relapse-free and overall survival.[8,23]

The alternative approach is a *supervised* analysis. Using a metric, such as clinical outcome, genes are sought that differ between patients who recur versus those who do not. This method is used to identify lesser numbers of individual genes whose expression is associated with prognosis and treatment response.[24,25]

GENOMIC CLASSIFIERS

Classifier Development

There is a large body of literature on prognostic factors for cancer patients; unfortunately, only a few are used in clinical practice. They are unlikely to be used unless they are therapeutically relevant, and most publications do not establish such therapeutic relevance. Most prognostic factor studies are conducted by use of a convenience sample of patients for whom tissue is available, and the cohort is often far too heterogeneous with regard to age, ER status, stage, and treatment to support therapeutically relevant conclusions.[26] There are many new classifiers in development, and it is useful to divide genomic classifier studies into developmental studies and validation studies:

- *Developmental studies* define the genes and the algorithms used in multigene classifiers and are analogous to phases I to II clinical trials.
- *Validation studies* are separate studies that are performed after developmental studies are complete, genes have been chosen, and cut-points have been

---

*"First-generation sequencing" refers to Sanger sequencing (capillary-based DNA sequencing). It uses radioactively or fluorescently labeled dideoxynucleotide triphosphates (ddNTPs) as DNA chain terminators. Various detection methods allow read-out of sequence according to the incorporation of each specific terminator.

optimized. Validation studies optimally are conducted in randomized clinical trial populations and use prespecified genes, algorithms, and analysis plans. These studies are analogous to phase III clinical trials.

In developmental studies, one significant concern is that the number of candidate genes studied by DNA expression arrays for use in the classifier is typically much larger than the number of cases available for analysis. In these studies, it is always possible to find genes or sets of genes that perfectly classify the data on which they were developed. This apparently *perfect* classification can be achieved even if there is no relationship between expression of any of the genes and outcome; this is called *false discovery*. Therefore, control for false discovery of genes and subsequent validation of the selected genes and gene expression classifier in a distinct validation study are necessary. "Internal" clinical validation may be accomplished by (1) splitting the study population into two populations, one used for training the model and the other used for testing the model; or (2) cross-validation that is based on repeated model development and testing on random data partitions. However, neither of these statistical methods provides true "independent" validation. Thus, these methods for *internal* validation do not constitute *external* validation of the classifier in a setting simulating broad clinical application.

ROADMAP FOR THE DEVELOPMENT OF GENOMIC CLASSIFIERS

Developmental and validation studies should be based on cohorts of patients that are sufficiently homogeneous for therapeutically relevant classifiers to be developed.[26] This is best achieved by studying patients who were included in a single, large, randomized clinical trial. Developmental studies should be sufficiently large so that they can incorporate either cross-validation or split-sample validation and demonstrate that the internally validated prediction error is statistically significantly less than would be expected by chance. Independent validation studies are essential before results are accepted into medical practice. Independent validation studies should apply the classifier completely prespecified, including cutoffs, by the developmental study and measure prediction accuracy.[27] The size of the validation study should be sufficient so that meaningful confidence intervals (CIs) on predictive accuracy and positive and negative predictive values can be reported. The size of the validation study should be sufficient so that the extent to which the classifier adds predictive accuracy to established prognostic factors can be meaningfully evaluated.

Prognostic and Predictive Signatures

The 70-gene assay of van't Veer and coworkers[24] from the Netherlands Cancer Institute was the first commercially available breast cancer multigene classifier, and it uses fresh tissue and gene expression arrays (MammaPrint; Agendia, Netherlands). This was followed by the 21-gene assay of Paik and colleagues[25] from the National Surgical Adjuvant Breast and Bowel Project (NSABP) to be commercially available; it uses formalin-fixed paraffin-embedded tissue and qPCR (Oncotype DX; Genomic Health, Redwood City, CA). Today, there are many other classifiers in the process of being commercialized or that are already on the market. These include a 50-gene assay from Parker and associates (PAM50; Nanostring, Seattle, WA),[28] a 2-gene ratio from Ma and coworkers (Ipsogen; France),[29] and a 76-gene classifier from Foekens and colleagues (Veridex, Raritan, NJ).[30] For the purposes of this discussion, we focus on the first two classifiers, which have been independently validated in more than one study, are currently being used clinically, and which are both being used in two large prospective trials in Europe (the MammaPrint assay in MINDACT [Microarray in Node-Negative Disease May Avoid Chemotherapy]) and the United States (the Onco*type* DX assay in TAILORx [Trial Assigning Individualized Options for Treatment]). Additional emerging classifiers are discussed in the following categories: (1) commercially available signatures, (2) stroma-based signatures, (3) pathway-based signatures, and (4) other gene-based predictive and prognostic tools.

Commercially Available Signatures

A NEW BREAST TAXONOMY: THE INTRINSIC SUBTYPES OF BREAST CARCINOMA

Perou and associates[8,31] and Sorlie and coworkers[23] first reported a molecular taxonomy of breast cancer based on variation in global gene expression patterns measured by DNA microarrays, using *unsupervised* statistical correlations in expression patterns. They demonstrated that breast carcinomas could be grouped into molecular subtypes that are distinguished by unique patterns of gene expression (*molecular subtypes*). Their seminal subtypes include luminal A and B (ER-positive), *HER2* (HER2-positive), and basal type (ER–/PR–/*HER2*– or "triple negative"). These types differ in disease outcome and therapeutic response (Figure 10-4).[23,28] In further studies using a *directed* or *supervised* approach, they identified and attempted to reconcile the definition of those subtypes and the accompanying differences in disease outcome. Perhaps most exciting about these elegant studies was the identification of at least two types of ER-positive breast carcinoma with differing outcomes (Figure 10-5). The luminal A subtype was characterized by a high expression of ER, GATA3, X-box binding protein trefoil factor 3, hepatocyte nuclear factor 3 alpha (also called FOXA1), and LIV-1, whereas the luminal B subgroup showed moderate expression of the genes expressed by the breast luminal cells and frequently higher proliferation and lower progesterone (PgR) levels. The basal type was characterized by expression of keratins 5 and 17 and by laminin and fatty acid binding protein 7. The *HER2* subgroup showed high expression of several genes from the *HER2* amplicon.

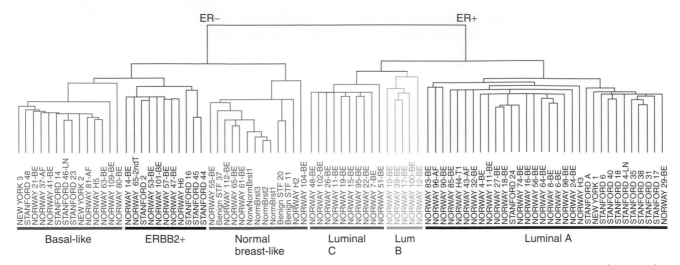

Basal-like   ERBB2+   Normal breast-like   Luminal C   Lum B   Luminal A

FIGURE 10-4 Gene expression patterns. Eight-five experimental samples representing 78 carcinomas, 3 benign tumors, and 4 normal tissues, analyzed by hierarchic clustering. The closer samples are together, the more similar are their expression profiles. The tumor specimens were divided into six subtypes based on differences in gene expression. Note differences in estrogen receptor–negative (ER–) and ER+. The cluster dendrogram shows the six subtypes of tumors from **left to right** (colored as): basal-like, *orange;* ERBB2+, *red;* normal breast–like, *green;* luminal subtype C, *light blue;* luminal subtype B, *yellow;* and luminal subtype A, *dark blue.*[23]

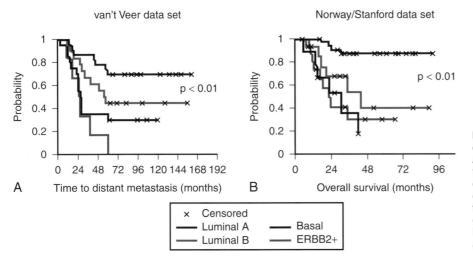

FIGURE 10-5 Kaplan-Meier analysis of disease outcome in two patient cohorts. **A,** Time to development of distant metastasis in the 97 cases from van't Veer and coworkers.[24] Patients were stratified according to the subtypes. **B,** Overall survival for 72 patients with locally advanced breast cancer in the Norway cohort. The normal-like tumor subgroup was omitted in both analyses.

TUMOR SUBTYPES ARE ASSOCIATED WITH SIGNIFICANT DIFFERENCE IN CLINICAL OUTCOME

In the previous work of Sorlie and coworkers,[23] the expression-based tumor subtypes were associated with a significant difference in overall survival as well as disease-free survival for the patients suffering from locally advanced breast cancer and belonging to the same treatment protocol. To investigate whether these subtypes were also associated with a significant difference in outcome in other patient cohorts, they performed a univariate Kaplan–Meier analysis with time to development of distant metastasis as a variable in the data set comprising the 97 sporadic tumors taken from van't Veer and coworkers.[24] They demonstrated that the probability of remaining disease-free was significantly different between the subtypes; patients with luminal A type tumors lived considerably longer before they developed distant disease, whereas the basal and *HER2* groups showed much shorter disease-free time intervals.

Luminal and basal tumor subtypes appear to be distinct biologic entities because the expression patterns have been shown to be detectable in other genomic studies of breast cancer. Sorlie and associates[32] have found strong evidence for the universality of a distinction between basal-like and luminal-like subtypes in three independent data sets comprising different patient populations whose gene expression profiles had been determined by using different microarray technology platforms.

The recently described claudin-low subtype has the genomic characteristics of a cancer stem cell–like phenotype CD44+/CD24–/low.[33,34]

MODIFIED INTRINSIC CLASSIFICATION DEFINITION (PAM50 ASSAY)

Microarray-based definitions are difficult to implement in clinical practice because addition of a new sample can result in a shift of the clustering algorithm. In order to address this issue, a quantitative RT-PCR based assay, PAM50, has been developed and commercialized. Initial studies have shown that the results of this assay are comparable with those obtained by "traditional" microarray methods.[28] A more recent analysis of a large retrospective cohort of patients treated with tamoxifen with long-term follow-up has demonstrated prognostic utility of an improved PAM50 assay that includes tumor size and proliferation.[35,36] Corresponding models using immunohistochemistry (IHC) markers alone could not identify a group with clinically significant favorable outcomes.[35]

Correlation of Breast Tumor Subtypes with Clinical and Pathologic Characteristics

The identification of molecular entities was followed with the analysis of the associated clinical and histologic features. The main associations noted with the basal-like subtype were that this group was associated with young age of onset of breast cancer, *BRCA1* positivity, p53 mutated status, and lack of expression ER, PgR, and *HER2* (triple negative). Nielsen and coworkers[37] were among the first to formulate an IHC-based definition to define the molecular groups using the expression of five IHC markers (ER, PgR, *HER2*, epidermal growth factor receptor [EGFR], and cytokeratin 5/6 [CK5/6]). A large retrospective analysis using this IHC definition confirmed the association of basal subtype with prognosis.[38] A number of different IHC definitions for molecular subtypes have been formulated.[39] One includes the use of CK5 antibody instead of the CK5/6 antibody. The definitions can be broadly divided into three categories: (1) those that define basal-like carcinoma (BLC) as a subset of triple-negative cancers, (2) those that are based on expression of basal markers irrespective of the tumor's ER, PgR, and *HER2* status,[39] and (3) those that consider triple-negative tumors to be synonymous with basal subtype. The entire topic of IHC definition of the *intrinsic classification* is controversial. The practical utility of classifying breast cancers into molecular subtypes is not clear at this time because, in most institutions, it does not alter the clinical management of the patients and, in the recent comparison with PAM50, did not appear to provide clinically useful prognostic information.[35] Detailed discussion of the IHC definitions and associated controversies is beyond the scope of this chapter and the readers are referred to a recent multiauthored review,[39] which suggests some practice guidelines. Chapter 20 also details this information as it applies to IHC.

Controversial Issues Related to Intrinsic Classification

BREAST TUMOR SUBTYPES AND REPRODUCIBLE DISTINCT BIOLOGIC ENTITIES A parsimonious interpretation of the reproducibility of several different patterns of gene expression is to regard each as representing a different biologic entity. One exciting hypothesis for the differences in these patterns may be that they originate from different mammary epithelial cell lineages. The findings that support this interpretation are breast tumor subtypes with patterns of gene expression similar to those of luminal epithelial cells (the cells that line the duct and give rise to the majority of breast cancers) and the basal epithelial cells (characterized by expression of CK18 and CK19 for luminal cells and CK5/6 and CK17 for basal cells). This concept has been recently challenged by work done using *BRCA* knock-down in mice. A proportion of breast cancers occurring in women with the *BRCA1* mutation that are phenotypically basal have been shown to be the result of downregulation of the ER pathway.[40] Many basal cancers simultaneously express genes of both luminal and basal/myoepithelial cells.[40] In addition, recent studies suggest that basal cancers may be derived from luminal progenitor cells rather than basal cells.[41] More recently, in an elegant set of experiments, Molyneux and colleagues[42] showed that tumors that develop from luminal cell progenitors in conditionally *BRCA1*-mutated mice do not have a "basal-like" phenotype.

CONSISTENCY OF THE DEFINITION OF THE INTRINSIC SUBTYPES Several papers have been published showing the utility of the intrinsic subtypes; however, many of these manuscripts cite different genes, gene sets, and subtypes. A close examination of these studies shows subtle differences in the definitions used. A recent study by Weigelt and associates[43–45] examined this issue and showed significant differences in the classification of a given tumor (as luminal or basal type) depending on the version of intrinsic classification definition used.

CONCORDANCE WITH IMMUNOHISTOCHEMISTRY DEFINITIONS The concordance of tumors identified as of a particular molecular subtype with that identified by immunohistochemical means is only modest.[43] As elegantly shown by Parker and associates,[28] the ER-negative tumors by IHC comprised 11% luminal, 32% *HER2*-enriched, 50% basal-like, and 7% normal-like tumors. More importantly, only 64% of the clinically *HER2*-positive (IHC or fluorescence in situ hybridization [FISH]) were classified as of molecular *HER2* subtype. However, it is important to note that the molecular *HER2* patients had a significantly worse outcome compared with other subtypes in patients with clinical *HER2*-positive tumors not treated with trastuzumab (Herceptin).

EXISTENCE OF SOME SUBTYPES IS CONTROVERSIAL The original "molecular portraits" classification identified three subtypes of luminal tumors (A, B, and C). Most of the recent work seems to disregard luminal C as a subtype. In addition, there is some controversy as to whether a "normal" subtype exists. The (unofficial) consensus is that it might represent an artifact of inadequate tumor in the sample being analyzed in the microarray studies.

INTRINSIC CLASSIFICATION AND PROLIFERATION Proliferation plays an important role in the prediction of behavior of tumors. Sotiriou and coworkers[46] asked the important question of what is the role of proliferation in determining the utility of the gene signatures. They compared the prognostic relevance of a number of commonly used signatures with and without the inclusion of genes that pertain to proliferation. They found that

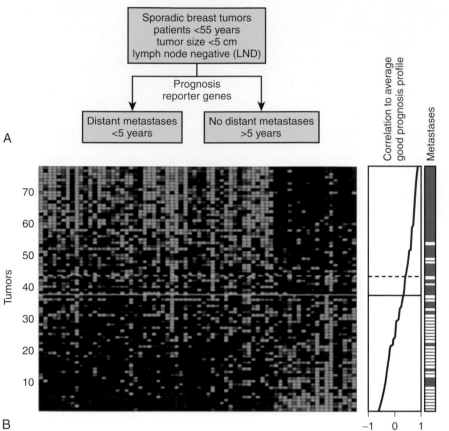

FIGURE 10-6 Supervised classification on prognosis signatures. **A,** Prognostic reporter genes identify optimally two types of disease outcome from 78 sporadic breast tumors into a poor-prognosis and a good-prognosis group. Each row represents a tumor and each column a gene. Genes are ordered according to their correlation coefficient with the two prognostic groups. The *solid line* represents the prognostic classifier with optimal accuracy and the *dashed line* with optimized sensitivity. Above the *dashed line* are patients with a good prognosis, and below, those with a poor prognosis. LND, lymph node dissection. **B,** The metastasis status for each patient is shown in the **right panel:** *white* indicates patients with metastases within 5 years and *blue* indicates those patients disease free for at least 5 years.

none of the gene signatures retained prognostic value if proliferation-related genes were excluded from the analysis.

MAMMAPRINT 70-GENE SIGNATURE

Breast Cancer Classifier: van't Veer and Coworkers[24]

The Netherlands group identified a 70-gene classifier developed using expression microarrays with approximately 25,000 human genes from fresh tissues obtained from primary breast tumors of 78 young female patients (age < 55 yr). Approximately 5000 genes were significantly regulated across the group of samples (P < .01 in more than five tumors). Unsupervised, hierarchical clustering identified two distinct groups, one with a poor prognosis with distant metastases and another good-prognosis group without progressive disease. Forty-four remained disease free for an interval of at least 5 years (good-prognosis group) and 34 patients who developed metastases within 5 years (poor-prognosis group) (Figure 10-6).

The 70-gene classifier was identified by using a three-step supervised classification method. The accuracy was improved until the optimal number of genes, 70, was identified. This classifier predicted correctly the actual outcome of disease for 65 out of the 78 patients (83%), with, respectively, 5 poor-prognosis and 8 good-prognosis patients assigned to the opposite category. An ideal threshold was established by optimizing the algorithm

so that no more than 10% of poor-prognosis patients were misclassified. This optimized sensitivity threshold resulted in 15 misclassifications: 3 poor-prognosis were classified as good and 12 good-prognosis tumors were classified as poor.

Upon analysis of the genes of the dominant expression signatures, the authors found that the ER-negative cases clustered together and there was a second group of associated lymphocytic infiltrate, including several genes expressed primarily by B and T lymphocytes. The up-regulated genes associated with a poor prognosis included those involved in cell cycle, invasion and metastasis, angiogenesis, and signal transduction (e.g., cyclin E_2, metalloproteinases [MMP] 9 and MMP1 and the vascular endothelial growth factor [VEGF] receptor FLT1). The prognosis classifier was validated in an additional independent set of 19 young, node-negative patients. This group consisted of 7 patients who remained disease free for at least 5 years and 12 patients who developed distant metastases within 5 years. The disease outcome was predicted by the 70-gene classifier and resulted in 2 out of 19 incorrect classifications using the optimized threshold.

The poor-prognosis signature according to this classifier indicates that, in women younger than 55 years who are diagnosed with lymph node–negative breast cancer and who will have a poor prognosis signature have a 28-fold odds ratio (OR) (95% CI 7–107, $P = 1.0 \times 10^{-8}$) for developing metastases. This classifier-provided prognostic information is additive to the traditional clinical and histopathologic prognostic factors: high grade

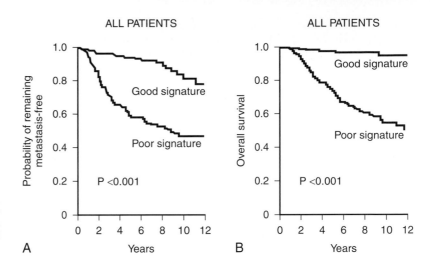

FIGURE 10-7 Validation of the 70-gene classifier. **A** and **B**, Kaplan-Meier analysis of the probability that a patient would remain free of distant metastases and the probability of overall survival among all patients.

(OR = 6.4, 95% CI 2.1–19, P = .0008), tumor size greater than 2 cm (OR = 4.4, 95% CI 1.7–11, P = .0028), angioinvasion (OR = 4.2, 95% CI 1.5–12, P = .01), age 40 years or older (OR = 3.7, 95% CI 0.9–6.6, P = .13), and ER negative (OR = 2.4, 95% CI 0.9–6.6, P = .13). Multivariate analysis that included all classic prognostic factors indicated that it was an independent factor in predicting outcome of disease (logistic regression OR = 18, 3.3–94, P = 1.4×10^{-4}).

Validation of the 70-Gene Classifier

The validation set consisted of 295 consecutive patients with primary breast carcinomas with stage I or II breast cancer and younger than 55 years of age.[7] Among these patients, 180 were found to have a poor-prognosis signature and 115 had a good-prognosis signature, and the mean (±SE [standard error]) overall 10-year survival rates were 54.6% ± 4.4% and 94.5% ± 2.6%, respectively. At 10 years, the probability of remaining free of distant metastases was 50.6% ± 4.5% in the group with a poor-prognosis signature and 85.2% ± 4.3% in the group with a good-prognosis signature (Figure 10-7). The prognosis profile was significantly associated with histologic grade $(P < .001)$, ER status $(P < .001)$, and age $(P > .001)$ but not with tumor size, extent of vascular invasion, the number of positive lymph nodes, or treatment.

Critical Issues Related to 70-Gene Classification

1. Frozen tissue requirement. The MammaPrint assay requires the collection of fresh frozen tissue for analysis. This can be difficult, labor intensive, and expensive. More importantly, it requires prior planning. It can also sometimes be difficult, in spite of best intentions, to obtain a representative sample of tumor owing to a variety of reasons including small tumor size, presence of a prior biopsy site, and peritumoral fibrosis.
2. Biologic relevance of the genes identified. The gene signature is based on the evaluation of 70 genes that were identified from a list of 5000 differentially expressed genes. The question was asked whether these genes pertain to important cellular

process and, therefore, would be used for targeted therapeutics. Ein-Dor and colleagues[47] attempted to analyze the prognostic value of the 70-gene set by selecting distinct sets of 70 genes from the original 5000 genes. When the prognostic impact of 10 such sets of 70 genes was analyzed, it was found that the prognostic value of any one of these 10 sets was identical. This indicates that the genes contained in the signature represent distinct biologic pathways but the resulting set of genes is not unique; it is strongly influenced by the subset of patients used for gene selection. Many equally predictive lists could have been produced from the same analysis. Three main properties of the data explain this sensitivity: (1) many genes are correlated with survival, (2) the differences between these correlations are small, and (3) the correlations fluctuate strongly when measured over different subsets of patients.

3. Utility in ER-negative patients. It has been noted that nearly all of the ER-negative patients fall into the poor-prognosis category. This raises questions as to the utility of the signature in the ER-negative patient population.
4. The 70-gene signature and proliferation. As discussed in the section on Intrinsic Classification, all the signatures available to date are heavily dependent on proliferation-related genes.[46]
5. Chemotherapy benefit. Knauer and associates recently analyzed the predictive value of the 70-gene signature in a series of previously analyzed 541 patients with early breast cancer treated with a variety of chemotherapies (CMF, anthracycline-containing regimens, and taxanes). Only 265 were lymph node negative. They found a significant and clinically meaningful benefit of adding chemotherapy to endocrine therapy in patients classified as "high risk" by the Mamma-Print assay. More importantly, there was no significant benefit for the addition of chemotherapy in patients classified as "low risk."[48] No formal interaction between the MammaPrint result and chemotherapy benefit was detected.

6. Cost-effectiveness analysis. Cost-effectiveness analysis of the 70-gene signature has been carried out comparing it with Adjuvant Online! and St. Gallen guidelines. The signature was shown to improve the quality-adjusted survival and had the highest probability of being cost-effective.[49]

Summary

This is the only U.S. Food and Drug Administration (FDA) 510(k) cleared test. It is intended for women who

- Are younger than age 61.
- Are in the two earliest stages of cancer (stages I and II).
- Have tumor size of 5 cm or smaller.
- Have no evidence that the cancer has spread to nearby lymph nodes (lymph node negative).

The 70-gene signature is currently being assessed in a prospective, phase III clinical trial coordinated by the European Organization for Research and Treatment of Cancer (EORTC), called the MINDACT trial (EORTC 10 041/BIG 3-04; http://www.eortc.be/services/unit/min dact/MINDACT websiteii.asp), in which 6000 patients will be profiled using the commercially available derivative of the 70-gene signature (MammaPrint) and have their clinicopathologic characteristics analysed. Patients with discordant results between the 70-gene signature and the clinicopathologic characteristics are being randomized to chemotherapy or not.

ONCO*TYPE* DX 21 GENE ASSAY

The 21-gene assay is a qPCR assay for FPET samples that is clinically validated to assess the risk of 10-year distant recurrence (DR) and the magnitude of chemotherapy benefit. The test is currently validated for women with early-stage ER-positive breast cancer who will be treated with 5 years of hormonal therapy. It is based on prior studies that have demonstrated the ability to reproducibly extract mRNA from fixed paraffin-embedded archival tissues up to 30 years in age, that have developed normalization strategies to account for increasing RNA degradation over time, and that have resolved issues of tumor heterogeneity and determined objective cutpoints for tumor manual microdissection.[12,50,51]

The assay was developed using a candidate gene approach, in which 250 were selected from the published literature, genomic databases, and experimental microarray data for breast cancer. The genes were tested in three independent studies including cases from NSABP B-20, in total, involving 447 patients.[10] Multivariate analyses indicated that panels of multiple genes had greater predictive power than any single gene. The data from all three studies were used to select a 21-gene panel (16 cancer-related genes and 5 reference genes) that strongly and consistently correlated with likelihood of DR. The 16 cancer-related genes are *Ki67*, *STK15*, *Survivin*, *CCNB1*, *MYBL2*, *GRB7*, *HER2*, *ER*, *PGR*, *BCL2*, *SCUBE2*, *MMP11*, *CTSL2*, *GSTM1*, *CD68*, and *BAG1* and the 5 reference genes are *ACTB*, *GAPDH*, *RPLPO*, *GUS*, and *TFRC*. The recurrence score (RS) calculation is as follows: RS = $+0.47 \times$ *HER2* group score $- 0.34 \times$ ER group score $+ 1.04 \times$ proliferation group score $+ 0.10 \times$ invasion group score $+ 0.05 \times$ CD68 $- 0.08 \times$ GSTM1 $- 0.07 \times$ BAG1. Although some of the coefficients are greater than others, each of the individual genes can greatly influence the individual RS. The RS is used to predict patient prognosis, scaled it ranges continuously from 0 to 100 and has been divided into three risk groups: (1) a low-risk score correlating with a risk of DR less than 10%, RS 0 to 18; (2) an intermediate-risk score correlating with a risk of DR between 10% and 20%, RS between 18 and 31; and (3) a high-risk score correlating with a risk of DR greater than 20%, RS 31 or greater.

Validation of the 21-Gene Assay

PREDICTION OF TAMOXIFEN BENEFIT: NSABP B-14 This clinical trial randomized patients with ER-positive breast lymph node–negative breast cancers to treatment with placebo or tamoxifen for 5 years. The trial used 668 node-negative patients with median follow-up of more than 14 years. The technical success rate of the 21-gene assay was 99%. The study met its prospectively defined end points: RSs were independent and highly significant predictors of recurrence-free survival and RS provided accuracy and precision in predicting likelihood of DR (P < .001). Importantly, there is a near-linear relationship between the numeric RS and the patient's actual risk of DR (Table 10-1).

PREDICTION OF CHEMOTHERAPY BENEFIT NSABP B-20 examined the performance of the 21-gene assay in tumor blocks from 651 patients enrolled from 1988 to 1993 in the tamoxifen alone and tamoxifen plus either CMF or MF chemotherapy treatment randomization arms of the NSABP Study B-20. Cox proportional hazards models for the global test of interaction between treatment effect (either tamoxifen alone or tamoxifen plus chemotherapy) and gene expression reveal that the RS is a significant predictor of chemotherapy benefit (P = .038). RS predicted the absolute risk of breast cancer death at 10 years (low RS = 2.8% [95% CI 1.7–3.9]; intermediate RS = 10.7% [95% CI 6.3–14.9]; high RS = 15.5% [95% CI 7.6–22.8]). These risk estimates were similar to those in the NSABP B-14 clinical validation study. More importantly, this study showed that patients with low RS tumors (RS < 18) derived minimal, if any, benefit from chemotherapy (an estimated increase in DRFS at 10 years of –1.1% ± 2.2%, mean ± SE). Patients with high-risk tumors (RS ≥ 31) had a large absolute benefit of chemotherapy (an absolute increase in DRFS at 10 years of 27.6% ± 8.0%, mean ± SE) (Figure 10-8).

KAISER PERMANENTE STUDY An additional validation study of 220 cases and 570 controls, conducted by the Northern California Kaiser Permanente in its community-based patient set, confirmed the results from the NSABP B-14 study, that the RS was statistically significantly associated with breast cancer survival in tamoxifen-treated patients with node-negative, ER-positive breast cancer (P = .0002). The risk of breast cancer death for patients in the low-risk group as determined by the RS (RS < 18) was 2.8% at 10 years. Moreover, over 50% of the patients were in the low-risk group.

| TABLE 10-1 | Multivariate Cox Proportional Analysis of Age, Tumor Size, Tumor Grade, and Recurrence Score in Relation to the Likelihood of Distant Recurrence* | | | |

	Analysis without RS[†]		Analysis with RS	
Variable	*P* Value	Hazard Ratio	*P* Value	Hazard Ratio
Age at surgery	.1	0.7	.22	0.76
Clinical tumor size	.13	1.35	.38	1.19
Tumor Grade				
Moderate	.04	1.87	.15	1.55
Poor	<.001	5.14	<.001	3.34
HER2 amplification	.89	1.04	.06	0.51
ER Protein				
50–99 fmol/mg	.23	0.71	.32	0.75
100–199 fmol/mg	.38	0.78	.72	0.9
>200 fmol/mg	.9	0.97	.94	1.02
RS			<.001	2.81

*Age at surgery was a binary variable (0 for an age of < 50 yr and 1 for an age of ≥ 50 yr); clinical tumor size was a binary variable (0 for a diameter of ≤ 2 cm and 1 for a diameter > 2 cm); grade was a binary variable (poorly differentiated relative to well differentiated and moderately differentiated relative to well differentiated); *HER2* amplification was a binary variable (0 for no amplification on fluorescence in situ hybridization and 1 for amplification); the amount of estrogen receptor protein was an ordinal variable, with the baseline level being 10 to 49 fmol/mg; and RS was a continuous variable, with the hazard ratio for distant recurrence calculated relative to an increment of 50 units.
[†]*P* < .001 and chi-square = 15.2 for the comparison with the analysis without the RS.
ER, estrogen receptor; RS, recurrence score.

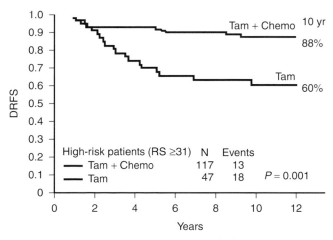

Tam vs Tam + Chemo – High Risk (RS ≥31)

FIGURE 10-8 Not all patients benefit equally from chemotherapy. Patients with low–recurrence score (RS) tumors derived minimal benefit from chemotherapy whereas patients with high-risk tumors had a 28% absolute benefit from chemotherapy as the 10-year Kaplan-Meier estimate for freedom from distant recurrence was improved from 60% to 88% by adding chemotherapy to tamoxifen in the high-risk group. Tam, tamoxifen.

It is notable that this genomic assay can identify a large cohort of patients who retain such a low risk of breast cancer death.

ATAC ("ARIMIDEX," TAMOXIFEN, ALONE OR IN COMBINATION) CLINICAL TRIAL (NODE POSITIVE AND NEGATIVE) To determine whether the RS provided independent information on risk of DR in the tamoxifen and anastrozole arms of the Arimidex, Tamoxifen, Alone or in Combination (ATAC) Trial, RNA was extracted from central pathology–reviewed patient samples from 1372 tumor blocks from postmenopausal patients with hormone receptor–positive primary breast cancer in the monotherapy (tamoxifen or anastrozole) arms of ATAC. For both lymph node–negative and lymph node–positive patients, the RS was significantly associated with time to DR in multivariate analyses *(P < .001 for N0 and P = .002 for N+).* The RS also showed significant prognostic value beyond that provided by Adjuvant! Online *(P < .001).* Nine-year DR rates in low- (RS < 18), intermediate- (RS = 18–30), and high-RS (RS ≥ 31) groups were 4%, 12%, and 25%, respectively, in N0 patients *(P < .001)* and 17%, 28%, and 49%, respectively, in N+ patients *(P < .001).* The prognostic value of RS was similar in anastrozole- and tamoxifen-treated patients. This study confirmed the performance of RS in postmenopausal hormone receptor–positive patients treated with tamoxifen in a large contemporary population and demonstrated that RS is an independent predictor of DR in both lymph node–negative and lymph node–positive hormone receptor–positive patients treated with anastrozole, adding value to estimates with standard clinicopathologic features.

Critical Issues Related to 21-Gene Assay

21-GENE ASSAY AND HISTOLOGIC GRADE There is a very strong correlation between histologic grade and RS. In the NASBP B-14 study, the hazard ratio for poor histologic grade was comparable with that obtained by RS. However, histologic grade is associated with significant subjectivity. The kappa value for concordance ranges from 0.8 to 0.5; this lack of consistency is one of the major reasons clinicians are wary about using grade in

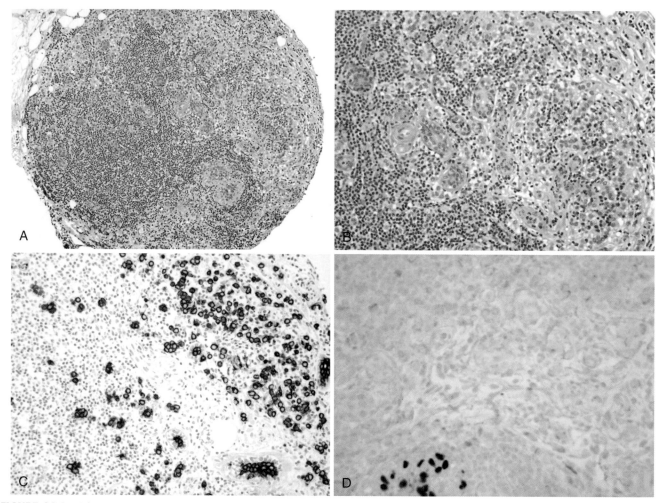

FIGURE 11-3 A breast core biopsy demonstrates a subtle invasive carcinoma with abundant intra- and peritumoral lymphocytic infiltrate (**A**, low power; **B**, high power). An AE1/3 immunostain confirms the epithelial nature of these infiltrating cells (**C**) and a p63 stain confirms absence of MECs around these infiltrating cells (**D**), establishing the diagnosis of invasive carcinoma.

IMMUNOHISTOCHEMISTRY OF PAPILLARY LESIONS

Papillary lesions range from benign papilloma to atypical papilloma to papillary carcinoma (in situ and invasive). There are several reports on the use of MEC markers to distinguish between different categories.[12,32–34] A papillary lesion could be classified as a papilloma if there is a uniform layer of MECs in the proliferating intraluminal component of the lesion, whereas the absence of MECs would be suggestive of a papillary carcinoma.[33] Some papillomas show the features of an "atypical papilloma," areas in which there is atypical ductal epithelial hyperplasia (ADH) that overgrows the papilloma.[35] These atypical areas lack MECs by immunoperoxidase examination.[36] Atypical papillomas and papillary carcinoma in situ also lose high-molecular-weight keratin immunostaining with 34βE12 and CK5/6.[37] The distinction between a papilloma, atypical papilloma, and papillary DCIS (either de novo or DCIS involving papilloma) is quite straightforward in the majority of cases and can be made using morphology and IHC staining (Figure 11-14). The more difficult and confusing area is the distinction between a "well-circumscribed papillary tumor" and an invasive carcinoma. The *well-circumscribed papillary*

tumor has been referred to by different names in the literature. The term *intracystic papillary carcinoma* has been used for a single mass-forming cystic lesion with malignant papillary proliferation.[38] *Papillary DCIS* is a term that has been used for more diffuse lesions.[39] The use of MEC markers to assess invasion in these lesions has yielded variable results. In an immunohistochemical study of papillary breast lesions, Hill and Yeh[32] found consistent staining pattern in cases originally diagnosed as papilloma or invasive papillary carcinoma, but found variable staining in cases diagnosed as intraductal papillary carcinomas. Of the nine intraductal papillary carcinomas in their series, four cases showed unequivocal basal MECs by IHC, one case showed partial discontinuous staining, and four cases were predominantly negative for basal MECs. The authors found that lesions originally classified as intraductal papillary carcinoma but lacked basal MECs by IHC were uniformly large, expansile, papillary lesions with pushing borders and a fibrotic rim. The authors hypothesized that such lesions form a part of the spectrum of progression intermediate between in situ and invasive disease and suggested that these lesions should be termed "encapsulated papillary carcinoma".[32] Collins and associates[40] have also favored such designation. In some recent reviews of

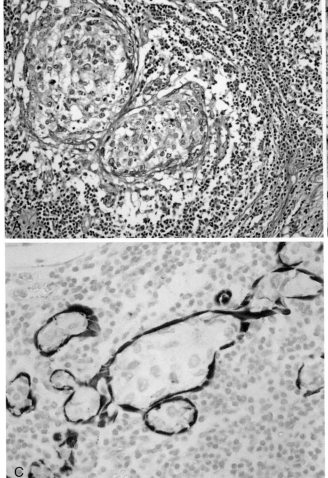

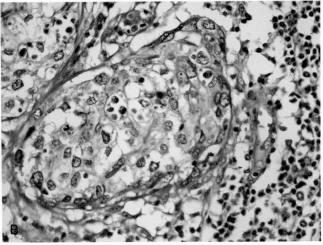

FIGURE 11-4 A ductal carcinoma in situ (DCIS; **A,** low power; **B,** high power) is heavily obscured with lymphocytes, but SMM-HC **(C)** clearly reflects the presence of MECs.

papillary lesions, an attempt has been made to classify the lesions in a uniform fashion using morphology and IHC. The papillary lesions are now classified as papilloma, papilloma with ADH (atypical papilloma), papilloma with DCIS, papillary DCIS, intracystic papillary carcinoma (encysted or encapsulated papillary carcinoma), solid-papillary carcinoma, and invasive papillary carcinoma.[36,41]

The problem in diagnosis arises from the fact that intracystic and solid-papillary carcinomas have the morphology of an in situ lesion, but most lesions lack the presence of MECs around the periphery (Figure 11-15). Because type IV collagen is an integral component of the BL that envelops normal and proliferative benign lesions, we recently studied its expression in intracystic papillary carcinoma and compared its expression with that of a variety of papillary lesions and invasive carcinoma.[42] We found a continuous strong collagen type IV staining around the periphery of intracystic papillary carcinomas (Figure 11-16) similar to benign lesions and DCIS, but generally a weak and discontinuous type staining around invasive carcinomas. Our results are very similar to a previous study regarding the usefulness of collagen type IV, published several years ago.[43] This pattern of staining supports the in situ nature of intracystic papillary carcinomas. Moreover, the clinical behavior of these lesions is more akin to in situ disease.[38,44–46]

A recent study, however, did not find the collagen IV stain helpful.[47] Regardless of collagen IV stain, intracystic papillary carcinomas and solid-papillary carcinomas are circumscribed papillary tumors that often lack basal MECs around the periphery, and in the absence of "frank" invasion, their behavior is similar to that of in situ carcinomas. However, it is extremely important to

KEY DIAGNOSTIC POINTS

Myoepithelial Cell Antibodies in Papillary Lesions

- The MECs are present in the proliferative cellular component of a papilloma, but are absent in the area of atypical ductal epithelial hyperplasia or DCIS.

- MECs are uniformly present around the periphery of the lesion in a papilloma, atypical papilloma, and papilloma with DCIS, and are often present around papillary DCIS, but are often absent at the periphery in intracystic and solid-papillary carcinomas.

- Caution is advised in diagnosing invasion based on MEC antibodies in a papillary lesion on a core biopsy. Recommend complete excision for assessing invasion.

DCIS, ductal carcinoma in situ; MECs, myoepithelial cells.

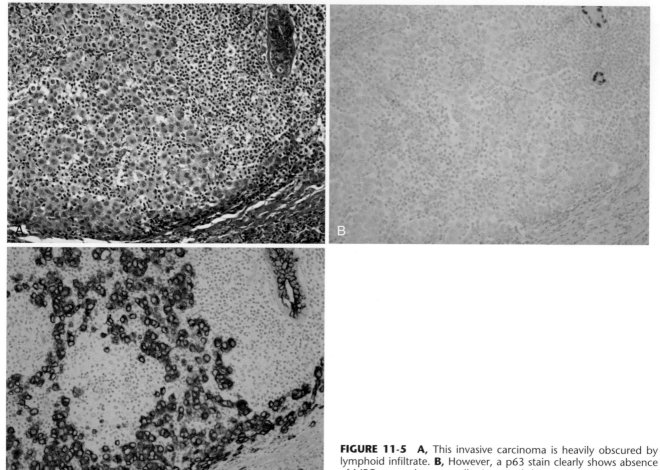

FIGURE 11-5 A, This invasive carcinoma is heavily obscured by lymphoid infiltrate. **B,** However, a p63 stain clearly shows absence of MECs around tumor cells. A normal duct serves as internal control. **C,** The tumor itself is highlighted by cytokeratin AE1/AE3.

analyze the resection specimen on these lesions in entirety by histologic evaluation owing to the not so infrequent presence of frank invasion (invasion into fat beyond the fibrotic rim) in the periphery of these lesions. We believe it is the presence of these minute foci of invasive carcinoma that is responsible for occasional metastatic disease reported with intracystic papillary carcinomas.[48] Given that SLN mapping procedure is not a highly morbid procedure, it should be offered to patients diagnosed with intracystic or solid-papillary carcinoma on core needle biopsy. The MEC staining pattern for each papillary lesion is summarized in Table 11-3.

PROLIFERATIVE DUCTAL EPITHELIAL LESIONS AND IN SITU CARCINOMAS

Differences in CK expression have been described between hyperplasia and DCIS.[49,50] The antibody 34βE12 recognizes CK1, CK5, CK10, and CK14, and these keratins are typically found in duct-derived epithelium and squamous epithelium. Normal breast MECs and luminal cells express 34βE12, as do proliferative duct epithelium of the usual type (Figure 11-17). The expression is generally lost in ADH.[51] DCIS is largely negative in 81% to 100% of cases for 34βE12 (see Figure 11-17), but it may show some positive cells. Most

DCISs are uniformly positive for cell adhesion molecule 5.2 (CAM5.2), reflecting a shift away from high-molecular weight-keratins to the more simple keratins 8 and 18. The 34βE12 immunostaining profile for DCIS and ADH is very similar and cannot be used to help distinguish DCIS from ADH but can be an aid to histomorphology in separating DCIS from florid ductal epithelial hyperplasia (DEH) in difficult cases. Clone D5/16B4 antibody CK5/6 is more specific for the DCIS morphology because it is largely completely negative in DCIS.[51] This expression of high-molecular-weight keratins (or basal keratins) in usual hyperplasia with loss in ADH and DCIS suggests that atypical lesions try to acquire a more "luminal" phenotype. Adding to the same theme, usual hyperplasia is generally negative or focally positive for estrogen receptor (ER), but atypical hyperplasia and low-/intermediate-grade DCIS are often more diffusely ER-positive. So, in a lesion with ambiguous morphology for ADH, a combination of CK5 and ER may be helpful in rendering a more definitive diagnosis. A CK5+ and ER low/negative immunophenotype of the proliferative component would favor usual hyperplasia, whereas the opposite (CK5–, ER+) profile would favor ADH/DCIS.[52] There are a few pitfalls for using these IHC stains for making a diagnosis of ADH/DCIS. First of all, this panel is not valid for columnar cell lesions because even benign columnar cell changes strongly

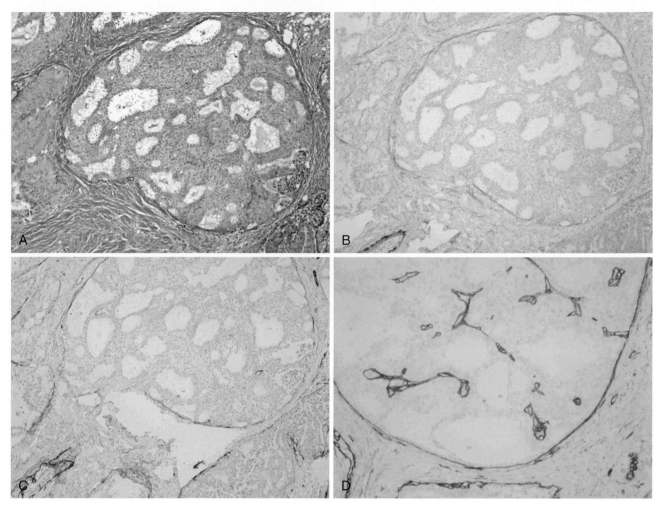

FIGURE 11-6 Approximately 5% of morphologically identifiable DCIS may not show MECs. This case of cribriform and papillary DCIS **(A)** shows lack of staining with p63 **(B)** and SMM-HC **(C). D,** Collagen type IV demonstrates strong continuous staining around tumor nests, confirming the in situ nature of the lesion.

KEY DIAGNOSTIC POINTS
Keratins in Proliferative and in Situ Lesions

- High-molecular-weight cytokeratin (CK) antibodies (34βE12, CK5/6, CK5) routinely intensely stain florid ductal hyperplasia of the breast, which may be useful in separating florid DEH in ducts or papillomas from ADH/DCIS.

- Both ADH and low-/intermediate-grade DCIS lack 34βE12, CK5, CK5/6 antibody staining and cannot be distinguished by IHC.

- Pitfall: Differential CK profiles are not valid for columnar cell lesions because even benign columnar cell changes strongly express ER.

- Pitfall: Apocrine DCIS or atypical apocrine lesions are generally negative for ER and may express CK5.

- Pitfall: Basal-like DCIS is almost always positive for CK5 and negative for ER.

DCIS, ductal carcinoma in situ; DEH, ductal epithelial hyperplasia; ER, estrogen receptor; IHC, immunohisto-chemistry.

express ER. Second, apocrine DCIS or atypical apocrine lesions (atypical apocrine adenosis) are generally negative for ER and may express CK5. Finally, the basal-like DCIS is almost always positive for CK5 and negative for ER. Therefore, CK5 and ER should be used in conjunction with defined morphologic criteria for diagnosing ADH/DCIS.

The diagnosis of atypia in papillary lesions is also very challenging. Fortunately, the same CK patterns of immunostaining hold up for the differential of ADH/DCIS in a papilloma versus a florid hyperplasia in a papilloma.[37]

TUMOR TYPE IDENTIFICATION BY IMMUNOHISTOCHEMISTRY

Cell Adhesion: Ductal versus Lobular Carcinoma

Based on cell cohesiveness, the two broad categories of breast carcinoma (invasive or in situ) are ductal and lobular types. DCIS increases the risk of invasive malignancy

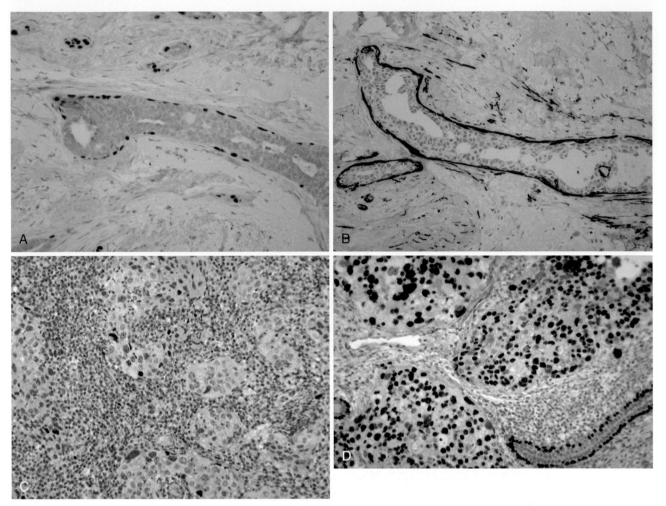

FIGURE 11-7 Pitfalls of p63 and SMM-HC. **A,** A p63 stain demonstrates apparent gaps in staining around the luminal epithelium of a duct within a radial scar. **B,** The same duct shows intense continuous staining with SMM-HC, but myofibroblastic cells in the background are also positive. **C,** A p63 stain on core biopsy shows staining of few tumor cells. **D,** A rare example of diffuse p63 staining of tumor cells.

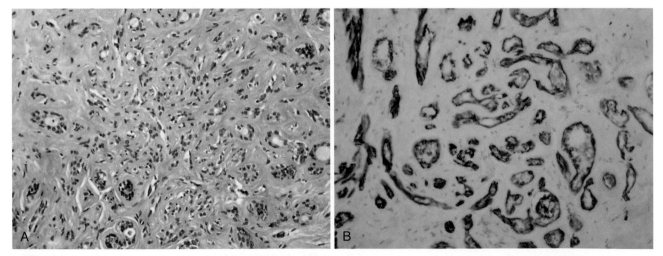

FIGURE 11-8 Sclerosing adenosis may simulate carcinoma **(A)** but demonstrates envelopment of cell nests by MECs with SMM-HC immunostaining **(B).**

at the local site whereas lobular carcinoma in situ (LCIS) is considered a marker of generalized increased risk of invasive malignancy, although some data suggest precursor properties for LCIS.[53–62] Invasive ductal carcinomas (IDCs) are often unifocal lesions compared with invasive lobular carcinoma, which are often multifocal and/or more extensive than what is estimated on clinical and mammographic examination.[63–65] Distant metastases from ductal carcinoma preferentially involve lung and brain, whereas metastases from lobular carcinoma

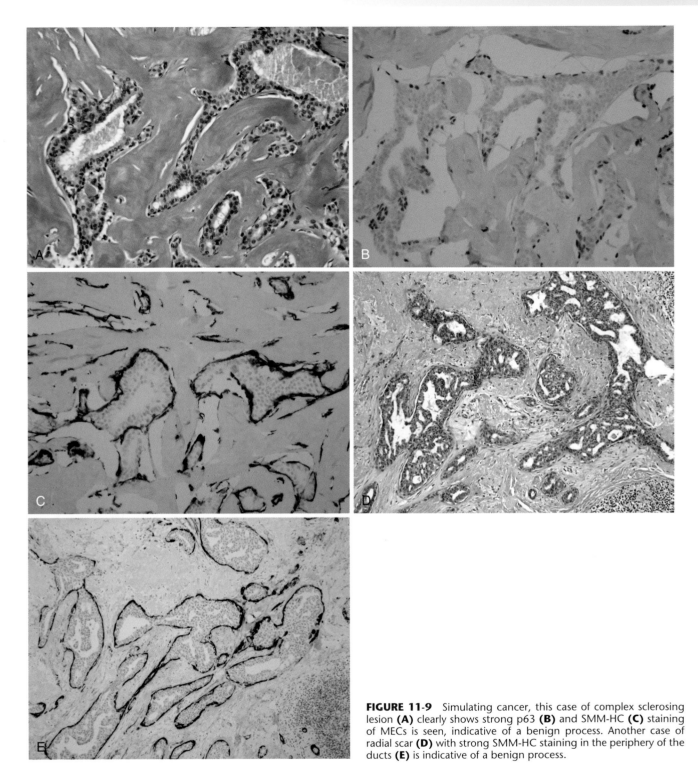

FIGURE 11-9 Simulating cancer, this case of complex sclerosing lesion **(A)** clearly shows strong p63 **(B)** and SMM-HC **(C)** staining of MECs is seen, indicative of a benign process. Another case of radial scar **(D)** with strong SMM-HC staining in the periphery of the ducts **(E)** is indicative of a benign process.

more often involve the peritoneum, bone, bone marrow, and visceral organs of gastrointestinal and gynecologic tracts.[66–69] In spite of the previously discussed differences, at present, with the combined multimodality therapy, there appears to be no difference in disease-free or overall survival between ductal and lobular carcinomas.[64,70,71] However, there are enough significant differences in patient preoperative evaluation and subsequent treatment that an accurate diagnosis is warranted at the time of core biopsy. At some breast cancer centers, a preoperative (before lumpectomy or mastectomy) magnetic resonance imaging (MRI) of the breast is performed to evaluate the extent of disease with a core biopsy diagnosis of invasive lobular carcinoma,[63,65,72,73] the rationale being that margins are more difficult to obtain from the surgeon's viewpoint. This probably has merit in selected patients pertaining to breast reconstruction. A core biopsy diagnosis of ductal versus lobular carcinoma is also important if the patient will be treated by neoadjuvant chemotherapy. Although there

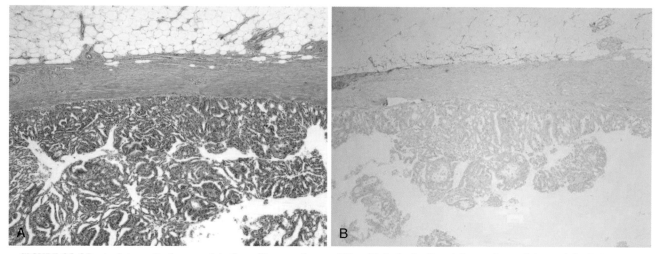

FIGURE 11-15 An intracystic (encapsulated) papillary carcinoma **(A)**, with lack of p63 staining at the periphery of the lesion **(B)**.

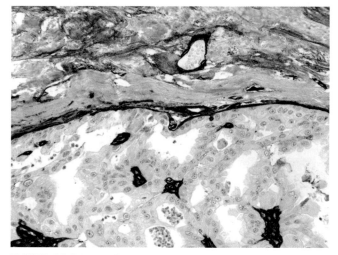

FIGURE 11-16 Another case of intracystic (encapsulated) papillary carcinoma demonstrates strong continuous collagen type IV staining.

Lobular Carcinoma Variants and Former Lobular Variants

PLEOMORPHIC LOBULAR CARCINOMA

Described by Bassler and Kronsbein in 1980[105] and further detailed by Weidner and Semple,[106] Eusebi and associates,[107] and Reis-Filho and coworkers,[108] the genetic, immunohistologic, and clinical features have been sufficiently detailed to recognize invasive pleomorphic lobular carcinoma (PLC) and pleomorphic lobular carcinoma in situ (PLCIS) as distinct clinicopathologic entities.[109–112] Based on cell cohesiveness, PLC and PLCIS are basically a subtype of lobular carcinoma. The histologically recognizable PLC and PLCIS are almost always ECAD– (or show aberrant staining) and demonstrate strong cytoplasmic immunoreactivity for p120.[113] Histologically, these show grade 3 nuclei with a dyshesive pattern of growth in both in situ and infiltrating varieties (Figure 11-22). The in situ component may be discovered

on mammograms as calcifications. The core biopsies demonstrate in situ dyshesive grade 3 nuclei with some cases showing comedonecrosis and calcification. Recently, a comprehensive analysis of 26 PLCs revealed a closer association between PLC and classic lobular carcinoma than between PLC and ductal carcinoma.[114] The authors analyzed 26 cases of PLC, 16 cases of classic lobular carcinoma, and 34 cases of IDC by IHC, array comparative genomic hybridization (a-CGH), fluorescent in situ hybridization (FISH), and chromogenic in situ hybridization (CISH). Comparative analysis of a-CGH data suggested the molecular features of PLC (ER+/PR+, ECAD–, 1q(+), 11q(–), 16p(+), and 16q(–)) were more closely related to those of classic ILC than IDC. However, PLCs also showed some molecular alterations that are more typical of high-grade IDC than ILC (p53 and *HER2* positivity in some cases, 8q(+), 17q24-q25(+), 13q(–) and amplification of 8q24, 12q14, 17q12 and 20q13). Some of these IDC-like alterations may be responsible for the aggressive biology of PLC.

Sneige and colleagues[115] studied 24 cases of PLCIS by IHC and found them to be universally positive for ER (100%). They also showed frequent p53 reactivity (25%) and moderate to high proliferative activity; *HER2* positivity was seen in 1 of 23 cases (4%). Of these 24 cases, 14 were associated with PLC, which showed similar IHC profile. Our experience with PLC and PLCIS is very similar. Although *HER2* overexpression/amplification may be seen in PLCs, the *HER2*+ rate is not very high as previously reported,[111] and PLCs are ER+ in the majority of cases, albeit expression levels may vary from case to case. Because there is a high likelihood for developing invasive carcinoma in the vicinity of PLCIS, these lesions should be managed similar to DCIS.

TUBULOLOBULAR CARCINOMA

Described originally by Fisher and associates in 1977[116] as a lobular growth pattern with tiny tubules and single-filing characteristic of lobular carcinoma. Subsequently,

TABLE 11-3	Papillary Lesions of the Breast Distribution of Myoepithelial Cells and Clinical Behavior	
Papillary Lesions	**MECs**	**Clinical Behavior**
Papilloma	Present within and around ducts	Benign
Papilloma with ADH/DCIS or papillary DCIS	Reduced/absent within, present around ducts	Risk for invasive malignancy
Encapsulated papillary carcinoma	Absent within, rare ± around ducts	Similar to DCIS, unless frankly invasive
Solid papillary carcinoma	Absent within, rare ± around ducts	Similar to DCIS, unless frankly invasive

ADH, atypical ductal hyperplasia; DCIS, ductal carcinoma in situ; MECs, myoepithelial cells.

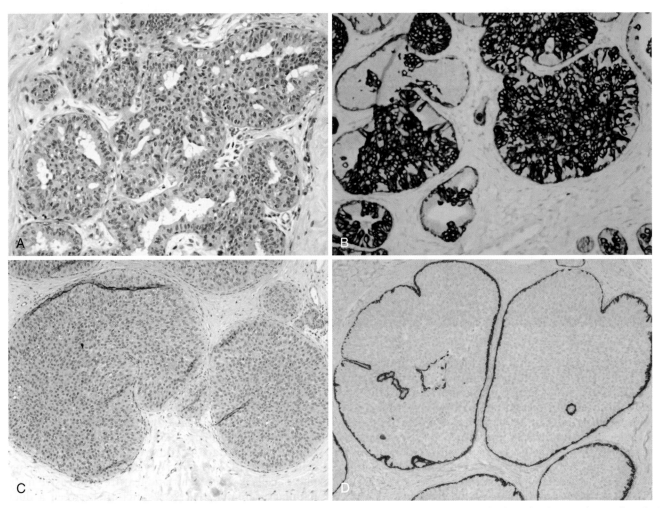

FIGURE 11-17 This case of florid duct hyperplasia **(A)** demonstrates strongly positive reactivity to high-molecular-weight cytokeratin-5 (CK5; **B**). In contrast to ductal hyperplasia, this solid variant of DCIS **(C)** is negative with CK5 **(D)**.

the prognosis was described as intermediate between that of pure tubular carcinoma and ILC.[117] This lesion had been categorized as a variant of ILC because of the small cells and characteristic ILC pattern of single-filing and targetoid infiltration.

Wheeler and coworkers,[118] as well as Esposito and colleagues,[119] documented uniform membranous ECAD immunostaining in the tubules and lobular-appearing components (Figure 11-23) and discovered that pure LCIS and mixed LCIS/DCIS predominate in these lesions. The combination of a small, rounded tubule profile with ILC-like patterns that is ECAD+ is a ductal immunoprofile.

HISTIOCYTOID CARCINOMA

The term *histiocytoid breast carcinoma (HBC)* was coined by Hood and associates[120] owing to tumor cells' resemblance to histiocytes. In 1983, Filotico and coworkers[121] described a case of lobular-appearing carcinoma with histiocytic features. Subsequent reports assumed that this variant was of lobular type by virtue of the characteristic infiltrating pattern. Only recently have immunohistologic studies been published on this rare entity. Gupta and colleagues,[122] reporting on type largest series, found that 8 of 11 cases lacked ECAD and 8 of 11 had LCIS. Three cases had ECAD,

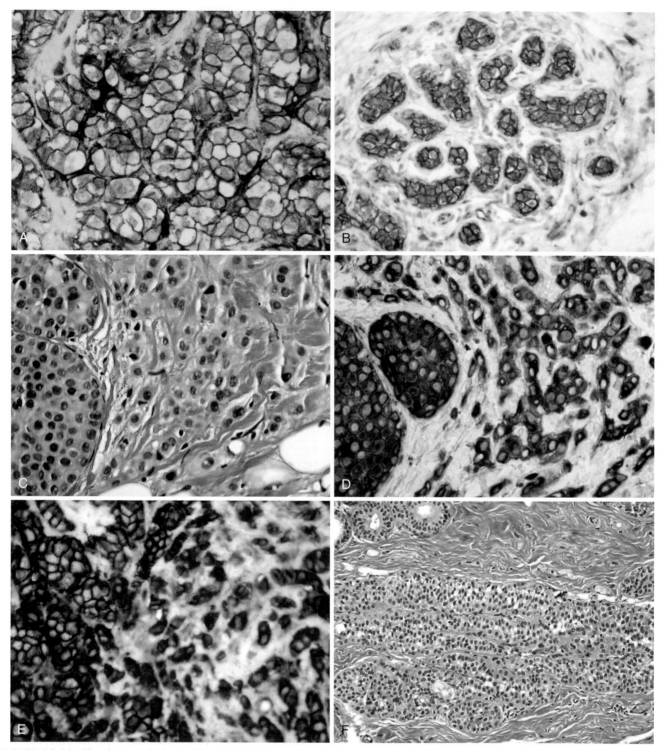

FIGURE 11-21 The dynamic biology of ECAD-p120 can be illustrated using a dual ECAD (brown)-p120 (red) stain. **A,** In this example of invasive ductal carcinoma, strong membranous reactivity (reddish-brown) is identified for both ECAD and p120. **B,** Similar reddish-brown membranous staining is identified in acinar cells within this lobule. An example of invasive lobular carcinoma and LCIS **(C)** demonstrates strong cytoplasmic immunoreactivity for p120 using a single-color stain **(D). E,** A dual ECAD-p120 stain demonstrates membranous ECAD and p120 (reddish-brown) immunoreactivity in the ductal component with lack of ECAD (absence of brown staining) but strong cytoplasmic p120 (red) staining in the lobular component in this example of mixed ductal and lobular carcinoma. The cells of lobular neoplasia **(F)** demonstrate strong cytoplasmic staining compared with membranous staining of normal duct cell with p120 **(G).**

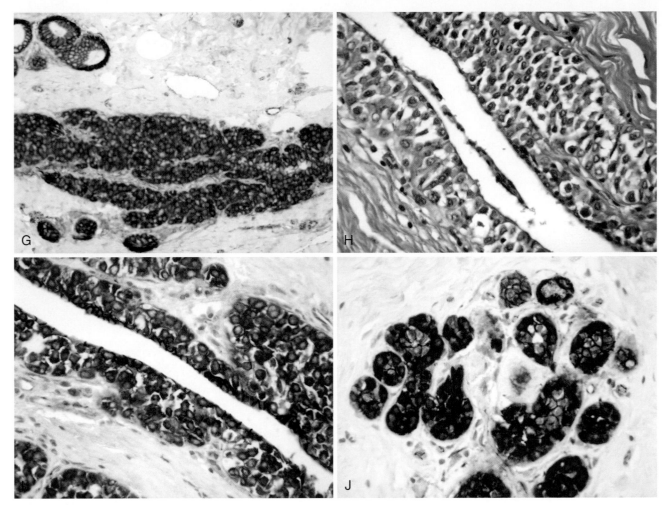

FIGURE 11-21, cont'd The cells of lobular neoplasia **(F)** demonstrate strong cytoplasmic staining compared with membranous staining of normal duct cell with p120 **(G). H,** Another example of LCIS with pagetoid extension into ducts. **I,** A dual ECAD-p120 stain shows a thin layer of residual luminal cells staining with ECAD (brown), and the duct largely replaced by LCIS cells demonstrates strong cytoplasmic reactivity (red) for p120. **J,** Another example of lobular neoplasia stained with dual ECAD-p120 stain demonstrates intense red cytoplasmic staining with p120.

characteristically "triple negative" and show expression of basal-type cytokeratin (CK5/6, CK14, CK17), epidermal growth factor receptor (EGFR), vimentin, and p53.[137,139] Often, a panel of basal-type CKs and EGFR in triple-negative tumors is used to identify basal-like carcinomas (Figure 11-25). The immunomarkers used to identify the basal-like variant are an example of "genomic application" of IHC. Based on the criteria established by the British Columbia group using gene expression profiling on some of their cases,[139] most studies in the literature have considered any reactivity for CK5/6 and/or EGFR in a triple-negative tumor as the definition for basal-like carcinoma. However, we have recently shown that the antibody to CK5 (clone XM26) is much more sensitive (but equally specific) than CK5/6 (clone D5/16B4) for identifying basal-like breast carcinomas.[140] Our immunohistochemical studies have also confirmed the existence of in situ carcinoma of basal phenotype.[141,142] Gene expression studies have consistently identified basal-like carcinomas to have poor prognosis.[136,143,144] These tumors occur in both pre- and postmenopausal patients;

however, identifying basal-like carcinoma in a young premenopausal patient may suggest the presence of hereditary breast and ovarian carcinoma syndrome.[145] Although there are no specific chemotherapeutic drugs currently available to treat these patients, data are emerging that it is important to recognize these tumors as therapies become more refined. For a more detailed discussion on morphology and immunohistology of basal-like breast carcinoma, see Chapter 20.

METAPLASTIC CARCINOMA—USE OF KERATINS, MELANOMA, AND VASCULAR MARKERS

Metaplastic carcinoma comprises a group of heterogeneous neoplasms that exhibit pure epithelial or a mixed epithelial and mesenchymal phenotype.[146,147] Diagnosis is not problematic when there is a recognizable component of metaplastic carcinoma (i.e., an obvious adenocarcinoma, adenosquamous or squamous cell carcinoma, osseous or chondroid differentiation). The most problematic cases are the ones that predominantly show spindle cell morphology without an obvious epithelial or

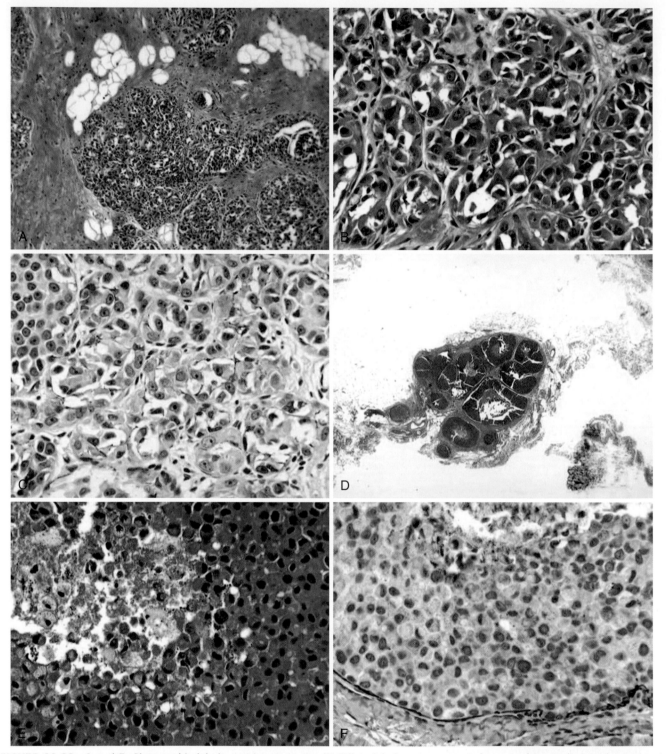

FIGURE 11-22 **A** and **B,** Pleomorphic lobular carcinoma in situ (PLCIS) in lobular arrangement shows nuclear grade 3 and prominent nucleoli. **C,** PLCIS is ECAD negative. **D,** Low magnification of PLCIS with comedonecrosis and calcification simulates DCIS. **E,** Note the dyshesion and plasmacytoid cellular features characteristic of PLCIS. **F,** ECAD is negative in PLCIS and positive in MECs.

DCIS component (Figure 11-26). This is usually the issue on a core biopsy rather than on an excision specimen. IHC stains can be helpful in this situation.[146] A panel composed of multiple keratin stains (CAM5.2, AE1/3, 34βE12, CK5, and CK7) and EMA is more useful than a single keratin.[148] Another sensitive and specific marker for metaplastic carcinoma is p63 and should always be included in the panel.[149,150] Vimentin expression in the tumor does not exclude a spindle cell carcinoma.[151,152] Vimentin expression has been found in 50% of hormone-independent cell lines and, because metaplastic carcinomas are usually negative for receptors, vimentin expression is actually expected.[153] If all the keratins, EMA, and p63 fail to show any immunoreactivity on

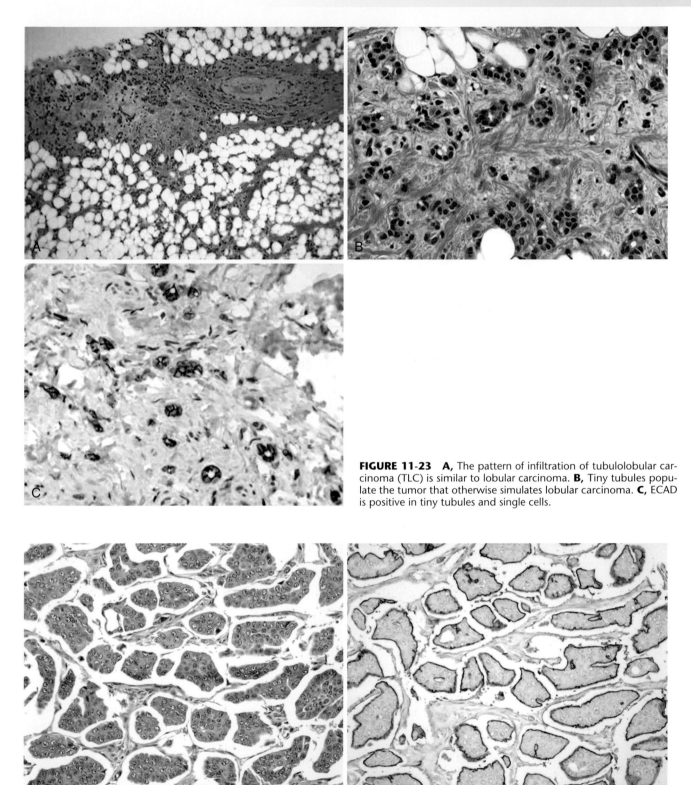

FIGURE 11-23 **A,** The pattern of infiltration of tubulolobular carcinoma (TLC) is similar to lobular carcinoma. **B,** Tiny tubules populate the tumor that otherwise simulates lobular carcinoma. **C,** ECAD is positive in tiny tubules and single cells.

FIGURE 11-24 An invasive micropapillary carcinoma of the breast **(A)** demonstrates "reverse polarity" of the neoplastic cells by epithelial membrane antigen (EMA) **(B).** Note the intense staining by EMA at the stroma-facing side of the cells.

a core biopsy, complete excision of the lesion should be recommended. In many cases, an epithelial component is present only focally. Although every effort should be made to prove an atypical spindle cell lesion to be a metaplastic carcinoma, it is important not to forget that melanomas and angiosarcomas can also occur in the breast. At least two melanoma markers should be performed. S100 is a very sensitive melanoma marker but has been reported to stain between 20% and 50% of metaplastic breast carcinomas and, therefore, is not

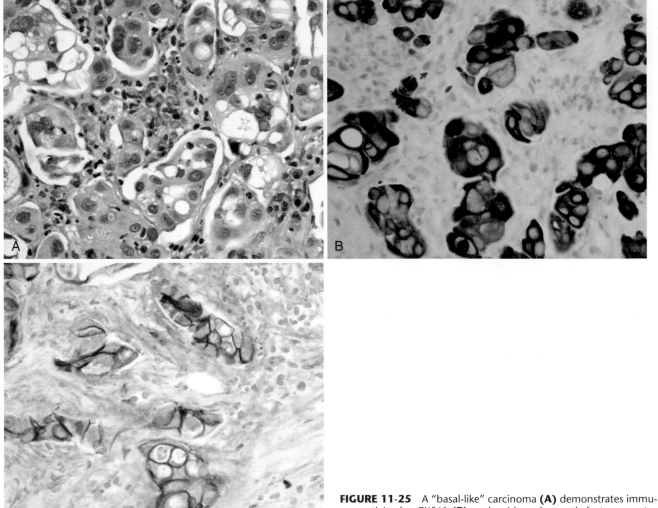

FIGURE 11-25 A "basal-like" carcinoma **(A)** demonstrates immunoreactivity for CK5/6 **(B)** and epidermal growth factor receptor (EGFR; **C**).

the best immunostain for this differential diagnosis.[154] Strong keratin reactivity or multiple keratin positivity would also exclude a melanoma. However, CAM5.2 positivity alone is not enough to exclude a melanoma unless it is strong and diffuse.[155,156]

Another significant malignant lesion with which metaplastic carcinoma can be confused is an angiosarcoma. These tumors may occur after radiation treatment or de novo. It is obvious to think about angiosarcoma in a malignant spindle or epithelioid lesion of the breast if there has been a prior history of radiation treatment. However, in the absence of such a clinical history, the lesion should be extensively examined by available IHC stains. More than one vascular marker should be used owing to the heterogeneous expression of vascular markers.[157] Of the three commonly used vascular markers (CD31, CD34, and Factor VIII), CD31 is generally considered to be the most specific, but occasional weak staining of carcinomas has been described.[158] We have also seen equivocal staining of carcinoma cells with CD31, likely because of "neovascularization" within the tumor. It is a diagnostic pitfall, especially in small samples. If CD34 is the only stain positive in malignant-appearing spindle cells, one should also consider

the possibility of the stromal component of phyllodes tumor. A diagnosis of a de novo primary angiosarcoma of the breast should be made only if there is unequivocal IHC staining for multiple vascular markers, negative staining for p63 and high-molecular-weight keratins, and appropriate histology of the lesion. In summary, a malignant spindle cell lesion is a metaplastic carcinoma unless proved otherwise. A panel comprising multiple keratins, EMA, p63, melanoma, and vascular markers is required in the workup of a malignant spindle cell lesion.

OTHER SPINDLE CELL NEOPLASMS (MYOEPITHELIAL AND MESENCHYMAL TUMORS)

Tumors of the breast in which MEC differentiation predominates include adenomyoepithelioma, myoepithelioma, and myoepithelial cell carcinoma (MECC).[159–162] Although the majority of adenomyoepitheliomas are benign, occasional tumors may exhibit aggressive behavior in the form of carcinoma or MECC.[163,164] The typical immunostaining pattern of the myoepithelial components of these tumors is strong cytoplasmic staining for 34βE12, CK5, and nuclear p63. Tumor

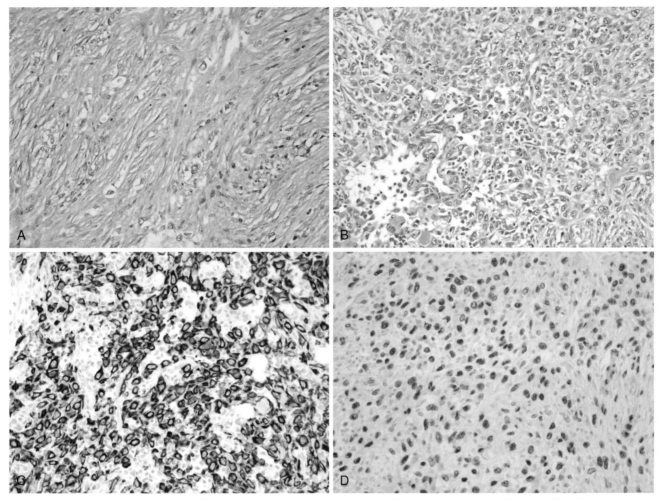

FIGURE 11-26 This predominantly spindle cell neoplasm **(A)** showed only a focal area of epithelioid malignant cells **(B).** The tumor was completely negative for AE1/3 and CAM5.2, but demonstrated staining for basal cytokeratins (CK5/6, CK14, CK17; **C)** and p63 **(D),** supporting the diagnosis of spindle cell metaplastic carcinoma.

cells are typically positive with S100 protein (90%) and may be positive with muscle markers such as calponin (86%), muscle-specific actin, desmin (14%), and alpha-smooth muscle actin (36%).[159,161] Occasional cells exhibit immunostaining with glial fibrillary acidic protein (GFAP). The presence of smooth muscle markers and immunostaining for GFAP is more in keeping with pure myoepithelial differentiation as opposed to metaplastic carcinomas (discussed previously), which are largely negative for these markers.[165,166] Expression of smooth muscle actin is very nonspecific and is not a definitive marker for muscle differentiation. Metaplastic carcinomas of the breast (carcinosarcoma, spindle cell carcinoma, sarcomatoid carcinoma) have an immunoprofile very similar to that of myoepithelial differentiation, because they regularly coexpress weak cytoplasmic CAM5.2 for low-molecular-weight keratins, strong cytoplasmic immunostaining for high-molecular-weight keratin 34βE12, CK5/6 or CK5, vimentin, and nuclear immunostaining for p63 (90%).[149] However, GFAP and SMM-HC are largely negative. Immunostaining with the muscle markers is most indicative of a pure myoepithelial neoplasm as opposed to a metaplastic carcinoma. The immunoprofile of metaplastic carcinoma is shared to a great degree with myoepithelial neoplasms, with some investigators suggesting that the MEC is the progenitor cell for metaplastic carcinomas.[154,167–169] Leibl and coworkers[154] demonstrated that the newly discovered experimental myoepithelial markers CD29 and 14-3-3 sigma stain metaplastic carcinomas, supplying further evidence of the myoepithelial nature of these tumors. The literature suggests that using the terms *myoepithelial carcinoma* versus *metaplastic carcinoma* is a matter of semantics and may not have any clinical significance.

Myoepithelial tumors need to be separated from the rare primary spindle cell sarcoma of the breast, which may include fibrosarcoma (vimentin-positive) leiomyosarcoma and rhabdomyosarcoma (positive with muscle markers), synovial sarcoma (positive with CK7 and CK19),[170] malignant nerve sheath tumors (S100+ and vimentin+), and malignant fibrous histiocytomas (vimentin-positive). Although each of these tumors may have characteristic light microscopic features, immunostaining patterns may be useful in the diagnostic distinction (Table 11-4). Primary liposarcomas (S100+) of the breast are rare tumors that may arise in a preexisting phyllodes tumor (CD34+ stroma).

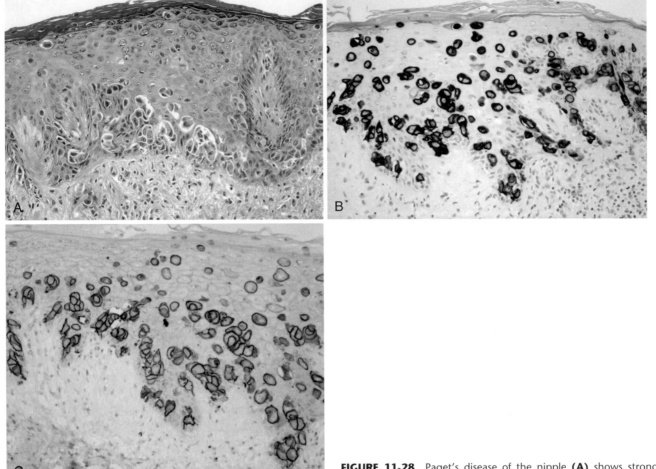

FIGURE 11-28 Paget's disease of the nipple **(A)** shows strong staining with antibodies to CK7 **(B)** and *HER2* **(C).**

for lymphatic space invasion; however, it is important to remember that lymphatic vessels are stained very intensely with D2-40 (see Figure 11-30C).

SENTINEL LYMPH NODE EXAMINATION

Historically, complete axillary lymph node dissections had been performed with lumpectomy or mastectomy specimens primarily for staging purposes, providing information that was used to determine adjuvant chemotherapy. The complete axillary lymph node dissection (CALND) may not change the course of the disease, although with removal of involved axillary nodes, the control of local recurrence in the axilla is easier. The morbidity associated with this procedure is substantial in terms of limitation of arm motion, arm pain, and chronic lymphedema.

The pioneering studies of sentinel lymph node metastasis (SLNM) originated with the study of melanoma patients; the goal was to spare these patients the morbidity of large regional lymph node dissections. Patients with melanomas who had SLN surgery were found to have a relatively orderly progression of lymph node metastases, with the SLN receiving the initial deposits of metastatic cells, followed by metastases in more distal lymph node groups. The same rationale is now being used for breast cancer patients.[200,201] The SLN is identified by injecting a radioisotope and blue dye before planned surgical excision. The SLN, identified by a combination of visual inspection for blue dye and intraoperative scanning for radioactivity, is harvested and submitted for pathologic study. The rationale is that, for patients who are SLN–, a further morbid procedure of axillary cleanout is unnecessary, but for SLN+, an axillary dissection is indicated for proper staging and possibly to provide better control for local recurrence. The controversy in this approach arises from several valid questions:

1. What is the natural history of micrometastatic (MM) disease in the axilla?
2. Is MM SLN disease an obligate pathway to clinically manifested local recurrence in the axilla?
3. Is MM SLN disease an indication for adjuvant chemotherapy?
4. How should the excised SLN be examined pathologically?
5. Does MM SLN disease affect overall survival?
6. What are the biologic parameters of MM disease that can predict the behavior of the disease in an individual patient?
7. Is it possible to recognize "benign transport" of epithelial elements in an SLN?

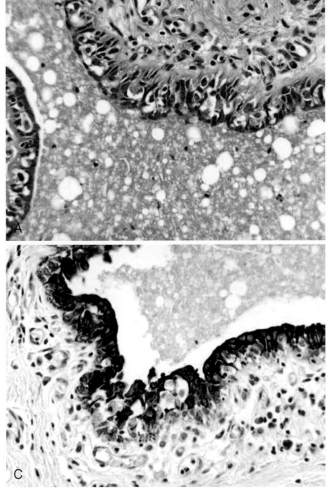

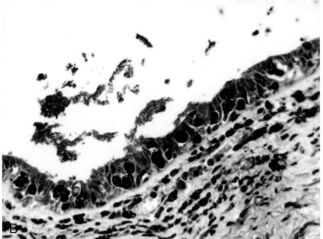

FIGURE 11-29 **A,** Duct ectasia with pseudopaget's of large ducts. Large clear cells intercalated in duct epithelium are CD68+ **(B)** and CK7– **(C).**

These are interesting and provocative questions for the care of the breast cancer patient. The American Joint Commission on Cancer defines *micrometastasis* as a cluster of cells that is no larger than 2 mm. Studies with more than 10 years of follow-up conclude that micrometastases are associated with a small but statistically significant decrease in tumor-free survival and overall survival when compared with truly node-negative cases,[202] but they are not an independent prognostic factor. The size of the metastatic deposit, taken together with tumor size and other factors, may additionally stratify patients at risk for further disease.

In most institutions, SLN biopsy with lumpectomy or mastectomy as indicated has become the standard of care.[203] The vast majority of SLN metastases are found in the first three SLNs that are submitted.[204]

Sentinel Lymph Node Immunohistochemistry

For the surgical pathologist, the appropriate triage and examination of the SLN is of utmost importance, but even here, some controversy exists. When the SLN mapping procedure began to be the standard of care a few years ago, the SLNs were histologically examined by multiple levels and CK stains on at least two levels. Since

then, more experience has been gained with the procedure and the reporting of SLNs. It was soon realized that the majority of micrometastases (metastases between 0.2 and 2 mm) can be identified by H&E alone and IHC for CK stains generally highlight isolated tumor cells (tumor cell aggregates ≤ 0.2 mm).[205] Although the exact clinical significance of isolated tumor cells, and even micrometastases, remains uncertain, studies have shown that they both are associated with non-SLN positivity in approximately 10% of cases, especially when the tumor size is larger than 1 cm (pT stage 1C or more).[206–209] In a study of 368 node-negative breast cancer patients with 20-year follow-up, Tan and colleagues[210] showed the prognostic significance of occult axillary node metastases and argued in favor of IHC on SLNs. In a recent prospective study of 3887 breast cancer patients, occult metastases (isolated tumor cells and micrometastases) were identified in 15.9% of patients.[211] Occult metastases were found to be an independent predictor of disease-free survival, overall survival, and distant disease-free interval. However, 5-year Kaplan-Meier estimates of overall survival among patients in whom occult metastases were detected and those without detectable metastases were 94.6% and 95.8%, respectively (i.e., the magnitude of difference in outcome at 5 years was small—only 1.2% age points).[211] Therefore, the authors rightfully concluded that additional tissue

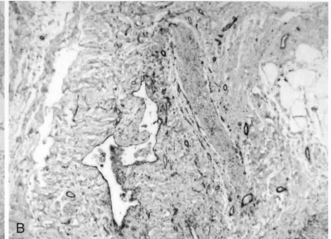

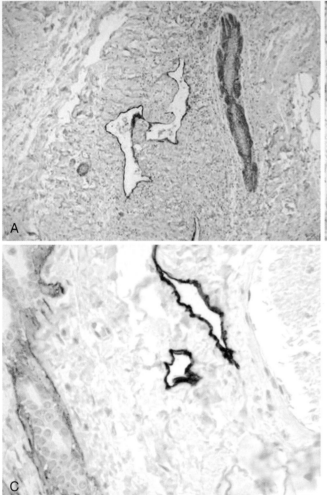

FIGURE 11-30 Immunohistochemical stain for D2-40 demonstrates selective staining of lymphatic endothelium **(A)** compared with CD31, which stains both lymphatic and vascular endothelium **(B). C,** A side-by-side comparison of lymphatic channel and a breast duct shows intense reactivity of lymphatic endothelium, but somewhat "smudgy" weak staining around the duct.

levels or CK IHC is not required for routine assessment of SLNs. However, the SLNs should be sectioned perpendicular to the longest axis at 2-mm intervals so as not to miss any macrometastases. We also agree with the conclusions of the latter study and follow a similar practice at our own institution.

If the primary breast carcinoma is of the ductal type, it would be difficult (but not impossible) to identify isolated tumor cells by H&E stain, and most pathologists would agree that they would be able to easily identify micrometastases (Figure 11-31A). Therefore, CK stains on SLNs do not add any significant information beyond H&E stain in a primary ductal cancer. However, there are significant differences when the primary breast tumor shows a lobular morphology. Owing to single cell infiltration, small (micro) metastases of lobular carcinoma (specially, the classic type) in a lymph node are extremely difficult to identify (see Figure 11-31B and C). Occasionally, CK stains would identify macrometastases, not readily apparent on H&E stain.[212] Cserni and associates[212] have reported that SLN positivity detected by IHC in lobular carcinomas was associated with further nodal metastases in 12 of 50 (24%) cases. Therefore, it is not unreasonable to do CK stains on SLNs in cases of lobular carcinoma and save some resources in cases of ductal carcinoma.

When performing CK immunostaining of SLNs, one should use a cocktail such as AE1/AE3 cocktail.[213] CAM5.2 is less desirable because of the manner in which it stains dendritic cells in the lymph node.[214] Micrometastatic cells occur in small clusters less than 2 mm in diameter within the lymph node or subcapsular sinus, and they need to be distinguished from the dendritic appearance of the interstitial reticulum cells of the lymph node, which are also keratin-positive.[215] It is uncertain if the site of lymph node micrometastasis (peripheral sinus versus parenchyma of lymph node) is clinically significant.

Aggregates of breast epithelial cells in the subcapsular sinus of axillary lymph nodes have been described by Carter and coworkers[216] as occurring as a result of "mechanical transport" after a breast biopsy. Some impugn the core biopsy itself or the breast massage that follows isotope/dye injection as sources of mechanical displacement of cells into the SLN.[217,218] Solitary keratin-positive cells may be transported to the SLN, and the histologic feature often associated with true benign transport is the association of CK+ cells with altered red blood cells and hemosiderin and macrophages (Figure 11-32). Diaz and colleagues[219] described benign epithelial tissue in skin dermal lymphatics and an SLN from a patient with pure DCIS. This lends morphologic

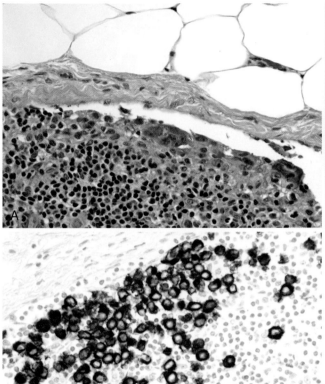

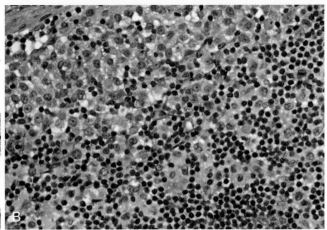

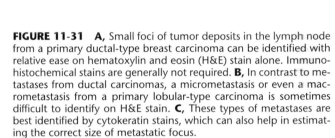

FIGURE 11-31 A, Small foci of tumor deposits in the lymph node from a primary ductal-type breast carcinoma can be identified with relative ease on hematoxylin and eosin (H&E) stain alone. Immunohistochemical stains are generally not required. **B,** In contrast to metastases from ductal carcinomas, a micrometastasis or even a macrometastasis from a primary lobular-type carcinoma is sometimes difficult to identify on H&E stain. **C,** These types of metastases are best identified by cytokeratin stains, which can also help in estimating the correct size of metastatic focus.

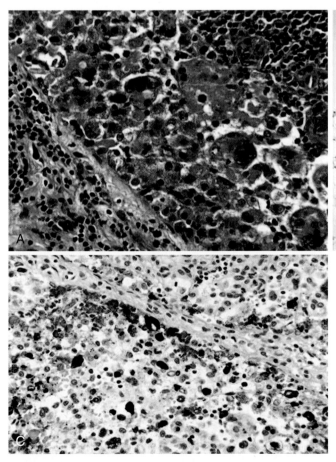

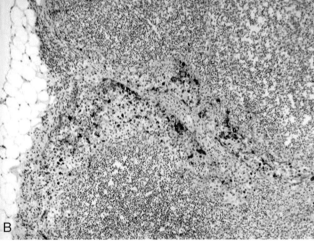

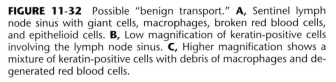

FIGURE 11-32 Possible "benign transport." **A,** Sentinel lymph node sinus with giant cells, macrophages, broken red blood cells, and epithelioid cells. **B,** Low magnification of keratin-positive cells involving the lymph node sinus. **C,** Higher magnification shows a mixture of keratin-positive cells with debris of macrophages and degenerated red blood cells.

documentation to the concept of "benign mechanical transport." The distinction between benign transport and "true" metastasis is easy if the cells in the lymph node appear "benign," but there is no objective way to distinguish benign transport from true metastasis when the cells appear cytologically malignant.

Intraoperative Molecular Testing of Sentinel Lymph Nodes

Recently, a few studies have shown the usefulness of intraoperative molecular tests in determining metastatic disease.[220,221] These are reverse-trancriptase polymerase chain reaction (RT-PCR) assays, which use a completely closed system and are fully automated from RNA extraction to final interpretation. One such assay, the Gene-Search Breast Lymph Node (BLN) Assay (Veridex LLC, Warren, NJ), was approved by the U.S. Food and Drug Administration (FDA) for axillary lymph node testing in July 2007. The GeneSearch BLN assay (Johnson & Johnson) is composed of a sample preparation kit, all reagents required for performing RT-PCR, and protocol software to be used with the Cepheid SmartCycler System (Sunnyvale, CA). According to the company, the test has been optimized for detecting metastatic disease larger than 0.2 mm. The test analyzes the expression of CK19 and mammaglobin genes. Some recent studies have shown high sensitivity, specificity, and positive and negative predictive values for the test.[221–224] Overall, this molecular assay is very much comparable with the frozen section examination, permanent sections, and even IHC. However, just like any other test, one should be aware of the false-positive and false-negative test results as well as the usefulness and pitfalls of a particular test. Because molecular tests are not morphologic assays, one has to be extremely careful with any sources of contamination. A cutting bench metastasis ("floater") can be easily recognized on an H&E-stained slide as such but will give a false-positive result by RT-PCR and there will be no definite way to identify this as an error. The SLNs identified in the axillary tail may contain a minute amount of breast tissue in the surrounding adipose tissue, which may also give a false-positive result. Therefore, lymph nodes should be completely trimmed of the adipose tissue before being sectioned for the molecular analysis. Moreover, fat interferes with the assay itself and this could be an issue when the SLN is diffusely replaced by adipose tissue. Occasionally, a benign epithelial inclusion (>0.2 mm) within the lymph node could also be a source of a false-positive result (Figure 11-33). Given the significance of the treatment decision based on a positive SLN result (complete axillary lymph node dissection, which cannot be undone) and several sources of false-positive result with molecular tests, we believe that currently, there are insufficient data to replace the morphologic methods with molecular assay. At present, we suggest that a positive molecular result should be confirmed by morphology by either frozen or permanent sections before a final decision is made. In contrast, a negative result is highly valuable given the very high negative predictive value of the molecular tests.

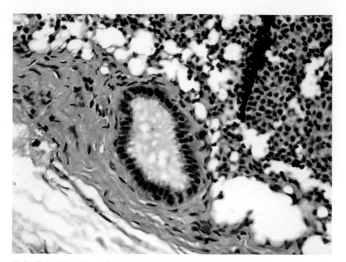

FIGURE 11-33 A benign epithelial glandular inclusion in an axillary lymph node as shown here may result in a false-positive molecular test for assessing micrometastatic disease.

KEY DIAGNOSTIC POINTS

Sentinel Lymph Node Micrometastatic Disease

- Section the lymph node perpendicular to the long axis at 2-mm intervals, examine with H&E and AE1/3 as indicated.

- For primary ductal carcinomas, AE1/3 keratin stain can be avoided.

- AE1/3 should always be performed for lobular carcinomas because even large tumor aggregates may be missed on H&E examination alone.

- The SLN procedure has been adopted as a standard of care in many institutions.

- Ninety-seven percent of all SLN metastases will be found in the first three SLN when multiple SLNs are submitted.

- Intraoperative molecular tests are comparable with morphologic examination, but there are potential sources of false-positive results.

- Molecular tests have very high negative predictive value that could be very useful for individual patient management.

H&E, hematoxylin and eosin; SLN, sentinel lymph node.

In fact, the company (J&J) abruptly discontinued the GeneSearch BLN assay in December 2009 owing to low adoption.

SYSTEMIC METASTASIS OF BREAST CARCINOMA

The diagnosis of breast carcinoma at a metastatic site requires a careful histologic examination, review of all prior case material, and immunohistologic evaluation of tumor cells. If the patient had a prior history of breast cancer, it is valuable to know whether it showed ductal or lobular morphology. Comparison with prior tumor is helpful in making the correct diagnosis in the majority of cases. Immunohistologic evaluation is mainly required in cases of carcinoma of unknown origin.[225] CK7 and CK20 have been generally used in this evaluation to narrow the differential diagnosis.[226,227] Breast carcinomas are generally CK7+ and CK20–; however, a similar CK profile is seen in lung, upper gastrointestinal tract, and gynecologic tract carcinomas.

GCDFP-15 has been used for several years as the most specific marker of breast carcinoma[228,229]; however, its sensitivity in formalin-fixed paraffin-embedded tissue is less than optimal.[228] Originally described by Pearlman and colleagues[230] and Haagensen and associates,[231] the prolactin-inducing protein identified by Murphy and coworkers[232] has the same amino acid sequence as GCDFP-15 and is found in abundance in breast cystic fluid and any cell type that has apocrine features.[229,233] The latter, in addition to breast, includes acinar structures in salivary glands, apocrine glands, and sweat glands and in Paget's disease of skin, vulva, and prostate.[229,234–237] Homologous-appearing carcinomas of the breast, skin adnexa, and salivary glands demonstrate a great deal of overlap immunostaining with GCDFP-15.[238] Aside from these immunoreactivities, most other carcinomas show no appreciable immunostaining. Breast carcinoma metastatic to the skin (or locally recurrent) may be difficult to distinguish from skin adnexal tumors.[239] Wick and colleagues,[240] in a study of the overlapping morphologic features of breast, salivary gland, and skin adnexal tumors, found that GCDFP-15 was infrequently found in eccrine sweat gland carcinomas, a paucity of CEA was found in breast carcinomas, and ERs were largely absent in salivary duct carcinomas. The positive predictive value and specificity for detection of breast carcinoma with GCDFP-15 have been reported up to 99%.[229] The sensitivity for the GCDFP-15 antibodies has been reported to be as high as 75% for tumors with apocrine differentiation,[229,239] but the overall sensitivity is 55% and only 23% for tumors without apocrine differentiation.[239] The sensitivity is even worse when it comes to core biopsy, because the pattern of staining for GCDFP-15 is often patchy.

Because the specificity of GCDFP-15 antibodies for breast carcinoma is so high, this antibody is often used in a screening panel in the appropriate clinical situation, which often turns out to be the presentation of a woman with metastasis of unknown primary or a new lung mass in a patient with a history of breast cancer. Others have demonstrated the utility and specificity of GCDFP-15 antibodies in the distinction of breast carcinoma metastatic in the lung.[241–243] However, a recent study by Striebel and coworkers[244] demonstrated GCDFP-15 immunoreactivity in 11 of 211 (5.2%) lung adenocarcinomas. This study again stresses the importance of a panel rather than an individual stain in determining site of origin of a metastatic tumor. On a similar note, Wilms' tumor protein 1 (WT1) (a specific marker of ovarian serous carcinoma) nuclear expression is seen in a subset of breast carcinoma that demonstrate mucinous differentiation. However, the expression is generally weak to moderate in contrast to ovarian serous carcinoma in which the expression is

generally strong and diffuse.[245] Another recent paper has shown reactivity for thyroid transcription factor 1 (TTF1) (thyroid and lung specific marker) in breast carcinomas. In a study of 546 primary breast carcinomas, Robens and associates[246] identified TTF1 reactivity in 13 (2.4%) cases using clone SPT24. The authors did not examine the other more popular clone 8G7G/1. However, only 3 cases showed diffuse strong reactivity, of which 2 were also positive for hormone receptors and hormone receptor data were not available on 1 case but it was a lobular carcinoma. Therefore, we believe that, if a panel approach is used, TTF1 reactivity in breast cancer should not pose a challenge in determining the primary site.

ER and PgR are very helpful in cases with a history of receptor-positive breast cancer; however, a large proportion of gynecologic tumors are also positive for hormone receptors. Hormone receptors have also been reported to be positive in nonbreast and nongynecologic sites.[247–249] However, diffuse strong expression is generally suggestive of a breast or gynecologic primary tumor.

Mammaglobin has been described to be a more sensitive marker than GCDFP-15 for diagnosis of breast carcinoma.[250,251] The mammaglobin gene is a member of the uteroglobin family that encodes a glycoprotein associated with breast epithelial cells. The immunostaining pattern is cytoplasmic, analogous to GCDFP-15. If the weak equivocal staining is disregarded (because it is not helpful in determining site of origin in "real life"), the sensitivity of mammaglobin is between 50% and 60% compared with less than 30% for GCDFP-15. We have seen that, even in cases positive for both GCDFP-15 and mammaglobin, the percentage of cells and intensity of staining are much higher with mammaglobin than with GCDFP-15 (Figure 11-34).[252] Some initial studies

---

KEY DIAGNOSTIC POINTS
Metastatic Breast Carcinoma

- Diagnostic confirmation requires use of a panel.
- Usual breast carcinoma immunoprofile is CK7+, GCDFP-15+, mammaglobin positive, ER+, CK20–, TTF-1–, WT1–.
- GCDFP-15 is the most specific marker of breast carcinoma; however, weak/equivocal staining is not helpful in the workup of a tumor of unknown origin.
- Mammaglobin is a more sensitive marker of breast carcinoma than GCDFP-15.
- Mammaglobin also stains endometrioid adenocarcinomas (≤40% cases) and rare melanomas.
- Salivary gland carcinomas and skin adnexal carcinomas have overlap staining with GCDFP-15 and mammaglobin.
- Up to 30% of breast carcinomas may be negative for both GCDFP-15 and mammaglobin.
- Novel markers such as NY-BR-1 (positive in breast carcinomas) and PAX8 (negative in breast tumors) are useful in distinguishing breast tumors from gynecologic tract primary tumors.

CK, cytokeratin; ER, estrogen receptor; GCDFP-15, gross cystic disease fluid protein-15.

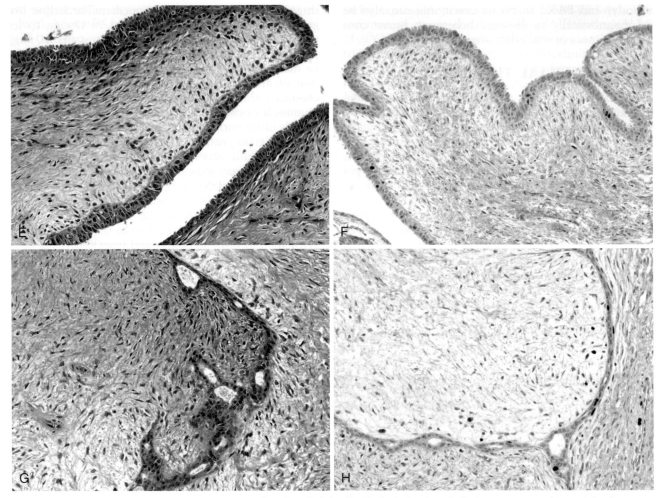

FIGURE 11-35, cont'd Note the numerous positive ductal epithelial cells. Similarly, benign phyllodes tumor may show minimal to no proliferative activity with Ki-67 as shown in **E** to **H. A–H,** *Courtesy Dr. Nicole N. Esposito, Tampa, FL.*

reliably differentiate between fibroadenomas and benign phyllodes tumors with low mitotic rates.[264] Molecular and chromosomal assays have also been utilized in distinguishing fibroadenomas from benign phyllodes with limited success.[265–268] A study examining mutations on a global scale using single nucleotide polymorphism (SNP) arrays reported at least one occurrence of loss of heterozygosity (LOH) in benign phyllodes tumors, whereas fibroadenomas most often had no LOH or very low fractional allelic losses (FALs).[269] However, cases designated as benign phyllodes tumors in this study included cases with mitotic rates of up to 5 per 10 high-power field and are thus more than likely borderline tumors by conventional criteria. Inclusion of such cases in the "benign" category likely inflated the FALs of the benign phyllodes study group. For practical purposes, the distinction between fibroadenoma and benign phyllodes is still best made using morphologic criteria.

Among the three categories of phyllodes tumor, the differences in stromal cell proliferation are more evident. Ki-67 labeling indices range from 1% to 5% in benign tumors, 6% to 16% in borderline tumors, and 12% to 50% in malignant tumors in published reports (Figure 11-36).[270–273] Similarly, tumor suppressor gene p53 is increasingly expressed with tumor grade, although less

consistently than Ki-67.[273–276] The expression of proteins with targeted therapy implications in phyllodes tumors have been explored. Chen and associates[277] first reported c-kit expression in the stroma of phyllodes tumors in 2000 and found c-kit expression to be preferentially expressed in histologically malignant phyllodes tumors. Since then, several additional studies have reported increased c-kit expression in malignant phyllodes tumors compared with benign and/or borderline tumors.[278–280] However, whether c-kit expression in these tumors infers susceptibility to the KIT-receptor tyrosine kinase inhibitor imatinib mesylate is doubtful, because activating c-kit mutations have yet to be reported. Of interest is a recent study by Djordjevic and Hanna[281] that suggest c-kit expression in fibroepithelial tumors is related to the presence of mast cells. The authors have argued against any appreciable true stromal cell c-kit staining in fibroepithelial tumors. EGFR has also recently been studied in phyllodes tumors, with most reports correlating increased stromal expression with tumor grade as well as chromosome 7 polysomy (Figure 11-37).[275,282,283] Once again, these immunohistochemical studies are of significant interest, but at a practical level, morphologic features of three grades of phyllodes tumor are equally distinctive. Moreover, assessment of prognosis in every

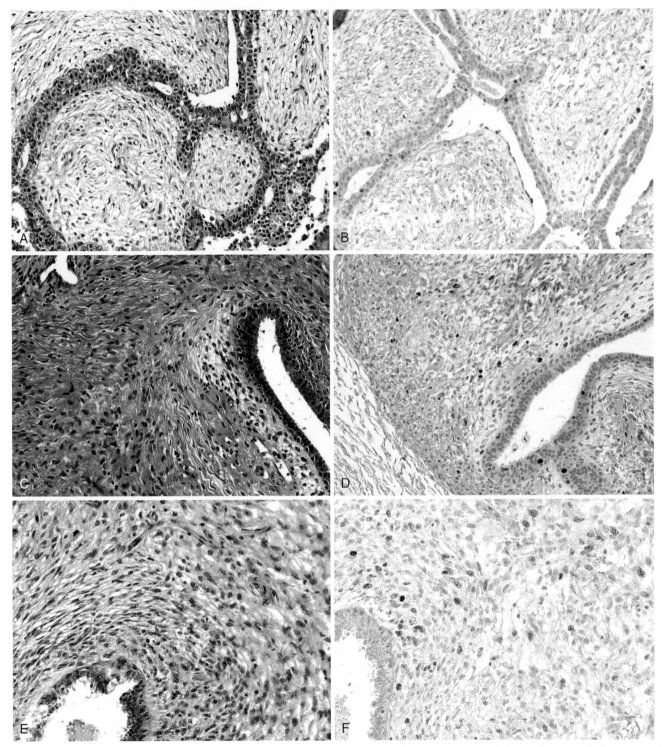

FIGURE 11-36 Ki-67 expression in benign **(A** and **B)**, borderline **(C** and **D)**, and malignant **(E** and **F)** phyllodes tumors of the breast. Labeling indexes as demonstrated by Ki-67 expression generally correlates linearly with tumor grade. **A–F,** *Courtesy Dr. Nicole N. Esposito, Tampa, FL.*

case of phyllodes tumor is extremely difficult regardless of the criteria used. Both morphologic criteria and immunohistochemical markers are far less than perfect in this regard.[270,272,273,276,278,284–288] However, at the current time, the factors most predictive of recurrence include histologic characteristics and status of surgical resection margins.[272,289–295]

Another fibroepithelial tumor to be considered here is the so-called periductal stromal tumor, initially described

by Burga and Tavassoli[296] as a distinct entity from phyllodes tumors, although histologically identical except lacking the intracanalicular or "leaflike" pattern. Like phyllodes tumors, however, the stromal cells express CD34, and thus, some have proposed they are best regarded as a phyllodes tumor variant that lacks the classic leaflike architecture rather than a distinct entity.[174,296]

Finally, a benign fibroepithelial lesion that may be challenging to diagnose on core biopsy is the so-called

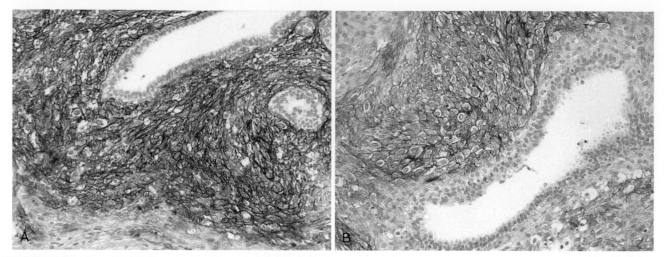

FIGURE 11-37 **A** and **B**, EGFR expression in two malignant phyllodes tumors. EGFR expression has been shown to be more commonly expressed in malignant phyllodes tumors and usually corresponds to polysomy 7 rather than EGFR amplification. **A** *and* **B**, *Courtesy Dr. Nicole N. Esposito, Tampa, FL.*

KEY DIAGNOSTIC POINTS

Fibroepithelial Tumors

- Phyllodes tumor stroma is CD34+, a finding that is useful in the workup of spindle cell lesion in a core biopsy.

- Ki-67 may supplement grading of phyllodes tumor in addition to morphology and counting of mitotic figures.

- Ki-67 proliferation index does not reliably distinguish between fibroadenoma and benign phyllodes tumor.

- Molecular analyses so far have also been inconclusive in distinguishing fibroadenomas from phyllodes tumors.

- Periductal stromal tumor is likely a variant of phyllodes tumor and also has CD34+ stroma.

myoid hamartoma. It can present as a mass-forming lesion with adenosis pattern and smooth muscle metaplasia of the stromal cells. The stromal cells are immunoreactive for vimentin and smooth muscle markers such as actin, desmin, SMM-HC, and caldesmon and are negative for S100 (Figure 11-38).[297,298]

SUMMARY

IHC has broad use in breast pathology. Diagnostically, determination of invasion, type of carcinoma, categorization of types of epithelial atypia, characterization of lymphatic space invasion and SLN status, and identification of breast carcinoma in metastatic sites are all fairly common practices. IHC, correctly performed and interpreted, enhances patient safety and ensures proper treatment regimens.

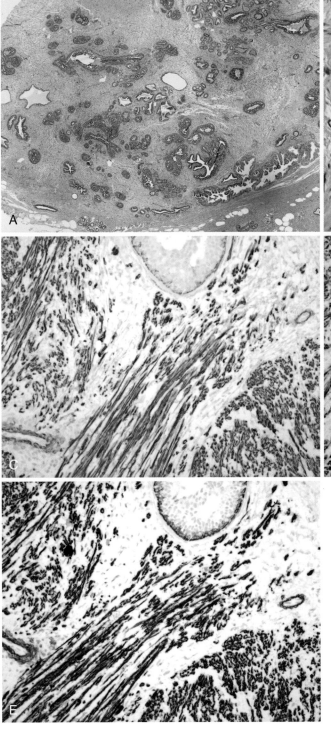

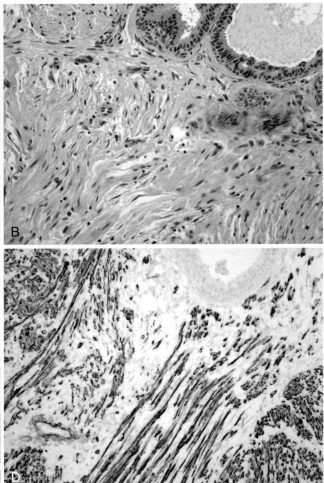

FIGURE 11-38 **A** and **B,** A well-circumscribed biphasic lesion with stromal smooth muscle metaplasia is consistent with the diagnosis of myoid hamartoma. The stromal smooth muscle metaplasia is positive for actin **(C),** H-caldesmon **(D),** and SMM-HC **(E).** Note that actin and SMM-HC also stain the blood vessels and MECs around the ducts.

REFERENCES

1. Joshi MG, Lee AK, Pedersen CA, et al. The role of immunocytochemical markers in the differential diagnosis of proliferative and neoplastic lesions of the breast. Mod Pathol 1996;9:57-62.

2. Rudland PS, Leinster SJ, Winstanley J, et al. Immunocytochemical identification of cell types in benign and malignant breast diseases: variations in cell markers accompany the malignant state. J Histochem Cytochem 1993;41:543-553.

3. Ahmed A. The myoepithelium in human breast carcinoma. J Pathol 1974;113:129-135.

4. Bussolati G. Actin-rich (myoepithelial) cells in lobular carcinoma in situ of the breast. Virchows Arch B Cell Pathol Incl Mol Pathol 1980;32:165-176.

5. Bussolati G, Botta G, Gugliotta P. Actin-rich (myoepithelial) cells in ductal carcinoma-in-situ of the breast. Virchows Arch B Cell Pathol Incl Mol Pathol 1980;34:251-259.

6. Bussolati G, Botto Micca FB, Eusebi V, Betts CM. Myoepithelial cells in lobular carcinoma in situ of the breast: a parallel immunocytochemical and ultrastructural study. Ultrastruct Pathol 1981;2:219-230.

7. Gould VE, Jao W, Battifora H. Ultrastructural analysis in the differential diagnosis of breast tumors. The significance of myoepithelial cells, basal lamina, intracytoplasmic lumina and secretory granules. Pathol Res Pract 1980;167:45-70.

8. Gusterson BA, Warburton MJ, Mitchell D, et al. Distribution of myoepithelial cells and basement membrane proteins in the normal breast and in benign and malignant breast diseases. Cancer Res 1982;42:4763-4770.

9. Dwarakanath S, Lee AK, Delellis RA, et al. S-100 protein positivity in breast carcinomas: a potential pitfall in diagnostic immunohistochemistry. Hum Pathol 1987;18:1144-1148.

10. Jarasch ED, Nagle RB, Kaufmann M, et al. Differential diagnosis of benign epithelial proliferations and carcinomas of the breast using antibodies to cytokeratins. Hum Pathol 1988;19:276-289.

11. Nagle RB, Bocker W, Davis JR, et al. Characterization of breast carcinomas by two monoclonal antibodies distinguishing myoepithelial from luminal epithelial cells. J Histochem Cytochem 1986;34:869-881.

12. Raju UB, Lee MW, Zarbo RJ, Crissman JD. Papillary neoplasia of the breast: immunohistochemically defined myoepithelial cells in the diagnosis of benign and malignant papillary breast neoplasms. Mod Pathol 1989;2:569-576.

13. Lele SM, Graves K, Gatalica Z. Immunohistochemical detection of maspin is a useful adjunct in distinguishing radial sclerosing lesion from tubular carcinoma of the breast. Appl Immunohistochem Mol Morphol 2000;8:32-36.

14. Mohsin SK, Zhang M, Clark GM, Allred DC. Maspin expression in invasive breast cancer: association with other prognostic factors. J Pathol 2003;199:432-435.

15. Navarro RL, Martins MT, de Araujo VC. Maspin expression in normal and neoplastic salivary gland. J Oral Pathol Med 2004;33:435-440.

16. Umekita Y, Yoshida H. Expression of maspin is up-regulated during the progression of mammary ductal carcinoma. Histopathology 2003;42:541-545.

17. Bocker W, Bier B, Freytag G, et al. An immunohistochemical study of the breast using antibodies to basal and luminal keratins, alpha-smooth muscle actin, vimentin, collagen IV and laminin. Part II: epitheliosis and ductal carcinoma in situ. Virchows Arch A Pathol Anat Histopathol 1992;421:323-330.

18. Bose S, Derosa CM, Ozzello L. Immunostaining of type IV collagen and smooth muscle actin as an aid in the diagnosis of breast lesions. Breast J 1999;5:194-201.

19. Gottlieb C, Raju U, Greenwald KA. Myoepithelial cells in the differential diagnosis of complex benign and malignant breast lesions: an immunohistochemical study. Mod Pathol 1990;3:135-140.

20. Gugliotta P, Sapino A, Macri L, et al. Specific demonstration of myoepithelial cells by anti-alpha smooth muscle actin antibody. J Histochem Cytochem 1988;36:659-663.

21. Raymond WA, Leong AS. Assessment of invasion in breast lesions using antibodies to basement membrane components and myoepithelial cells. Pathology 1991;23:291-297.

22. Gimona M, Herzog M, Vandekerckhove J, Small JV. Smooth muscle specific expression of calponin. FEBS Lett 1990;274:159-162.

23. Werling RW, Hwang H, Yaziji H, Gown AM. Immunohistochemical distinction of invasive from noninvasive breast lesions: a comparative study of p63 versus calponin and smooth muscle myosin heavy chain. Am J Surg Pathol 2003;27:82-90.

24. Winder SJ, Walsh MP. Calponin: thin filament-linked regulation of smooth muscle contraction. Cell Signal 1993;5:677-686.

25. Titus MA. Myosins. Curr Opin Cell Biol 1993;5:77-81.

26. Strasser P, Gimona M, Moessler H, et al. Mammalian calponin. Identification and expression of genetic variants. FEBS Lett 1993;330:13-18.

27. Barbareschi M, Pecciarini L, Cangi MG, et al. p63, a p53 homologue, is a selective nuclear marker of myoepithelial cells of the human breast. Am J Surg Pathol 2001;25:1054-1060.

28. Kaufmann O, Fietze E, Mengs J, Dietel M. Value of p63 and cytokeratin 5/6 as immunohistochemical markers for the differential diagnosis of poorly differentiated and undifferentiated carcinomas. Am J Clin Pathol 2001;116:823-830.

29. Bhargava R, Dabbs DJ. Use of immunohistochemistry in diagnosis of breast epithelial lesions. Adv Anat Pathol 2007;14:93-107.

30. Eusebi V, Foschini MP, Betts CM, et al. Microglandular adenosis, apocrine adenosis, and tubular carcinoma of the breast. An immunohistochemical comparison. Am J Surg Pathol 1993;17:99-109.

31. Lee KC, Chan JK, Gwi E. Tubular adenosis of the breast. A distinctive benign lesion mimicking invasive carcinoma. Am J Surg Pathol 1996;20:46-54.

32. Hill CB, Yeh IT. Myoepithelial cell staining patterns of papillary breast lesions: from intraductal papillomas to invasive papillary carcinomas. Am J Clin Pathol 2005;123:36-44.

33. Papotti M, Eusebi V, Gugliotta P, Bussolati G. Immunohistochemical analysis of benign and malignant papillary lesions of the breast. Am J Surg Pathol 1983;7:451-461.

34. Saddik M, Lai R. CD44s as a surrogate marker for distinguishing intraductal papilloma from papillary carcinoma of the breast. J Clin Pathol 1999;52:862-864.

35. Raju U, Vertes D. Breast papillomas with atypical ductal hyperplasia: a clinicopathologic study. Hum Pathol 1996;27:1231-1238.

36. Collins LC, Schnitt SJ. Papillary lesions of the breast: selected diagnostic and management issues. Histopathology 2008;52:20-29.

37. Rabban JT, Koerner FC, Lerwill MF. Solid papillary ductal carcinoma in situ versus usual ductal hyperplasia in the breast: a potentially difficult distinction resolved by cytokeratin 5/6. Hum Pathol 2006;37:787-793.

38. Carter D, Orr SL, Merino MJ. Intracystic papillary carcinoma of the breast. After mastectomy, radiotherapy or excisional biopsy alone. Cancer 1983;52:14-19.

39. Carter D. Intraductal papillary tumors of the breast: a study of 78 cases. Cancer 1977;39:1689-1692.

40. Collins LC, Carlo VP, Hwang H, et al. Intracystic papillary carcinomas of the breast: a reevaluation using a panel of myoepithelial cell markers. Am J Surg Pathol 2006;30:1002-1007.

41. Mulligan AM, O'Malley FP. Papillary lesions of the breast: a review. Adv Anat Pathol 2007;14:108-119.

42. Esposito NN, Dabbs DJ, Bhargava R. Are encapsulated papillary carcinomas of the breast in situ or invasive? A basement membrane study of 27 cases. Am J Clin Pathol 2009;131:228-242.

43. Barsky SH, Siegal GP, Jannotta F, Liotta LA. Loss of basement membrane components by invasive tumors but not by their benign counterparts. Lab Invest 1983;49:140-147.

44. Leal C, Costa I, Fonseca D, et al. Intracystic (encysted) papillary carcinoma of the breast: a clinical, pathological, and immunohistochemical study. Hum Pathol 1998;29:1097-1104.

45. Lefkowitz M, Lefkowitz W, Wargotz ES. Intraductal (intracystic) papillary carcinoma of the breast and its variants: a clinicopathological study of 77 cases. Hum Pathol 1994;25:802-809.

46. Solorzano CC, Middleton LP, Hunt KK, et al. Treatment and outcome of patients with intracystic papillary carcinoma of the breast. Am J Surg 2002;184:364-368.

47. Wynveen CA, Nehhozina T, Akram M, et al. Intracystic papillary carcinoma of the breast: an in situ or invasive tumor? Results of immunohistochemical analysis and clinical follow-up. Am J Surg Pathol 2011;35:1-14.

48. Mulligan AM, O'Malley FP. Metastatic potential of encapsulated (intracystic) papillary carcinoma of the breast: a report of 2 cases with axillary lymph node micrometastases. Int J Surg Pathol 2007;15:143-147.

49. Masood S, Sim SJ, Lu L. Immunohistochemical differentiation of atypical hyperplasia vs. carcinoma in situ of the breast. Cancer Detect Prev 1992;16:225-235.

50. Moinfar F, Man YG, Lininger RA, et al. Use of keratin 35betaE12 as an adjunct in the diagnosis of mammary intraepithelial neoplasia-ductal type—benign and malignant intraductal proliferations. Am J Surg Pathol 1999;23:1048-1058.

51. Lacroix-Triki M, Mery E, Voigt JJ, et al. Value of cytokeratin 5/6 immunostaining using D5/16 B4 antibody in the spectrum of proliferative intraepithelial lesions of the breast. A comparative study with 34betaE12 antibody. Virchows Arch 2003;442:548-554.

52. Grin A, O'Malley FP, Mulligan AM. Cytokeratin 5 and estrogen receptor immunohistochemistry as a useful adjunct in identifying atypical papillary lesions on breast needle core biopsy. Am J Surg Pathol 2009;33:1615-1623.

53. Cangiarella J, Guth A, Axelrod D, et al. Is surgical excision necessary for the management of atypical lobular hyperplasia and lobular carcinoma in situ diagnosed on core needle biopsy?: a report of 38 cases and review of the literature. Arch Pathol Lab Med 2008;132:979-983.

54. Chuba PJ, Hamre MR, Yap J, et al. Bilateral risk for subsequent breast cancer after lobular carcinoma-in-situ: analysis of surveillance, epidemiology, and end results data. J Clin Oncol 2005;23:5534-5541.

55. Crisi GM, Mandavilli S, Cronin E, Ricci Jr A. Invasive mammary carcinoma after immediate and short-term follow-up for lobular neoplasia on core biopsy. Am J Surg Pathol 2003;27:325-333.

56. Elsheikh TM, Silverman JF. Follow-up surgical excision is indicated when breast core needle biopsies show atypical lobular hyperplasia or lobular carcinoma in situ: a correlative study of 33 patients with review of the literature. Am J Surg Pathol 2005;29:534-543.

57. Fisher ER, Costantino J, Fisher B, et al. Pathologic findings from the National Surgical Adjuvant Breast Project (NSABP) Protocol B-17. Five-year observations concerning lobular carcinoma in situ. Cancer 1996;78:1403-1416.

58. Fisher ER, Land SR, Fisher B, et al. Pathologic findings from the National Surgical Adjuvant Breast and Bowel Project: twelve-year observations concerning lobular carcinoma in situ. Cancer 2004;100:238-244.

59. Leonard GD, Swain SM. Ductal carcinoma in situ, complexities and challenges. J Natl Cancer Inst 2004;96:906-920.

60. Li CI, Malone KE, Saltzman BS, Daling JR. Risk of invasive breast carcinoma among women diagnosed with ductal carcinoma in situ and lobular carcinoma in situ, 1988-2001. Cancer 2006;106:2104-2112.

61. Maluf H, Koerner F. Lobular carcinoma in situ and infiltrating ductal carcinoma: frequent presence of DCIS as a precursor lesion. Int J Surg Pathol 2001;9:127-131.

62. Winchester DP, Jeske JM, Goldschmidt RA. The diagnosis and management of ductal carcinoma in-situ of the breast. CA Cancer J Clin 2000;50:184-200.

63. Bedrosian I, Mick R, Orel SG, et al. Changes in the surgical management of patients with breast carcinoma based on preoperative magnetic resonance imaging. Cancer 2003;98:468-473.

64. Molland JG, Donnellan M, Janu NC, et al. Infiltrating lobular carcinoma—a comparison of diagnosis, management and outcome with infiltrating duct carcinoma. Breast 2004;13:389-396.

65. Munot K, Dall B, Achuthan R, et al. Role of magnetic resonance imaging in the diagnosis and single-stage surgical resection of invasive lobular carcinoma of the breast. Br J Surg 2002;89:1296-1301.

66. Borst MJ, Ingold JA. Metastatic patterns of invasive lobular versus invasive ductal carcinoma of the breast. Surgery 1993;114:637-641:discussion 641–642.

67. Harris M, Howell A, Chrissohou M, et al. A comparison of the metastatic pattern of infiltrating lobular carcinoma and infiltrating duct carcinoma of the breast. Br J Cancer 1984;50:23-30.

68. Jain S, Fisher C, Smith P, et al. Patterns of metastatic breast cancer in relation to histological type. Eur J Cancer 1993;29A:2155-2157.

69. Tham YL, Sexton K, Kramer R, et al. Primary breast cancer phenotypes associated with propensity for central nervous system metastases. Cancer 2006;107:696-704.

70. Arpino G, Bardou VJ, Clark GM, Elledge RM. Infiltrating lobular carcinoma of the breast: tumor characteristics and clinical outcome. Breast Cancer Res 2004;6:R149-156.

71. Mersin H, Yildirim E, Gulben K, Berberoglu U. Is invasive lobular carcinoma different from invasive ductal carcinoma? Eur J Surg Oncol 2003;29:390-395.

72. Kneeshaw PJ, Turnbull LW, Smith A, Drew PJ. Dynamic contrast enhanced magnetic resonance imaging aids the surgical management of invasive lobular breast cancer. Eur J Surg Oncol 2003;29:32-37.

73. Schelfout K, Van Goethem M, Kersschot E, et al. Preoperative breast MRI in patients with invasive lobular breast cancer. Eur Radiol 2004;14:1209-1216.

74. Cocquyt VF, Blondeel PN, Depypere HT, et al. Different responses to preoperative chemotherapy for invasive lobular and invasive ductal breast carcinoma. Eur J Surg Oncol 2003;29:361-367.

75. Cristofanilli M, Gonzalez-Angulo A, Sneige N, et al. Invasive lobular carcinoma classic type: response to primary chemotherapy and survival outcomes. J Clin Oncol 2005;23:41-48.

76. Mathieu MC, Rouzier R, Llombart-Cussac A, et al. The poor responsiveness of infiltrating lobular breast carcinomas to neoadjuvant chemotherapy can be explained by their biological profile. Eur J Cancer 2004;40:342-351.

77. Tubiana-Hulin M, Stevens D, Lasry S, et al. Response to neoadjuvant chemotherapy in lobular and ductal breast carcinomas: a retrospective study on 860 patients from one institution. Ann Oncol 2006;17:1228-1233.

78. Acs G, Lawton TJ, Rebbeck TR, et al. Differential expression of E-cadherin in lobular and ductal neoplasms of the breast and its biologic and diagnostic implications. Am J Clin Pathol 2001;115:85-98.

79. Gamallo C, Palacios J, Suarez A, et al. Correlation of E-cadherin expression with differentiation grade and histological type in breast carcinoma. Am J Pathol 1993;142:987-993.

80. Moll R, Mitze M, Frixen UH, Birchmeier W. Differential loss of E-cadherin expression in infiltrating ductal and lobular breast carcinomas. Am J Pathol 1993;143:1731-1742.

81. Berx G, Cleton-Jansen AM, Nollet F, et al. E-cadherin is a tumour/invasion suppressor gene mutated in human lobular breast cancers. EMBO J 1995;14:6107-6115.

82. Berx G, Cleton-Jansen AM, Strumane K, et al. E-cadherin is inactivated in a majority of invasive human lobular breast cancers by truncation mutations throughout its extracellular domain. Oncogene 1996;13:1919-1925.

83. Vos CB, Cleton-Jansen AM, Berx G, et al. E-cadherin inactivation in lobular carcinoma in situ of the breast: an early event in tumorigenesis. Br J Cancer 1997;76:1131-1133.

84. Handschuh G, Candidus S, Luber B, et al. Tumour-associated E-cadherin mutations alter cellular morphology, decrease cellular adhesion and increase cellular motility. Oncogene 1999;18:4301-4312.

85. Goldstein NS, Bassi D, Watts JC, et al. E-cadherin reactivity of 95 noninvasive ductal and lobular lesions of the breast. Implications for the interpretation of problematic lesions. Am J Clin Pathol 2001;115:534-542.

86. De Leeuw WJ, Berx G, Vos CB, et al. Simultaneous loss of E-cadherin and catenins in invasive lobular breast cancer and lobular carcinoma in situ. J Pathol 1997;183:404-411.

87. Gonzalez MA, Pinder SE, Wencyk PM, et al. An immunohistochemical examination of the expression of E-cadherin, alpha- and beta/gamma-catenins, and alpha2- and beta1-integrins in invasive breast cancer. J Pathol 1999;187:523-529.

88. Aberle H, Schwartz H, Kemler R. Cadherin-catenin complex: protein interactions and their implications for cadherin function. J Cell Biochem 1996;61:514-523.

89. Aghib DF, McCrea PD. The E-cadherin complex contains the src substrate p120. Exp Cell Res 1995;218:359-369.

90. Gooding JM, Yap KL, Ikura M. The cadherin-catenin complex as a focal point of cell adhesion and signalling: new insights from three-dimensional structures. Bioessays 2004;26:497-511.

91. Piepenhagen PA, Nelson WJ. Defining E-cadherin–associated protein complexes in epithelial cells: plakoglobin, beta- and gamma-catenin are distinct components. J Cell Sci 1993;104:751-762.

92. Reynolds AB, Daniel J, McCrea PD, et al. Identification of a new catenin: the tyrosine kinase substrate p120cas associates with E-cadherin complexes. Mol Cell Biol 1994;14:8333-8342.

93. Yap AS, Niessen CM, Gumbiner BM. The juxtamembrane region of the cadherin cytoplasmic tail supports lateral clustering, adhesive strengthening, and interaction with p120ctn. J Cell Biol 1998;141:779-789.

94. Shibamoto S, Hayakawa M, Takeuchi K, et al. Association of p120, a tyrosine kinase substrate, with E-cadherin/catenin complexes. J Cell Biol 1995;128:949-957.

95. Davis MA, Ireton RC, Reynolds AB. A core function for p120-catenin in cadherin turnover. J Cell Biol 2003;163:525-534.

96. Noren NK, Liu BP, Burridge K, Kreft B. p120 catenin regulates the actin cytoskeleton via Rho family GTPases. J Cell Biol 2000;150:567-580.

97. Dabbs DJ, Bhargava R, Chivukula M. Lobular versus ductal breast neoplasms: the diagnostic utility of p120 catenin. Am J Surg Pathol 2007;31:427-437.

98. Berx G, Van Roy F. The E-cadherin/catenin complex: an important gatekeeper in breast cancer tumorigenesis and malignant progression. Breast Cancer Res 2001;3:289-293.

99. Berx G, Nollet F, van Roy F. Dysregulation of the E-cadherin/catenin complex by irreversible mutations in human carcinomas. Cell Adhes Commun 1998;6:171-184.

100. Karabakhtsian RG, Johnson R, Sumkin J, Dabbs DJ. The clinical significance of lobular neoplasia on breast core biopsy. Am J Surg Pathol 2007;31:717-723.

101. Goldstein NS. Does the level of E-cadherin expression correlate with the primary breast carcinoma infiltration pattern and type of systemic metastases? Am J Clin Pathol 2002;118:425-434.

102. Goldstein NS, Kestin LL, Vicini FA. Clinicopathologic implications of E-cadherin reactivity in patients with lobular carcinoma in situ of the breast. Cancer 2001;92:738-747.

103. Jacobs TW, Pliss N, Kouria G, Schnitt SJ. Carcinomas in situ of the breast with indeterminate features: role of E-cadherin staining in categorization. Am J Surg Pathol 2001;25:229-236.

104. Lehr HA, Folpe A, Yaziji H, et al. Cytokeratin 8 immunostaining pattern and E-cadherin expression distinguish lobular from ductal breast carcinoma. Am J Clin Pathol 2000;114:190-196.

105. Bassler R, Kronsbein H. Disseminated lobular carcinoma—a predominantly pleomorphic lobular carcinoma of the whole breast. Pathol Res Pract 1980;166:456-470.

106. Weidner N, Semple JP. Pleomorphic variant of invasive lobular carcinoma of the breast. Hum Pathol 1992;23:1167-1171.

107. Eusebi V, Magalhaes F, Azzopardi JG. Pleomorphic lobular carcinoma of the breast: an aggressive tumor showing apocrine differentiation. Hum Pathol 1992;23:655-662.

108. Reis-Filho JS, Simpson PT, Jones C, et al. Pleomorphic lobular carcinoma of the breast: role of comprehensive molecular pathology in characterization of an entity. J Pathol 2005;207:1-13.

109. Bentz JS, Yassa N, Clayton F. Pleomorphic lobular carcinoma of the breast: clinicopathologic features of 12 cases. Mod Pathol 1998;11:814-822.

110. Frolik D, Caduff R, Varga Z. Pleomorphic lobular carcinoma of the breast: its cell kinetics, expression of oncogenes and tumour suppressor genes compared with invasive ductal carcinomas and classical infiltrating lobular carcinomas. Histopathology 2001;39:503-513.

111. Middleton LP, Palacios DM, Bryant BR, et al. Pleomorphic lobular carcinoma: morphology, immunohistochemistry, and molecular analysis. Am J Surg Pathol 2000;24:1650-1656.

112. Radhi JM. Immunohistochemical analysis of pleomorphic lobular carcinoma: higher expression of p53 and chromogranin and lower expression of ER and PgR. Histopathology 2000;36:156-160.

113. Dabbs DJ, Kaplai M, Chivukula M, et al. The spectrum of morphomolecular abnormalities of the E-cadherin/catenin complex in pleomorphic lobular carcinoma of the breast. Appl Immunohistochem Mol Morphol 2007;15:260-266.

114. Simpson PT, Reis-Filho JS, Lambros MB, et al. Molecular profiling pleomorphic lobular carcinomas of the breast: evidence for a common molecular genetic pathway with classic lobular carcinomas. J Pathol 2008;215:231-244.

115. Sneige N, Wang J, Baker BA, et al. Clinical, histopathologic, and biologic features of pleomorphic lobular (ductal-lobular) carcinoma in situ of the breast: a report of 24 cases. Mod Pathol 2002;15:1044-1050.

116. Fisher ER, Gregorio RM, Redmond C, Fisher B. Tubulolobular invasive breast cancer: a variant of lobular invasive cancer. Hum Pathol 1977;8:679-683.

117. Green I, McCormick B, Cranor M, Rosen PP. A comparative study of pure tubular and tubulolobular carcinoma of the breast. Am J Surg Pathol 1997;21:653-657.

118. Wheeler DT, Tai LH, Bratthauer GL, et al. Tubulolobular carcinoma of the breast: an analysis of 27 cases of a tumor with a hybrid morphology and immunoprofile. Am J Surg Pathol 2004;28:1587-1593.

119. Esposito NN, Chivukula M, Dabbs DJ. The ductal phenotypic expression of the E-cadherin/catenin complex in tubulolobular carcinoma of the breast: an immunohistochemical and clinicopathologic study. Mod Pathol 2007;20:130-138.

120. Hood CI, Font RL, Zimmerman LE. Metastatic mammary carcinoma in the eyelid with histiocytoid appearance. Cancer 1973;31:793-800.

121. Filotico M, Trabucco M, Gallone D, et al. Histiocytoid carcinoma of the breast. A problem of differential diagnosis for the pathologist. Report of a case. Pathologica 1983;75:429-433.

122. Gupta D, Croitoru CM, Ayala AG, et al. E-cadherin immunohistochemical analysis of histiocytoid carcinoma of the breast. Ann Diagn Pathol 2002;6:141-147.

123. Reis-Filho JS, Fulford LG, Freeman A, Lakhani SR. Pathologic quiz case: a 93-year-old woman with an enlarged and tender left breast. Histiocytoid variant of lobular breast carcinoma. Arch Pathol Lab Med 2003;127:1626-1628.

124. Luna-More S, Gonzalez B, Acedo C, et al. Invasive micropapillary carcinoma of the breast. A new special type of invasive mammary carcinoma. Pathol Res Pract 1994;190:668-674.

125. Siriaunkgul S, Tavassoli FA. Invasive micropapillary carcinoma of the breast. Mod Pathol 1993;6:660-662.

126. Li YS, Kaneko M, Sakamoto DG, et al. The reversed apical pattern of MUC1 expression is characteristic of invasive micropapillary carcinoma of the breast. Breast Cancer 2006;13:58-63.

127. Nassar H, Pansare V, Zhang H, et al. Pathogenesis of invasive micropapillary carcinoma: role of MUC1 glycoprotein. Mod Pathol 2004;17:1045-1050.

128. Guo X, Chen L, Lang R, et al. Invasive micropapillary carcinoma of the breast: association of pathologic features with lymph node metastasis. Am J Clin Pathol 2006;126:740-746.

129. Nassar H. Carcinomas with micropapillary morphology: clinical significance and current concepts. Adv Anat Pathol 2004;11:297-303.

130. Nassar H, Wallis T, Andea A, et al. Clinicopathologic analysis of invasive micropapillary differentiation in breast carcinoma. Mod Pathol 2001;14:836-841.

131. Pettinato G, Manivel CJ, Panico L, et al. Invasive micropapillary carcinoma of the breast: clinicopathologic study of 62 cases of a poorly recognized variant with highly aggressive behavior. Am J Clin Pathol 2004;121:857-866.

132. Walsh MM, Bleiweiss IJ. Invasive micropapillary carcinoma of the breast: eighty cases of an underrecognized entity. Hum Pathol 2001;32:583-589.

133. Acs G, Esposito NN, Rakosy Z, et al. Invasive ductal carcinomas of the breast showing partial reversed cell polarity are associated with lymphatic tumor spread and may represent part of a spectrum of invasive micropapillary carcinoma. Am J Surg Pathol 2010;34:1637-1646.

134. Paterakos M, Watkin WG, Edgerton SM, et al. Invasive micropapillary carcinoma of the breast: a prognostic study. Hum Pathol 1999;30:1459-1463.

135. Perou CM, Sorlie T, Eisen MB, et al. Molecular portraits of human breast tumours. Nature 2000;406:747-752.
136. Sorlie T, Perou CM, Tibshirani R, et al. Gene expression patterns of breast carcinomas distinguish tumor subclasses with clinical implications. Proc Natl Acad Sci U S A 2001;98:10869-10874.
137. Livasy CA, Karaca G, Nanda R, et al. Phenotypic evaluation of the basal-like subtype of invasive breast carcinoma. Mod Pathol 2006;19:264-271.
138. Bhargava R, Chivukula M, Carter GJ, Dabbs DJ. E-cadherin and p120 catenin expression in basal-like invasive breast carcinoma [abstract 118]. Mod Pathol 2007;20(Suppl 2):30A.
139. Nielsen TO, Hsu FD, Jensen K, et al. Immunohistochemical and clinical characterization of the basal-like subtype of invasive breast carcinoma. Clin Cancer Res 2004;10:5367-5374.
140. Bhargava R, Beriwal S, McManus K, Dabbs DJ. CK5 is more sensitive than CK5/6 in identifying the "basal-like" phenotype of breast carcinoma. Am J Clin Pathol 2008;130:724-730.
141. Bryan BB, Schnitt SJ, Collins LC. Ductal carcinoma in situ with basal-like phenotype: a possible precursor to invasive basal-like breast cancer. Mod Pathol 2006;19:617-621.
142. Dabbs DJ, Chivukula M, Carter G, Bhargava R. Basal phenotype of ductal carcinoma in situ: recognition and immunohistologic profile. Mod Pathol 2006;19:1506-1511.
143. Carey LA, Perou CM, Livasy CA, et al. Race, breast cancer subtypes, and survival in the Carolina Breast Cancer Study. JAMA 2006;295:2492-2502.
144. van de Rijn M, Perou CM, Tibshirani R, et al. Expression of cytokeratins 17 and 5 identifies a group of breast carcinomas with poor clinical outcome. Am J Pathol 2002;161:1991-1996.
145. Sorlie T, Tibshirani R, Parker J, et al. Repeated observation of breast tumor subtypes in independent gene expression data sets. Proc Natl Acad Sci U S A 2003;100:8418-8423.
146. Carter MR, Hornick JL, Lester S, Fletcher CD. Spindle cell (sarcomatoid) carcinoma of the breast: a clinicopathologic and immunohistochemical analysis of 29 cases. Am J Surg Pathol 2006;30:300-309.
147. Davis WG, Hennessy B, Babiera G, et al. Metaplastic sarcomatoid carcinoma of the breast with absent or minimal overt invasive carcinomatous component: a misnomer. Am J Surg Pathol 2005;29:1456-1463.
148. Adem C, Reynolds C, Adlakha H, et al. Wide spectrum screening keratin as a marker of metaplastic spindle cell carcinoma of the breast: an immunohistochemical study of 24 patients. Histopathology 2002;40:556-562.
149. Koker MM, Kleer CG. p63 expression in breast cancer: a highly sensitive and specific marker of metaplastic carcinoma. Am J Surg Pathol 2004;28:1506-1512.
150. Tse GM, Tan PH, Chaiwun B, et al. p63 is useful in the diagnosis of mammary metaplastic carcinomas. Pathology 2006;38:16-20.
151. Ellis IO, Bell J, Ronan JE, et al. Immunocytochemical investigation of intermediate filament proteins and epithelial membrane antigen in spindle cell tumours of the breast. J Pathol 1988;154:157-165.
152. Wargotz ES, Norris HJ. Metaplastic carcinomas of the breast. III. Carcinosarcoma. Cancer 1989;64:1490-1499.
153. Sommers CL, Walker-Jones D, Heckford SE, et al. Vimentin rather than keratin expression in some hormone-independent breast cancer cell lines and in oncogene-transformed mammary epithelial cells. Cancer Res 1989;49:4258-4263.
154. Leibl S, Gogg-Kammerer M, Sommersacher A, et al. Metaplastic breast carcinomas: are they of myoepithelial differentiation? Immunohistochemical profile of the sarcomatoid subtype using novel myoepithelial markers. Am J Surg Pathol 2005;29:347-353.
155. Miettinen M, Franssila K. Immunohistochemical spectrum of malignant melanoma. The common presence of keratins. Lab Invest 1989;61:623-628.
156. Zarbo RJ, Gown AM, Nagle RB, et al. Anomalous cytokeratin expression in malignant melanoma: one- and two-dimensional Western blot analysis and immunohistochemical survey of 100 melanomas. Mod Pathol 1990;3:494-501.
157. Pusztaszeri MP, Seelentag W, Bosman FT. Immunohistochemical expression of endothelial markers CD31, CD34, von Willebrand factor, and Fli-1 in normal human tissues. J Histochem Cytochem 2006;54:385-395.
158. Miettinen M, Lindenmayer AE, Chaubal A. Endothelial cell markers CD31, CD34, and BNH9 antibody to H- and Y-antigens—evaluation of their specificity and sensitivity in the diagnosis of vascular tumors and comparison with von Willebrand factor. Mod Pathol 1994;7:82-90.
159. Chen PC, Chen CK, Nicastri AD, Wait RB. Myoepithelial carcinoma of the breast with distant metastasis and accompanied by adenomyoepitheliomas. Histopathology 1994;24:543-548.
160. Foschini MP, Eusebi V. Carcinomas of the breast showing myoepithelial cell differentiation. A review of the literature. Virchows Arch 1998;432:303-310.
161. Thorner PS, Kahn HJ, Baumal R, et al. Malignant myoepithelioma of the breast. An immunohistochemical study by light and electron microscopy. Cancer 1986;57:745-750.
162. Young RH, Clement PB. Adenomyoepithelioma of the breast. A report of three cases and review of the literature. Am J Clin Pathol 1988;89:308-314.
163. Schurch W, Potvin C, Seemayer TA. Malignant myoepithelioma (myoepithelial carcinoma) of the breast: an ultrastructural and immunocytochemical study. Ultrastruct Pathol 1985;8:1-11.
164. Tavassoli FA. Myoepithelial lesions of the breast. Myoepitheliosis, adenomyoepithelioma, and myoepithelial carcinoma. Am J Surg Pathol 1991;15:554-568.
165. Hornick JL, Fletcher CD. Myoepithelial tumors of soft tissue: a clinicopathologic and immunohistochemical study of 101 cases with evaluation of prognostic parameters. Am J Surg Pathol 2003;27:1183-1196.
166. Hornick JL, Fletcher CD. Cutaneous myoepithelioma: a clinicopathologic and immunohistochemical study of 14 cases. Hum Pathol 2004;35:14-24.
167. Dunne B, Lee AH, Pinder SE, et al. An immunohistochemical study of metaplastic spindle cell carcinoma, phyllodes tumor and fibromatosis of the breast. Hum Pathol 2003;34:1009-1015.
168. Popnikolov NK, Ayala AG, Graves K, Gatalica Z. Benign myoepithelial tumors of the breast have immunophenotypic characteristics similar to metaplastic matrix-producing and spindle cell carcinomas. Am J Clin Pathol 2003;120:161-167.
169. Reis-Filho JS, Milanezi F, Paredes J, et al. Novel and classic myoepithelial/stem cell markers in metaplastic carcinomas of the breast. Appl Immunohistochem Mol Morphol 2003;11:1-8.
170. Smith TA, Machen SK, Fisher C, Goldblum JR. Usefulness of cytokeratin subsets for distinguishing monophasic synovial sarcoma from malignant peripheral nerve sheath tumor. Am J Clin Pathol 1999;112:641-648.
171. Damiani S, Miettinen M, Peterse JL, Eusebi V. Solitary fibrous tumour (myofibroblastoma) of the breast. Virchows Arch 1994;425:89-92.
172. Julien M, Trojani M, Coindre JM. Myofibroblastoma of the breast. Report of 8 cases [in French]. Ann Pathol 1994;14:143-147.
173. Wargotz ES, Weiss SW, Norris HJ. Myofibroblastoma of the breast. Sixteen cases of a distinctive benign mesenchymal tumor. Am J Surg Pathol 1987;11:493-502.
174. Lee AH. Recent developments in the histological diagnosis of spindle cell carcinoma, fibromatosis and phyllodes tumour of the breast. Histopathology 2008;52:45-57.
175. Chaudary MA, Millis RR, Lane EB, Miller NA. Paget's disease of the nipple: a ten year review including clinical, pathological, and immunohistochemical findings. Breast Cancer Res Treat 1986;8:139-146.
176. Yim JH, Wick MR, Philpott GW, et al. Underlying pathology in mammary Paget's disease. Ann Surg Oncol 1997;4:287-292.
177. Anderson JM, Ariga R, Govil H, et al. Assessment of Her-2/Neu status by immunohistochemistry and fluorescence in situ hybridization in mammary Paget disease and underlying carcinoma. Appl Immunohistochem Mol Morphol 2003;11:120-124.
178. Haerslev T, Krag Jacobsen G. Expression of cytokeratin and erbB-2 oncoprotein in Paget's disease of the nipple. An immunohistochemical study. APMIS 1992;100:1041-1047.
179. Lammie GA, Barnes DM, Millis RR, Gullick WJ. An immunohistochemical study of the presence of c-erbB-2 protein in Paget's disease of the nipple. Histopathology 1989;15:505-514.

180. Wolber RA, Dupuis BA, Wick MR. Expression of c-erbB-2 oncoprotein in mammary and extramammary Paget's disease. Am J Clin Pathol 1991;96:243-247.

181. Meissner K, Riviere A, Haupt G, Loning T. Study of neu-protein expression in mammary Paget's disease with and without underlying breast carcinoma and in extramammary Paget's disease. Am J Pathol 1990;137:1305-1309.

182. Tani EM, Skoog L. Immunocytochemical detection of estrogen receptors in mammary Paget cells. Acta Cytol 1988;32:825-828.

183. Fu W, Lobocki CA, Silberberg BK, et al. Molecular markers in Paget disease of the breast. J Surg Oncol 2001;77:171-178.

184. Gillett CE, Bobrow LG, Millis RR. S100 protein in human mammary tissue—immunoreactivity in breast carcinoma, including Paget's disease of the nipple, and value as a marker of myoepithelial cells. J Pathol 1990;160:19-24.

185. Lundquist K, Kohler S, Rouse RV. Intraepidermal cytokeratin 7 expression is not restricted to Paget cells but is also seen in Toker cells and Merkel cells. Am J Surg Pathol 1999;23:212-219.

186. Marucci G, Betts CM, Golouh R, et al. Toker cells are probably precursors of Paget cell carcinoma: a morphological and ultrastructural description. Virchows Arch 2002;441:117-123.

187. Zeng Z, Melamed J, Symmans PJ, et al. Benign proliferative nipple duct lesions frequently contain CAM 5.2 and anti-cytokeratin 7 immunoreactive cells in the overlying epidermis. Am J Surg Pathol 1999;23:1349-1355.

188. Yao DX, Hoda SA, Chiu A, et al. Intraepidermal cytokeratin 7 immunoreactive cells in the non-neoplastic nipple may represent interepithelial extension of lactiferous duct cells. Histopathology 2002;40:230-236.

189. Bader AA, Tio J, Petru E, et al. T1 breast cancer: identification of patients at low risk of axillary lymph node metastases. Breast Cancer Res Treat 2002;76:11-17.

190. Barth A, Craig PH, Silverstein MJ. Predictors of axillary lymph node metastases in patients with T1 breast carcinoma. Cancer 1997;79:1918-1922.

191. Chadha M, Chabon AB, Friedmann P, Vikram B. Predictors of axillary lymph node metastases in patients with T1 breast cancer. A multivariate analysis. Cancer 1994;73:350-353.

192. Gajdos C, Tartter PI, Bleiweiss IJ. Lymphatic invasion, tumor size, and age are independent predictors of axillary lymph node metastases in women with T1 breast cancers. Ann Surg 1999;230:692-696.

193. Van den Eynden GG, Van der Auwera I, Van Laere SJ, et al. Distinguishing blood and lymph vessel invasion in breast cancer: a prospective immunohistochemical study. Br J Cancer 2006;94:1643-1649.

194. Amparo RS, Angel CD, Ana LH, et al. Inflammatory breast carcinoma: pathological or clinical entity? Breast Cancer Res Treat 2000;64:269-273.

195. Bonnier P, Charpin C, Lejeune C, et al. Inflammatory carcinomas of the breast: a clinical, pathological, or a clinical and pathological definition? Int J Cancer 1995;62:382-385.

196. Le MG, Arriagada R, Contesso G, et al. Dermal lymphatic emboli in inflammatory and noninflammatory breast cancer: a French-Tunisian joint study in 337 patients. Clin Breast Cancer 2005;6:439-445.

197. Kahn HJ, Marks A. A new monoclonal antibody, D2-40, for detection of lymphatic invasion in primary tumors. Lab Invest 2002;82:1255-1257.

198. Kaiserling E. Immunohistochemical identification of lymph vessels with D2-40 in diagnostic pathology [in German]. Pathologe 2004;25:362-374.

199. Kahn HJ, Bailey D, Marks A. Monoclonal antibody D2-40, a new marker of lymphatic endothelium, reacts with Kaposi's sarcoma and a subset of angiosarcomas. Mod Pathol 2002;15:434-440.

200. Steinhoff MM. Axillary node micrometastases: detection and biologic significance. Breast J 1999;5:325-329.

201. Mansi JL, Gogas H, Bliss JM, et al. Outcome of primary-breast-cancer patients with micrometastases: a long-term follow-up study. Lancet 1999;354:197-202.

202. Nasser IA, Lee AK, Bosari S, et al. Occult axillary lymph node metastases in "node-negative" breast carcinoma. Hum Pathol 1993;24:950-957.

203. Bass SS, Lyman GH, McCann CR, et al. Lymphatic mapping and sentinel lymph node biopsy. Breast J 1999;5:288-295.

204. Dabbs DJ, Johnson R. The optimal number of sentinel lymph nodes for focused pathologic examination. Breast J 2004;10:186-189.

205. Klevesath MB, Bobrow LG, Pinder SE, Purushotham AD. The value of immunohistochemistry in sentinel lymph node histopathology in breast cancer. Br J Cancer 2005;92:2201-2205.

206. Dabbs DJ, Fung M, Landsittel D, et al. Sentinel lymph node micrometastasis as a predictor of axillary tumor burden. Breast J 2004;10:101-105.

207. den Bakker MA, van Weeszenberg A, de Kanter AY, et al. Non-sentinel lymph node involvement in patients with breast cancer and sentinel node micrometastasis: too early to abandon axillary clearance. J Clin Pathol 2002;55:932-935.

208. Kamath VJ, Giuliano R, Dauway EL, et al. Characteristics of the sentinel lymph node in breast cancer predict further involvement of higher-echelon nodes in the axilla: a study to evaluate the need for complete axillary lymph node dissection. Arch Surg 2001;136:688-692.

209. Mignotte H, Treilleux I, Faure C, et al. Axillary lymph-node dissection for positive sentinel nodes in breast cancer patients. Eur J Surg Oncol 2002;28:623-626.

210. Tan LK, Giri D, Hummer AJ, et al. Occult axillary node metastases in breast cancer are prognostically significant: results in 368 node-negative patients with 20-year follow-up. J Clin Oncol 2008;26:1803-1809.

211. Weaver DL, Ashikaga T, Krag DN, et al. Effect of occult metastases on survival in node-negative breast cancer. N Engl J Med 2011;364:412-421.

212. Cserni G, Bianchi S, Vezzosi V, et al. The value of cytokeratin immunohistochemistry in the evaluation of axillary sentinel lymph nodes in patients with lobular breast carcinoma. J Clin Pathol 2006;59:518-522.

213. Czerniecki BJ, Scheff AM, Callans LS, et al. Immunohistochemistry with pancytokeratins improves the sensitivity of sentinel lymph node biopsy in patients with breast carcinoma. Cancer 1999;85:1098-1103.

214. Doglioni C, Dell'Orto P, Zanetti G, et al. Cytokeratin-immunoreactive cells of human lymph nodes and spleen in normal and pathological conditions. An immunocytochemical study. Virchows Arch A Pathol Anat Histopathol 1990;416:479-490.

215. Iuzzolino P, Bontempini L, Doglioni C, Zanetti G. Keratin immunoreactivity in extrafollicular reticular cells of the lymph node. Am J Clin Pathol 1989;91:239-240.

216. Carter BA, Jensen RA, Simpson JF, Page DL. Benign transport of breast epithelium into axillary lymph nodes after biopsy. Am J Clin Pathol 2000;113:259-265.

217. Diaz NM, Cox CE, Ebert M, et al. Benign mechanical transport of breast epithelial cells to sentinel lymph nodes. Am J Surg Pathol 2004;28:1641-1645.

218. Diaz NM, Vrcel V, Centeno BA, Muro-Cacho C. Modes of benign mechanical transport of breast epithelial cells to axillary lymph nodes. Adv Anat Pathol 2005;12:7-9.

219. Diaz NM, Mayes JR, Vrcel V. Breast epithelial cells in dermal angiolymphatic spaces: a manifestation of benign mechanical transport. Hum Pathol 2005;36:310-313.

220. Hughes SJ, Xi L, Raja S, et al. A rapid, fully automated, molecular-based assay accurately analyzes sentinel lymph nodes for the presence of metastatic breast cancer. Ann Surg 2006;243:389-398.

221. Viale G, Dell'Orto P, Biasi MO, et al. Comparative evaluation of an extensive histopathologic examination and a real-time reverse-transcription-polymerase chain reaction assay for mammaglobin and cytokeratin 19 on axillary sentinel lymph nodes of breast carcinoma patients. Ann Surg 2008;247:136-142.

222. Blumencranz P, Whitworth PW, Deck K, et al. Scientific Impact Recognition Award. Sentinel node staging for breast cancer: intraoperative molecular pathology overcomes conventional histologic sampling errors. Am J Surg 2007;194:426-432.

223. Mansel RE, Goyal A, Douglas-Jones A, et al. Detection of breast cancer metastasis in sentinel lymph nodes using intra-operative real time GeneSearch BLN Assay in the operating room: results of the Cardiff study. Breast Cancer Res Treat 2009;115:595-600.

224. Martin Martinez MD, Veys I, Majjaj S, et al. Clinical validation of a molecular assay for intra-operative detection of metastases in breast sentinel lymph nodes. Eur J Surg Oncol 2009;35: 387-392.

225. DeYoung BR, Wick MR. Immunohistologic evaluation of metastatic carcinomas of unknown origin: an algorithmic approach. Semin Diagn Pathol 2000;17:184-193.

226. Rubin BP, Skarin AT, Pisick E, et al. Use of cytokeratins 7 and 20 in determining the origin of metastatic carcinoma of unknown primary, with special emphasis on lung cancer. Eur J Cancer Prev 2001;10:77-82.

227. Tot T. Adenocarcinomas metastatic to the liver: the value of cytokeratins 20 and 7 in the search for unknown primary tumors. Cancer 1999;85:171-177.

228. Perry A, Parisi JE, Kurtin PJ. Metastatic adenocarcinoma to the brain: an immunohistochemical approach. Hum Pathol 1997;28:938-943.

229. Wick MR, Lillemoe TJ, Copland GT, et al. Gross cystic disease fluid protein-15 as a marker for breast cancer: immunohistochemical analysis of 690 human neoplasms and comparison with alpha-lactalbumin. Hum Pathol 1989;20:281-287.

230. Pearlman WH, Gueriguian JL, Sawyer ME. A specific progesterone-binding component of human breast cyst fluid. J Biol Chem 1973;248:5736-5741.

231. Haagensen Jr DE, Mazoujian G, Holder Jr WD, et al. Evaluation of a breast cyst fluid protein detectable in the plasma of breast carcinoma patients. Ann Surg 1977;185:279-285.

232. Murphy LC, Lee-Wing M, Goldenberg GJ, Shiu RP. Expression of the gene encoding a prolactin-inducible protein by human breast cancers in vivo: correlation with steroid receptor status. Cancer Res 1987;47:4160-4164.

233. Mazoujian G, Parish TH, Haagensen Jr DE. Immunoperoxidase localization of GCDFP-15 with mouse monoclonal antibodies versus rabbit antiserum. J Histochem Cytochem 1988;36:377-382.

234. Mazoujian G, Margolis R. Immunohistochemistry of gross cystic disease fluid protein (GCDFP-15) in 65 benign sweat gland tumors of the skin. Am J Dermatopathol 1988;10:28-35.

235. Mazoujian G, Pinkus GS, Davis S, Haagensen Jr DE. Immunohistochemistry of a gross cystic disease fluid protein (GCDFP-15) of the breast. A marker of apocrine epithelium and breast carcinomas with apocrine features. Am J Pathol 1983;110:105-112.

236. Swanson PE, Pettinato G, Lillemoe TJ, Wick MR. Gross cystic disease fluid protein-15 in salivary gland tumors. Arch Pathol Lab Med 1991;115:158-163.

237. Viacava P, Naccarato AG, Bevilacqua G. Spectrum of GCD-FP-15 expression in human fetal and adult normal tissues. Virchows Arch 1998;432:255-260.

238. Ormsby AH, Snow JL, Su WP, Goellner JR. Diagnostic immunohistochemistry of cutaneous metastatic breast carcinoma: a statistical analysis of the utility of gross cystic disease fluid protein-15 and estrogen receptor protein. J Am Acad Dermatol 1995;32:711-716.

239. Mazoujian G, Bodian C, Haagensen Jr DE, Haagensen CD. Expression of GCDFP-15 in breast carcinomas. Relationship to pathologic and clinical factors. Cancer 1989;63:2156-2161.

240. Wick MR, Ockner DM, Mills SE, et al. Homologous carcinomas of the breasts, skin, and salivary glands. A histologic and immunohistochemical comparison of ductal mammary carcinoma, ductal sweat gland carcinoma, and salivary duct carcinoma. Am J Clin Pathol 1998;109:75-84.

241. Fiel MI, Cernaianu G, Burstein DE, Batheja N. Value of GCDFP-15 (BRST-2) as a specific immunocytochemical marker for breast carcinoma in cytologic specimens. Acta Cytol 1996;40:637-641.

242. Kaufmann O, Deidesheimer T, Muehlenberg M, et al. Immunohistochemical differentiation of metastatic breast carcinomas from metastatic adenocarcinomas of other common primary sites. Histopathology 1996;29:233-240.

243. Raab SS, Berg LC, Swanson PE, Wick MR. Adenocarcinoma in the lung in patients with breast cancer. A prospective analysis of the discriminatory value of immunohistology. Am J Clin Pathol 1993;100:27-35.

244. Striebel JM, Dacic S, Yousem SA. Gross cystic disease fluid protein-(GCDFP-15): expression in primary lung adenocarcinoma. Am J Surg Pathol 2008;32:426-432.

245. Domfeh AB, Carley AL, Striebel JM, et al. WT1 immunoreactivity in breast carcinoma: selective expression in pure and mixed mucinous subtypes. Mod Pathol 2008;21:1217-1223.

246. Robens J, Goldstein L, Gown AM, Schnitt SJ. Thyroid transcription factor-1 expression in breast carcinomas. Am J Surg Pathol 2010;34:1881-1885.

247. Dabbs DJ, Landreneau RJ, Liu Y, et al. Detection of estrogen receptor by immunohistochemistry in pulmonary adenocarcinoma. Ann Thorac Surg 2002;73:403-405:discussion 406.

248. Nash JW, Morrison C, Frankel WL. The utility of estrogen receptor and progesterone receptor immunohistochemistry in the distinction of metastatic breast carcinoma from other tumors in the liver. Arch Pathol Lab Med 2003;127:1591-1595.

249. Wallace ML, Longacre TA, Smoller BR. Estrogen and progesterone receptors and anti-gross cystic disease fluid protein 15 (BRST-2) fail to distinguish metastatic breast carcinoma from eccrine neoplasms. Mod Pathol 1995;8:897-901.

250. Ciampa A, Fanger G, Khan A, et al. Mammaglobin and CRxA-01 in pleural effusion cytology: potential utility of distinguishing metastatic breast carcinomas from other cytokeratin 7-positive/cytokeratin 20-negative carcinomas. Cancer 2004;102:368-372.

251. Han JH, Kang Y, Shin HC, et al. Mammaglobin expression in lymph nodes is an important marker of metastatic breast carcinoma. Arch Pathol Lab Med 2003;127:1330-1334.

252. Bhargava R, Beriwal S, Dabbs DJ. Mammaglobin vs GCDFP-15: an immunohistologic validation survey for sensitivity and specificity. Am J Clin Pathol 2007;127:103-113.

253. Jager D, Filonenko V, Gout I, et al. NY-BR-1 is a differentiation antigen of the mammary gland. Appl Immunohistochem Mol Morphol 2007;15:77-83.

254. Woodard AH, Yu J, Dabbs DJ, et al. NYBR1 expression in breast and gynecologic tract carcinomas [abstract]. Mod Pathol 2011;24(suppl 1):72A(Abstract 291). 100th Annual Meeting of United States and Canadian Academy of Pathology. February 26-March 4, 2011. San Antonio, TX.

255. Chivukula M, Dabbs DJ, O'Connor S, Bhargava R. PAX 2: a novel müllerian marker for serous papillary carcinomas to differentiate from micropapillary breast carcinoma. Int J Gynecol Pathol 2009;28:570-578.

256. Yu J, Woodard AH, Florea AV, et al. PAX-8 expression in gynecologic and breast carcinomas [abstract]. Mod Pathol 2011;24 (suppl 1):272A(Abstract 1156). 100th Annual Meeting of United States and Canadian Academy of Pathology. February 26-March 4, 2011. San Antonio, TX.

257. Noguchi S, Aihara T, Motomura K, et al. Demonstration of polyclonal origin of giant fibroadenoma of the breast. Virchows Arch 1995;427:343-347.

258. Noguchi S, Motomura K, Inaji H, et al. Clonal analysis of fibroadenoma and phyllodes tumor of the breast. Cancer Res 1993;53:4071-4074.

259. Aranda FI, Laforga JB, Lopez JI. Phyllodes tumor of the breast. An immunohistochemical study of 28 cases with special attention to the role of myofibroblasts. Pathol Res Pract 1994;190:474-481.

260. Auger M, Hanna W, Kahn HJ. Cystosarcoma phyllodes of the breast and its mimics. An immunohistochemical and ultrastructural study. Arch Pathol Lab Med 1989;113:1231-1235.

261. Yeh IT, Francis DJ, Orenstein JM, Silverberg SG. Ultrastructure of cystosarcoma phyllodes and fibroadenoma. A comparative study. Am J Clin Pathol 1985;84:131-136.

262. Pietruszka M, Barnes L. Cystosarcoma phyllodes: a clinicopathologic analysis of 42 cases. Cancer 1978;41:1974-1983.

263. Jacobs TW, Chen YY, Guinee Jr DG, et al. Fibroepithelial lesions with cellular stroma on breast core needle biopsy: are there predictors of outcome on surgical excision? Am J Clin Pathol 2005;124:342-354.

264. Umekita Y, Yoshida H. Immunohistochemical study of MIB1 expression in phyllodes tumor and fibroadenoma. Pathol Int 1999;49:807-810.

265. Lae M, Vincent-Salomon A, Savignoni A, et al. Phyllodes tumors of the breast segregate in two groups according to genetic criteria. Mod Pathol 2007;20:435-444.

266. Lu YJ, Birdsall S, Osin P, et al. Phyllodes tumors of the breast analyzed by comparative genomic hybridization and association of increased 1q copy number with stromal overgrowth and recurrence. Genes Chromosomes Cancer 1997;20:275-281.

267. Ojopi EP, Rogatto SR, Caldeira JR, et al. Comparative genomic hybridization detects novel amplifications in fibroadenomas of the breast. Genes Chromosomes Cancer 2001;30:25-31.

268. Polito P, Cin PD, Pauwels P, et al. An important subgroup of phyllodes tumors of the breast is characterized by rearrangements of chromosomes 1q and 10q. Oncol Rep 1998;5:1099-1102.

269. Wang ZC, Buraimoh A, Iglehart JD, Richardson AL. Genome-wide analysis for loss of heterozygosity in primary and recurrent phyllodes tumor and fibroadenoma of breast using single nucleotide polymorphism arrays. Breast Cancer Res Treat 2006;97:301-309.

270. Kleer CG, Giordano TJ, Braun T, Oberman HA. Pathologic, immunohistochemical, and molecular features of benign and malignant phyllodes tumors of the breast. Mod Pathol 2001;14:185-190.

271. Kuenen-Boumeester V, Henzen-Logmans SC, Timmermans MM, et al. Altered expression of p53 and its regulated proteins in phyllodes tumours of the breast. J Pathol 1999;189:169-175.

272. Niezabitowski A, Lackowska B, Rys J, et al. Prognostic evaluation of proliferative activity and DNA content in the phyllodes tumor of the breast: immunohistochemical and flow cytometric study of 118 cases. Breast Cancer Res Treat 2001;65:77-85.

273. Shpitz B, Bomstein Y, Sternberg A, et al. Immunoreactivity of p53, Ki-67, and c-erbB-2 in phyllodes tumors of the breast in correlation with clinical and morphologic features. J Surg Oncol 2002;79:86-92.

274. Millar EK, Beretov J, Marr P, et al. Malignant phyllodes tumours of the breast display increased stromal p53 protein expression. Histopathology 1999;34:491-496.

275. Suo Z, Nesland JM. Phyllodes tumor of the breast: EGFR family expression and relation to clinicopathological features. Ultrastruct Pathol 2000;24:371-381.

276. Tse GM, Putti TC, Kung FY, et al. Increased p53 protein expression in malignant mammary phyllodes tumors. Mod Pathol 2002;15:734-740.

277. Chen CM, Chen CJ, Chang CL, et al. CD34, CD117, and actin expression in phyllodes tumor of the breast. J Surg Res 2000;94:84-91.

278. Esposito NN, Mohan D, Brufsky A, et al. Phyllodes tumor: a clinicopathologic and immunohistochemical study of 30 cases. Arch Pathol Lab Med 2006;130:1516-1521.

279. Sawyer EJ, Poulsom R, Hunt FT, et al. Malignant phyllodes tumours show stromal overexpression of c-myc and c-kit. J Pathol 2003;200:59-64.

280. Tse GM, Putti TC, Lui PC, et al. Increased c-kit (CD117) expression in malignant mammary phyllodes tumors. Mod Pathol 2004;17:827-831.

281. Djordjevic B, Hanna WM. Expression of c-kit in fibroepithelial lesions of the breast is a mast cell phenomenon. Mod Pathol 2008;21:1238-1245.

282. Kersting C, Kuijper A, Schmidt H, et al. Amplifications of the epidermal growth factor receptor gene (EGFR) are common in phyllodes tumors of the breast and are associated with tumor progression. Lab Invest 2006;86:54-61.

283. Tse GM, Lui PC, Vong JS, et al. Increased epidermal growth factor receptor (EGFR) expression in malignant mammary phyllodes tumors. Breast Cancer Res Treat 2009;114:441-448.

284. Feakins RM, Mulcahy HE, Nickols CD, Wells CA. p53 expression in phyllodes tumours is associated with histological features of malignancy but does not predict outcome. Histopathology 1999;35:162-169.

285. Inoshita S. Phyllodes tumor (cystosarcoma phyllodes) of the breast. A clinicopathologic study of 45 cases. Acta Pathol Jpn 1988;38:21-33.

286. Khan SA, Badve S. Phyllodes tumors of the breast. Curr Treat Options Oncol 2001;2:139-147.

287. Kuijper A, de Vos RA, Lagendijk JH, et al. Progressive deregulation of the cell cycle with higher tumor grade in the stroma of breast phyllodes tumors. Am J Clin Pathol 2005;123:690-698.

288. Shabahang M, Franceschi D, Sundaram M, et al. Surgical management of primary breast sarcoma. Am Surg 2002;68:673-677:discussion 677.

289. Asoglu O, Ugurlu MM, Blanchard K, et al. Risk factors for recurrence and death after primary surgical treatment of malignant phyllodes tumors. Ann Surg Oncol 2004;11:1011-1017.

290. Ben Hassouna J, Damak T, Gamoudi A, et al. Phyllodes tumors of the breast: a case series of 106 patients. Am J Surg 2006;192:141-147.

291. Chen WH, Cheng SP, Tzen CY, et al. Surgical treatment of phyllodes tumors of the breast: retrospective review of 172 cases. J Surg Oncol 2005;91:185-194.

292. Cheng SP, Chang YC, Liu TP, et al. Phyllodes tumor of the breast: the challenge persists. World J Surg 2006;30:1414-1421.

293. Hawkins RE, Schofield JB, Fisher C, et al. The clinical and histologic criteria that predict metastases from cystosarcoma phyllodes. Cancer 1992;69:141-147.

294. Kapiris I, Nasiri N, A'Hern R, et al. Outcome and predictive factors of local recurrence and distant metastases following primary surgical treatment of high-grade malignant phyllodes tumours of the breast. Eur J Surg Oncol 2001;27:723-730.

295. Tan PH, Jayabaskar T, Chuah KL, et al. Phyllodes tumors of the breast: the role of pathologic parameters. Am J Clin Pathol 2005;123:529-540.

296. Burga AM, Tavassoli FA. Periductal stromal tumor: a rare lesion with low-grade sarcomatous behavior. Am J Surg Pathol 2003;27:343-348.

297. Garfein CF, Aulicino MR, Leytin A, et al. Epithelioid cells in myoid hamartoma of the breast: a potential diagnostic pitfall for core biopsies. Arch Pathol Lab Med 1996;120:676-680.

298. Mathers ME, Shrimankar J. Lobular neoplasia within a myoid hamartoma of the breast. Breast J 2004;10:58-59.

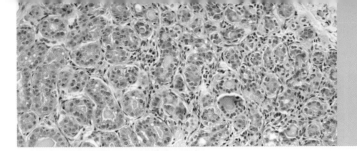

Fibroepithelial Lesions

Nicole N. Esposito

FIBROADENOMA

Fibroadenomas are benign tumors that arise from the epithelium and stroma of the terminal ductal-lobular unit. They represent the most common benign breast tumor, occurring in 25% of asymptomatic women, and the most common lesion diagnosed in premenopausal women.[1-3]

Whether fibroadenomas are hormonally responsive is uncertain. In one of the first reports that studied 450 cases of fibroadenomas, the authors concluded fibroadenomas are hormonally responsive based on the following observations: (1) their easy producability in male animals when estrogen is present, (2) their prevalence in prepubertal females, when "small but steady estrogen breast secretions occur for 3 to 5 years before menstrual onset," (3) their growth during the latter two trimesters of pregnancy, (4) generation or growth of fibroadenomas with "injection of repeated small doses of estrogen into monkeys" rather than high doses given over shorter periods, and (5) the presence of estrogen in these lesions.[4] These findings were supported by an additional early report published in 1940, which found estrogen injections in male monkeys transplanted with "adenofibromas" of the breast resulted in tumor growth.[5] In contrast, in a study of fibroadenomas from premenopausal women, no difference in proliferation was observed in fibroadenomas sampled in the luteal versus the secretory menstrual phases.[6] These authors concluded that fibroadenomas are not influenced by endocrine cyclic changes, but rather rely on paracrine factors for growth and involution, like neoplasms.

Whether fibroadenomas represent a hyperplastic or neoplastic growth is uncertain. One study found a high incidence of chromosome 21 monosomy in breast fibroadenomas[7]; however, this genetic abnormality has also been reported in epithelial hyperplasia.[8] In another study of 13 fibroadenomas, either no fractional allelic losses or a very low incidence of loss of heterozygosity was observed using single nucleotide polymorphism (SNP) array analysis,[9] thus suggesting that these lesions represent nonclonal or hyperplastic growths rather than neoplasms. In contrast, a study by Noguchi and coworkers[10] reported fibroadenomas were monoclonal neoplasms, although only three fibroadenomas were included in this study, which further found the same allele of the androgen receptor was inactivated in fibroadenomas and phyllodes tumor diagnosed in the same patients. The authors thus concluded that phyllodes tumors have the same origin as fibroadenomas.

Clinical Presentation and Imaging Features

Fibroadenomas are more common in premenopausal women, most frequent in women of 20 to 30 years of age, but may be present at any age.[6] Fibroadenomas usually present as a well-defined, mobile mass on physical examination or a well-defined solid, hypoechoic mass on ultrasound (Figure 12-1).[11]

Gross Pathology

Fibroadenomas are grossly well-circumscribed masses with smooth or lobulated contours. When sectioned, they typically show a "bulging," tan-white cut surface (Figure 12-2). They range in size from less than a centimeter and can grow to over 4 cm in greatest dimension. Such larger tumors, however, are more common in adolescent females.[12]

Some fibroadenomas, particularly if histologically myxoid, can show a gelatinous cut surface or may be partially cystic.

mitotic figures can be observed. Cellular fibroadenomas may grow to reach large sizes; when larger than 5 cm or more than 500 g the term *giant fibroadenoma* has been used. Giant fibroadenomas are uncommon and represent 0.5% to 2% of all fibroadenomas.[23,24] They are more common in young African American women and have been postulated to result from abnormal estrogen exposure, as evidenced by their increased frequency during pubescence and pregnancy.[25]

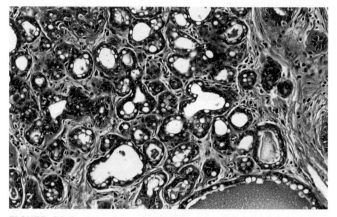

FIGURE 12-8 Lactating adenoma demonstrates typical secretory change.

Ultrastructural studies of fibroadenomas have characterized the stromal cells as fibroblastic, and fewer have noted myoid or myofibroblastic differentiation.[26] Electron microscopy will demonstrate varying amounts of microfilaments, 5 to 7 nm in diameter (actin-type filaments); the reported absence of a dense body in some cases, however, suggests that fibroadenoma stromal cells may be variants of myofibroblasts.[27–29] The stromal cells in fibroadenomas, reflective of their fibroblastic and/or myofibroblastic differentiation, are positive for actin and CD34 by immunohistochemistry and have also been reported to be variably CD10+, which has been traditionally used by some in breast pathology as a myoepithelial cell marker.[30,31]

Multinucleated stromal giant cells have been infrequently described in benign breast stroma, and were originally described by Rosen.[32] In his report, the giant cells were visible at low (×10) magnification, were dispersed rather than aggregated, demonstrated scanty cytoplasm and hyperchromatic nuclei, and were not associated with adjacent carcinoma. Similarly, multinucleated stromal giant cells have been reported in fibroadenomas. Although the multinucleated giant cells are often pleomorphic, the stroma in these cases generally lack mitotic activity and are thought to be of no clinical significance. The presence of mitoses, especially atypical mitotic figures, should raise suspicion of

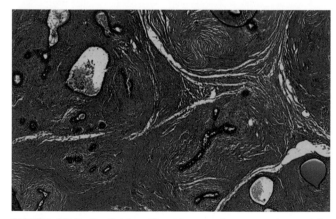

FIGURE 12-9 Hyalinizing fibroadenoma forms a micronodular pattern.

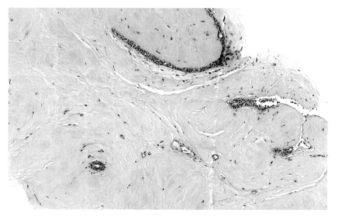

FIGURE 12-10 Pale, dense collagenous matrix.

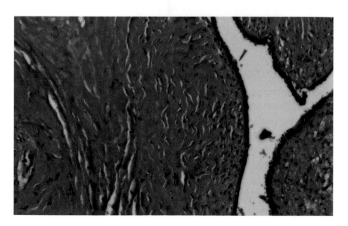

FIGURE 12-11 High-power view of a hyalinizing fibroadenoma shows densely collagenous stroma.

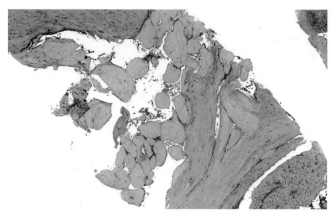

FIGURE 12-12 Fragmentation during core biopsy of a hyalinizing fibroadenoma can simulate a sclerosed papilloma.

a phyllodes tumor, although both usual and atypical mitotic figures have been reported in otherwise benign fibroadenomas.[33–37] Rarely, fibroadenomas demonstrate necrosis, which is often a result of spontaneous infarction.[38]

The stroma in fibroadenomas may show differentiation other than that of fibroblasts or myofibroblasts. Although it has been reported that most fibroepithelial lesions with adipocytic differentiation represent phyllodes tumor, it is not infrequent to encounter benign adipocytes in fibroadenomatous stroma in routine practice (Figure 12-16).[39]

Carcinoma may arise in or extend to involve fibroadenomas. Lobular neoplasia in the form of lobular carcinoma in situ (LCIS) more commonly arises in fibroadenomas than does ductal neoplasia, with more than

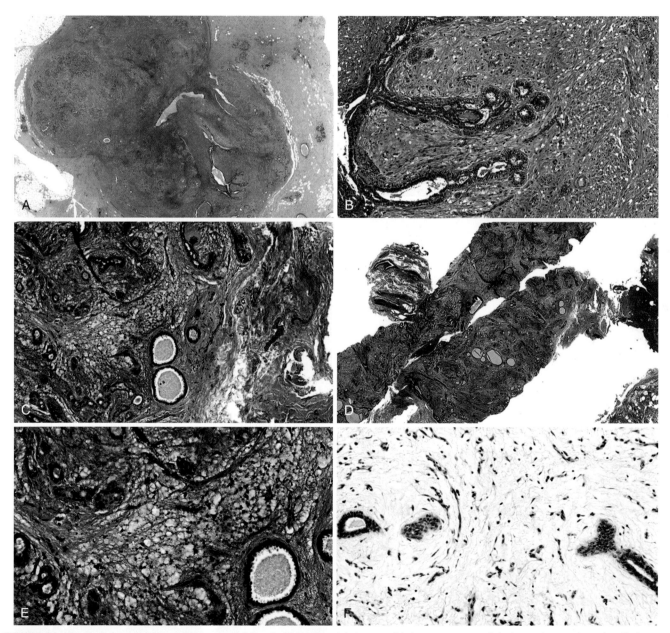

FIGURE 12-13   A–F, Myxoid fibroadenomas exhibit pale blue, myxoid stroma with homogenous cellularity and smooth and well-circumscribed borders. Note the lack of periductal condensation, cellular atypia, and mitoses, useful distinguishing factors when considering phyllodes tumors in the differential diagnosis.

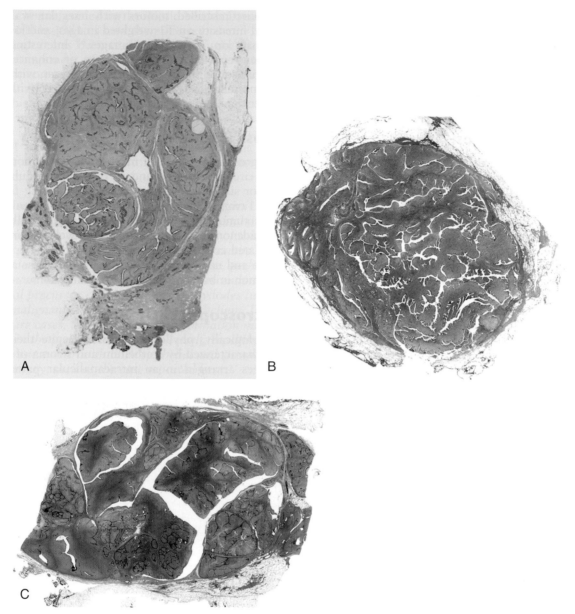

FIGURE 12-20 A–C, Low-power views of benign phyllodes tumors show fairly well-circumscribed borders and prominent intracanalicular growth patterns. The presence of stromal heterogeneity in cellularity is apparent.

stroma compresses the ductal component, such that they form cleftlike spaces (Figure 12-20). A pericanalicular pattern may be focally present (Figure 12-21A). The epithelium is often very hyperplastic and can otherwise demonstrate metaplasias seen in fibroadenomas and in benign breast tissue.

Benign phyllodes tumors show pushing, lobulated borders and moderate stromal cellularity. Periductal condensation of the stroma is often present (Figure 12-22; see also Figure 12-21B–E). The stroma is mildly to focally moderately atypical and is often characterized by euchromatic or hyperchromatic spindle cells with scant cytoplasm, evidence of their fibroblastic and/or myofibroblastic differentiation (Figure 12-23). Mitotic figures are infrequent; when present, they rarely exceed 1 to 2 per 10 high-power fields and are often located in the zones of periductal condensation surrounding ducts.

Benign phyllodes tumors can be difficult to distinguish from fibroadenomas (Figure 12-24). However, they typically demonstrate heterogeneity in stromal cellularity and mitotic activity, although the absence of stromal mitoses does not exclude a benign phyllodes tumor. On core biopsy, they can show fragmentation and simulate a papillary lesion (Figure 12-25).

Borderline phyllodes tumors have variable morphologies but, overall, demonstrate a relatively expanded stromal compartment and pronounced intracanalicular growth pattern compared with benign tumors (Figure 12-26). Mitotic figures range from 3 to 5 per 10 high-power fields. Like benign phyllodes tumors, the stroma shows variable degrees of cellularity throughout the lesion and may be prominently myxoid (Figure 12-27). Tumor borders may be pushing or focally infiltrative (Figure 12-28).

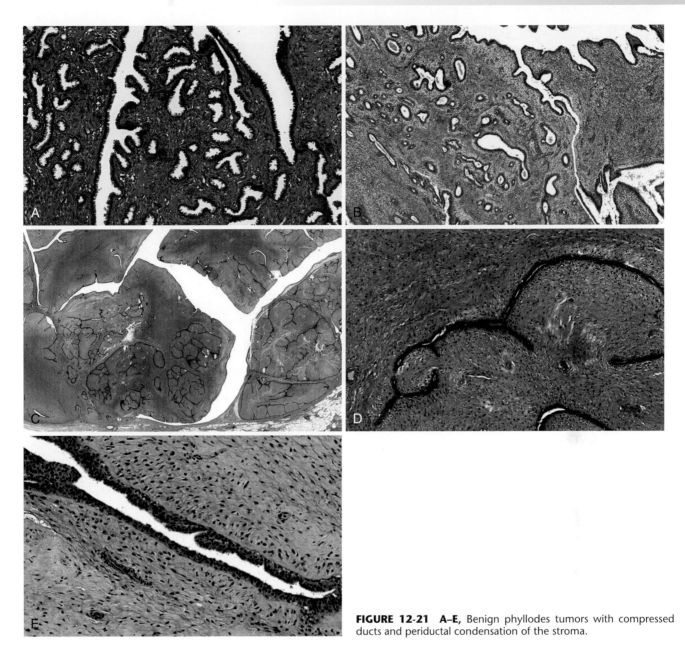

FIGURE 12-21   A–E, Benign phyllodes tumors with compressed ducts and periductal condensation of the stroma.

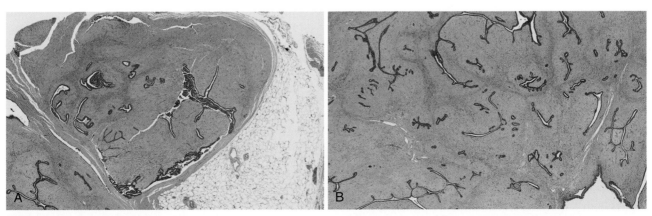

FIGURE 12-22   A and **B,** Although periductal stromal condensation is usually present throughout phyllodes tumors, they can show a lack of such changes, mimicking fibroadenoma.

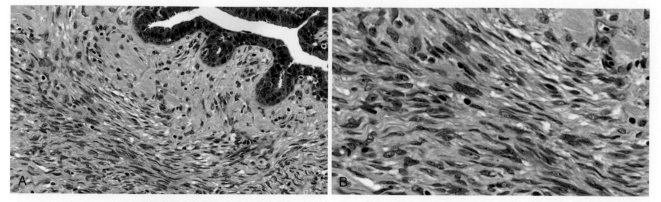

FIGURE 12-23 **A** and **B,** Mild stromal cell atypia in a benign phyllodes tumor.

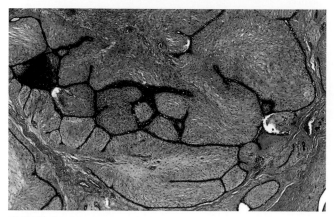

FIGURE 12-24 Benign phyllodes tumor lacking periductal condensation and hypercellularity simulates a fibroadenoma. Other areas of the tumor showed typical phyllodes tumor morphology.

Malignant phyllodes tumors demonstrate expanded stroma with brisk mitotic activity and significant cellular atypia (Figure 12-29). Mitoses are generally greater than 5 per 10 high-power field. *Stromal overgrowth,* defined as stroma accompanying a single 40× field, is a feature almost strictly confined to the malignant phenotype and often correlates with sarcomatous overgrowth. In frankly malignant phyllodes tumors with stromal overgrowth, heterologous differentiation, such as osteosarcomatous, chondrosarcomatous, or liposarcomatous elements, may be found (Figure 12-30). Stromal overgrowth may be so prominent that the appearance may

KEY PATHOLOGIC FEATURES

Phyllodes Tumors

- **Gross:** Well-circumscribed and lobulated if benign; malignant tumors may show grossly infiltrative margins, necrosis, and/or hemorrhage.

- **Microscopic:** Biphasic neoplasms with compressed ducts forming a "leaflike" or intracanalicular growth pattern; stroma is variably cellular and mitotically active.

- **Immunohistochemistry:** Largely noncontributory; expression of Ki-67 and p53 correlate with tumor grade.

- **Differential diagnosis:** Fibroadenoma, periductal stromal sarcoma.

mimic a primary breast sarcoma (Figures 12-31 and 12-32); in such cases, it is of utmost importance to diligently search for the presence of epithelium to establish the biphasic nature of the neoplasm.

Treatment and Prognosis

Standard therapy includes mastectomy or wide local excision, depending on the degree of malignancy and tumor size. Axillary lymph node sampling is currently not routinely performed because the rate of lymph node metastases is less than 1%. Rather, like most sarcomas, metastases are via the hematogenous route and are strictly composed of the sarcomatous element of the primary breast tumor. The most common metastatic sites are lung and bone.[72–75] Overall recurrent and visceral metastatic rates range from 8% to 40% and 1% to 21%, respectively. Unlike infiltrating ductal and lobular carcinomas, in which the utility of adjuvant treatment is well known, the role of postoperative radiotherapy and chemotherapy remains to be fully established in the treatment of phyllodes tumors.[76–78]

Although the gold standard of determination of tumor behavior relies on histopathologic examination at the light microscopic level by pathologists in the vast majority of cases, stratification of phyllodes tumors into prognostic categories does not consistently predict behavior. As a result, numerous histomorphologic, immunohistochemical, and molecular studies have been published with the aim of outperforming histologic grade in determining prognosis. In one study of 239 phyllodes tumors with a mean follow-up of 7.9 years, tumor necrosis and fibroproliferation, defined as the presence of "fibroadenomatoid" nodules in the surrounding breast, and positive surgical margins of resection were associated with a higher actuarial local recurrence rate in univariate analysis. However, only fibroproliferation and necrosis remained important predictors of local recurrence in multivariate analysis.[79] In contrast, Tan and associates[80] found negative margin status reduced recurrence hazards by 51.7% in multivariate analysis in their study of 335 phyllodes tumors. The importance of "adequate" resection margins, defined as a tumor to resection margin distance of greater than 1 cm, has also been shown to be significantly associated with a lower recurrence rate in numerous additional studies.[81–87]

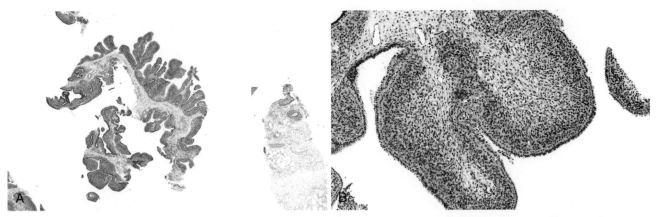

FIGURE 12-25 **A** and **B,** Core biopsy of a phyllodes tumor with fragmentation of the lesion simulates a papillary neoplasm.

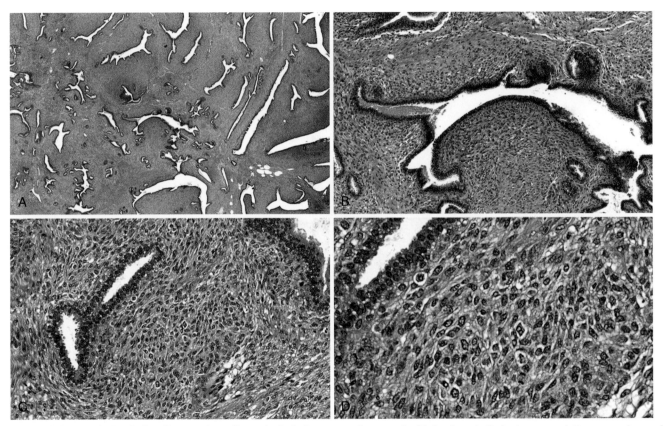

FIGURE 12-26 **A–D,** Borderline (low-grade malignant) phyllodes tumor. Compared with benign phyllodes tumors, relative expansion and hypercellularity of the stroma are evident.

Besides adequate resection margins, stromal overgrowth in phyllodes tumors has been associated with increased recurrent rates as well as increased risk of metastatic disease. In a study of 101 phyllodes tumors with relatively long follow-up, patients with stromal overgrowth had significantly lower 5- and 10-year survival rates than patients without stromal overgrowth.[88] Reports by Kario and coworkers[89] and Hawkins and colleagues[71] also demonstrated the presence of stromal overgrowth correlated with more aggressive clinical and histopathologic features. It is important to note, however, that almost all of the cases reported with stromal overgrowth correlated with a malignant phenotype

histologically, emphasizing the association of stromal overgrowth with malignancy.

Immunohistochemical studies examining proliferative markers, expression of tumor suppressor genes, and expression of proteins with targeted therapy implications have also been performed. Several studies have examined the proliferative rate of phyllodes tumors using Ki-67 as a surrogate marker, with most reports demonstrating increased Ki-67 stromal expression with increasing tumor grade.[87,90,91] However, consistent correlations between Ki-67 proliferation indices and patient outcomes have not been demonstrated. Similarly, studies examining the expression

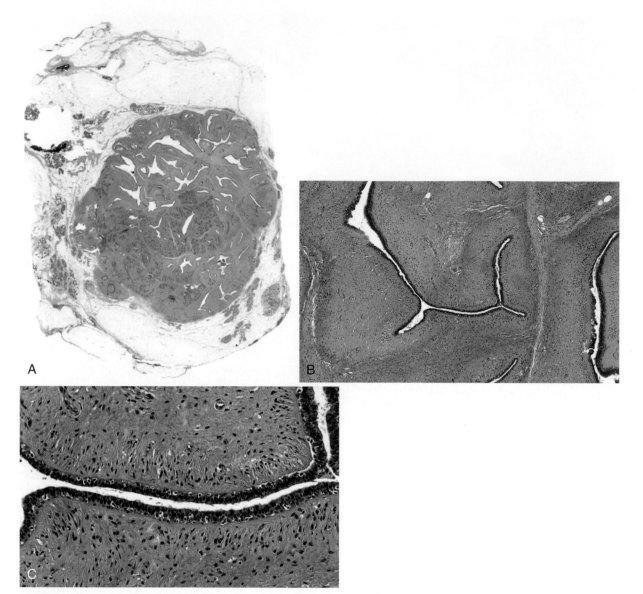

FIGURE 12-27   A–C, Phyllodes tumor with diffuse myxoid change. Note the stromal expansion and periductal condensation.

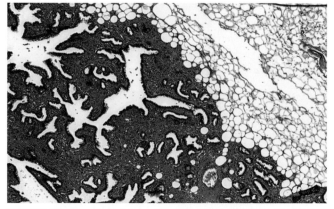

FIGURE 12-28 Phyllodes tumor with focal infiltration of adjacent adipose tissue.

of p53 by immunohistochemistry have correlated its expression with tumor grade but inconsistently with prognosis.[92–94]

Overexpression of the c-kit oncogene, which encodes a tyrosine-kinase transmembrane receptor protein, characterizes gastrointestinal stromal tumors (GISTs) that, like phyllodes tumors, show a spectrum of behavior from benign to malignant. The finding of c-kit overexpression in GISTs led to the development of targeted therapy with the KIT-receptor tyrosine-kinase inhibitor, imatinib mesylate (STI-571). c-kit expression in phyllodes tumors has also been reported,[95–98] although some authors purport such expression is the result of mast cell immunoreactivity rather than neoplastic stromal cell expression.[99] c-kit expression, when present, is preferentially expressed in malignant tumors; however, reports have failed to associate tumor behavior with c-kit expression. Furthermore, activating c-kit mutations, despite its possible protein expression, have been

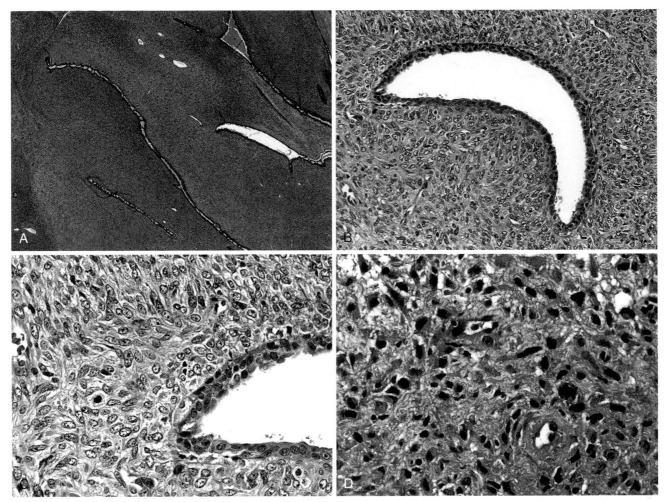

FIGURE 12-29 A–D, Malignant phyllodes tumors. The stroma is prominent and demonstrates significant nuclear atypia, pleomorphism, and mitotic activity.

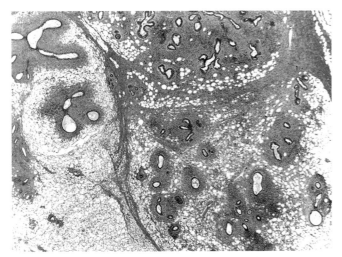

FIGURE 12-30 Malignant phyllodes tumor with liposarcomatous differentiation.

rarely reported, suggesting the probable lack of any predictive response from imatinib mesylate.

Another protein with targeted therapy implications studied in phyllodes tumor is the epidermal growth factor receptor (EGFR or *HER1)*. Tumors with mutations in the tyrosine kinase domain of the EGFR gene and concomitant EGFR overexpression have been shown to respond to tyrosine kinase inhibitors, such as gefitinib and erlotinib.[100] Kersting and associates[101] reported EGFR expression in stromal tumor cells in 19% of phyllodes tumors overall and in 75% of histologically malignant tumors. Furthermore, they found EGFR overexpression correlated with either whole gene or intron 1 amplification. Any potential relationship between EGFR expression and/or amplification and patient prognosis, however, could not be analyzed because none of the tumors recurred or metastasized. Such studies to date are lacking, and thus, whether EGFR stromal expression is prognostically significant remains to be investigated.

Differential Diagnosis

The main differential diagnosis of phyllodes tumors is fibroadenoma, and can be especially diagnostically challenging on core or fine-needle aspiration (FNA) biopsies. In a study of 112 cases of fibroepithelial lesions diagnosed on biopsy, statistically significant parameters associated with a phyllodes tumor diagnosis included increased stromal cellularity, pleomorphism, stromal overgrowth, fragmentation (defined as fragments of

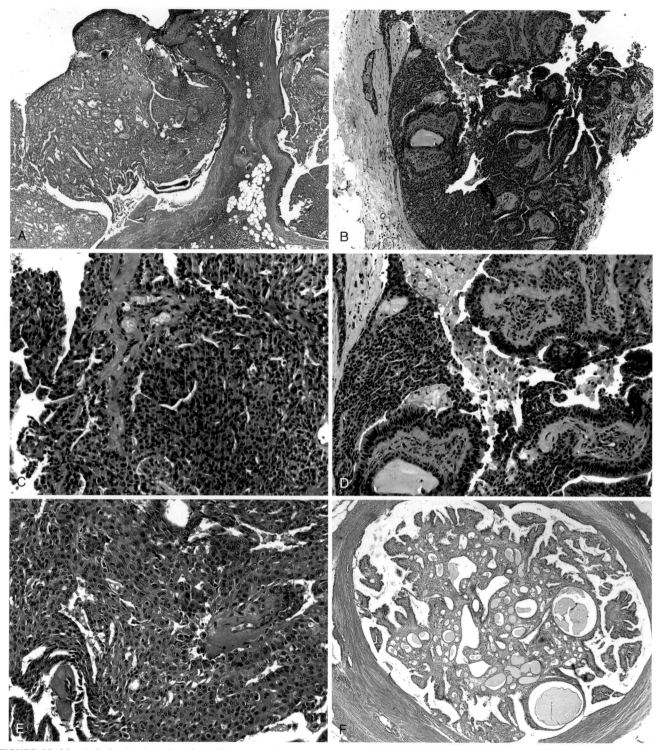

FIGURE 13-10   A–F, Benign intraductal papillomas involved by variable degrees of usual ductal hyperplasia and florid ductal hyperplasia. These more complex papillomas show irregular, "slitlike" lumina and microacini and lack cellular monotony.

necessitate complete excision, management of benign papillomas is less defined. Whereas two studies reported benign follow-up excisions after a diagnosis of benign papilloma on biopsy,[35,36] another reported a final diagnosis of atypical ductal hyperplasia or carcinoma in 26% of cases.[31] Similar results were reported in a study of 101 benign papillomas (without adjacent atypia or carcinoma) diagnosed on core biopsy in which 18.8%

and 8.9% of cases were upgraded to atypical ductal hyperplasia and DCIS, respectively.[3] Similarly, Bernik and associates[37] reported a final diagnosis of atypia and carcinoma in 28% and 9%, respectively, of patients diagnosed with a benign papilloma on core biopsy.

In a relatively large study that reported follow-up on women with papillomas on biopsy and no surgical excision, 28.5% had normal mammograms, and 8.3% had

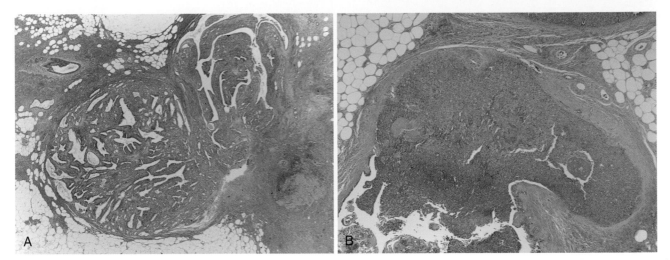

FIGURE 13-11 **A** and **B,** Low-power views of sclerosing intraductal papillomas. Sclerosis surrounding the papillomas distorts the lesional borders.

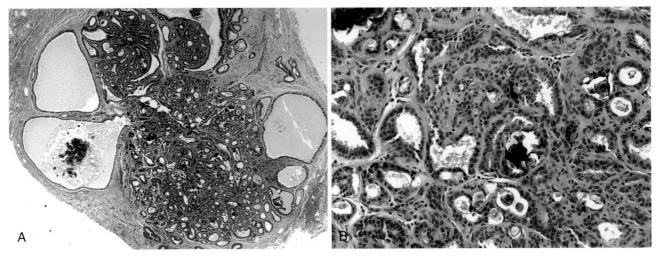

FIGURE 13-12 **A** and **B,** Sclerosing intraductal papilloma with microcalcification.

abnormal mammograms (Breast Imaging Reporting and Data System [BIRADS] 0 or 4).[3] The remaining patients had no follow-up or a "probably normal" mammogram. Another study reported a 95% 5-year freedom from repeat ipsilateral breast sampling in women who did not undergo excision of benign papillomas on biopsy, although 2 patients in this group were diagnosed with malignancy at 48 and 59 months after the original biopsy.[38] These data suggest patients without residual mammographic abnormalities after biopsy may not necessarily require excision.

Differential Diagnosis

PAPILLARY HYPERPLASIA

Papillary hyperplasia is a form of usual ductal hyperplasia. It differs from a papilloma in that it is formed by a vascular stalk rather than a fibrovascular stalk. It also lacks any form of hierarchical branching often seen in intraductal papillomas. Similar to simple papillomas, papillary hyperplasia is composed of myoepithelial cells covered by a single layer of ductal epithelial cells (Figure 13-13).

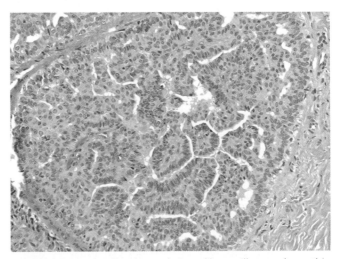

FIGURE 13-13 Papillary hyperplasia, unlike papillomas, shows thin vascular cores and lacks complex hierarchical branching.

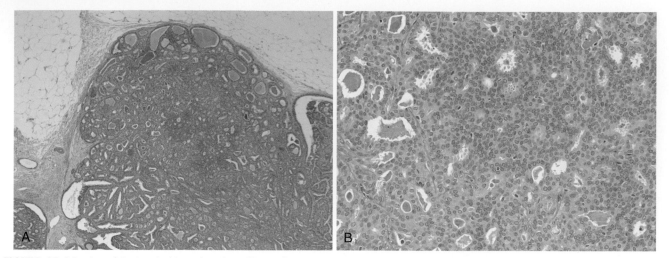

FIGURE 13-14 **A** and **B,** Atypical intraductal papilloma demonstrates an area of atypical cells showing monotonous, low-grade cytology and cribriform architecture.

ATYPICAL PAPILLOMA

The term *atypical papilloma,* synonymous with *intraductal papilloma with atypia,* refers to an intraductal papilloma involved by variable amounts of atypical ductal hyperplasia. Unlike usual or florid ductal hyperplasia, atypia in papillomas can be identified by a monotonous proliferation of epithelial cells forming either solid sheets, cribriform architecture with "punched-out" lumina, or atypical micropapillary projections (Figures 13-14 to 13-16). Immunohistochemistry can be useful in highlighting atypical foci within papillomas. Cytokeratin 5/6 will be absent or attenuated in areas of atypical ductal hyperplasia, in contrast to usual ductal hyperplasia in which high-weight-molecular cytokeratin demonstrates a typical "mosaic" pattern of immunoreactivity. Estrogen receptor immunohistochemistry shows a reverse pattern, with strong and intense staining in atypical foci and either absent or weak, patchy staining in areas of usual ductal hyperplasia.[39–43]

Although treatment of atypical papillomas is less controversial than papillomas without atypia, disagreement as to its proper clinical management persists. A study by Bernik and colleagues[37] suggested patients with single atypical papillomas have a greater likelihood of recurrence or malignancy and, thus, necessitate additional surgery, whereas a study performed in the United Kingdom concluded complete excision was not necessary for patients with atypical papillomas.[26,44] The risk of carcinoma, nevertheless, has been consistently reported to be higher when a papilloma with atypia versus without atypia is present on biopsy, underscoring the importance of noting atypia within a papilloma.[35,36,45–49]

PAPILLARY DUCTAL CARCINOMA IN SITU

DCIS with a papillary growth pattern must be differentiated from a papilloma. The distinction between these two lesions was first described in detail by a 1962 report by Kraus and Neubecker.[19] In their report, they described the stroma of the papillary stalks in DCIS as "thin and relatively inconspicuous" with frequent

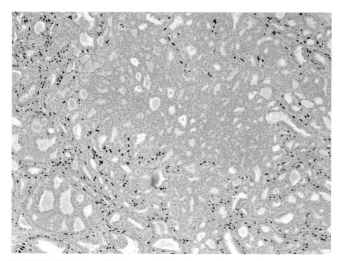

FIGURE 13-15 p63 immunohistochemical stain shows a lack of myoepithelial cells in the area of atypia.

epithelial hyperplasia. This results in a low-power appearance of a more "blue" appearing lesion whereas benign papillomas have a relative "pink" low-power appearance. Papillomas show variable stalk widths but are almost always thicker and more collagenized. The cells lining the fronds of papillary DCIS are atypical epithelial cells devoid of myoepithelium. Papillary DCIS may show low- or intermediate-grade but rarely high-grade cytology. The cells of papillary DCIS are monotonous, demonstrate hyperchromatic nuclei, and are often columnar in shape. Myoepithelial cells are absent, except at the periphery (Figure 13-17). Papillary DCIS is most often associated with carcinomas of the "low-grade" pathway, because they are often seen in association with invasive carcinomas exhibiting mucinous, lobular, tubular, or papillary differentiation, of low or intermediate grade with absent lymphatic invasion, and high estrogen receptor expression.[50,51]

Papillomas involved by DCIS are thought to be histologically distinct from papillary DCIS.[52] DCIS in papillomas will show partial involvement of the papilloma,

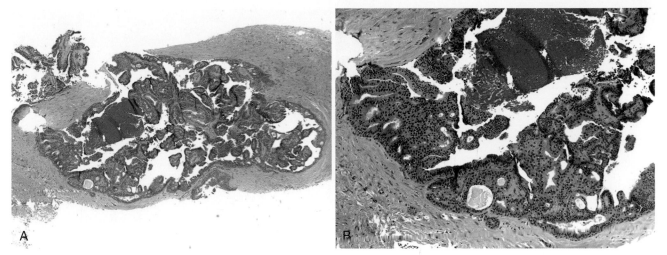

FIGURE 13-16 **A** and **B,** Atypical intraductal papilloma on core needle biopsy. Note the atypical, monotonous cellular proliferation partially involving the lesion. Atypia in papillomas is important to identify on core biopsy because it significantly increases the risk of an upgraded diagnosis on subsequent excisions.

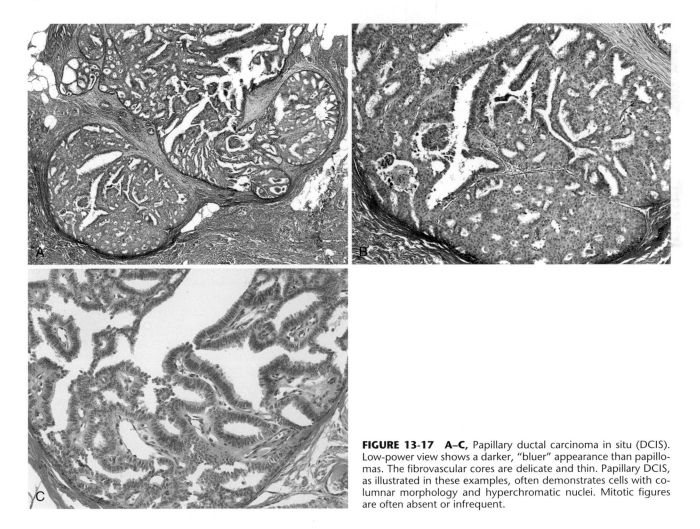

FIGURE 13-17 **A–C,** Papillary ductal carcinoma in situ (DCIS). Low-power view shows a darker, "bluer" appearance than papillomas. The fibrovascular cores are delicate and thin. Papillary DCIS, as illustrated in these examples, often demonstrates cells with columnar morphology and hyperchromatic nuclei. Mitotic figures are often absent or infrequent.

but the essential scaffolding of the papilloma is evident adjacent to and surrounding the area of DCIS. Some authors enforce size criteria in differentiating a papilloma involved by DCIS versus a papilloma with atypia. Page and colleagues[29] categorized a lesion as papilloma with DCIS when the papilloma shows "any area of uniform histology and cytology consistent with non-comedo DCIS" that is greater than 3 mm in size. If such areas measure less than 3 mm, a diagnosis of papilloma with atypia or atypical papilloma is made.[29] In contrast, Tavassoli[42] defines DCIS involving a papilloma when the atypical population of cells involves "at least a third

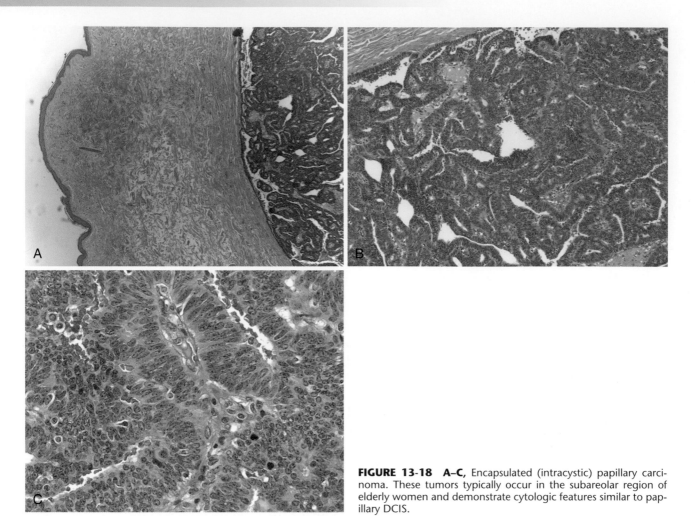

FIGURE 13-18 A–C, Encapsulated (intracystic) papillary carcinoma. These tumors typically occur in the subareolar region of elderly women and demonstrate cytologic features similar to papillary DCIS.

but less than 90% of the lesion." Finally, others render a diagnosis of a papilloma involved by DCIS when the "atypical proliferation in the papilloma shows all the combined architectural and cytological features of DCIS regardless of its extent."[52,53]

ENCAPSULATED (INTRACYSTIC, ENCYSTED) PAPILLARY CARCINOMA

Encapsulated papillary carcinoma (EPC) of the breast, synonymous with "intracystic" or "encysted" papillary carcinoma, is traditionally considered to be a variant of DCIS.[52] It represents approximately 0.5% to 2% of all breast cancers and typically occurs in postmenopausal women.[54] These tumors are typically well circumscribed and demonstrate cytologic features akin to papillary DCIS. Unlike the majority of papillary DCISs, however, EPCs lack myoepithelium at the periphery, leading some authors to conclude that they are invasive carcinomas with an expansile growth pattern and metastatic potential.[54,55] EPCs have been shown, however, to demonstrate linear, continuous basement membrane at their leading edges, which others have suggested support their in situ nature.[56]

EPCs are often located in the central, subareolar region, in postmenopausal women.[28,43] They are histologically akin to papillary DCIS, demonstrating a delicate papillary architecture lined by epithelial cells only.

The epithelium is most commonly columnar in morphology with hyperchromatic nuclei and infrequent mitotic figures. Immunohistochemistry will demonstrate a lack of myoepithelial cells both within and at the periphery of the tumoral masses, whereas these lesions are almost uniformly diffusely and strongly positive for estrogen receptor expression (Figures 13-18 to 13-20).

As stated previously, whether EPCs represent in situ or invasive lesions is controversial. A study examining 27 encapsulated papillary carcinomas showed they exhibit a continuous and linear basement membrane with collagen type IV immunohistochemistry in 65% of cases, in contrast to the absent or discontinuous basement membrane pattern demonstrated by all invasive carcinomas studied.[56] The same study showed all patients with "pure" EPC (no associated frankly invasive carcinoma) in whom axillary lymph node sampling was performed were node-negative, except for 1 case positive for micrometastasis in one of four nodes. The authors thus concluded, based on the pattern of collagen type IV staining and clinical data, that EPCs most likely represent in situ carcinomas. In contrast, a study by Wynveen and coworkers[57] of 13 pure EPCs, 8 EPCs with or indeterminate for microinvasion, and 19 EPCs with invasion, reported discontinuous collagen IV staining in 89% of cases, a positive sentinel lymph node rate of 11%, and local recurrence in 10% of patients. The

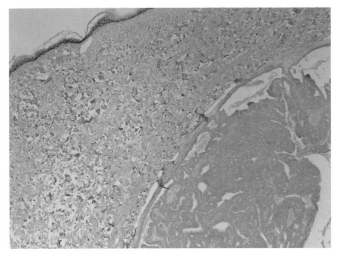

FIGURE 13-19 Myoepithelial cell markers, as shown here with p63 immunohistochemical stain, will be absent within and at the periphery of encapsulated papillary carcinomas. Note the positive internal control in the overlying epidermal cells.

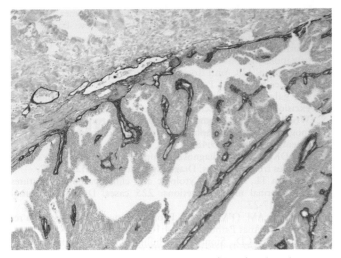

FIGURE 13-20 Collagen type IV immunohistochemistry in an encapsulated papillary carcinoma. Some authors have shown encapsulated papillary carcinomas are surrounded by complete basement membranes, suggesting these lesions may represent in situ rather than invasive carcinomas.

TABLE 13-1	**Histologic and Immunohistochemical Features for Differentiating among Papillary Lesions of the Breast**		
	Intraductal Papilloma	**Papillary DCIS**	**Encapsulated (Intracystic) Papillary Carcinoma**
Fibrovascular stalks	Variable thickness; commonly hyalinized or sclerotic	Thin and delicate	Thin and delicate
Cell types	Myoepithelial and epithelial cells	Epithelial cells only	Epithelial cells only
Nuclear atypia	Absent	Present	Present
Mitoses	Rare, if any	Present	Present
Estrogen receptor	Patchy, weakly positive	Commonly diffusely and strongly positive	Commonly diffusely and strongly positive
p63 and calponin/actin immunohistochemistry	Highlights myoepithelial cells lining fibrovascular stalks and at lesional borders	Absent myoepithelial cells lining fibrovascular cores; usually present at lesional borders although may be absent in some cases	Complete absence of myoepithelial cells, including at leading edges of tumor

DCIS, ductal carcinoma in situ.

authors thus suggested EPCs constitute a "spectrum of intraductal and [invasive carcinoma], with predominance of the latter."[57] Of note, however, is the lack of data regarding specimen handling in cases that were associated with lymph node metastasis and/or recurrence; specifically, lack of information on how much tissue from the specimen was submitted raises the possibility of an occult, unsampled frankly invasive carcinoma. It is thus imperative in cases of apparent "pure" EPC, as with any form of in situ carcinoma, to carefully examine the gross specimen and aggressively sample specimens to exclude an invasive carcinoma.

SUMMARY

In summary, intraductal papillomas of the breast represent 8% to 10% of all benign breast lesions and are commonly encountered in routine practice. They may be central or peripheral and are defined by their fibrovascular stalks projecting intraluminally and lined by both myoepithelial and ductal epithelial cells. Whether these lesions should be excised if diagnosed on biopsy is controversial. They must be distinguished from papillary DCIS and EPCs. A summary of the key histologic and immunohistochemical features distinguishing among these papillary lesions is shown in Table 13-1.

REFERENCES

1. Di Cristofano C, et al. Papillary lesions of the breast: a molecular progression? Breast Cancer Res Treat 2005;90:71-76.
2. Gendler LS, et al. Association of breast cancer with papillary lesions identified at percutaneous image-guided breast biopsy. Am J Surg 2004;188:365-370.
3. Rizzo M, et al. Surgical follow-up and clinical presentation of 142 breast papillary lesions diagnosed by ultrasound-guided core-needle biopsy. Ann Surg Oncol 2008;15:1040-1047.
4. Batori M, et al. Papillomatosis and breast cancer: a case report and a review of the literature. Eur Rev Med Pharmacol Sci 2000;4:99-103.

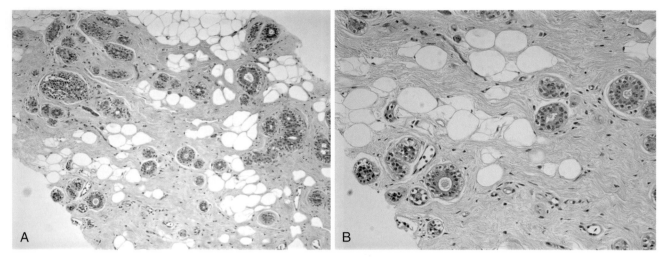

FIGURE 14-18 A and **B,** In this example of sclerosing adenosis, distinct epithelial and myoepithelial layers are visible on routine stain.

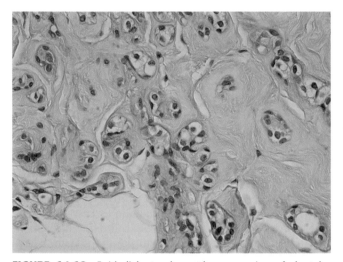

FIGURE 14-19 Epithelial atrophy and compression of ductules results in prominent myoepithelial cells with clear cytoplasm and small dark nuclei, along with luminal obliteration.

described as clusters and single cells with abundant granular to focally vacuolated cytoplasm, enlarged pleomorphic nuclei with irregular nuclear membranes, granular chromatin, and prominent nucleoli.[10] In a small series of three cases, the cytologic features were summarized as being frequently cellular, with small compact cell clusters, variable background naked nuclei and foam cells, and some individual cells. The nuclei often had prominent nucleoli and anisonucleosis, but a conspicuous lack of hyperchromatism, highlighted by the authors as a useful feature in differentiating this lesion from a malignant process.[11]

TUBULAR ADENOSIS

Tubular adenosis is an uncommon variant. In a study of six cases of tubular adenosis by Lee and coworkers,[12] tubular adenosis was described as a haphazard proliferation of elongated, narrow, sometimes branching tubules. Depending on the plane of section, they may appear as elongated tubules or round ductules

(Figure 14-35). With increasing sclerosis, the glandular lumina are less prominent and may be compressed, as in sclerosing adenosis (Figure 14-36). The tubules do not maintain a lobulocentric distribution and may be difficult to distinguish from infiltrating carcinoma, especially tubular carcinoma, owing to this infiltrative appearance. The tubules may be somewhat crowded but generally show a small amount of intervening stroma. The epithelial cells are small and round, with pale cytoplasm, and they lack the comma shape and "apical snouts" of tubular carcinoma. Immunohistochemical stains for myoepithelial cells, such as p63 or smooth muscle myosin heavy chain (SMM-HC), demonstrate an intact myoepithelial layer. Luminal secretions may be present.

BLUNT DUCT ADENOSIS

The morphologic features of blunt duct adenosis, an uncommon form of adenosis, are not as well defined as other variants of adenosis. The proliferation consists of small nests, arranged in a lobular configuration. Small and sometimes dilated lumina are identified within the nests (Figure 14-37). The cells are small with round to ovoid nuclei, and myoepithelial cells with more hyperchromatic nuclei may be prominent. Apocrine metaplasia may also be seen within the nests.

KEY PATHOLOGIC FEATURES

Adenosis

- **Gross:** Lobular mass, granularity, or firm dense white tissue with small cystic spaces.

- **Microscopic:** Lobulocentric proliferation of small ductules that may show hyperplasia, sclerosis with epithelial atrophy, or apocrine cytologic features. Associated microcalcifications are common.

- **Immunohistochemistry:** Preservation of myoepithelial cells can be demonstrated with stains for smooth muscle myosin heavy chain (SMM-HC) or p63.

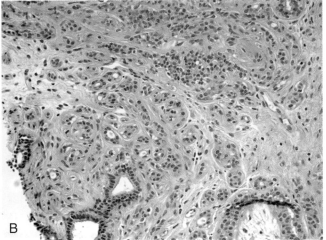
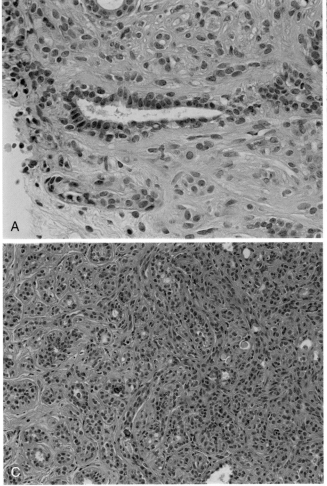

FIGURE 14-20 A-C, Small, compressed ductules of sclerosing adenosis with epithelial atrophy and an infiltrative appearance.

Treatment and Prognosis

Adenosis is a benign histologic diagnosis most frequently made when associated microcalcifications are identified on screening mammogram and represents part of the spectrum of fibrocystic change. Adenosis that is not involved by other more advanced lesions requires no additional treatment. If adenosis is diagnosed on needle core biopsy and the finding is not considered to be concordant with the mammographic or ultrasound findings, excision of the area for further examination is generally recommended. Some have recommended excision of atypical apocrine adenosis when identified on needle core biopsy,[9] similar to the common practice of excision when atypical ductal or atypical lobular hyperplasia is identified on needle core biopsy. Adenosis involved by in situ carcinoma or identified in association with invasive carcinoma should be treated based on the extent or stage of carcinoma.

Adenosis as a risk factor for the development of subsequent carcinoma has been addressed in numerous studies and appears to be associated with a small, but independent, increased risk. Some studies have included adenosis and sclerosing adenosis in a more general category of proliferative disease without atypia, because the risk for development of subsequent carcinoma is

significantly higher for atypical hyperplasia than for other categories of breast disease. The calculated relative risk of subsequent carcinoma has ranged from 1.7 to 5.0, with numerous studies showing a relative risk between 1.7 and 2.5.[13-20] Ashbeck and colleagues[21] reported a hazard ratio for subsequent breast carcinoma in patients with a diagnosis of adenosis of 2.28, with increases to 2.72 and 2.81 when adjusted for other low-risk diagnoses and breast density, ethnicity, and family history, respectively. The hazard ratio was 3.53 for women older than 55 years. More recently, in a nested case-control study of 1239 women within a large multicenter cohort of women, Kabat and associates[22] reported no increased risk of breast cancer in women with a previous breast biopsy diagnosis of sclerosing adenosis.

In a clinicopathologic study of 37 women with atypical apocrine adenosis, the relative risk of developing carcinoma was 5.5 (95% confidence interval [CI] 1.9–16) overall, and the relative risk was 14 (95% CI 4.1–48) in women older than age 60 at the time of breast biopsy.[23] Because cases with concomitant atypical ductal hyperplasia were not excluded, this study may overestimate the risk posed by atypical apocrine adenosis alone. Carter and Rosen[24] identified 51 patients with atypical apocrine metaplasia involving sclerosing lesions of

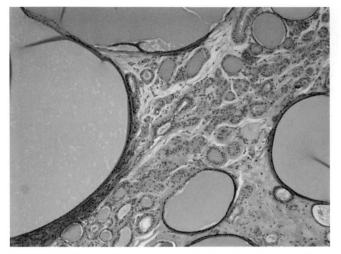

FIGURE 14-25 Small round glands of adenosis adjacent to fibrocystic change.

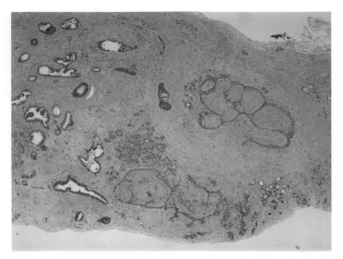

FIGURE 14-26 Needle core biopsy of fibroadenoma with proliferation of small ductules of sclerosing adenosis in the center of the image.

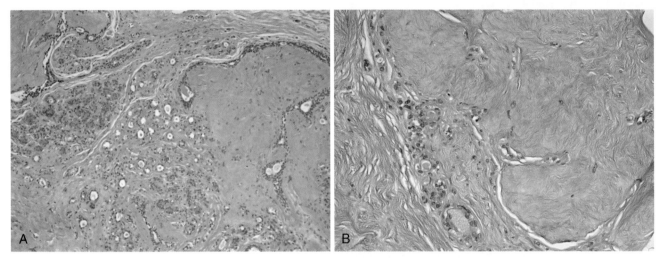

FIGURE 14-27 **A** and **B,** Sclerosing adenosis involving a fibroadenoma.

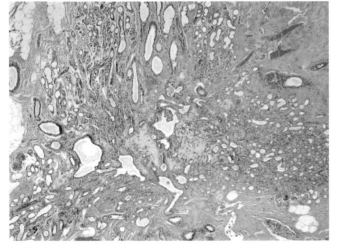

FIGURE 14-28 Sclerosing adenosis as a conspicuous component of this radial sclerosing lesion with central stromal elastosis.

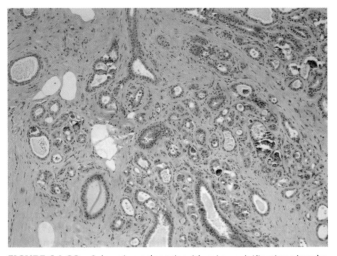

FIGURE 14-29 Sclerosing adenosis with microcalcifications involving a radial sclerosing lesion.

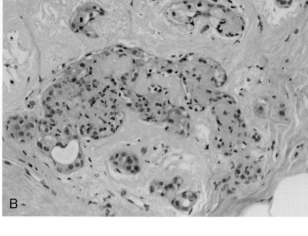

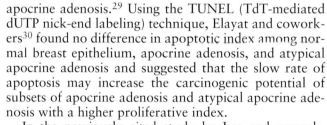

FIGURE 14-30 A-C, Collagenous spherulosis and stromal elastosis in sclerosing adenosis.

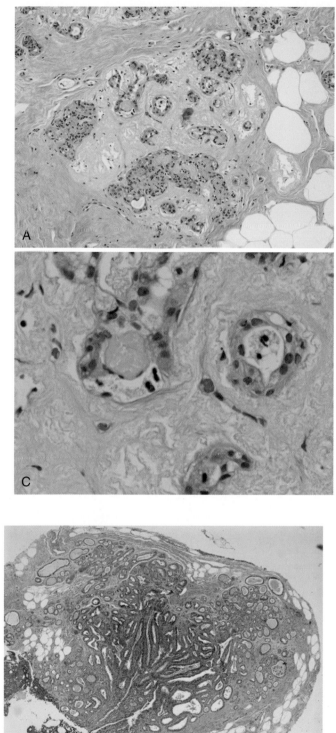

FIGURE 14-31 Columnar cell change in sclerosing adenosis.

A fluorescence in situ hybridization study of apocrine metaplasia and apocrine adenosis found no amplification of the c-myc gene, suggesting that this genetic alteration constitutes a late event in the pathogenesis of breast carcinomas.[28] A study of cell cycle markers and proliferative fraction found no significant difference between expression in apocrine adenosis and atypical apocrine adenosis.[29] Using the TUNEL (TdT-mediated dUTP nick-end labeling) technique, Elayat and coworkers[30] found no difference in apoptotic index among normal breast epithelium, apocrine adenosis, and atypical apocrine adenosis and suggested that the slow rate of apoptosis may increase the carcinogenic potential of subsets of apocrine adenosis and atypical apocrine adenosis with a higher proliferative index.

In the previously cited study by Lee and coworkers,[12] two of five patients with tubular adenosis showed involvement by ductal carcinoma in situ, although the association of tubular adenosis and in situ and invasive carcinoma has not been adequately studied. In a case report of tubular adenosis identified in association with adenoid cystic carcinoma of the breast, comparative genomic hybridization demonstrated several gross copy number changes within the component of tubular adenosis, suggesting genomic instability of unknown significance.[31]

Differential Diagnosis

The differential diagnosis of adenosis and its variants includes invasive carcinoma, particularly well-differentiated carcinoma such as tubular carcinoma, and carcinoma in situ (lobular or ductal) involving adenosis.

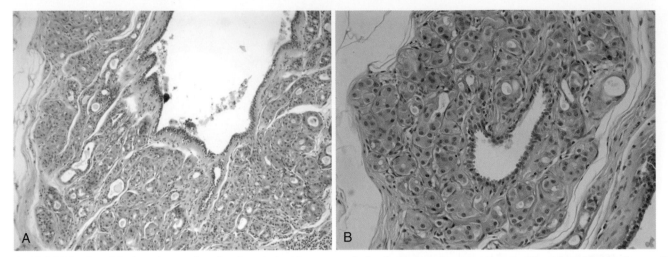

FIGURE 14-32 **A** and **B,** Apocrine cytology in adenosis. In this case, small glands of adenosis surround ducts. The cells making up the small glands have abundant eosinophilic cytoplasm and round dark nuclei, with some obliteration of lumina.

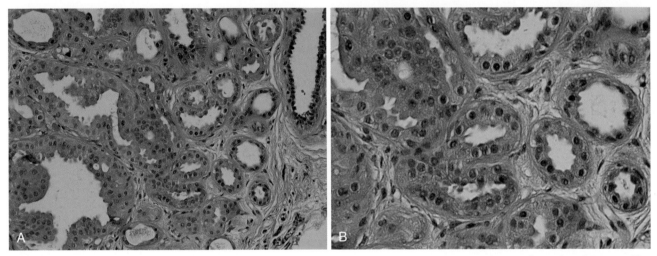

FIGURE 14-33 **A,** Apocrine cytology in adenosis. The cells forming the ductules have eosinophilic cytoplasm and round nuclei. Some dilated glands to the left of the image show epithelial hyperplasia. **B,** The apocrine cells have abundant eosinophilic cytoplasm, round nuclei, and small, mostly single, nucleoli.

Sclerosing adenosis can mimic invasive carcinoma, ductal or lobular, both at low-power and at high-power examination. At low power, sclerosing adenosis can have an infiltrative appearance, particularly when it extends into adjacent adipose tissue. The often swirling proliferation of small cells can also be mistaken for invasive lobular carcinoma. This can be especially problematic on needle core biopsy, which can make the lobulocentric distribution more difficult to identify than on resection specimens. At high power, sclerosing adenosis can be confused with invasive carcinoma when the lobules become compressed with epithelial atrophy, imparting the appearance of single cells. Ultrastructural analysis of sclerosing adenosis and tubular carcinoma shows significant differences between the two lesions, including prominent, often multilayered myoepithelial cells and basal lamina in the former and absent myoepithelial cells and prominent microvilli in the latter.[32]

Atypical ductal and lobular hyperplasia and in situ carcinoma (ductal or lobular) may involve adenosis. These proliferations can be difficult to distinguish from invasive carcinoma when expansile growth suggests a solid sheet of tumor cells or when small ductules involved by the cytologically abnormal cells of in situ carcinoma appear to infiltrate surrounding stroma or adipose tissue. These foci may be the only in situ carcinoma identified in a breast lesion or may be seen in association with carcinoma identified elsewhere.

Involvement of adenosis by LCIS is more common than involvement by DCIS.[33] When LCIS involves adenosis, the ductules are completely filled by a proliferation with characteristic features of lobular carcinoma, including dyscohesive cells with small eccentric nuclei (Figure 14-38). Signet-ring cells may also be identified, a helpful clue to the presence of involvement by a lobular proliferation. Distention of the ductules is common, but not necessary for the diagnosis, nor is involvement of all ductules in a given focus of sclerosing adenosis.[34] Architectural assessment at low power is important in the distinction from invasive carcinoma because the

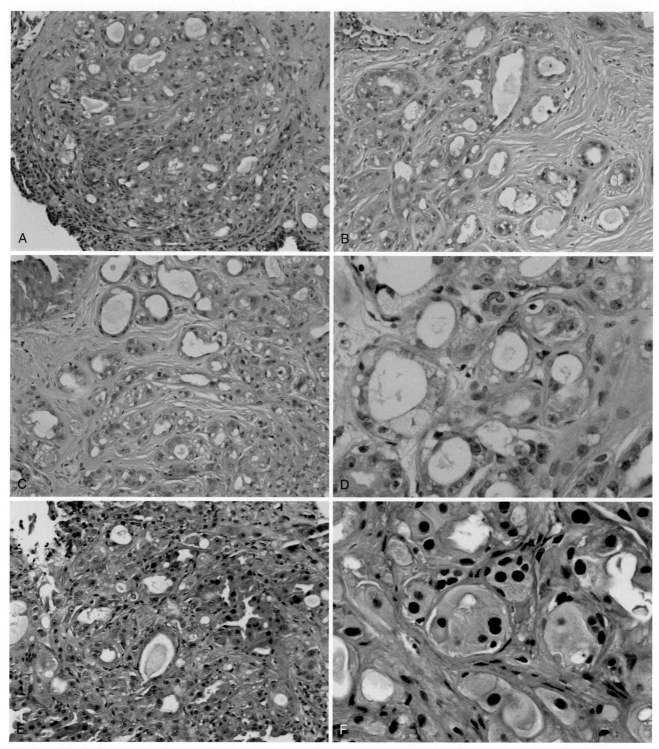

FIGURE 14-34 **A-C,** Apocrine adenosis with apocrine cytologic features and prominent cytoplasmic vacuolation. **D-F,** Atypical apocrine adenosis.

lobulocentric distribution will be preserved even when the ductules are expanded by neoplastic cells. Myoepithelial cells may be seen at the periphery of the involved ductules, but these are generally difficult to identify in these cellular lesions on routine stains. Immunohistochemical stains show a pattern similar to that seen in LCIS not involving adenosis, in which myoepithelial cells can be highlighted with usual myoepithelial

markers, and the neoplastic epithelial cells involving the ductules will not express E-cadherin (Figure 14-39).

DCIS involving adenosis maintains the same identifying architectural features as LCIS involving adenosis, but the cells filling and expanding the ductules have characteristics of DCIS, including more cytologic atypia (usually) and more prominent cell borders, along with comedonecrosis in high-grade lesions.

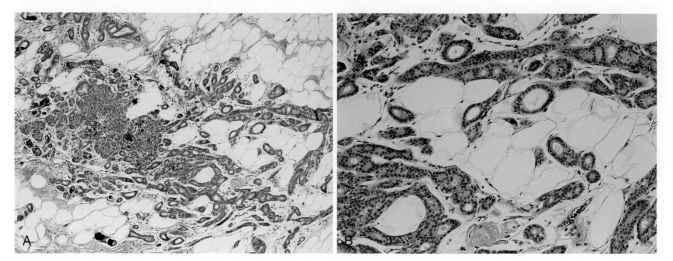

FIGURE 14-35 **A** and **B**, Tubular adenosis. Haphazard proliferation of elongated, branching tubules, many with open lumina, and associated microcalcifications.

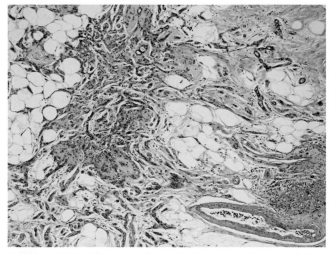

FIGURE 14-36 Tubular adenosis. Haphazard proliferation of elongated, branching tubules, many with compressed lumina, extending into adjacent adipose tissue. This example is associated with infiltrating lobular carcinoma, pleomorphic type (lower right corner of image).

Periductal elastosis, rather than randomly distributed stromal elastosis, has also been suggested as a useful feature for identifying involvement of adenosis by in situ carcinoma.[6] Calcifications may be associated with either DCIS or LCIS involving adenosis. It can be difficult to recognize invasive carcinoma in association with or arising from in situ carcinoma involving adenosis. Invasive carcinoma usually disrupts the lobulocentric architecture, but isolated cells may be difficult to identify. Eusebi and colleagues[35] studied seven cases of in situ carcinoma involving adenosis (two cases with DCIS, five cases with LCIS) and found that a continuous staining of the basement membrane with periodic acid–Schiff (PAS), along with staining of myoepithelial cells with actin, was helpful in distinguishing invasive from in situ carcinoma involving adenosis.

Tubular adenosis may be distinguished from tubular carcinoma by the shape of the ductules because tubular carcinoma tends to show angulated ductules, whereas the ductules of tubular adenosis are round or elongated. Lack of desmoplastic stroma is also a helpful feature in recognizing tubular adenosis. Preservation of the myoepithelial layer is the most helpful feature and can be demonstrated with immunohistochemical stains for SMM-HC and p63.

Blunt duct adenosis may be confused with lobular neoplasia owing to the lobular architecture and solid nests of cells. Higher-power examination shows that the cells exhibit cohesion and a less monotonous appearance than lobular neoplasia. In addition, lumen formation is not characteristic of lobular neoplasia.

Apocrine adenosis involving a sclerosing lesion can be difficult to distinguish from invasive carcinoma, owing to the overall increase in cellularity as well as the cellular enlargement characteristic of apocrine lesions. These changes are most troublesome at low power and when elastotic stroma imparts the appearance of desmoplasia. Immunohistochemical stains for myoepithelial cells should be very helpful with this differential diagnosis.

Nerve and perineural invasion has been described by benign epithelial elements consistent with adenosis. Davies[36] identified perineural invasion in 3.8% of cases studied, and Taylor and Norris[37] identified perineural invasion in 2.0% of 1000 cases of sclerosing adenosis in a series of consecutive biopsies diagnosed as sclerosing adenosis. Although not common, it is important to be aware of such lesions because subsequent surgical specimens and follow-up data from the study patients showed no evidence of invasive breast carcinoma. The explanation for this finding is not clear, although the infiltrative capacity of the epithelium in sclerosing adenosis may enable invasion of nerves as well as adjacent stroma and adipose tissue. Perineural invasion by adenosis is not thought to be related to mechanical manipulation by previous biopsy or surgery because there was very little history to support this possibility in the cases studied.[37]

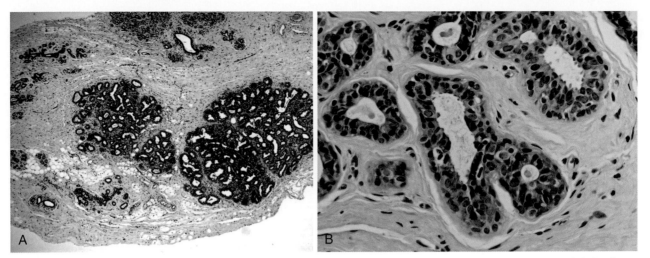

FIGURE 14-37 Blunt duct adenosis. **A,** Proliferation of small ductules. See also Figure 18-9. **B,** Prominent myoepithelial cells.

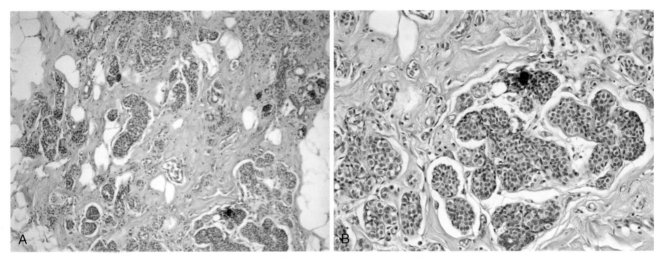

FIGURE 14-38 LCIS involving sclerosing adenosis. **A,** Proliferation of small bland cells filling and focally expanding the glands of sclerosing adenosis. **B,** The cells have a dyscohesive appearance and uniform, round central nuclei.

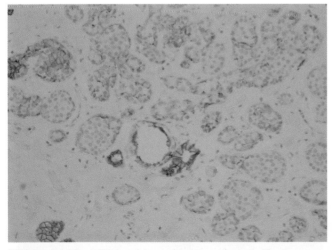

FIGURE 14-39 LCIS involving sclerosing adenosis. The immuno-histochemical stain for E-cadherin highlights residual ductal epithelial cells but is not expressed by the lobular proliferation.

Benign inclusions resembling adenosis have been identified in an axillary lymph node in a patient with invasive ductal carcinoma. The epithelial cells showed atypia with prominent nucleoli, but a distinct basal layer suggestive of myoepithelial cells was identified on routine staining.[38] Although rare, it is important to distinguish these lesions from metastatic carcinoma. This uncommon finding also argues against reliance on immunohistochemical stains for diagnosis of micrometastases in sentinel lymph node biopsies.

MICROGLANDULAR ADENOSIS

MGA is believed to have been first described by McDivitt and associates[39] as a proliferation of small glands mimicking tubular carcinoma. It is an uncommon lesion, benign in its uncomplicated form, and consisting of a proliferation of round glands composed of a single layer of epithelial cells, without an accompanying myoepithelial cell layer. This lesion is of clinical importance owing to a strong association with in situ and invasive carcinoma of the triple-negative type, necessitating thorough microscopic examination and complete excision in its management.

Clinical Presentation

MGA has been diagnosed in women with a wide age range, although they tend to be of middle age and somewhat older than women diagnosed with sclerosing adenosis. The lesion is often identified incidentally in breasts biopsied or excised for benign disease, such as fibrocystic change, but when extensive, may present as a palpable mass. The firm consistency and nodularity may be suspicious for invasive carcinoma on clinical examination. The mass may be painful and has been described as changing in size with various phases of the menstrual cycle.[40] MGA may be multifocal. Carcinoma arising in MGA usually presents as a palpable mass.

Clinical Imaging

Data are limited regarding the mammographic appearance of uncomplicated MGA. In one study of three cases, including one with a palpable mass, calcifications were the only abnormality detected, and these calcifications were detected in only one case.[41] In a case report

of carcinoma arising in MGA, mammogram showed a round, circumscribed, high-density mass containing pleomorphic calcifications. Ultrasound examination of the same lesion showed a hypoechoic mass with posterior acoustic enhancement.[42]

Gross Pathology

MGA is an infiltrative proliferation that does not have a characteristic appearance on gross examination. Breast tissue may appear normal or show an ill-defined nodularity, firmness, or mass. Reports have also described a thickening or plaquelike lesion.[40,42] Associated fibrocystic change may impart the most obvious changes seen grossly.

In cases of carcinoma arising in atypical microglandular adenosis (AMGA), Koenig and coworkers[43] described the gross appearance of cases without invasion (DCIS) as either ill defined, dense, white-tan areas without discrete masses (five cases) or a grossly apparent nodule or mass (three cases). Of the cases of invasive carcinoma arising in AMGA, there was a grossly apparent mass in 10/11 cases. In another study of carcinoma arising in MGA, there was no grossly distinct tumor in most specimens.[44]

Microscopic Pathology

MGA is composed of a poorly circumscribed proliferation of small glands that infiltrate the surrounding stroma and adipose tissue in a haphazard manner (Figure 14-40). The proliferation generally does not maintain a lobulocentric distribution, although clustering reminiscent of a lobule has been described.[45] The glands may be so closely packed that they resemble a solid sheet of small cells at low power, but distinct acini are obvious on closer inspection. The glands are round and uniform and are similar in size or slightly larger than a normal lobular acinus. The glands are composed of a single layer of cuboidal epithelial cells with vacuolated clear or eosinophilic cytoplasm (Figures 14-41 and 14-42). Examples with eosinophilic cytoplasm may also exhibit prominent apocrine cytoplasmic granularity

---

KEY CLINICAL FEATURES
Microglandular Adenosis

- Haphazard proliferation of round glands composed of a single layer of epithelial cells, without an accompanying myoepithelial cell layer.

- Uncommon lesion.

- Usually discovered incidentally, but may form a nodular mass when extensive.

- Carcinoma arising in microglandular adenosis usually presents as a mass.

- Benign when uncomplicated; carcinoma arising in microglandular adenosis may have a more favorable prognosis.

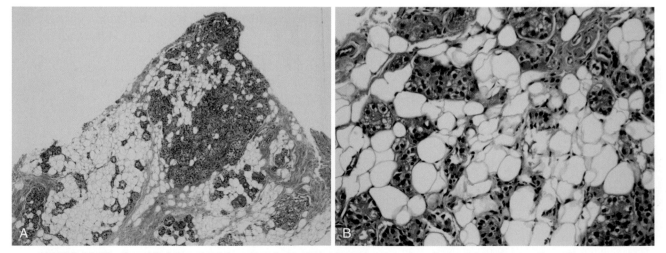

FIGURE 14-40 A and **B,** Microglandular adenosis. Haphazard proliferation of small glands into surrounding adipose tissue.

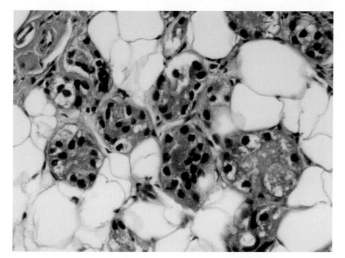

FIGURE 14-41 Microglandular adenosis. Only one cell layer is visible. Cytoplasm is amphophilic and shows prominent vacuolation.

(Figure 14-43). The nuclei are small and round with fine chromatin and inconspicuous nucleoli. Nuclear hyperchromatism and mitotic figures are absent. The lumina are generally open and often contain densely eosinophilic, PAS-positive, diastase-resistant and mucicarmine-positive secretion. A PAS or reticulin stain may also highlight the continuous basement membrane surrounding the glands, as will laminin or collagen type IV immunohistochemical stains (Figure 14-44). Myoepithelial cells are not identified on routine stains or immunohistochemical stains that highlight myoepithelial cells, such as SMM-HC or p63 (Figures 14-45 and 14-46). The luminal secretions may occasionally be basophilic and may show calcifications. The epithelial cells express cytokeratins (CKs), S100, epidermal growth factor receptor (EGFR), and cathepsin D by immunohistochemistry (Figure 14-47).[41,44] Epithelial membrane antigen (EMA) is usually negative but may show focal membranous staining and has been reported as having intense reactivity in AMGA and DCIS (Figure 14-48).[41,42,45] Gross

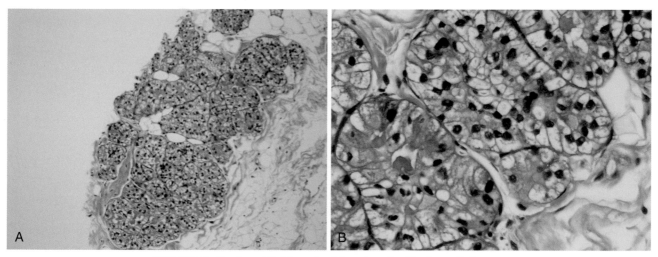

FIGURE 14-42 **A** and **B,** Microglandular adenosis with clear cell change.

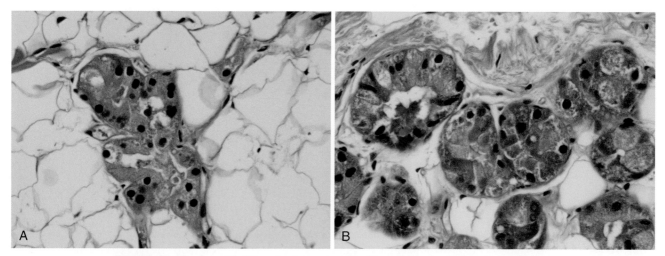

FIGURE 14-43 **A** and **B,** Microglandular adenosis with prominent cytoplasmic granularity.

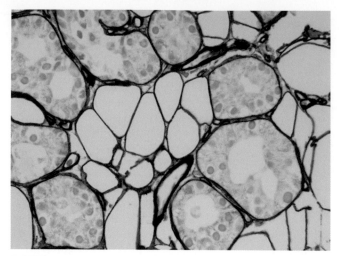

FIGURE 14-44 Microglandular adenosis. Immunohistochemical stain for collagen type IV highlights the basement membrane.

cystic disease fluid protein-15 (GCDFP-15) is negative.[45] The vast majority of MGA, AMGA, and carcinoma arising in MGA are negative for estrogen receptor (ER), progesterone receptor (PgR), and *HER2*/neu, that is, "triple negative" (Figures 14-49 and 14-50).

Fine-needle aspiration biopsy of MGA reveals sparse cellularity, with a monotonous population of medium-sized cells, vacuolated clear cytoplasm, and round uniform nuclei with small nucleoli, with no naked nuclei of myoepithelial origin in the background.[46]

A diagnosis of AMGA consists of larger, more irregularly shaped glands along with cytologic atypia, including increased nuclear size and hyperchromasia, nuclear pleomorphism, nuclear membrane irregularities, and more prominent nucleoli (Figure 14-51).[43] Increased complexity of the proliferation, including luminal bridging and some coalescence of the glands, may be identified (Figure 14-52). The glands may extend into adjacent adipose tissue, mimicking invasive carcinoma

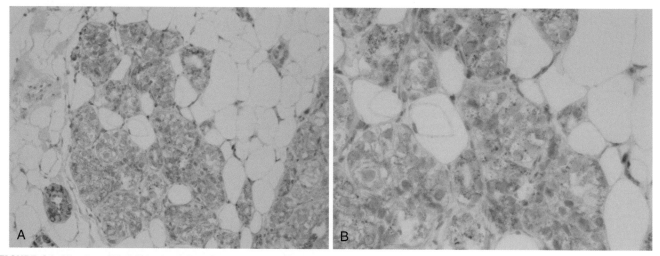

FIGURE 14-45 **A** and **B,** Microglandular adenosis. Immunohistochemical stain for p63 shows some cytoplasmic positivity, but the nuclear staining characteristic of myoepithelial cells is absent.

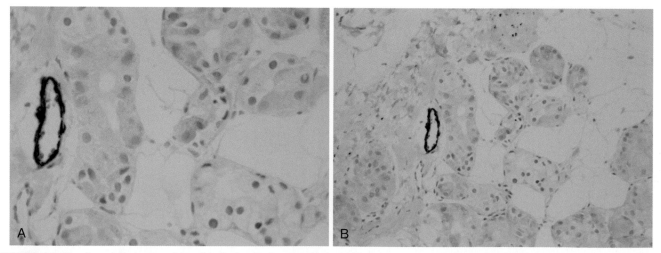

FIGURE 14-46 **A** and **B,** Immunohistochemical stain for smooth muscle myosin heavy chain (SMM-HC) is negative in microglandular adenosis.

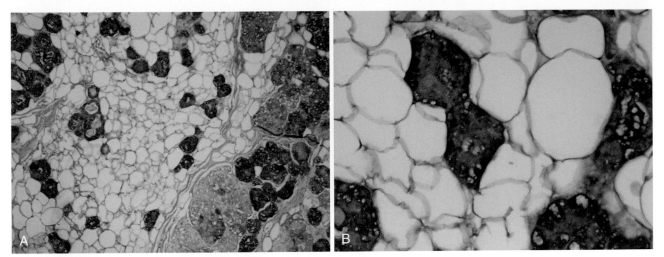

FIGURE 14-47 **A** and **B,** Immunohistochemical stain for S100 highlights the glands of microglandular adenosis.

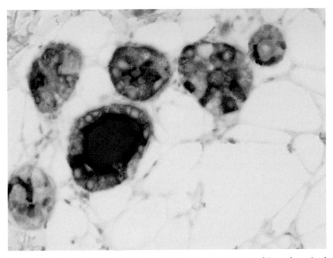

FIGURE 14-48 Microglandular adenosis. Immunohistochemical stain for epithelial membrane antigen (EMA) shows some cytoplasmic and luminal positivity, but membrane staining is not observed.

(Figure 14-53). Occasional mitotic figures may be present. DCIS arising in MGA or AMGA may be diagnosed when severe cytologic atypia, necrosis, or expansive proliferation of the cells is identified. DCIS is generally of solid type, with or without comedonecrosis, although cribriform architecture may also be observed. Residual MGA of usual type or AMGA is helpful in distinguishing DCIS from invasive carcinoma because myoepithelial cells will be absent from this lesion. A desmoplastic stromal or inflammatory response may also be present.

Invasive carcinoma arising in association with MGA is poorly differentiated and may form solid, coalescent nodules of tumor cells or small nests with an alveolar pattern. Clear cell change and cytoplasmic granularity akin to that described in uncomplicated MGA may be identified, along with cartilagenous metaplasia. Basal-like, acinic-like, sarcomatoid, and adenoid cystic patterns have also been described.[41] It can be difficult to identify the extent of carcinoma when it arises in association with MGA, because MGA often extends beyond the carcinoma.

Treatment and Prognosis

MGA is a benign proliferation, but a number of cases of carcinoma arising in MGA have been reported, suggesting a significantly increased risk for development of carcinoma in this lesion. Complete excision and close clinical follow-up of MGA and AMGA is recommended. In one report, a patient treated with breast conservation surgery for carcinoma arising in MGA developed recurrent carcinoma 10 years after incomplete resection of MGA.[42] In another, AMGA recurred as invasive carcinoma 8 years after incomplete excision of the lesion.[41] Carcinoma arising in MGA should be treated based on the stage of the carcinoma, although it has been noted that, because the lesion can extend beyond what is apparent clinically or on gross examination, mastectomy is usually necessary.[44] Carcinoma arising in association with MGA seems to have a relatively favorable prognosis, despite the high-grade features of many of the carcinomas examined, but the case numbers are somewhat small.

The association of MGA and carcinoma is well established, but it is the presence of transitional patterns, such as AMGA, that suggests MGA as a substrate

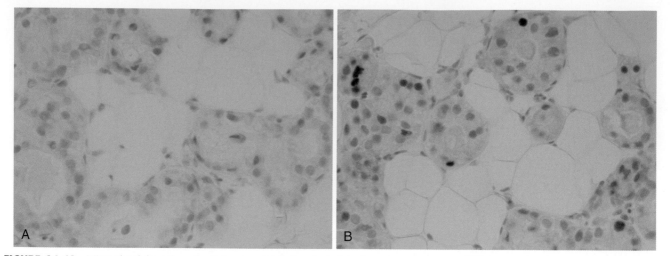

FIGURE 14-49 Microglandular adenosis. **A,** Immunohistochemical stain for estrogen receptor (ER) is negative. **B,** Immunohistochemical stain for progesterone receptor (PgR) shows focal nuclear staining.

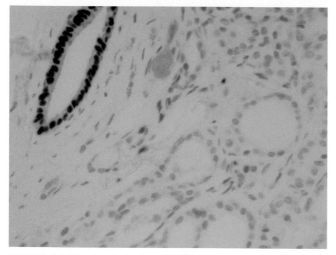

FIGURE 14-50 Atypical microglandular adenosis (AMGA): Immunohistochemical stain for ER is negative.

for the development of carcinoma.[47] In a study of carcinoma arising in MGA, 14 of 60 cases of MGA had associated carcinoma. In addition, 13 of the 14 cases showed carcinoma present in association with MGA at the time of diagnosis. This study also noted that both clinical and gross pathologic measurement of tumor size was underestimated owing to microscopic extension of MGA (both benign and involved by carcinoma) beyond the palpable and grossly visible lesion.[44] In addition to transitional patterns identified by routine histopathologic examination, molecular evidence of clonal evolution from uncomplicated MGA to invasive carcinoma also exists. In a case report of a 74-year-old woman with coexistent MGA, AMGA, and high-grade infiltrating ductal carcinoma of no special type, array comparative genomic hybridization studies performed on all three components demonstrated similar genomic profiles, including low-level copy number changes with increasing complexity in AMGA and infiltrating ductal carcinoma.[48] Shin and colleagues[49] studied 17 cases of

MGA or AMGA using laser-capture microdissection and high-resolution comparative genomic hybridization along with chromogenic in situ hybridization for MYC. Seven of 12 cases of uncomplicated MGA had copy number changes, whereas 9 of 12 cases of AMGA had copy number changes. The most common genetic alterations in uncomplicated MGA were 2q+, 5q−, 8q+, and 14q−, and the most common copy number changes in AMGA were 1q+, 5q−, 8q+, 14q−, and 15q−. This study demonstrated concordance in genetic profiles between MGA and carcinoma arising in MGA, along with strong overlap in genetic profiles from different lesions (MGA, AMGA, carcinoma in situ, and invasive carcinoma) from the same patient, with evidence of increased genetic instability in more advanced lesions.

These studies also suggested that MGA is a nonobligate precursor of breast carcinoma with a basal-like (triple-negative) phenotype, based on the results of immunohistochemical stains and studying the molecular alterations previously attributed to this phenotype. MGA, AMGA, and invasive carcinoma were ER−, PgR−, and *HER2*/neu−, and each component also showed strong expression of CK8/18, along with focal CK5/6, CK14, and CK17.[48] Expression of p53 and Ki-67 by immunohistochemistry has been variable, with some studies demonstrating variable or negative expression in uncomplicated MGA with a higher percentage of intense, uniform staining in AMGA and carcinoma arising in MGA.[41,44] More studies are needed to evaluate this connection.

Differential Diagnosis

The main differential diagnostic considerations of MGA include sclerosing adenosis and well-differentiated invasive carcinoma, such as tubular carcinoma.

MGA can be distinguished from adenosis by several histopathologic features. MGA does not generally maintain a lobulocentric distribution and infiltrates surrounding stroma and adipose tissue in a haphazard fashion. Although myoepithelial cells can be difficult

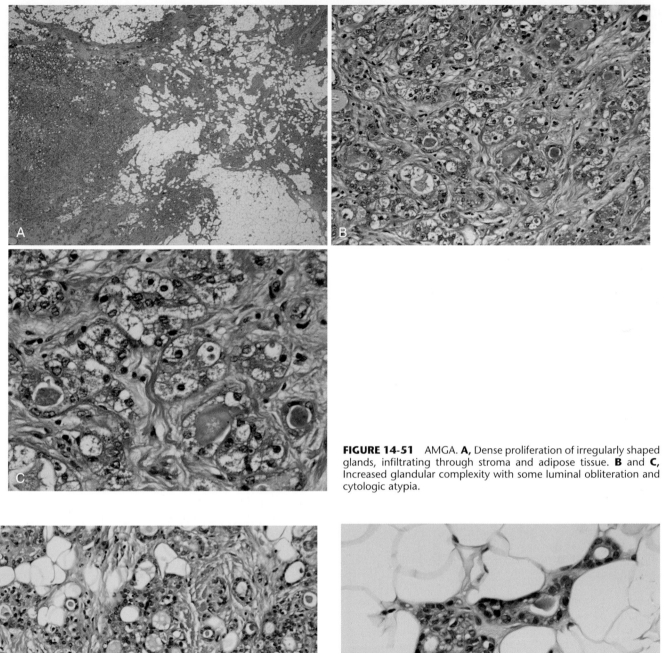

FIGURE 14-51 AMGA. **A,** Dense proliferation of irregularly shaped glands, infiltrating through stroma and adipose tissue. **B** and **C,** Increased glandular complexity with some luminal obliteration and cytologic atypia.

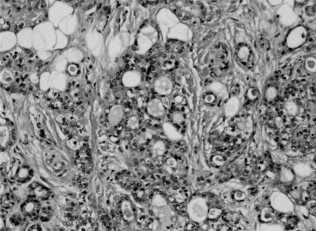

FIGURE 14-52 AMGA. Luminal bridging and coalescence of glandular structures.

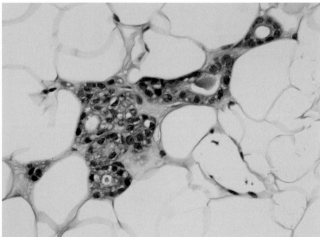

FIGURE 14-53 AMGA. Involvement of adipose tissue by glands with single cell layer and cytologic atypia.

to identify in cases of adenosis with prominent sclerosis, two distinct layers may be visible on routine stains, and immunohistochemical stains for myoepithelial cells should reveal their presence in difficult cases.

Some of the challenges previously described in distinguishing tubular carcinoma from sclerosing adenosis apply when MGA is in the differential diagnosis, with the added challenge that myoepithelial cells are absent in both tubular carcinoma and MGA. Other features, however, help to distinguish the two lesions. The glands of MGA are round, whereas the glands of tubular carcinoma are characteristically angulated and have open lumina. The epithelial cells of tubular carcinoma have at least mild nuclear atypia and pleomorphism, commonly have apical snouts, and are more likely than MGA to have amphophilic or basophilic, rather than densely eosinophilic, luminal secretions.[45] In addition, the stroma of MGA is relatively acellular, whereas the stroma involved by tubular carcinoma is cellular and often elastotic. In difficult cases, immunohistochemistry may be helpful because the epithelial cells of tubular carcinoma are positive for ER and EMA, whereas the cells of MGA are negative for these markers.

AMGA and carcinoma in situ involving MGA can be extremely difficult to distinguish from invasive carcinoma owing to the absence of myoepithelial cells, haphazard distribution, and involvement of surrounding adipose tissue. Clues to these diagnoses include uncomplicated MGA in the vicinity and demonstration of a continuous basement membrane. Using a PAS stain, Shui and Yang[50] demonstrated the lack of a continuous basement membrane in invasive carcinoma arising in MGA. This can be helpful in differentiating invasive carcinoma from AMGA and carcinoma in situ because immunohistochemical stains for myoepithelial cells do not help to differentiate in situ from invasive lesions in these cases. Determination of the extent of invasive carcinoma for staging purposes in cases with foci of uncomplicated MGA, AMGA, and carcinoma in situ can be very difficult owing to the lack of myoepithelial cells in uncomplicated MGA and more advanced lesions. Another recent case report used the Ki-67 proliferative index (PI) in an attempt to quantify the proportion of invasive carcinoma in a mass composed of uncomplicated MGA, AMGA, carcinoma in situ, and invasive carcinoma arising in MGA because the uncomplicated MGA had a PI less than 5%, AMGA had a PI ranging from 10% to 20%, and the Ki-67 stain was positive in approximately 80% of the cells in the invasive component.[51] The invasive component may also show stromal desmoplasia, a marked lymphocytic reaction, a lack of PAS-positive luminal secretions, and the glands may have a more angular contour.[51] The difficulty in assessing surgical margins in cases with in situ and invasive carcinoma as well as AMGA was addressed by Salarieh and Sneige,[52] who suggested the use of an S100 immunohistochemical stain to delineate resection margins free of the lesion.

SUMMARY

Adenosis is a common entity, presenting in a substantial number of breast samples. Challenges in discriminating adenosis and its variants from carcinoma arise in small biopsies and spindle cell cellular variants or when apocrine or neoplastic lesions involve adenosis. Immunohistology with myoepithelial cell antibodies is often discriminatory in these situations.

REFERENCES

1. Foote FW, Stewart FW. Comparative studies of cancerous versus noncancerous breasts. Ann Surg 1945;121:6-53.
2. Nielsen NS, Nielsen BB. Mammographic features of sclerosing adenosis presenting as a tumour. Clin Radiol 1986;37:371-373.
3. DiPiro PJ, Gulizia JA, Lester SC, Meyer JE. Mammographic and sonographic appearances of nodular adenosis. AJR Am J Roentgenol 2000;175:31-34.
4. Gunhan-Bilgen I, Memis A, Ustun EE, et al. Sclerosing adenosis: mammographic and ultrasonographic findings with clinical and histopathological correlation. Eur J Radiol 2002;44:232-238.
5. Heller EL, Fleming JC. Fibrosing adenomatosis of the breast. Am J Clin Pathol 1950;20:141-146.
6. Nielsen BB. Adenosis tumour of the breast—a clinicopathological investigation of 27 cases. Histopathology 1987;11:1259-1275.
7. Cho EY, Oh YL. Fine needle aspiration cytology of sclerosing adenosis of the breast. Acta Cytol 2001;45:353-359.
8. Simpson J, Page D, Dupont W. Apocrine adenosis—a mimic of mammary carcinoma. Surg Pathol 1990;3:289-299.
9. O'Malley FP, Bane AL. The spectrum of apocrine lesions of the breast. Adv Anat Pathol 2004;11:1-9.
10. Kaufman D, Sanchez M, Mizrachy B, Jaffer S. Cytologic findings of atypical adenosis of the breast. A case report. Acta Cytol 2002;46:369-372.
11. Watanabe K, Nomura M, Hashimoto Y, et al. Fine-needle aspiration cytology of apocrine adenosis of the breast: report on three cases. Diagn Cytopathol 2007;35:296-299.
12. Lee KC, Chan JK, Gwi E. Tubular adenosis of the breast. A distinctive benign lesion mimicking invasive carcinoma. Am J Surg Pathol 1996;20:46-54.
13. Bodian CA, Perzin KH, Lattes R, et al. Prognostic significance of benign proliferative breast disease. Cancer 1993;71:3896-3907.
14. Carter CL, Corle DK, Micozzi MS, et al. A prospective study of the development of breast cancer in 16,692 women with benign breast disease. Am J Epidemiol 1988;128:467-477.
15. Dupont WD, Page DL. Risk factors for breast cancer in women with proliferative breast disease. N Engl J Med 1985;312:146-151.
16. Hartmann LC, Sellers TA, Frost MH, et al. Benign breast disease and the risk of breast cancer. N Engl J Med 2005;353:229-237.
17. Hutchinson WB, Thomas DB, Hamlin WB, et al. Risk of breast cancer in women with benign breast disease. J Natl Cancer Inst 1980;65:13-20.
18. Jensen RA, Page DL, Dupont WD, Rogers LW. Invasive breast cancer risk in women with sclerosing adenosis. Cancer 1989;64:1977-1983.
19. Kodlin D, Winger EE, Morgenstern NL, Chen U. Chronic mastopathy and breast cancer. A follow-up study. Cancer 1977;39:2603-2607.
20. Krieger N, Hiatt RA. Risk of breast cancer after benign breast diseases. Variation by histologic type, degree of atypia, age at biopsy, and length of follow-up. Am J Epidemiol 1992;135:619-631.
21. Ashbeck EL, Rosenberg RD, Stauber PM, Key CR. Benign breast biopsy diagnosis and subsequent risk of breast cancer. Cancer Epidemiol Biomarkers Prev 2007;16:467-472.
22. Kabat GC, Jones JG, Olson N, et al. A multi-center prospective cohort study of benign breast disease and risk of subsequent breast cancer. Cancer Causes Control 2010;21:821-828.
23. Seidman JD, Ashton M, Lefkowitz M. Atypical apocrine adenosis of the breast: a clinicopathologic study of 37 patients with 8.7-year follow-up. Cancer 1996;77:2529-2537.
24. Carter DJ, Rosen PP. Atypical apocrine metaplasia in sclerosing lesions of the breast: a study of 51 patients. Mod Pathol 1991;4:1-5.
25. Wells CA, McGregor IL, Makunura CN, et al. Apocrine adenosis: a precursor of aggressive breast cancer? J Clin Pathol 1995;48:737-742.
26. Celis JE, Moreira JM, Gromova I, et al. Characterization of breast precancerous lesions and myoepithelial hyperplasia in sclerosing adenosis with apocrine metaplasia. Mol Oncol 2007;1:97-119.
27. Selim AG, Ryan A, El-Ayat GA, Wells CA. Loss of heterozygosity and allelic imbalance in apocrine adenosis of the breast. Cancer Detect Prev 2001;25:262-267.
28. Selim AG, El-Ayat G, Naase M, Wells CA. c-myc oncoprotein expression and gene amplification in apocrine metaplasia and apocrine change within sclerosing adenosis of the breast. Breast 2002;11:466-472.
29. Elayat G, Selim AG, Wells CA. Cell cycle alterations and their relationship to proliferation in apocrine adenosis of the breast. Histopathology 2009;54:348-354.

30. Elayat G, Selim AG, Wells CA. Cell turnover in apocrine metaplasia and apocrine adenosis of the breast. Ann Diagn Pathol 2010;14:1-7.

31. Da Silva L, Buck L, Simpson PT, et al. Molecular and morphological analysis of adenoid cystic carcinoma of the breast with synchronous tubular adenosis. Virchows Arch 2009;454:107-114.

32. Jao W, Recant W, Swerdlow MA. Comparative ultrastructure of tubular carcinoma and sclerosing adenosis of the breast. Cancer 1976;38:180-186.

33. Oberman HA, Markey BA. Noninvasive carcinoma of the breast presenting in adenosis. Mod Pathol 1991;4:31-35.

34. Fechner RE. Lobular carcinoma in situ in sclerosing adenosis. A potential source of confusion with invasive carcinoma. Am J Surg Pathol 1981;5:233-239.

35. Eusebi V, Foschini MP, Betts CM, et al. Microglandular adenosis, apocrine adenosis, and tubular carcinoma of the breast. An immunohistochemical comparison. Am J Surg Pathol 1993;17:99-109.

36. Davies JD. Neural invasion in benign mammary dysplasia. J Pathol 1973;109:225-231.

37. Taylor HB, Norris HJ. Epithelial invasion of nerves in benign diseases of the breast. Cancer 1967;20:2245-2249.

38. Chen YB, Magpayo J, Rosen PP. Sclerosing adenosis in sentinel axillary lymph nodes from a patient with invasive ductal carcinoma: an unusual variant of benign glandular inclusions. Arch Pathol Lab Med 2008;132:1439-1441.

39. McDivitt R, Stewart F, Berg J. Tumors of the Breast. Bethesda, MD: AFIP; 1968; p. 91.

40. Rosen PP. Microglandular adenosis. A benign lesion simulating invasive mammary carcinoma. Am J Surg Pathol 1983;7: 137-144.

41. Khalifeh I, Albarracin C, Wu Y, et al. Clinical, histopathologic, biologic/molecular features of microglandular adenosis with transition into in-situ and invasive carcinoma. Mod Path 2007;20(Suppl 2):38A.

42. Resetkova E, Flanders DJ, Rosen PP. Ten-year follow-up of mammary carcinoma arising in microglandular adenosis treated with breast conservation. Arch Pathol Lab Med 2003;127:77-80.

43. Koenig C, Dadmanesh F, Bratthauer GL, Tavassoli FA. Carcinoma arising in microglandular adenosis: an immunohistochemical analysis of 20 intraepithelial and invasive neoplasms. Int J Surg Pathol 2000;8:303-315.

44. James BA, Cranor ML, Rosen PP. Carcinoma of the breast arising in microglandular adenosis. Am J Clin Pathol 1993;100:507-513.

45. Clement PB, Azzopardi JG. Microglandular adenosis of the breast—a lesion simulating tubular carcinoma. Histopathology 1983;7:169-180.

46. Gherardi G, Bernardi C, Marveggio C. Microglandular adenosis of the breast: fine-needle aspiration biopsy of two cases. Diagn Cytopathol 1993;9:72-76.

47. Rosenblum MK, Purrazzella R, Rosen PP. Is microglandular adenosis a precancerous disease? A study of carcinoma arising therein. Am J Surg Pathol 1986;10:237-245.

48. Geyer FC, Kushner YB, Lambros MB, et al. Microglandular adenosis or microglandular adenoma? A molecular genetic analysis of a case associated with atypia and invasive carcinoma. Histopathology 2009;55:732-743.

49. Shin SJ, Simpson PT, Da Silva L, et al. Molecular evidence for progression of microglandular adenosis (MGA) to invasive carcinoma. Am J Surg Pathol 2009;33:496-504.

50. Shui R, Yang W. Invasive breast carcinoma arising in microglandular adenosis: a case report and review of the literature. Breast J 2009;15:653-656.

51. Lee YH, Dai YC, Lin IL, Tu CW. Young-aged woman with invasive ductal carcinoma arising in atypical microglandular adenosis: a case report. Pathol Int 2010;60:685-689.

52. Salarieh A, Sneige N. Breast carcinoma arising in microglandular adenosis: a review of the literature. Arch Pathol Lab Med 2007;131:1397-1399.

Nipple Adenoma (Florid Papillomatosis of the Nipple)

Sandra J. Shin

INTRODUCTION

An uncommon variant of intraductal papilloma that involves the nipple, florid papillomatosis was first described as a clinicopathologic entity in 1955 by Jones.[1] Alternative terms for this entity include "nipple adenoma,"[2-4] "erosive adenomatosis,"[5-9] "syringomatous adenoma," "superficial papillary adenomatosis,"[10] and "papillary adenoma."[11] The spectrum of clinicopathologic features related to its unique location and heterogenous histopathology make florid papillomatosis of the nipple a distinctive entity.

NIPPLE ADENOMA

Clinical Presentation

The nipple location as well as proliferative histopathology of florid papillomatosis gives rise to an interesting constellation of clinical manifestations. Almost all but a few examples from a supernumerary nipple originate in the nipple proper.[7,12] Nipple discharge is the most common presenting symptom and reported to occur in 65% to 70% of patients.[13] The discharge is often bloody but can also be serous or serosanguineous. Nipple discharge can be intermittent or constant with symptomatic exacerbation just prior to menses.[7,14] In some instances, a mass or discrete indurated area in or under the nipple can be visibly appreciated or palpated. On palpation, the tumor is typically adherent to the overlying skin but freely movable from the underlying breast tissue.[7] The nipple itself can appear enlarged, thickened, swollen, or rarely, retracted. In conjunction with these findings, the overlying nipple skin may be eroded, ulcerated, reddened, scaly, crusty, and/or thickened. Such dermatoses of the nipple can be misdiagnosed as eczema or inflammatory skin disorders and, thus, initially (mis)treated with topical medication. If the surface of the nipple is clinically involved, the entity is usually mistaken for Paget's disease. Alternatively, the skin can be intact but hyperplastic. In such instances when the skin's surface is intact but a tumor is evident, the clinical suspicion is that of a papillary lesion (i.e., papilloma). Patients can experience localized pain, itching, or a burning sensation. Coexisting axillary lymphadenopathy does not occur. Typically, florid papillomatosis of the nipple is not considered in the clinical differential diagnosis because even the most experienced clinicians will see it only a few times in their professional careers.[12]

The majority of patients are women who are in their fifth decade of life at the time of diagnosis.[15,16] However, florid papillomatosis of the nipple has been reported to occur in younger patients in their first decade of life[6,17] as well as older patients including an 89-year-old woman.[18] This tumor uncommonly arises in men (<5%), and in a minority of these cases, coexistent invasive and/or in situ duct carcinoma has been reported arising within florid papillomatosis.[19,20] There is one report of a man developing florid papillomatosis after long-term treatment with diethylstilbestrol for prostatic carcinoma.[21]

There is no predisposition in laterality. Bilateral or incidental cases are rare.[15,19,22,23] Most individuals seek medical attention shortly (months) after developing clinical symptoms; however, some patients harbor the lesion for many (>10) years.[8,14,19] Patients who present with nipple ulceration or erosion are more likely to seek medical attention sooner owing to the alarming nature of the symptoms. Likewise, clinicians are more suspicious of a malignancy (i.e., Paget's disease) when patients present in this fashion.

The etiology of florid papillomatosis is unknown and largely understudied. Possible causes such as trauma has been entertained but are not confirmed.[24] The overall incidence of florid papillomatosis of the nipple in the general population as well as in patients with breast cancer is unknown.[2] Furthermore, this entity has not been found to be a proven risk factor in the development of carcinoma or more frequently found in those with a family history of breast cancer.

The coexistence of florid papillomatosis of the nipple and ipsilateral or contralateral mammary carcinoma has been reported in retrospective studies of breast specimens performed for carcinoma and range in frequency from 1.2% to 16.5% in these studies.[15,16,19,25,26] These tumors were found to occur independently with sufficient distance and intervening breast parenchyma.

Even more uncommon is the occurrence of carcinoma arising from preexisting florid papillomatosis of the nipple. To date, there are eight reported such cases, three of which occurred in men.[4,19,20,27] The apparently high frequency of carcinoma associated with florid papillomatosis in men is most likely due to their shared predisposition to arise in the central, subareolar region of the breast, and as such, the notion that florid papillomatosis has precancerous potential in men has not been substantiated. Interestingly, all of these patients had invasive or in situ carcinoma exclusively of the ductal type with or without concurrent Paget's disease. An occasional case of closely approximated florid papillomatosis with severely atypical duct hyperplasia and invasive duct carcinoma has been also reported.[2]

Clinical Imaging

A tailored imaging evaluation with multiple modalities may be necessary to accurately diagnose an abnormality of the nipple-areolar complex. Owing to x-ray overpenetration, the nipple-areolar complex can be poorly depicted on conventional mammograms, and supplemental mammographic views with spot compression and magnification are often needed. In fact, several reports of this entity state that mammogram done at the time of workup showed no abnormalities.[28] If visible, a circumscribed nodule with a smooth margin can be seen in the nipple in some cases.[29] By ultrasound, a hypoechoic nodule with or without posterior echo enhancement can be seen.[30,31] Contrast-enhanced magnetic resonance imaging (MRI) may be further employed in cases for which there is substantial suspicion of undiagnosed malignancy. In particular, MRI is useful in distinguishing extent of involvement limited to the retroareolar tissue or into (or arising from) the nipple-areolar complex.[30] MRI findings of florid papillomatosis of the nipple have not been well described.[29,32] Owing to the varying histologic components of this entity, the findings by MRI can be heterogeneous. By one report, early rim enhancement with prolonged strong rim enhancement on dynamic contrast-enhanced images was observed and thought to correlate with the presence of vessels and fibrosis.[29] However, rim enhancement is not specific for florid papillomatosis of the nipple because it can also be seen in invasive carcinomas with some frequency. In addition, MRI has been described to show early enhancement with washout of the internal portion in rare cases.[32] Needless to say, additional radiologic-histologic correlative studies are needed to better define the imaging features of this entity.

Gross Pathology

On cut section, a mass is appreciated in most cases. Mass-forming examples have been described as firm, solid, or rubbery with cut surfaces that are white or variations of white (yellow, gray).[23,29,33] The tumor is characteristically unencapsulated.[33] The surface of the tumor can be uneven and the tumor borders are usually ill-defined.[33] Gross tumor sizes have reportedly ranged from 0.5 cm to 4.0 cm in greatest dimension.[7,12,34]

Microscopic Pathology

Florid papillomatosis of the nipple is characteristically a proliferative lesion in which the proliferative component is in the form of papillary duct hyperplasia and/or adenosis. The lesion is composed of two layers, an epithelium and a myoepithelium, both of which can be demonstrated by immunohistochemistry. Secondary sclerosis may or may not be present in any individual example. In cases of marked sclerosis, the distortion of participating glands ensues that can lead to the appearance of a pseudoinvasive growth pattern. In most cases, the surface squamous epithelium is in continuity with the columnar epithelium of lesional cells and can even be seen within superficially located squamous cysts.[18]

An effort has been made to subclassify this lesion into histologic subgroups, namely sclerosing papillomatosis, papillomatosis, adenosis, and mixed proliferative patterns.[19] There is no known relationship among these histologic subtypes to specific prognoses and/or pathogenesis. Nevertheless, it has been noted that the clinical presentation of lesions with the sclerosing papillomatosis pattern is distinctive from the other subgroups in that a discrete tumor in the nipple and serous nipple discharge were common signs and symptoms whereas ulceration is infrequent. The clinical suspicion in this subgroup is usually that of a papilloma and not Paget's disease.[19,35]

Papillary duct hyperplasia can be exuberant with or without distortion due to concurrent surrounding stromal proliferation (Figure 15-1). The proliferative process can be arranged in papillary, solid-papillary, and/or glandular structures (Figure 15-2). As with other benign ductal proliferations, the myoepithelial layer can be focally hyperplastic, and at other times, if located in a particularly sclerotic area, can be attenuated or even focally absent by immunohistochemistry. When florid, some ducts involved by papillary duct hyperplasia contain focal central necrosis and/or epithelial mitoses (Figure 15-3). These features are not to be considered "atypical" and likely attributable to the characteristically proliferative nature of this lesion. However, such features may lead to a misdiagnosis of carcinoma by the inexperienced. Squamous cysts and/or apocrine metaplasia can also be present in association with this entity (Figure 15-4). Hyperplastic glandular tissue may replace the squamous epithelium overlying the nipple's skin surface. In other cases, the overlying epidermis can show squamous hyperplasia.

An adenomatous pattern can be the dominant characteristic in cases in which papillary duct hyperplasia is less prominent. Typically, adenosis is seen as closely packed but orderly arranged glandular structures (Figure 15-5).

Concurrent hyperplasia of the myoepithelium is not uncommon. Peripherally located lesional glands can exhibit a syringomatous appearance in rare cases.[19] More commonly than not, the proliferative growth pattern of any individual case is composed of a mixture of papillary duct hyperplasia and adenosis (Figure 15-6).

Identifying intraductal carcinoma in florid papillomatosis of the nipple can be problematic. The difficulty lies in the fact that epithelial hyperplasia is a common feature of any individual case, and when sufficiently florid, these areas can exhibit cytologic atypia with associated epithelial mitoses and/or luminal necrosis that can be mistaken for intraductal carcinoma. The ductal hyperplasia can also exhibit cribriform or micropapillary patterns, which further raise the suspicion of atypia or carcinoma. Immunostains for myoepithelial markers may be of some value in detecting intraductal carcinoma arising in florid papillomatosis in instances of absent or weak attenuated staining in the former; however, importantly, a similar staining pattern can be seen in heavily sclerotic areas of usual florid papillomatosis (Figure 15-7). The presence of concurrent invasive carcinoma and/or Paget's disease greatly aids in this diagnostic dilemma (Figure 15-8). As discussed in greater detail elsewhere (see Chapters 11 and 27), various immunostains such as those against cytokeratin 7 (CK7), estrogen receptor (ER), and/or *HER2*/neu can help detect Paget's cells in the overlying epidermis of the nipple. Neither invasive nor in situ lobular carcinoma has been reported to have arisen in preexisting florid papillomatosis of the nipple, although the reason for this is uncertain, because the latter, in particular, is known to arise from or involve other benign epithelial proliferative lesions in the breast such as sclerosing adenosis or papillomas with reasonable frequency.

Florid papillomatosis of the nipple has been rarely studied by molecular techniques. Manavi and colleagues[13] studied 10 examples by polymerase chain reaction (PCR) and dot-blot hybridization and confirmed the absence of low-, intermediate-, and high-risk human papillomavirus (HPV) (6/11,16,18) as well as weak c-cerbB-2 protein expression in all cases.

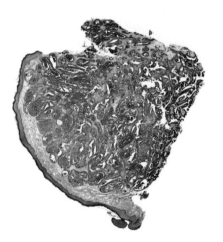

FIGURE 15-1 Florid papillomatosis of the nipple with a predominantly papillary and solid-papillary growth pattern. The overlying skin is spared from this proliferative process.

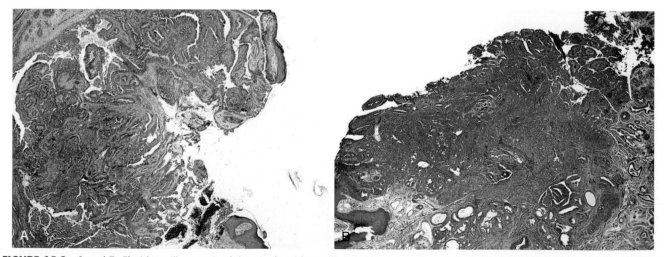

FIGURE 15-2 **A** and **B,** Florid papillomatosis of the nipple with papillary and solid-papillary growth patterns with involvement and erosion of the overlying skin.

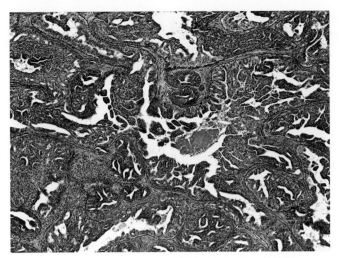

FIGURE 15-3 Central necrosis and/or epithelial mitoses are not atypical features when found in florid papillomatosis of the nipple.

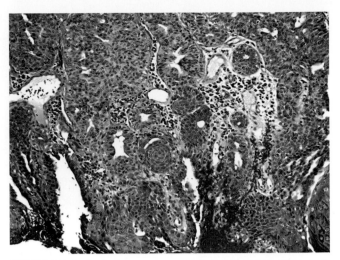

FIGURE 15-4 Foci of squamous metaplasia in florid papillomatosis of the nipple.

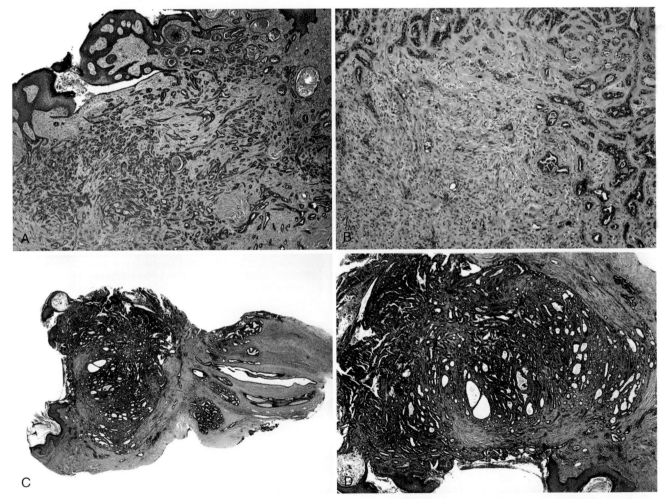

FIGURE 15-5 **A,** Florid papillomatosis of the nipple demonstrates an adenosis growth pattern with notable stromal sclerosis. **B,** Higher magnification shows foci of squamous metaplasia. **C,** Another example with a predominantly adenosis architectural pattern and ulceration of the overlying skin. **D,** Higher magnification shows areas of stromal sclerosis within this proliferative lesion.

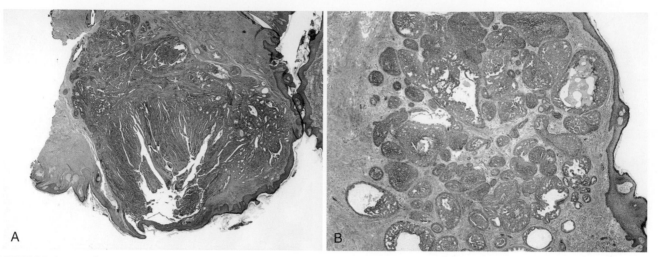

FIGURE 15-6 **A** and **B,** Most examples of florid papillomatosis of the nipple show a mixed proliferative growth pattern with varying degrees of papillary duct hyperplasia and adenosis.

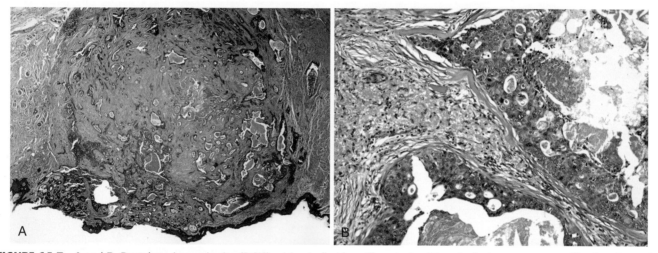

FIGURE 15-7 **A** and **B,** Ductal carcinoma in situ (DCIS) arising in florid papillomatosis of the nipple. Low-power magnification shows the overall structure of florid papillomatosis of the nipple with a predominant adenosis pattern and significant stromal sclerosis. However, higher magnification reveals cytologically malignant glands with central necrosis. Myoepithelial immunostains demonstrated the presence of an intact myoepithelium around neoplastic glands (not shown).

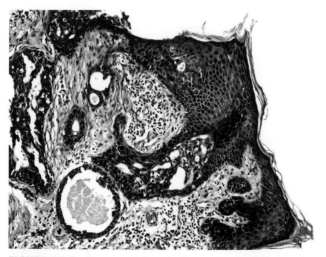

FIGURE 15-8 Concurrent Paget's disease was identified in the example in Figure 15-7.

Treatment and Prognosis

Simple, complete excision constitutes definitive treatment and usually requires removal of the nipple in larger lesions.[36] Earlier attempts to extirpate only the tumor have led to damaged lactiferous ducts or a misshapen nipple.[23] Several reports in the literature describe adequate surgical treatment with conservation of the nipple.[36,37] An alternative method using cryosurgery has been described.[28,38] For clinically early cases, Mohs' microsurgery can lead to complete removal as well as minimize deformation of the remaining portions of the nipple.[28,39,40] In children, enucleation or local excision with preservation of the main lactiferous duct has been found to provide sufficient treatment.[33] As a general rule, the extent of local surgery should be predicated on the size of the tumor to be excised.[3] Although local recurrence of florid papillomatosis may occur after incomplete excision,[16,41] many patients experience

KEY PATHOLOGIC FEATURES
Nipple Adenoma

- **Gross:** Firm, unencapsulated mass with variably defined tumor borders. Cut surface is typically some variation of white.

- **Microscopic:** Predominantly composed of papillary duct hyperplasia or adenosis with varying degrees of sclerosis. A mixture of these two patterns is common.

- **Immunohistochemistry:** Epithelial and myoepithelial markers highlight respective layers in this benign proliferative lesion.

- **Other special studies:** None.

- **Differential diagnosis:** Papilloma, subareolar sclerosing duct hyperplasia, syringomatous adenoma, adenomyoepithelioma, low-grade adenosquamous carcinoma, sweat gland tumors (syringadenoma papilliferum, hidradenoma papilliferum).

an asymptomatic postoperative course. Mastectomy should be reserved for only those clinical scenarios in which concurrent carcinoma is present.

Differential Diagnosis

Arriving at the correct diagnosis relies heavily upon the size of the biopsy material that is being histologically interpreted. A skin punch or incisional wedge biopsy is commonly employed as an initial diagnostic procedure. Although the diagnosis of florid papillomatosis can be made on such limited material, the possibility of carcinoma arising in the lesion cannot be excluded with certainty. Some instances of initial sampling by fine-needle aspiration have reported the advantages of such a modality in recognizing the benignity of this lesion, which subsequently prevented unnecessary and overaggressive surgery.[42]

Morphologically, this entity should be distinguished from papilloma, adenomyoepithelioma, subsclerosing duct hyperplasia, adenosis tumor, syringomatous adenoma, and low-grade adenosquamous carcinoma. Dermatologic entities such as hidradenoma papilliferum and syringadenoma papilliferum should also be considered.[18,24] Immunohistochemical stains per se are not useful in making the primary diagnosis of florid papillomatosis but can be of value in diagnosing (or excluding) carcinoma arising in this entity.

Direct connection and transition with the overlying epidermis of the nipple is a helpful clue that distinguishes florid papillomatosis from morphologic mimics, particularly papillomas, adenomyoepithelioma, subsclerosing duct hyperplasia, and adenosis tumor, which do not grow in this fashion. Like florid papillomatosis, low-grade adenosquamous carcinoma can show squamous differentiation including keratin cysts; however, it more commonly arises in the peripheral breast parenchyma rather than the central, retroareolar/nipple region. In a study comparing florid papillomatosis with sweat gland tumors, it was found that the presence of superficial keratocysts, intraluminal giant cells, intraductal papillomatosis, and the absence of thin or broad papillae were

particularly supportive of the former.[18] In contrast, the epithelial hyperplasia in sweat gland tumors rarely mimicked florid papillomatosis. In syringadenoma papilliferum, the epithelial hyperplasia was prominent but only as a lacelike network bridging adjacent papillae, whereas in hidradenoma papilliferum, this feature was uncommon.[18] Examples of florid papillomatosis with a predominant adenomatous pattern could resemble that of syringadenoma papilliferum.[34] Finally, single cells may spill into the overlying epidermis in florid papillomatosis of the nipple. These should not be mistaken for Paget's cells, although they are CK7+. Careful microscopic examination will reveal that the cells are not cytologically malignant, do not contain mucin, and will typically be negative with *HER2* by immunohistochemistry, whereas 80% of Paget's cells will be *HER2* 3+ by immunohistochemistry.

SUMMARY

The nipple adenoma/florid papillomatosis of the nipple is a rare lesion that must not be mistaken for duct carcinoma or papillary carcinoma. Excision alone is curative, and there is no currently known risk factor for development of carcinoma, although occasionally the lesion may be associated with severe atypia or carcinoma.

REFERENCES

1. Jones DB. Florid papillomatosis of the nipple ducts. Cancer 1955;8:315-319.
2. Jones MW, Tavassoli FA. Coexistence of nipple duct adenoma and breast carcinoma: a clinicopathologic study of five cases and review of the literature. Mod Pathol 1995;8:633-636.
3. Goldman RL, Cooperman H. Adenoma of the nipple: a benign lesion simulating carcinoma clinically and pathologically. Am J Surg 1970;119:322-325.
4. Gudjónsdótter A, Hägerstrand I, Östberg G. Adenoma of the nipple with carcinomatous development. Acta Path Microbiol Scand 1971;79:767-780.
5. La Gal Y, Gros CM, Bader P. L'adenomatose erosive du mamelon. Ann Anat Pathol (Paris) 1959;112:1427-1428.
6. Albers SE, Barnard M, Thorne P, et al. Erosive adenomatosis of the nipple in an eight-year-old girl. J Am Acad Dermatol 1999;40:834-837.
7. Bourlond J, Bourlond-Reinert L. Erosive adenomatosis of the nipple. Dermatol 1992;185:319-324.
8. Diaz NM, Palmer JO, Wick MR. Erosive adenomatosis of the nipple: histology, immunohistology, and differential diagnosis. Mod Pathol 1992;5:179-184.
9. Pratt-Thomas HR. Erosive adenomatosis of the nipple. J So Carolina Med Assoc 1968;64:37-40.
10. Montemarano AD, James WD. Superficial papillary adenomatosis of the nipple: a case report and review of the literature. J Am Acad Dermatol 1995;33:871-875.
11. Bashioum RW, Shank J, Kaye V, et al. Papillary adenoma of the nipple. Plastic Reconstr Surg 1992;90:1077-1078.
12. de Souza LJ, Sarker SK, Chinoy RF. Adenoma of the nipple. Indian J Cancer 1978;15:5-7.
13. Manavi M, Baghestanian M, Kucera E, et al. Papilloma virus and c-erbB-2 expression in diseases of the mammary nipple. Anticancer Res 2001;21:797-803.
14. Taylor HB, Robertson AG. Adenomas of the nipple. Cancer 1965;18:995-1002.
15. Handley RS, Thackray AC. Adenoma of nipple. Br J Cancer 1962;15:187-194.
16. Perzin KH, Lattes R. Papillary adenoma of the nipple (florid papillomatosis, adenoma, adenomatosis): a clinicopathologic study. Cancer 1972;29:997-1009.

17. Miller G, Bemier L. Adenomatose erosive du mamelon. Can J Surg 1965;8:261-266.
18. Brownstein MH, Phelps RG, Magnin PH. Papillary adenoma of the nipple: analysis of fifteen new cases. J Am Acad Dermatol 1985;12:707-715.
19. Rosen PP, Caicco JA. Florid papillomatosis of the nipple: a study of 51 patients, including nine with mammary carcinoma. Am J Surg Pathol 1986;10:87-101.
20. Burdick C, Rinehart RM, Matsumoto T, et al. Nipple adenoma and Paget's disease in a man. Arch Surg 1965;91:835-838.
21. Waldo ED, Sidhu GS, Hu AW. Florid papillomatosis of the male nipple after diethystilbesterol therapy. Arch Pathol 1975;99:364-366.
22. Kono S, Kurosumi M, Simooka H, et al. Nipple adenoma found in a mastectomy specimen: report of a case with special regard to the proliferation pattern. Breast Cancer 2007;14:234-238.
23. Bergdahl L, Bergman F, Rais O, et al. Bilateral adenoma of nipple. Acta Chir Scand 1971;137:583-586.
24. Higginbotham LH, Mikhail GR. Erosive adenomatosis of the nipple. J Dermatol Surg Oncol 1986;11:514-516.
25. Fisher ER, Gregorio RM, Fisher R, et al. The pathology of invasive breast cancer: a syllabus derived from findings of the National Surgical Adjuvant Breast Project (Protocol No. 4). Cancer 1975;36:1.
26. Nichols FS, Dockerty MD, Judd ES. Florid papillomatosis of the nipple. Surg Gynecol Obstet 1958;107:474.
27. Bhagavan BS, Patchefsky A, Koss LG. Florid subareolar duct papillomatosis (nipple adenoma) and mammary carcinoma: report of three cases. Hum Pathol 1973;4:289-295.
28. Lee H-J, Chung K-Y. Erosive adenomatosis of the nipple: conservation of nipple by Mohs micrographic surgery. J Am Acad Dermatol 2002;47:578-580.
29. Matsubayashi RN, Adachi A, Yasumori K, et al. Adenoma of the nipple: correlation of magnetic resonance imaging findings with histologic features. J Comput Assist Tomogr 2006;30:148-150.
30. Da Costa D, Taddese A, Cure ML, et al. Common and unusual diseases of the nipple-areolar complex. Radiographics 2007;27:S65-S77.
31. Fornage BD, Faroux MJ, Pluot M, et al. Nipple adenoma simulating carcinoma: misleading clinical, mammographic, sonographic and cytologic findings. J Ultrasound Med 1991;10:55-57.
32. Buadu AA, Buadu LD, Murakami J, et al. Enhancement of the nipple-areolar-complex on contrast-enhanced MR imaging of the breast. Breast Cancer 1998;5:285-289.
33. Sugai M, Murata K, Kimura N, et al. Adenoma of the nipple in an adolescent. Breast Cancer 2002;9:254-256.
34. Doctor VM, Sirsat MV. Florid papillomatosis (adenoma) and other benign tumors of the nipple and areola. Br J Cancer 1970;25:1-9.
35. Healy CE, Dijkstra B, Walsh M, et al. Nipple adenoma: a differential diagnosis for Paget's disease. Breast J 2003;9:325-326.
36. Sadanaga N, Kataoka A, Mashino K, et al. An adequate treatment for the nipple adenoma. J Surg Oncol 2000;74:171-172.
37. Ku B-S, Kwon O-E, Kim D-C, et al. A case of erosive adenomatosis of nipple treated with total excision using purse-string suture. Dermatol Surg 2006;32:1093-1096.
38. Kuflik EG. Erosive adenomatosis of the nipple treated with cryosurgery. J Am Acad Dermatol 1998;38:270-271.
39. Van Mierlo PL, Geelen GM, Neumann HA. Mohs micrographic surgery for an erosive adenomatosis of the nipple. Dermatol Surg 1998;24:681-683.
40. Kowal R, Miller CJ, Elenitsas R, et al. Eroded patch on the nipple of a 57-year-old woman. Arch Dermatol 2008;144:933-938.
41. Lewis HM, Ovitz MC, Golitz LE. Erosive adenomatosis of the nipple. Arch Dermatol 1976;112:1427-1428.
42. Kijima Y, Matsukita S, Yoshinaka H, et al. Adenoma of the nipple: report of a case. Breast Cancer 2006;13:95-99.

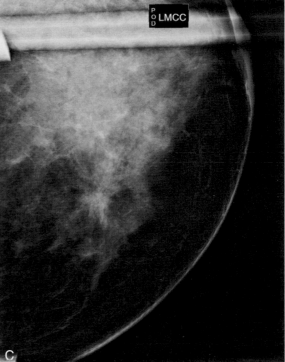

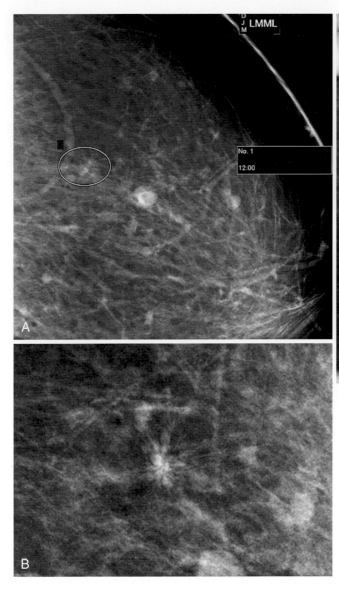

FIGURE 16-1 Mammographic features. **A,** Radial scar (RS) presents as a stellate lesion *(circle)* with indistinct borders interdigitating with surrounding fat in the mediolateral view. The center is often translucent but opacity may be seen, as shown here. **B,** A higher-magnification view shows a heterogeneous center with both density and lucency. Note that the spicules are elongated and of variable length rather than short, as is often the case in invasive cancers. **C,** This stellate lesion is well developed and measured more than 10 mm in craniocaudal view and represents an example of a complex sclerosing lesion. The center is relatively homogeneous and dense and the spicules are long and irregular.

cells and composed of elastic and collagen fibers. The "spoke" area is the one with compressed and often angulated tubular structures. The peripheral "tire" zone is not quite uniform or circumscribed and usually appears irregular, depending on the type and extent of proliferative lesions (Figure 16-3).

In the evolving RS, the axle is not present, creating a central sclerotic zone and an expanded, irregular/infiltrating peripheral zone. The key to diagnostic evaluation and reaching a correct diagnosis is to recognize this pattern at low power. Once the architectural pattern of RS is established, each of these zones can be studied more carefully at higher magnification. The central "axle" zone always shows a mixture of collagen and elastic fibers (Figure 16-4). The appearance of this sclerotic area is quite typical, with collagen tissue being hypocellular and intimately admixed with elastic fibers. The collagen is usually densely eosinophilic, very much like a well-developed scar. The elastosis takes the form of either smooth or often finely granular pale pink to light blue material in hematoxylin and eosin (H&E) sections (Figure 16-5). In tissues processed in alcohol

or rapid tissue processors, elastic fibers may appear as dense, ribbon-like, sometimes broken fibers, which most likely represent an artifact (Figure 16-6). Usually, this zone of RS lacks any inflammatory cells or vascular proliferation.

The intermediate "spoke" zone consists of either collapsed or open but compressed tubular structures. This area needs to be differentiated from invasive tubular carcinoma. The epithelial component varies from a single-file pattern to well-formed simple glands. The myoepithelial cells are often quite attenuated and difficult to recognize, raising the suspicion of well-differentiated invasive carcinoma. Although uncommon, the tubules in this zone may be associated with calcifications (Figures 16-7 and 16-8). Other changes in epithelium, such as apocrine metaplasia, or hyperplasia are not characteristic in this zone of RS. In some cases, an expanded central fibroelastotic zone abuts the peripheral zone (Figure 16-9).

In most cases, it is the epithelial proliferation in the dilated spaces in the peripheral "tire" zone that catches one's attention at scanning magnification. The periphery

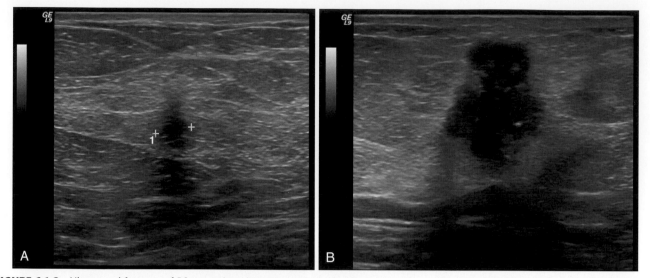

FIGURE 16-2 Ultrasound features of RS versus invasive cancer. **A,** This hypoechoic mass is taller than it is wide with very irregular borders. No internal heterogeneity in echotexture is seen. There is prominent shadowing underneath the lesion. **B,** Invasive cancer shares several sonographic features with RS, such as irregular borders and shadowing. However, in contrast, the irregular edges are short and stubby, thus giving a more rounded appearance. There is often heterogeneous echoing in invasive cancer with a few calcifications, which appear as intense white areas.

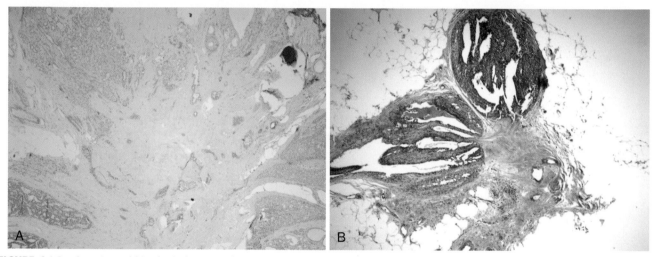

FIGURE 16-3 Overview of histologic features of RS. **A,** On low power, RS shows three zones with different histologic appearances. The central zone is mostly acellular with collagen and elastic fibers, the intermediate zone has compressed tubules, and the peripheral zone has epithelial proliferation. **B,** This microscopic RS was incidentally sampled in a core needle biopsy. Note that the central and peripheral zones are overlapping and the peripheral dilated spaces contain minimal epithelial proliferation.

of an RS interdigitates with the surrounding fatty breast stroma, enhancing its "infiltrating" appearance (Figures 16-10 and 16-11).

Some entrapment of single and small clusters of benign adipose tissue is often seen. The most common finding is simple columnar cell change involving most of the spaces, followed by variable degrees of apocrine metaplasia and columnar cell hyperplasia, with or without microcalcifications. It is important to rule out flat epithelial atypia (FEA) when columnar cell proliferation is recognized at low power (Figures 16-12 and 16-13).

Once the epithelial proliferation starts to pile up in the lumen, the suspicion of either atypical hyperplasia or in situ carcinoma rises. However, in most cases, the epithelial proliferation comprises usual ductal hyperplasia

(UDH) of variable degree. The mixed cell types, epithelial streaming, and a moderate amount of cytoplasm in these benign cells often impart a relatively hypochromatic low-power appearance (Figure 16-14).

The diagnostic criteria for atypical ductal hyperplasia (ADH) and ductal carcinoma in situ (DCIS) are similar to those used in the settings without an RS (Figure 16-15).

RS can also be seen in association with lobular neoplasia (i.e., atypical lobular hyperplasia [ALH] and lobular carcinoma in situ [LCIS]). One of the challenges is the presence of sclerosing adenosis in the peripheral zone of an RS with secondary involvement by lobular neoplasia. Close attention to typical cytologic features of lobular neoplasia cells should help in the correct identification of these lesions (Figure 16-16).

Treatment and Prognosis

The clinical management of patients who are found to have an RS can be divided into two pathways—immediate and long term. The former refers to a situation in which RS either contains an in situ or invasive cancer or the epithelial proliferation is so complex that the possibility of malignancy cannot be reliably ruled out based on a small sample, such as core needle biopsy. The long-term management becomes a concern when RS is found to have a premalignant lesion that poses increased risk of malignancy for an individual patient.

A stellate lesion seen on an imaging study prompts a core needle biopsy. Then, even a diagnosis of RS without malignancy often triggers an excisional biopsy to remove the entire abnormality to rule out any remaining possibility of cancer. However, if malignancy is found on a needle biopsy, a planned cancer surgery can

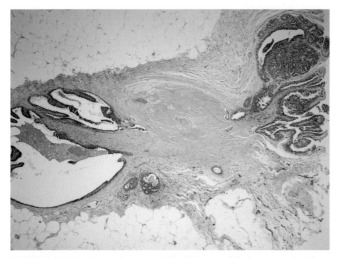

FIGURE 16-4 Central zone of RS. This small lesion sampled in a core needle biopsy displays the characteristic appearance of a central zone containing a dense collagenous core surrounded by a rim of pale blue elastic fibers.

be performed. The clinical management of RS is based on a fairly consistent body of literature showing a substantial risk associated with missing cancers, if only a needle biopsy is performed.[17,23,26–28,30,31,38] In a series of 126 cases, Sloane and Mayers[3] reported an incidence of 8% to 17% for ADH and DCIS and 1% to 6% for invasive cancer in RS. They found ADH and invasive cancer was unlikely in RS less than 6 mm in size and in patients younger than 40 years old and those older than 60 years old. They noted a higher rate of malignancy in mammographically detected RS than in the lesions found incidentally in biopsies performed for another

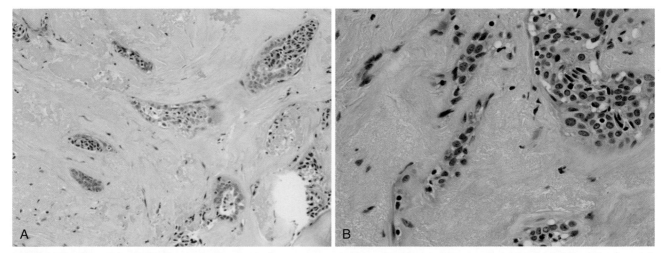

FIGURE 16-5 Elastosis in RS. **A,** The elastic fibers typically appear as pale blue, ropy fibers in hematoxylin and eosin (H&E) sections, merging into the intermediate zone containing compressed ductal structures. **B,** In certain cases, the immature elastic fibers have a granular to powdery microscopic texture.

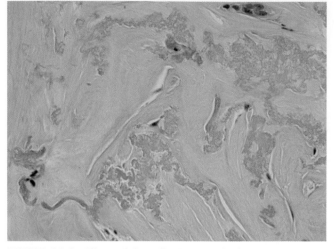

FIGURE 16-6 Effects of tissue fixation on RS. This tissue was processed on a rapid tissue processor employing microwave technology. This type of processing can make the elastic fibers appear darker and coarser than tissue processed in traditional processors.

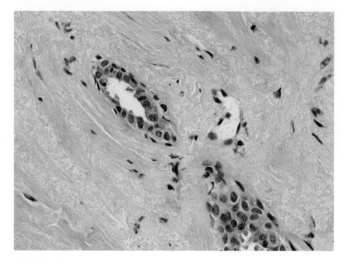

FIGURE 16-7 Intermediate zone of RS. This zone transitions from the fibroelastotic center and contains compressed tubular structures that can mimic well-differentiated invasive carcinoma. In this instance, the myoepithelial layer is obvious, which makes the distinction between RS and cancer.

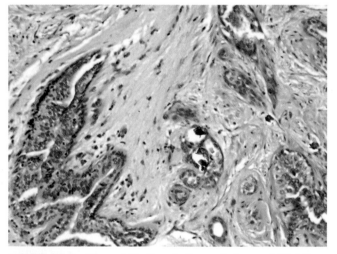

FIGURE 16-8 Microcalcifications in the central area of RS. Microcalcifications are uncommon in the trapped epithelium in the intermediate zone of RS with small tubular structures.

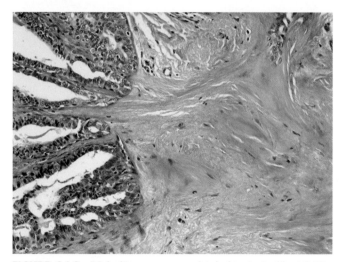

FIGURE 16-9 RS lacking compressed tubules. In incidental RSs, typically measuring less than 5 mm, it is not uncommon to see the fibroelastotic core merging with dilated ductal spaces in the periphery. These lesions can be identified in digital mammograms and can provide correlation with imaging.

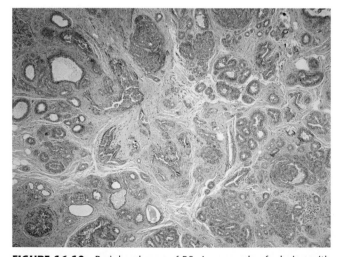

FIGURE 16-10 Peripheral zone of RS. An example of a lesion with a prominent and expanded peripheral zone with large, dilated spaces showing a wide range of proliferative lesions. Note the absence of central paucicellular core.

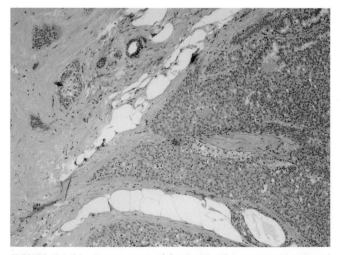

FIGURE 16-11 Entrapment of fat in RS. The peripheral zone of RS interdigitates with surrounding benign fatty breast stroma, corresponding to elongated spicules seen on mammogram.

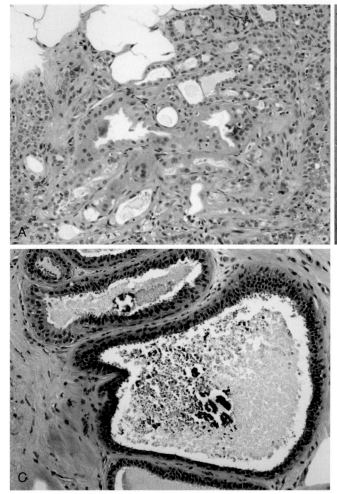

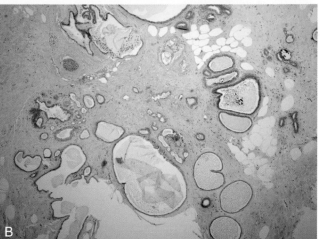

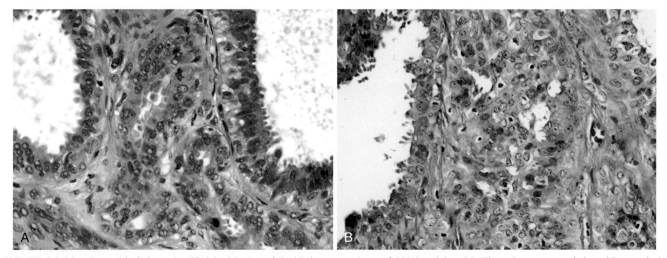

FIGURE 16-12 Benign proliferative changes in RS. The peripheral zone of RS displays a spectrum of benign proliferative changes. **A,** Apocrine metaplasia typically occurs in dilated spaces with a single layer of epithelial cells, often called *microcysts*. Sclerosing adenosis is a common finding in the peripheral zone of RS. This high-magnification view shows a combination of sclerosing adenosis and apocrine metaplasia (apocrine adenosis). **B** and **C,** Columnar cell change without atypia is one of the most common early proliferative changes in this location.

FIGURE 16-13 Flat epithelial atypia (FEA) in RS. **A** and **B,** High-power views of FEA involving RS. There is some usual ductal hyperplasia (UDH) in a nearby space.

reason, although this was partly related to the size of the lesion. These studies suggest that, in cases in which the differential diagnosis between a benign epithelial proliferation in an RS and a malignancy remains doubtful, an excision of the lesion should be considered. Conversely, a series of 80 cases studied at M.D. Anderson Cancer Center suggested that extensive sampling by

9- and 11-gauge needles, in conjunction with close correlation between imaging and pathologic findings, can spare an open surgical biopsy in the majority of patients with RS.[39]

The issue of long-term follow-up in patients with an RS without malignancy remains controversial, that is, is RS by itself a risk factor for developing breast

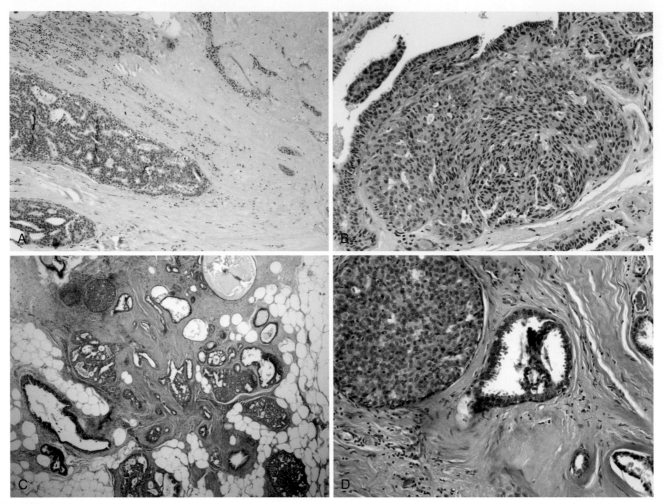

FIGURE 16-14 UDH in RS. **A,** The fibroelastosis from the central area of this RS can be seen next to a ductal space with moderate UDH. This example illustrates the mixed cell type with myoepithelial cells containing clear cytoplasm. **B,** The peripheral, irregular spaces with cellular streaming are the hallmark of UDH. **C,** A low-power view of an RS shows UDH, focally extending into the intermediate zone of the lesion. **D,** UDH appears hypochromatic compared with columnar cell hyperplasia.

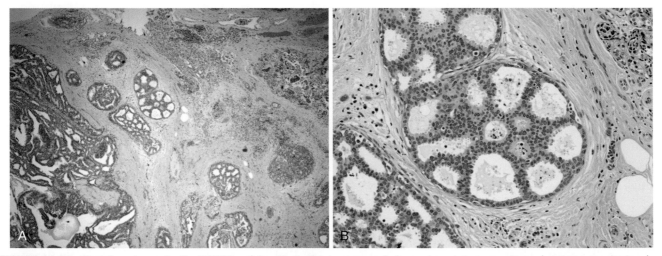

FIGURE 16-15 Ductal carcinoma in situ (DCIS) involving RS. **A,** This is an example from a lumpectomy specimen showing extensive involvement of an RS by DCIS. The *right upper corner* shows changes related to previous core needle biopsy. **B,** DCIS shows rigid cribriform architecture with monotonous cells and early cell necrosis.

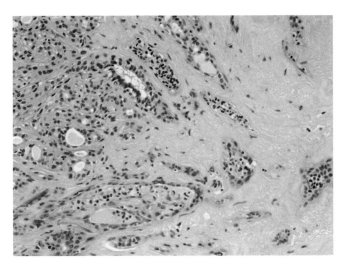

FIGURE 16-16 Lobular neoplasia in RS. This lesion shows sclerosing adenosis at the periphery with secondary involvement by atypical lobular hyperplasia (ALH).

cancer? Two small studies examined RS as a risk factor for breast cancer. Finoglio and Lattes[6] studied 54 cases, although nearly one half of them were lost to follow-up, which was only 6.3 years. They did not note an increased risk for breast cancer after finding RS in their patients. Anderson and Gram[11] reported an incidence rate of 1.7% in their database. They found that, after a follow-up of 19.5 years with 32 cases of RS, only 1 patient developed breast cancer. Both these retrospective studies concluded that RS is a benign lesion and does not require long-term follow-up after excision.

Subsequently, RS has been examined as a risk factor for breast cancer in three large databases in the United States, which are well known for studying the breast cancer risk associated with other premalignant breast lesions. In the Nurses' Health Study, Jacobs and coworkers[40] studied 1396 women followed for a median of 12 years. They reported an incidence of 7.1% and relative risk (RR) of cancer after RS as 1.8. They also found that not only was this risk independent but it was additive to the risk associated with other well-established premalignant lesions, such as ADH. Unlike the study by Sloane and Mayers,[3] they did not find any association between the risk for cancer and either the number or the size of RS. Sanders and colleagues[20] reported their experience of RS in the Nashville Breast Cohort. They reported an incidence of 9.2% and had a mean follow-up of 20.4 years. In this database, RS increased the risk of invasive breast cancer minimally (RR 1.11). It was noted that, in most cases, RS was found to be associated with other proliferative breast disease and RS by itself did not pose a significant risk for either in situ or invasive cancer. The authors suggested that, if RS is recognized in a needle biopsy, follow-up should be determined by the presence and extent of atypical hyperplasia. The third important study by Berg and colleagues[21] evaluated RS in the Mayo Clinic breast disease database. They reported an incidence of 4.7% and the mean follow-up was 17 years. Their conclusion, which was similar to that by Sanders and colleagues,[20]

was that RS did not elevate the risk of breast cancer above and beyond the presence of other proliferative breast disease. Overall, the results of these studies may appear conflicting, but it is possible that the risk imposed by RS is minimal and probably of short duration. Dupont and associates[41] have reported similar trends in the risk associated with atypical hyperplasia, which decreased or approached that of the general population with time. Therefore, it seems that it is the presence of other proliferative breast disease, in particular atypical hyperplasia, that raises concerns in long-term patient management.

In summary, if RS is found incidentally in a breast biopsy (i.e., typically ≤ 4 mm), and it is not associated with atypical hyperplasia within either the RS or the adjacent breast tissue, no excisional biopsy is needed, provided there is otherwise complete correlation between the imaging and the histologic findings. The presence of atypical hyperplasia in or outside an RS should be managed in the same fashion as cases without an RS.

Differential Diagnosis

The histopathologic assessment of stellate lesions described previously can also be used in the differential diagnoses commonly encountered in evaluation of these lesions. This includes situations in which an invasive carcinoma either mimics an RS or arises in association with an RS. Similarly, proliferative breast disease arising in or secondarily involving an RS can be systematically studied.

The main differential diagnosis of lesions mimicking or involving the central part of an RS includes well-differentiated invasive carcinomas, particularly tubular carcinoma and low-grade adenosquamous carcinoma. Most of the literature has addressed the issue of well-differentiated invasive ductal or tubular carcinoma. It is often difficult to make this distinction. The key low-power feature of invasive carcinomas, including tubular carcinoma, is lack of radial orientation of individual glands. In RS, the compressed or open small glandular spaces may have an angulated appearance, but they are fairly well aligned to each other and point out to the periphery, like the spokes in a bicycle wheel. Conversely, the glands in tubular carcinoma are haphazardly arranged. For example, if a line is drawn through the long axis of each of the glands in a carcinoma, they end up intersecting each other. Another useful feature is to look at the interface of these glands with the surrounding adipose tissue. In some cases, invasive cancer and RS occur in close proximity (Figures 16-17 and 16-18).

Invariably, cancers show individual glands infiltrating adipose tissue. Immunostains for myoepithelial markers are very useful in this differential diagnosis and resolve most cases rather easily (Figure 16-19).

Over the years, the search for a perfect marker for myoepithelial cells has remained somewhat elusive. A detailed discussion about sensitivity and specificity of such markers is beyond the scope of this chapter (see Chapter 11). In current practice, four markers are most commonly used, often in some sort of combination.

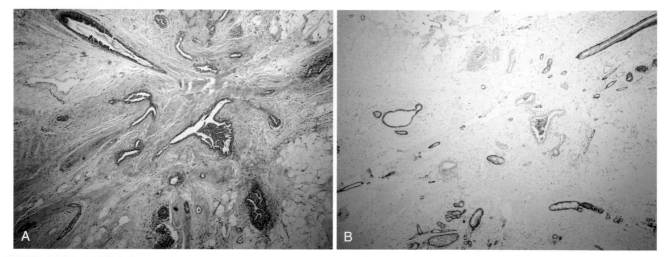

FIGURE 16-20 Pitfalls in interpreting immunostains in RS. **A,** An incidental lesion from a lumpectomy in a 53-year-old patient with an invasive ductal carcinoma, elsewhere in the specimen. Immunostains for myoepithelial cells were done to confirm the lesion as an RS. **B,** Smooth muscle myosin–heavy chain (SMM-HC) immunostain failed to highlight myoepithelial layer in some of the glands, and this was considered a second focus of invasive tumor. A close attention to histology on H&E sections shows two layers in all the ductal structures.

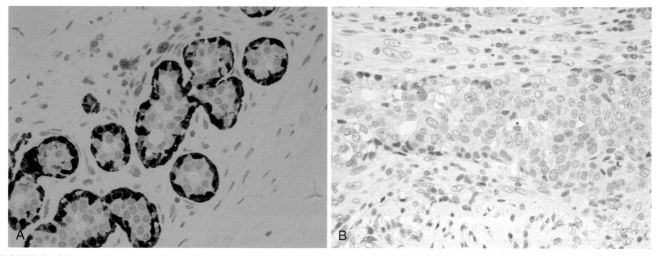

FIGURE 16-21 Use of immunostain cocktail. **A,** Some laboratories use a cocktail of p63 (brown nuclear stain) and SMM-HC (red cytoplasmic stain) in the workup. This example is from normal breast tissue. **B,** Invasive cancer lacks staining with this cocktail.

Collagen IV or laminin stains are very helpful to confirm the invasive nature of these glands in this setting (Figure 16-22).

The differential diagnoses of lesions in the peripheral zone of an RS include UDH, ADH, and DCIS. The same diagnostic criteria used to identify these lesions elsewhere in the breast also apply to these lesions in association with an RS. UDH shows swirling, pink cells with random mild polymorphism admixed with dark staining myoepithelial cells with clear cytoplasm. ADH on low power appears blue on H&E sections due to hyperchromasia of the nuclei and increased nuclear-cytoplasmic ratio. The architecture is more rigid and the cells look monotonous. Low-grade DCIS shows features similar to ADH. The recognition of high-grade DCIS is usually not problematic. Immunostains for high-molecular-weight CK or CK5/6 can be helpful in differentiating UDH from ADH or low-grade DCIS but should be interpreted with caution. UDH shows diffuse staining with a mosaic pattern, in contrast to ADH and DCIS, which tend to lack immunostaining for these markers. The other important lesions often seen with RS include columnar cell change or hyperplasia and FEA. The latter shows nuclear pleomorphism and loss of polarity, which is not seen in columnar cell change or hyperplasia. Lastly, a search for lobular neoplasia (ALH and LCIS) should be undertaken. Use of E-cadherin stain can assist in confirming the diagnosis of lobular neoplasia.

If RS is seen in a core biopsy, a careful histological review to rule out in situ or invasive cancer should be performed, in addition to reviewing the imaging studies. If any doubts remain, the pathology report should clearly document the need for an excisional biopsy.

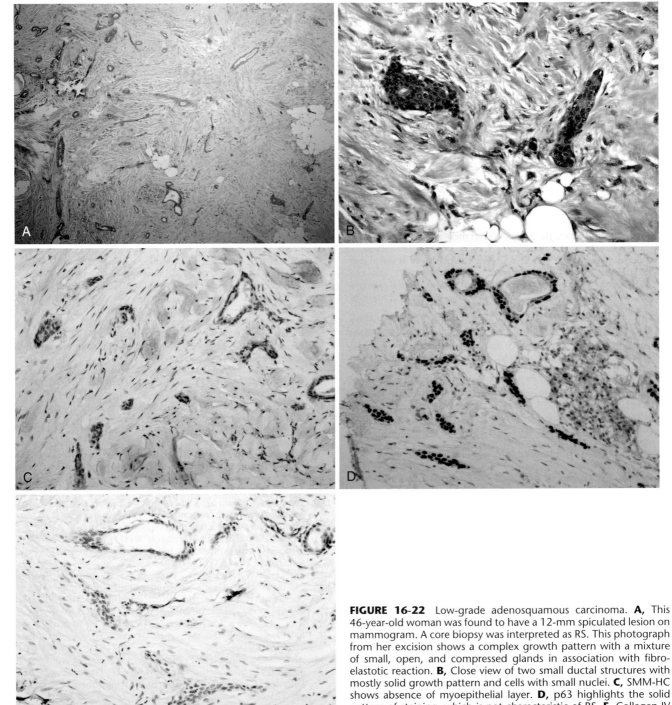

FIGURE 16-22 Low-grade adenosquamous carcinoma. **A,** This 46-year-old woman was found to have a 12-mm spiculated lesion on mammogram. A core biopsy was interpreted as RS. This photograph from her excision shows a complex growth pattern with a mixture of small, open, and compressed glands in association with fibro-elastotic reaction. **B,** Close view of two small ductal structures with mostly solid growth pattern and cells with small nuclei. **C,** SMM-HC shows absence of myoepithelial layer. **D,** p63 highlights the solid pattern of staining, which is not characteristic of RS. **E,** Collagen IV stain demonstrates lack of basal lamina. The blood vessels serve as internal controls.

SUMMARY

The diagnosis of RS can be challenging. It is imperative to be able to differentiate the small, less than 4 mm incidental RS-like lesions from the stellate lesions that patients present with on imaging. If RS is found incidentally in a breast biopsy (typically ≤ 4-mm) and it is not associated with atypical hyperplasia, no excisional biopsy is needed, provided there is otherwise complete correlation between the imaging and the histologic findings.

REFERENCES

1. Hamperl H. [Radial scars (scarring) and obliterating mastopathy (author's transl)]. Virchows Arch A Pathol Anat Histol 1975;369:55-68.
2. Page DL, Anderson TJ. Radial scar/complex sclerosing lesion. In Page DL, Anderson TJ, eds. Diagnostic Histopathology of the Breast. Edinburgh: Churchill Livingstone; 1987; pp. 112-113.
3. Sloane JP, Mayers MM. Carcinoma and atypical hyperplasia in radial scars and complex sclerosing lesions: importance of lesion size and patient age. Histopathology 1993;23:225-231.

Gross Pathology

Adenomyoepitheliomas of the breast have been well documented in the English language literature (Figure 17-1).[26] Some of these tumors are described as either myoepithelioma or leiomyosarcoma.[1,27] Yet the bulk of the English language literature indicates that adenomyoepitheliomas present as breast masses (on average 2–3 cm) in the same age range as for patients with breast carcinoma. They are firm to rubbery, generally

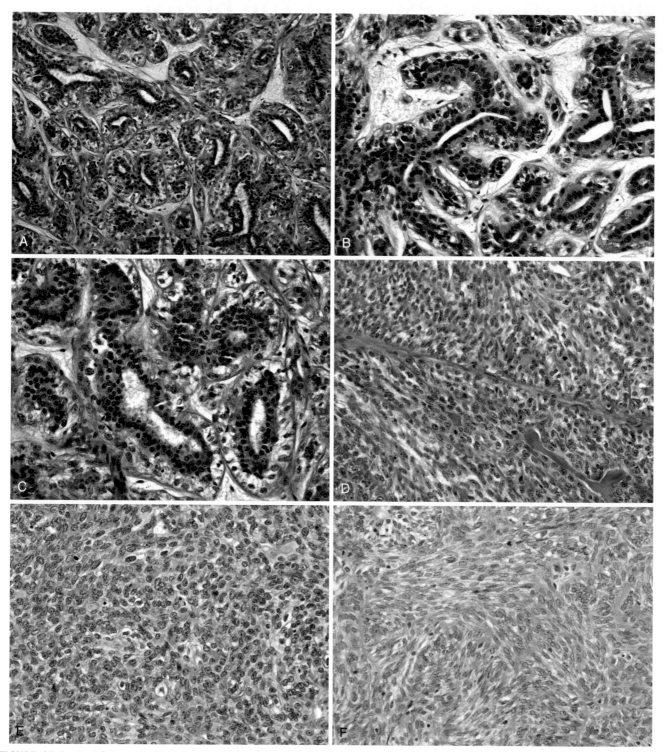

FIGURE 17-1 A, Adenomyoepithelioma, predominantly epithelial type. **B,** Higher magnification shows biphasic epithelial-myoepithelial architecture. **C,** Duct luminal epithelial cells surrounded by clear myoepithelial cells. **D,** Dispersed form of sclerosing adenosis imparts a pseudoinvasive pattern (also called tubular adenosis). **E,** Higher-power magnification of dispersed form of sclerosing adenosis. **F,** Sometimes, the myoepithelial cells of sclerosing adenosis become quite spindled.

circumscribed, but can mimic carcinoma grossly. Malignant transformation into myoepithelial carcinoma will show infiltrative borders.

Microscopic Pathology

Adenomyoepitheliomas have a biphasic cytoarchitecture composed of tubular structures lined by duct luminal epithelial cells, surrounded by myoepithelial cells that have spindle cell or polygonal cell shapes (often with clear cytoplasm). The myoepithelial cells may predominate, necrosis may be present, and mitotic activity can be brisk, measuring up to 10 mitotic figures per 10 high-power fields. Epithelial proliferation may include regions of papillary proliferation, including apocrine metaplasia. It is helpful to keep in mind that adenomyoepithelioma and intraductal papilloma represent opposite ends of a spectrum of intraductal proliferations of the breast. Malignant transformation may take the form of myoepithelial carcinoma, leiomyosarcoma, or undifferentiated overgrowth.

Treatment and Prognosis

The majority of adenomyoepitheliomas have been considered benign, but they can recur locally. Rosen[20] described 18 cases and emphasized that, in most, myoepithelial cells were polygonal and had clear cytoplasm. Myoid spindle cell differentiation was rarely prominent but was present focally in most cases. In addition, Rosen believed his cases to be benign breast tumors that could be treated adequately with complete local excision. Weidner and Levine[24] described two cases of spindle cell adenomyoepitheliomas that followed a benign course. These spindle cell tumors were well circumscribed and showed no necrosis, cytologic atypia, or mitotic activity, which suggests a benign rather than a malignant course. There was no associated adenosis, although areas of proliferative fibrocystic change were adjacent to foci of intraductal carcinoma in one case. Tavassoli's study[23] of 27 adenomyoepitheliomas confirmed that these tumors are composed of two populations of cells, tubular cells and spindled or epithelioid myoepithelial cells with clear, pink, or amphophilic cytoplasm. Only 2 of the 27 cases recurred and none metastasized; however, 9 of the 27 patients had mastectomy, 8 with excision of axillary nodes, because of an overdiagnosis of carcinoma.

However, Loose and colleagues[25] reported six cases including two malignant examples, one of which metastasized to the lung and brain after multiple local recurrences and caused death. Both malignant examples had high mitotic rates (11–14 per 10 high-power fields) and cytologically malignant cells. The metastasizing example showed the biphasic features of typical adenomyoepithelioma; the other showed spindle cell morphology in the malignant "sarcomatous" component. Another report by Van Dorpe and coworkers[28] described rare cases of adenomyoepithelioma giving rise to carcinomas with epithelial, myoepithelial, or mixed epithelial and myoepithelial differentiation. Carcinomas arising in adenomyoepithelioma range from low grade to high grade, 15 cases have been reported in the literature, and they add a 36-year-old woman with a very rare AdCC arising in a tubular adenomyoepithelioma. Moreover, Rasbridge and Millis[29] described the clinicopathologic features of 7 cases of adenomyoepithelioma of the breast with features suggestive of malignancy. There was a high incidence of local tumor recurrence in 2 cases as high-grade infiltrating carcinoma of the breast of no special type ("ductal," grade III). One patient died as the result of a clinically diagnosed cerebral metastasis. Histologic examination of the primary breast tumors reveals two main patterns: (1) tumors consisting in part of typical adenomyoepitheliomas but that merge with areas of obviously invasive malignant cells and (2) neoplasms that have the overall architecture of an adenomyoepithelioma but that, on close examination, are found to contain foci of cellular atypia and increased mitotic activity. The two patterns of tumor exhibit the same clinical behavior and should be distinguished from adenomyoepitheliomas, which are cytologically bland throughout. The authors have encountered a few of the latter, which we believe could be considered "malignant" adenomyoepitheliomas (Figures 17-2 and 17-3).

Differential Diagnosis

Because of the marked differences in tumor aggressiveness and therapy, typical adenomyoepithelioma should be clearly distinguished from the spindle cell variant of metaplastic breast carcinoma (see Chapter 25). Moreover, closely related examples of "malignant myoepithelioma" or "myoepithelial carcinoma" or "adenomyoepithelioma with undifferentiated carcinoma" are scattered throughout the literature.[18,19,23,25,30] Yet histologic, ultrastructural, and immunohistochemical features of some malignant adenomyoepitheliomas or myoepithelial carcinoma overlap greatly with those reported for the spindle cell variant of metaplastic breast carcinoma—indeed, the distinctions between these malignant entities is poorly defined, arbitrary, and not likely reproducible. As described in the subsequent discussion of spindle cell breast carcinoma, these lesions show myoepithelial differentiation, and their distinction may have more academic than practical value. A peculiar ductal carcinoma in situ (DCIS) variant has been described that is characterized by the intraductal growth of carcinoma cells having clear cell and spindle cell myoepithelial differentiation.[31]

Invasive ductal carcinoma of not otherwise specified (NOS) type lacks a spindle component, but the epithelial component of an adenomyoepithelioma with the spindle cell component can be mistaken for invasive carcinoma in a desmoplastic stroma. Adding to this pitfall, if apocrine metaplasia is present, it may exhibit immunoreactivity for *HER2*/neu.

Finally, less well developed benign myoepithelial lesions are encountered such as myoepitheliosis (periductal proliferation of eosinophilic myoepithelial cells) or adenomyoepithelial adenosis (periductal proliferation of clear myoepithelial cells).

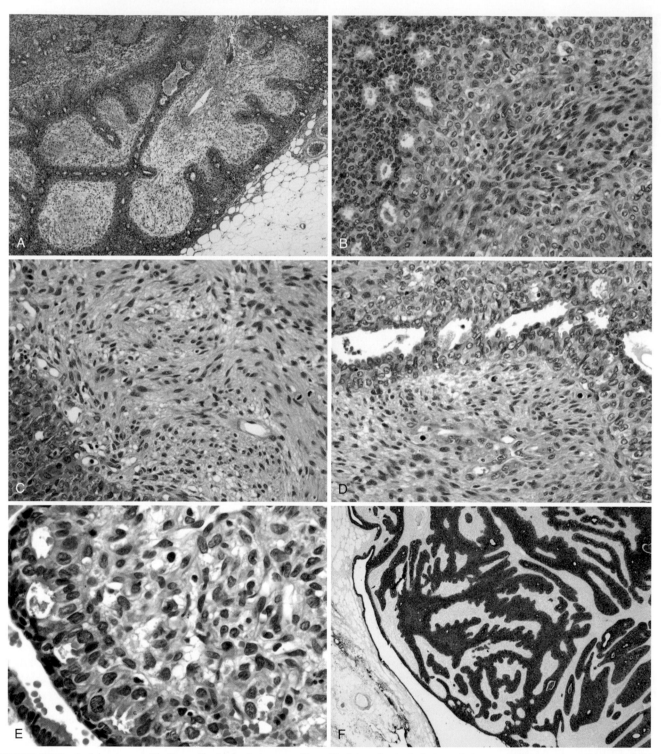

FIGURE 17-2 **A,** Adenomyoepithelioma-like biphasic tumor with epithelial and spindled stromal elements. **B,** Note the mild atypia of the epithelial and stromal cells. **C** and **D,** Mitotic activity of stromal cells. **E,** Hypercellular spindle cell stroma. **F,** Keratin highlights adenomatous component.

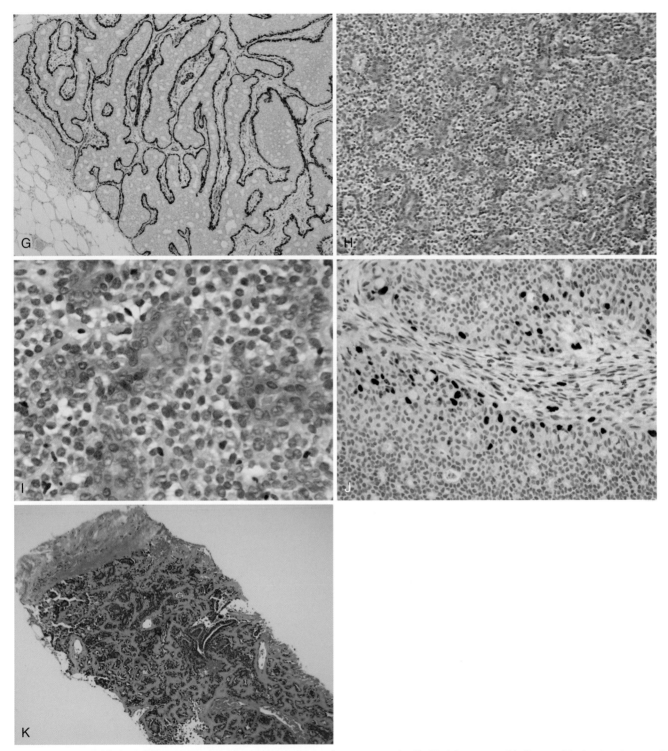

FIGURE 17-2, cont'd G, Calponin decorates myoepithelial layer and some stromal cells. **H,** Adenomyoepithelioma with dominant myoepithelial cells between tubular glands. **I,** Higher magnification of **H** for myoepithelial cells. **J,** Ki-67 highlights proliferating cells in adenomatous and stromal areas. **K,** Adenomyoepithelioma on core biopsy. Note circumscription and metachromatic matrix.

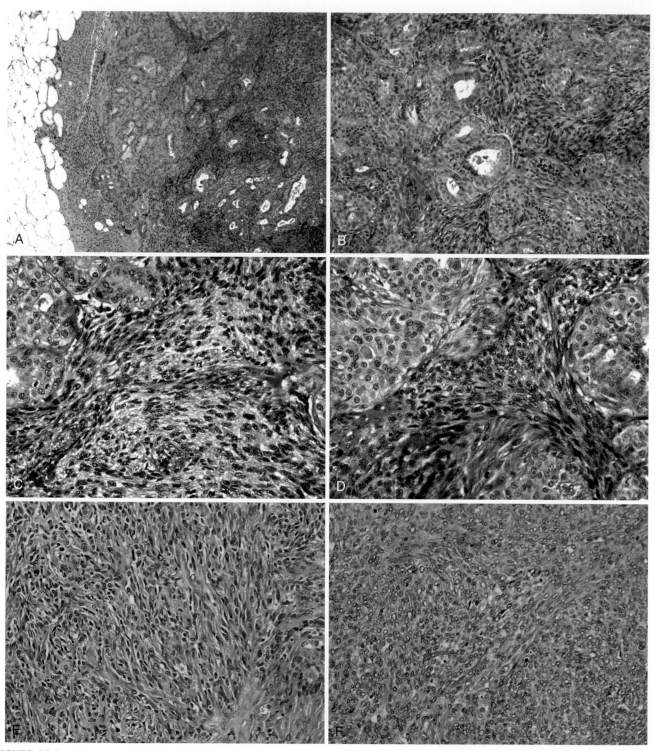

FIGURE 17-3 **A,** Atypical ("malignant") adenomyoepithelioma with epithelial glandular and spindled stromal elements. **B,** Note the mild atypia of the epithelial and hypercellular and hyperchromatic stromal cells. **C** and **D,** Note hypercellularity (high N/C ratios) and mitotic activity of stromal cells. **E,** Myoepithelial carcinoma (MC) shows a spindle pattern. **F,** Here, MC shows a cellular sarcomatous pattern.

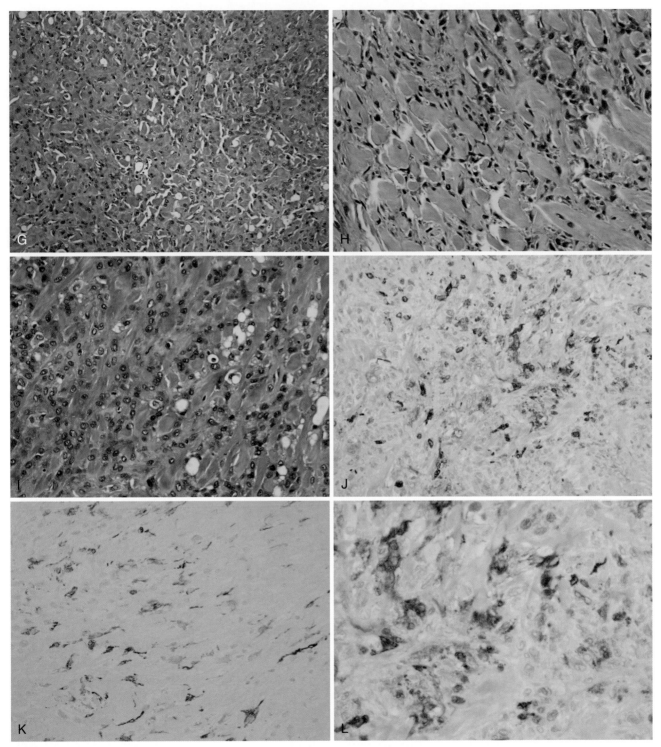

FIGURE 17-3, cont'd G, Hyaline stroma is characteristic of MC. **H,** Hyaline stroma can be keloid-like and is characteristic of MC. **I,** Epithelioid areas of MC show cytologic atypia. **J,** Actin typically decorates MC. **K,** Pankeratin cocktail commonly shows positive cytoplasm in MC. **L,** Desmin is often patchy in MC.

Continued

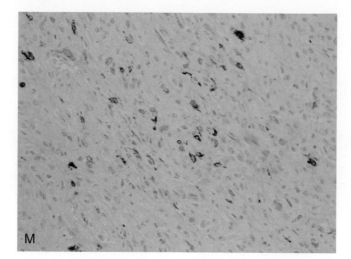

FIGURE 17-3, cont'd M, Cytokeratin 5 shows patchy cytoplasmic reactivity.

KEY PATHOLOGIC FEATURES

Adenomyoepithelioma

- Biphasic epithelial/myoepithelial proliferation, begins as intraductal proliferation.
- Benign lesions lack atypia and increased mitoses.
- IHC may highlight myoepithelial population (p63, SMM-HC, calponin, muscle actin).
- Increased mitoses, marked atypia, and spindle cell overgrowth are hallmarks of malignant transformation. Malignant transformation may involve epithelial cell, myoepithelial cells, or both.
- Differential diagnosis includes pleomorphic adenoma, spindle cell metaplastic carcinoma (myoepithelial carcinoma).

IHC, immunohistochemistry; SMM-HC, smooth muscle myosin–heavy chain.

MYOFIBROBLASTOMA

Clinical Presentation

Myofibroblastoma of breast, a tumor showing myofibroblastic differentiation without epithelial features, simulates spindle cell adenomyoepithelioma and other spindle tumors of the breast (Figure 17-4).[32] Myofibroblastomas have a predilection for occurring in men, but they are benign tumors in either sex.

Clinical Imaging

Myofibroblastoma, like adenomyoepithelioma, may be palpable (especially in men) depending on size and location. Occasionally, they are seen as masses on mammographic imaging.

Gross Pathology

Wargotz and associates[32] reported 16 cases of myofibroblastoma of the breast. Eleven of the 16 patients were men, and the average age at presentation was

---

KEY CLINICAL FEATURES

Myofibroblastoma

- Dominant occurrence in males.
- Palpable but may be discovered on imaging.
- Benign, requires excision only.

---

63 years. Fourteen were treated by local excision and 2 by simple mastectomy. None of the lesions recurred or metastasized. The tumors were grossly nodular and well demarcated from the surrounding mammary tissue.

Microscopic Pathology

Microscopic examination showed the lesions to be formed by uniform, slender, bipolar spindle cells haphazardly arranged in fascicular clusters separated by broad bands of hyalinized collagen.[32] Ducts and lobules are not engulfed by the neoplasm. Ultrastructural examination of four lesions identified a predominance of myofibroblasts. Immunoreactivity for S100 protein and cytokeratin was absent in the 10 tumors examined, but desmin immunoreactivity was focally present in 3 lesions. Others have reported examples of myofibroblastoma that have been quite vascular and/or having infiltrating borders.[32] Cellular examples of the angiolipoma of the breast could also simulate the spindle cell variant of adenomyoepithelioma or myofibroblastoma and even angiosarcoma.[33]

KEY PATHOLOGIC FEATURES

Myofibroblastoma

- Circumscribed mass.
- Slender, bland spindle cells, rare mitotic figures.
- Spindle cells may infiltrate adipose and incorporate fat into the mass.
- Keratin-negative, patchy-positive possible with actins/desmin.
- Differential diagnosis: adenomyoepithelioma, spindle cell sarcomas.

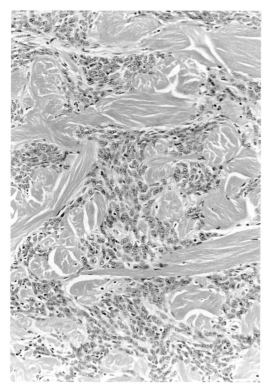

FIGURE 17-4 Myofibroblastoma of breast shows spindle cell and densely collagenase stroma. Mast cells are often quite prominent.

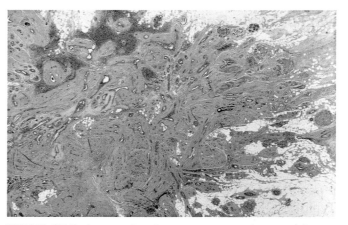

FIGURE 17-5 Low-grade adenosquamous carcinoma of breast. Note the invasive quality of the peripheral glandular elements, simulating a radial scar. The pattern is essentially that of invasive microcystic adnexal carcinoma of skin.

ADENOID CYSTIC CARCINOMA

Of the malignant breast tumors showing myoepithelial differentiation, AdCC deserves extensive discussion in this chapter. AdCC of the breast closely resembles AdCC of salivary gland origin, but it is much less common in the breast, accounting for only approximately 0.1% of all breast carcinomas.[34–39] Electron microscopic studies have revealed the same diverse cell types in mammary AdCC that are encountered in AdCC arising in the salivary glands. This likely reflects the common ectodermal "sweat gland" origin of both breast and salivary gland, and it seems that there should be even more overlap in the patterns of tumors arising in both locations, but this is not usually the case. Other salivary gland–like tumors arising within the breast are very uncommon.

Indeed, breast glands and salivary glands are tubuloacinar exocrine glands that can manifest as tumors with similar morphologic features but that differ in incidence and clinical behavior depending on whether they are primary in breast or salivary glands. Salivary gland–like tumors of the breast are of two types: tumors with myoepithelial differentiation and those devoid of myoepithelial differentiation. The first and more numerous group comprises a spectrum of lesions ranging from bona fide benign, such as benign adenomyoepithelioma and pleomorphic adenoma, to low-grade malignant, such as AdCC, low-grade adenosquamous carcinoma (Figure 17-5), and adenomyoepithelioma, to high-grade malignant lesions such as metaplastic breast carcinoma (also called malignant myoepithelioma). A second group comprises lesions that have only recently been recognized, such as acinic cell carcinoma, oncocytic carcinoma of the breast, and the rare mucoepidermoid carcinoma.[40]

Clinical Presentation

AdCC occurs in adult women of the same age group as for mammary carcinoma (i.e., mean ages 50–63 yr; range 25–80 yr).[35,36,38–44] AdCC usually presents as discrete, firm masses. Uncommonly, they are detected by mammography.[43] They can present "acutely" but some have been present for 10 years or more.[42] Occasionally, AdCC may be found as an incidental finding in the breast.

Clinical Imaging

AdCC presents as a mass lesion that may be palpable, depending on size and location. Occasional discovery is made by mammographic imaging.

KEY CLINICAL FEATURES
Adenoid Cystic Carcinoma of Breast

- Mean age 50s.
- Most often seen on imaging studies as a malignant-appearing mass.
- May be observed as an incidental finding.
- Complete excision with margins necessary.
- Aggressive behavior is rare, but may metastasize to lung, bone, and other areas.

Gross Pathology

Sizes varies from 0.2 to 12 cm with most between 1 and 3 cm.[36,41,43] They are usually circumscribed, but cystic areas occur.[43] They may be gray, pale yellow, tan, or pink.

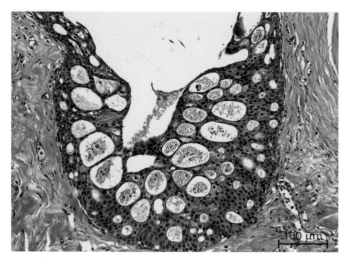

FIGURE 18-25 DCIS with proliferation of monotonous neoplastic cells with cribriform growth pattern. In such a lesion, architecture and cell type are diagnostic and do not need confirmation by immunostains.

diagnosis may be even more difficult if the lesion is small or if only a limited amount of material is available (needle core biopsy). However, even for such lesions, the fundamental principles of the constituent cells, discussed previously, hold true. The CK5/14 mosaic pattern is indicative of UDH whereas intermediate-grade DCIS shows a distinct CK5/14–, CK8/18+ phenotype. In conventional histology, such features may be virtually unrecognizable (compare, e.g., Figures 18-26A, 18-27A, and 18-28A). In such a crucial situation, any tool that allows analysis of the cellular constituents of a given lesion in a more objective way is most welcome.

Micropapillary Epithelial Hyperplasia versus Micropapillary Ductal Carcinoma In Situ

Malignant micropapillae of DCIS are usually composed of monotonous cells with low-grade nuclei. The micropapillae vary greatly in size and shapes but are often long and slender at the base and bulbous at the tips. Sometimes, the neoplastic cells of the micropapillae have

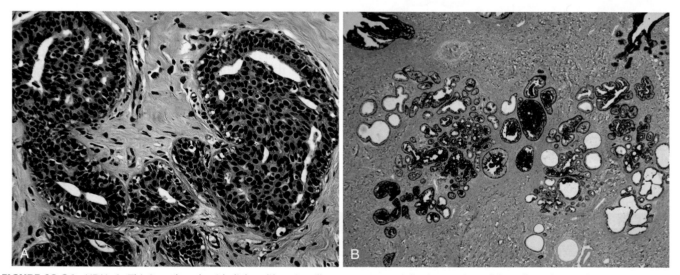

FIGURE 18-26 UDH. **A,** This intraductal epithelial proliferation illustrates some cytologic variation of the cells and some fenestration, which, however, is difficult to interpret. **B,** Immunostain for CK5 demonstrates the mosaic pattern of the proliferative process.

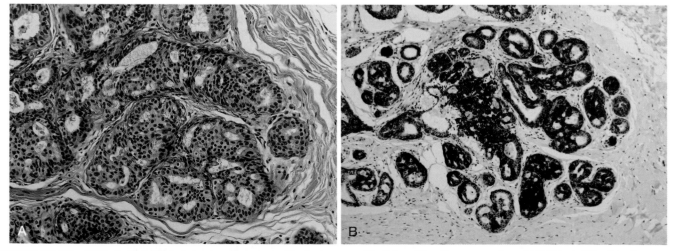

FIGURE 18-27 UDH. **A,** This H&E-stained section again illustrates an epithelial proliferation suggestive of UDH but difficult to interpret. **B,** CK5/14 immunostains show a mosaic pattern, thus indicating UDH.

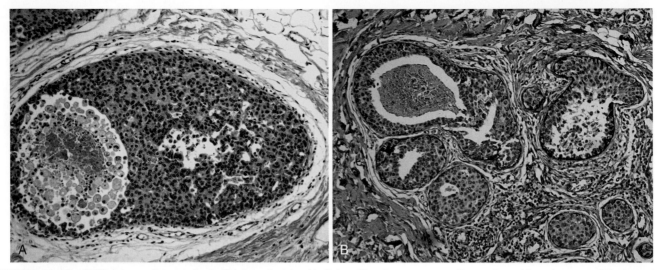

FIGURE 18-28 DCIS, intermediate grade. **A,** This intraductal epithelial proliferation may cause diagnostic problems because of the irregular placement of the cells and fenestrations. **B,** CK5 immunostain illustrates the lack of expression of basal keratins in the tumor cells, and thus, the lesion has to be classified as a ductal neoplasia (surrounding myoepithelial cells show staining for CK5). Immunostain for CK5 demonstrates the mosaic pattern of the proliferative process.

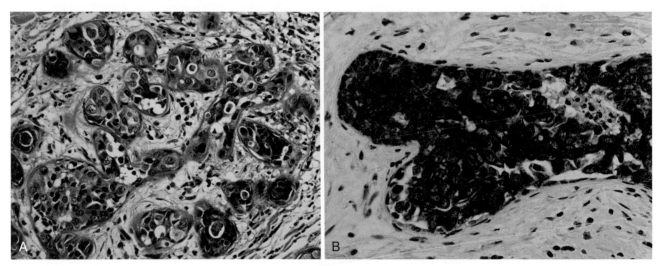

FIGURE 18-29 DCIS, high grade. **A,** Enlarged lobule shows solid epithelial proliferation displaying highly atypical and hyperchromatic nuclei and early comedo necrosis with apoptotic cells indicative of DCIS, high grade. **B,** CK5/6 immunostain demonstrates the intensive expression of basal keratins in nearly all cells.

smaller or somewhat more hyperchromatic nuclei in the basal population compared with the bulbous periphery of micropapillae.

Hyperplastic micropapillae usually contain crowded cells of different sizes and shapes often with hyperchromatic nuclei, and hyperplastic papillae tend to lack the slender base and bulbous tip, being uniformly thin. The distinction between these lesions in small biopsies may be difficult and sometimes arbitrary, but it is important for patient management purposes. In difficult cases, CK5/14 immunostaining is helpful (Figure 18-30).

Although spindling of cells may sometimes be extensive in UDH, it is rarely seen throughout the entire lesion. In the event of any unusual-looking spindle cell proliferation, therefore, the lesion should be examined for areas that are more diagnostic and clearly contain features of UDH. The presence of only one type of spindle cell in a lesion should raise the suspicion of DCIS, spindle type. In our experience, CK5/14 helps in this differential diagnostic setting because staining of DCIS, spindle-cell type, is negative, whereas UDH is positive.

Usual Ductal Hyperplasia versus Lobular Neoplasia

Occasional cases of UDH may show more uniform cells with bland nuclei and solid growth pattern, and the differential diagnosis in these cases should, therefore, include lobular neoplasia. Classic-type lobular neoplasia is CK5/14−. Additional immunostains may confirm the diagnosis of lobular neoplasia by demonstration of loss of E-cadherin adhesion molecules in cells.

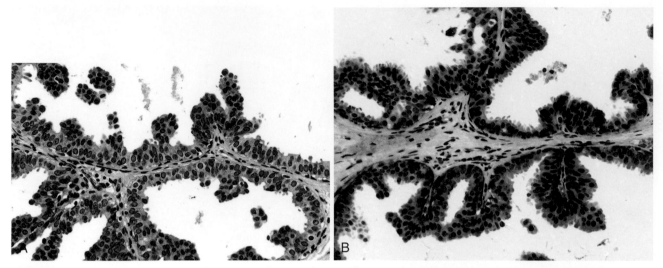

FIGURE 18-30 Ductal neoplasia, low grade, micropapillary. **A,** This view illustrates the club-shaped micropapillations with uniform distribution of cells and nuclei, clearly indicating the neoplastic process. **B,** Immunostain for CK5/6 demonstrated a lack of staining of the tumor cells for basal keratins.

USUAL DUCTAL HYPERPLASIAS AND THEIR BENIGN COUNTERPARTS

Usual Ductal Hyperplasia versus Adenomyoepithelioma

It is not uncommon for the proliferating cells of UDH to acquire a spindle cell shape, possibly leading to a false diagnosis of adenomyoepithelioma. As discussed previously, the cells of UDH differentiate along the glandular pathway and do not, therefore, express myoepithelial markers. Thus, smooth muscle actin immunohistochemistry is of great help in making a correct diagnosis.

Cytokeratin 5/14+ Clonal Intraductal Epithelial Proliferations

Exceptionally rare cases of intraductal epithelial proliferations with a homogeneous CK5/14 positivity with or without CK8/18 expression may be observed. Their clinical significance is currently unknown.

SUMMARY

Hyperplasia within the FCC comprises an important range of morphologic variants that require recognition for proper patient management. Immunohistochemistry may be used as an adjunct in difficult lesions. Careful study of imaging, morphology, and adjunctive studies should yield a proper diagnosis.

REFERENCES

1. Bartow SA, Pathak DR, Black WC, et al. Prevalence of benign, atypical, and malignant breast lesions in populations at different risk for breast cancer. A forensic autopsy study. Cancer 1987;60:2751-2760.
2. Frantz VK, Pickren JW, Melcher GW, Auchincloss H. Incidence of chronic cystic disease in so-called "normal breasts": a study based on 225 postmortem examinations. Cancer 1951;4: 762-783.
3. Silverberg SG, Chitale AR, Levitt SH. Prognostic implications of fibrocystic dysplasia in breast removed for mammary carcinoma. Cancer 1972;29:574-580.
4. Drukker BH, deMendonca WC. Fibrocystic change and fibrocystic disease of the breast. Obstet Gynecol Clin North Am 1987;14:685-702.
5. Fiorica JV. Fibrocystic changes. Obstet Gynecol Clin North Am 1994;21:445-452.
6. Hutter RVP. Consensus meeting. Is fibrocystic disease of the breast precancerous. Arch Pathol 1986;110:171-173.
7. Hockenberger SJ. Fibrocystic breast disease: every woman is at risk. Plast Surg Nurs 1993;13:37-40.
8. Vorherr H. Fibrocystic breast disease: pathophysiology, pathomorphology, clinical picture, and management. Am J Obstet Gynecol 1986;154:161-179.
9. Wellings SR, Alpers CE. Apocrine cystic metaplasia: subgross pathology and prevalence in cancer-associated versus random autopsy breasts. Hum Pathol 1987;18:381-386.
10. Geschickter CF. Diseases of the Breast. Diagnosis-Pathology-Treatment. 2nd ed. Philadelphia: JB Lippincott; 1945.
11. Kier LC, Kickey RC, Keettel WC, et al. Endocrine relationships in benign lesions of the breast. Ann Surg 1952;135:669-671.
12. Sitruk-Ware R, Sterkers N, Mauvais-Jarvis P. Benign breast disease I: hormonal investigation. Obstet Gynecol 1979;53: 457-460.
13. Heywang-Kobrunner SH, Dershaw DD, Scheer I. Cysts; inflammatory conditions. In Diagnostic Breast Imaging. Stuttgart, Germany: Thieme; 2001.
14. Lanyi M. Diagnosis and Differential Diagnosis of Breast Calcifications. Berlin: Springer; 1986.
15. Tot T, Tabar L, Dean PB. Practical Breast Pathology. Stuttgart, Germany and New York: 2002.
16. Pearlman WH, Gueriguian JL, Sawyer ME. A specific progesterone-binding component of human breast cyst fluid. J Biol Chem 1973;248:5736-5741.
17. Azzopardi JG. Problems in Breast Pathology. 1st ed. London: WB Saunders; 1979.
18. Eusebi V, Millis RR, Cattani MG, et al. Apocrine carcinoma of the breast. A morphologic and immunocytochemical study. Am J Pathol 1986;123:532-541.
19. Viacava P, Naccarato AG, Bevilacqua G. Apocrine epithelium of the breast: does it result from metaplasia? Virchows Arch 1997;431:205-209.
20. Ahmed A. Apocrine metaplasia in cystic hyperplastic mastopathy. Histochemical and ultrastructural observations. J Pathol 1975;115:211-214.
21. Page DL, Vander Zwaag R, Rogers LW, et al. Relation between component parts of fibrocystic disease complex and breast cancer. J Natl Cancer Inst 1978;61:1055-1060.
22. Haagensen DE Jr, Mazoujian G, Dilley WG, et al. Breast gross cystic disease fluid analysis. I. Isolation and radioimmunoassay for a major component protein. J Natl Cancer Inst 1979;62:239-247.

23. Mazoujian G, Pinkus GS, Davis S, Haagensen DE Jr. Immuno-histochemistry of a gross cystic disease fluid protein (GCDFP-15) of the breast. A marker of apocrine epithelium and breast carcinomas with apocrine features. Am J Pathol 1983;110:105-112.

24. Pagani A, Sapino A, Eusebi V, et al. PIP/GCDFP-15 gene expression and apocrine differentiation in carcinomas of the breast. Virchows Arch 1994;425:459-465.

25. Tavassoli FA. Pathology of the Breast. Norwalk, CT: Appleton & Lange; 1999.

26. Gonzalez JE, Caldwell RG, Valaitis J. Calcium oxalate crystals in the breast. Pathology and significance. Am J Surg Pathol 1991;15:586-591.

27. Bonser GM, Dossett JA, Jull JW. Human and Experimental Breast Cancer. London: Pitman Medical; 1961.

28. Schnitt SJ. The diagnosis and management of pre-invasive breast disease: flat epithelial atypia—classification, pathologic features and clinical significance. Breast Cancer Res 2003;5:263-268.

29. Schnitt SJ, Vincent-Salomon A. Columnar cell lesions of the breast. Adv Anat Pathol 2003;10:113-124.

30. Dawson EK. Sweat gland carcinoma of the breast. Edinb Med J 1932;39:409-438.

31. Foote FW, Stewart FW. Comparative studies of cancerous versus non-cancerous breasts. Basic morphologic characteristics. Ann Surg 1945;121:6-53.

32. Geschickter CF. The early literature of chronic cystic mastitis. Bull Inst Hist Med 1939;2:249-257.

33. Haagensen CD. The relationship of gross cystic disease of the breast and carcinoma. Ann Surg 1977;185:375-376.

34. Hutter RV. Goodbye to "fibrocystic disease." N Engl J Med 1985;312:179-181.

35. Love SM, Gelman RS, Silen W. Sounding board: fibrocystic "disease" of the breast—a nondisease? N Engl J Med 1982;3(07):1010-1014.

36. Page DL, Dupont WD. Are breast cysts a premalignant marker? Eur J Cancer Clin Oncol 1986;22:635-636.

37. Page DL, Kasami M, Jensen RA. Hypersecretory hyperplasia with atypia in breast biopsies. What is the proper level of clinical concern? Pathol Case Rev 1996;1:36-40.

38. Haagensen CD, Bodian C, Haagensen DE. Breast Carcinoma—Risk and Detection. Philadelphia: WB Saunders; 1981.

39. Dixon JM, McDonald C, Elton RA, Miller WR. Risk of breast cancer in women with palpable breast cysts: a prospective study. Edinburgh Breast Group. Lancet 1999;353:1742-1745.

40. Wells CA, McGregor IL, Makunura CN, et al. Apocrine adenosis: a precursor of aggressive breast cancer? J Clin Pathol 1995;48:737-742.

41. Agnantis NJ, Mahera H, Maounis N, Spandidos DA. Immuno-histochemical study of ras and myc oncoproteins in apocrine breast lesions with and without papillomatosis. Eur J Gynaecol Oncol 1992;13:309-315.

42. Washington C, Dalbegue F, Abreo F, et al. Loss of heterozygosity in fibrocystic change of the breast: genetic relationship between benign proliferative lesions and associated carcinomas. Am J Pathol 2000;157:323-329.

43. Jones C, Damiani S, Wells D, et al. Molecular cytogenetic comparison of apocrine hyperplasia and apocrine carcinoma of the breast. Am J Pathol 2001;158:207-214.

44. Celis JE, Gromov P, Moreira JM, et al. Apocrine cysts of the breast: biomarkers, origin, enlargement, and relation with cancer phenotype. Mol Cell Proteomics 2006;5:462-483.

45. De Potter CR, Foschini MP, Schelfhout AM, et al. Immunohistochemical study of neu protein overexpression in clinging in situ duct carcinoma of the breast. Virchows Arch A Pathol Anat Histopathol 1993;422:375-380.

46. Eusebi V, Feudale E, Foschini MP, et al. Long-term follow-up of in situ carcinoma of the breast. Semin Diagn Pathol 1994;11:223-235.

47. Rosen PP. Rosen's Breast Pathology. 2nd ed. Philadelphia: Lippincott Williams & Wilkins; 2001.

48. Ironside JW, Guthrie W. The galactocoele: a light- and electron-microscopic study. Histopathol 1985;9:457-467.

49. Page DL, Anderson TJ, Rogers LW. Epithelial hyperplasia. In Page DL, Anderson TJ, eds. Diagnostic Histopathology of the Breast. Edinburgh: Churchill Livingstone; 1988; pp. 120-156.

50. Tavassoli FA, Norris HJ. A comparison of the results of long-term follow-up for atypical intraductal hyperplasia and intraductal hyperplasia of the breast. Cancer 1990;65:518-529.

51. Haagensen CD. Anatomy of the mammary glands. In Haagensen CD, ed. Diseases of the Breast. 3rd ed. Philadelphia: WB Saunders; 1986; pp. 1-46.

52. McDivitt RW, Holleb AI, Foote F-WJ. Prior breast disease in patients treated for papillary carcinoma. Arch Pathol 1968;85:117-124.

53. Tavassoli FA. Ductal intraepithelial neoplasia (IDH, AIDH and DCIS). Breast Cancer 2000;7:315-320.

54. Black MM, Speer FD. Nuclear structure in cancer tissues. Surg Gynaecol Obstet 1957;105:97-105.

55. Cutler SJ, Black MM, Mork T, et al. Further observations on prognostic factors in cancer of the female breast. Cancer 1969;24:653-667.

56. Deng G, Lu Y, Zlotnikov G, et al. Loss of heterozygosity in normal tissue adjacent to breast carcinomas. Science 1996;274:2057-2059.

57. Gobbi H, Dupont WD, Simpson JF, et al. Transforming growth factor-beta and breast cancer risk in women with mammary epithelial hyperplasia. J Natl Cancer Inst 1999;91:2096-2101.

58. Goldstein NS, Murphy T. Intraductal carcinoma associated with invasive carcinoma of the breast. A comparison of the two lesions with implications for intraductal carcinoma classification systems. Am J Clin Pathol 1996;106:312-318.

59. Ohuchi N, Abe R, Takahashi T, et al. Three-dimensional atypical structure in intraductal carcinoma differentiating from papilloma and papillomatosis of the breast. Breast Cancer Res Treat 1985;5:57-65.

60. Tham KT, Dupont WD, Page DL, et al. Micro-papillary hyperplasia with atypical features in female breasts, resembling gynecomastia. In Fenoglio-Preiser M, Wolff M, Rilke F (eds): Progress in Surgical Pathology. Heidelberg, Germany: Springer; 1989; pp. 101-109.

61. Elston CW, Ellis IO. The Breast. 1st ed. Edinburgh: Harcourt Brace & Company Ltd; 1998.

62. Rosen PP, Holmes G, Lesser ML, et al. Juvenile papillomatosis and breast carcinoma. Cancer 1985;55:1345-1352.

63. Rosen PP, Kimmel M. Juvenile papillomatosis of the breast. A follow-up study of 41 patients having biopsies before 1979 [see comments]. Am J Clin Pathol 1990;93:599-603.

64. McDivitt R, Stewart FW, Berg JW. Atlas of Tumour Pathology. Washington, DC: Armed Forces Institute of Pathology; 1968.

65. Fenoglio C, Lattes R. Sclerosing papillary proliferations in the female breast. A benign lesion often mistaken for carcinoma. Cancer 1974;33:691-700.

66. Eusebi V, Millis RR. Epitheliosis, infiltrating epitheliosis, and radial scar. Semin Diagn Pathol 2010;27:5-12.

67. Böcker WJ, Bier B, Freytag G, et al. An immunohistochemical study of the breast using antibodies to basal and luminal keratins, alpha-smooth muscle actin, vimentin, collagen IV and laminin. Part I: normal breast and benign proliferative lesions. Virchows Archiv A 1992;421:315-322.

68. Böcker WJ, Bier B, Freytag G, et al. An immunohistochemical study of the breast using antibodies to basal and luminal keratins, alpha-smooth muscle actin, vimentin, collagen IV and laminin. Part II: epitheliosis and ductal carcinoma in situ. Virchows Archiv A 1992;421:323-330.

69. Jarasch E-D, Nagle RB, Kaufmann M, et al. Differential diagnosis of benign epithelial proliferations and carcinomas of the breast using antibodies to cytokeratins. Hum Pathol 1988;19:276-289.

70. Nagle RB, Bocker W, Davis JR, et al. Characterization of breast carcinomas by two monoclonal antibodies distinguishing myoepithelial from luminal epithelial cells. J Histochem Cytochem 1986;34:869-881.

71. Boecker W, Moll R, Poremba C, et al. Common adult stem cells in the human breast give rise to glandular and myoepithelial cell lineages: a new cell biological concept. Lab Invest 2002;82:737-746.

72. Lacroix-Triki M, Mery E, Voigt JJ, et al. Value of cytokeratin 5/6 immunostaining using D5/16 B4 antibody in the spectrum of proliferative intraepithelial lesions of the breast. A comparative study with 34betaE12 antibody. Virchows Arch 2003;442:548-554.

73. Dabbs DJ, Chivukula M, Carter G, Bhargava R. Basal phenotype of ductal carcinoma in situ: recognition and immunohistologic profile. Mod Pathol 2006;19:1506-1511.

74. Allred DC, O'Connell P, Fuqua SAW, et al. Immunohistochemical studies of early breast cancer evolution. Breast Cancer Res Treat 1994;32:13-18.

75. Siziopikou KP, Prioleau JE, Harris JR, Schnitt SJ. bcl-2 expression in the spectrum of preinvasive breast lesions. Cancer 1996;77:499-506.

76. Umekita Y, Takasaki T, Yoshida H. Expression of p53 protein in benign epithelial hyperplasia, atypical ductal hyperplasia, non-invasive and invasive mammary carcinoma: an immunohistochemical study. Virchows Arch 1994;424:491-494.

77. Done SJ, Arneson NC, Ozcelik H, et al. p53 mutations in mammary ductal carcinoma in situ but not in epithelial hyperplasias. Cancer Res 1998;58:785-789.

78. Stark A, Hulka BS, Joens S, et al. HER-2/neu amplification in benign breast disease and the risk of subsequent breast cancer. J Clin Oncol 2000;18:267-274.

79. Alle KM, Henshall SM, Field AS, Sutherland RL. Cyclin D1 protein is overexpressed in hyperplasia and intraductal carcinoma of the breast. Clin Cancer Res 1998;4:847-854.

80. Mommers EC, van Diest PJ, Leonhart AM, et al. Expression of proliferation and apoptosis-related proteins in usual ductal hyperplasia of the breast. Hum Pathol 1998;29:1539-1545.

81. Weinstat SD, Merino MJ, Manrow RE, et al. Overexpression of cyclin D mRNA distinguishes invasive and in situ breast carcinomas from non-malignant lesions. Nature Med 1995;1:1257-1260.

82. Parham DM, Jankowski J. Transforming growth factor alpha in epithelial proliferative diseases of the breast. J Clin Pathol 1992;45:513-516.

83. Shaaban AM, Sloane JP, West CR, Foster CS. Breast cancer risk in usual ductal hyperplasia is defined by estrogen receptor-alpha and Ki-67 expression. Am J Pathol 2002;160:597-604.

84. Roger P, Sahla ME, Makela S, et al. Decreased expression of estrogen receptor beta protein in proliferative preinvasive mammary tumors. Cancer Res 2001;61:2537-2541.

85. Lakhani SR, Slack DN, Hamoudi RA, et al. Detection of allelic imbalance indicates that a proportion of mammary hyperplasia of usual type are clonal, neoplastic proliferations. Lab Invest 1996;74:129-135.

86. O'Connell P, Fischbach K, Hilsenbeck S, et al. Loss of heterozygosity at D14S62 and metastatic potential of breast cancer [see comments]. J Natl Cancer Inst 1999;91:1391-1397.

87. Kaneko M, Arihiro K, Takeshima Y, et al. Loss of heterozygosity and microsatellite instability in epithelial hyperplasia of the breast. J Exp Ther Oncol 2002;2:9-18.

88. Maitra A, Wistuba II, Washington C, et al. High-resolution chromosome 3p allelotyping of breast carcinomas and precursor lesions demonstrates frequent loss of heterozygosity and a discontinuous pattern of allele loss. Am J Pathol 2001;159:119-130.

89. Boecker W, Moll R, Dervan P, et al. Usual ductal hyperplasia of the breast is a committed stem (progenitor) cell lesion distinct from atypical ductal hyperplasia and ductal carcinoma in situ. J Pathol 2002;198:458-467.

90. Dupont WD, Page DL. Risk factors for breast cancer in women with proliferative breast disease. N Engl J Med 1985;312:146-151.

91. Werner M, Mattis A, Aubele M, et al. 20q13.2 amplification in intraductal hyperplasia adjacent to in situ and invasive ductal carcinoma of the breast. Virchows Arch 1999;435:469-472.

92. Gong G, DeVries S, Chew KL, et al. Genetic changes in paired atypical and usual ductal hyperplasia of the breast by comparative genomic hybridization. Clin Cancer Res 2001;7:2410-2414.

93. Jones C, Merrett S, Thomas VA, et al. Comparative genomic hybridization analysis of bilateral hyperplasia of usual type of the breast. J Pathol 2003;199:152-156.

94. Noguchi S, Aihara T, Koyama H, et al. Clonal analysis of benign and malignant human breast tumors by means of polymerase chain reaction. Cancer Lett 1995;90:57-63.

95. Diallo R, Schaefer KL, Poremba C, et al. Monoclonality in normal epithelium and in hyperplastic and neoplastic lesions of the breast. J Pathol 2001;193:27-32.

96. Mommers EC, Page DL, Dupont WD, et al. Prognostic value of morphometry in patients with normal breast tissue or usual ductal hyperplasia of the breast. Int J Cancer 2001;95:282-285.

97. Koukoulis GK, Virtanen I, Korhonen M, et al. Immunohistochemical localization of integrins in the normal, hyperplastic, and neoplastic breast. Correlations with their functions as receptors and cell adhesion molecules. Am J Pathol 1991;139:787-799.

98. Sloane JP. Biopsy Pathology of the Breast. 2nd ed. Vol 24. London: Arnold; 2001.

99. Moinfar F, Man YG, Lininger RA, et al. Use of keratin 35betaE12 as an adjunct in the diagnosis of mammary intraepithelial neoplasia-ductal type—benign and malignant intraductal proliferations. Am J Surg Pathol 1999;23:1048-1058.

100. Otterbach F, Bankfalvi A, Bergner S, et al. Cytokeratin 5/6 immunohistochemistry assists the differential diagnosis of atypical proliferations of the breast. Histopathol 2000;37:232-240.

101. Raju U, Crissman JD, Zarbo R, Gottlieb C. Epitheliosis of the breast. An immunohistochemical characterization and comparison to malignant intraductal proliferations of the breast. Am J Surg Pathol 1990;14:939-947.

102. Schnitt SJ, Conolly JL, Tavassoli FA, et al. Interobserver reproducibility in the diagnosis of ductal proliferative breast lesions using standardized criteria. Am J Surg Pathol 1992;16:1133-1143.

103. Buerger H, Otterbach F, Simon R, et al. Comparative genomic hybridization of ductal carcinoma in situ of the breast-evidence of multiple genetic pathways. J Pathol 1999;187:396-402.

104. Dupont WD, Parl FF, Hartmann WH, et al. Breast cancer risk associated with proliferative breast disease and atypical hyperplasia [see comments]. Cancer 1993;71:1258-1265.

105. Schnitt SJ. Benign breast disease and breast cancer risk: morphology and beyond. Am J Surg Pathol 2003;27:836-841.

106. Bodian CA, Perzin KH, Lattes R, Hoffmann P. Reproducibility and validity of pathologic classifications of benign breast disease and implications for clinical applications [see comments]. Cancer 1993;71:3908-3913.

107. Bodian CA, Perzin KH, Lattes R, et al. Prognostic significance of benign proliferative breast disease. Cancer 1993;71:3896-3907.

108. Kodlin D, Winger EE, Morgenstern NL, Chen U. Chronic mastopathy and breast cancer. A follow-up study. Cancer 1977;39:2603-2607.

109. Page DL, Dupont WD, Rogers LW, Rados AM. Atypical hyperplastic lesions of the female breast. A long-term follow-up study. Cancer 1985;55:2698-2708.

110. Carter CL, Corle DK, Micozzi MS, et al. A prospective study of the development of breast cancer in 16,692 women with benign breast disease. Am J Epidemiol 1988;128:467-477.

111. Fitzgibbons PL, Henson DE, Hutter RV. Benign breast changes and the risk for subsequent breast cancer: an update of the 1985 consensus statement. Cancer Committee of the College of American Pathologists. Arch Pathol Lab Med 1998;122:1053-1055.

112. London SJ, Connolly JL, Schnitt SJ, Colditz GA. A prospective study of benign breast disease and the risk of breast cancer [published erratum appears in JAMA 1992;267:1780]. JAMA 1992;267:941-944.

113. McDivitt RW, Stevens JA, Lee NC, et al. Histologic types of benign breast disease and the risk for breast cancer. Cancer 1992;69:1408-1414.

114. Dehner LP. The continuing evolution of our understanding of juvenile papillomatosis of the breast [editorial; comment]. Am J Clin Pathol 1990;93:713.

115. Rohan TE, Hartwick W, Miller AB, Kandel RA. Immunohistochemical detection of c-erbB-2 and p53 in benign breast disease and breast cancer risk. J Natl Cancer Inst 1998;90:1262–1269.

116. Bratthauer GL, Moinfar F, Stamatakos MD, et al. Combined E-cadherin and high molecular weight cytokeratin immunoprofile differentiates lobular, ductal, and hybrid mammary intraepithelial neoplasias. Hum Pathol 2002;33:620-627.

Columnar Cell Alterations, Flat Epithelial Atypia, and Atypical Ductal Epithelial Hyperplasia

David J. Dabbs

INTRODUCTION

The intent of this chapter is to present the diagnostic criteria, differential diagnosis, immunohistology, clinical relevance, clinical risk, and molecular-genetic alterations associated with the spectrum of columnar cell alterations of the breast.

COLUMNAR CELL ALTERATIONS AND FLAT EPITHELIAL ATYPIA

Alterations of the terminal duct lobular unit (TDLU) by the spectrum of columnar cell changes (CCCs) have been known for well over 100 years. This spectrum of simple CCCs and CCC with atypical cytology has generated a wide variety of different pathologic designations (Table 19-1), including "abnormal involution,"[1] "adenoid cystic change of senile parenchymatous hypertrophy,"[2] "hyperplastic unfolded lobules,"[3] "low-grade clinging carcinoma,"[4] "columnar alteration with prominent apical

snouts,"[5] "atypical cystic lobules,"[6] "enlarged lobular units with columnar alteration (ELUCAs),"[7] "hyperplastic enlarged lobular units (HELUs),"[8] and "flat DIN1a."[9,10]

There is a renewed interest in these lesions because they now come across the pathologist's microscope frequently as a result of abnormal calcifications seen on screening mammography. The variety of different names, taken together, describes the salient microscopic features that have attracted the attention of so many pathologists. These alterations involve replacement of the normal TDLU acinar cells with columnar cells, which may on occasion appear atypical, may be cystically dilated, are often enlarged, and may have apical cellular "snouts."

There is emerging evidence that the spectrum of CCCs, which includes the entity of flat epithelial atypia (FEA) at one end, are related morphologically, cytologically, and by molecular alterations to atypical ductal epithelial hyperplasia (ADH) and low-grade ductal carcinoma in situ (DCIS). Indeed, CCC, FEA, and ADH are commonly seen on the same microscopic slide and are considered to be precursor lesions in the low-grade estrogen-dependent pathways of ductal/lobular neoplasia.[11–14] It is important for pathologists to recognize and accurately classify the spectrum of these cellular changes because they affect patient management.

TABLE 19-1	Terminology Previously Applied to Flat Epithelial Atypia of the Breast
Clinging carcinoma[4]	
Atypical cystic lobules[6]	
Columnar alteration with prominent apical snouts and secretions with atypia[32]	
Columnar cell change with atypia[5]	
Columnar cell hyperplasia with atypia[5]	
Hypersecretory hyperplasia with atypia[64]	
Pretubular hyperplasia[64]	
Ductal intraepithelial neoplasia of the flat monomorphic type[71]	

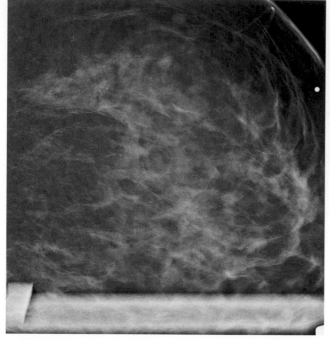

FIGURE 19-1 Typical appearance of microcalcifications with flat epithelial atypia (FEA).

Clinical Presentation

The vast majority of patients with CCC and FEA are found to have calcifications on mammographic screening.[5,10,15–26] The observed mammographic calcifications are almost invariably seen to be intimately involved with CCC and FEA on microscopic sections of breast core biopsies ("determinate calcifications"). The calcifications are often irregular, within the lumen, and sometimes associated with flocculent intraluminal secretion material. On rare occasions, there may be marked dilatation of ducts with eosinophilic material simulating thyroid follicles.[10] The epithelium should be scrutinized in these areas, because this type of luminal content is rarely seen with fibrocystic change. Less commonly, columnar cell–related lesions (CCLs) may be seen in a breast biopsy in which the calcifications are seen in other areas of the breast tissue ("nondeterminate calcifications").

Clinical Imaging

Patients with CCLs are found to have calcifications on screening mammography. CCL ranks fifth among the common findings associated with mammographic calcifications, behind fibrocystic change, fibroadenoma,

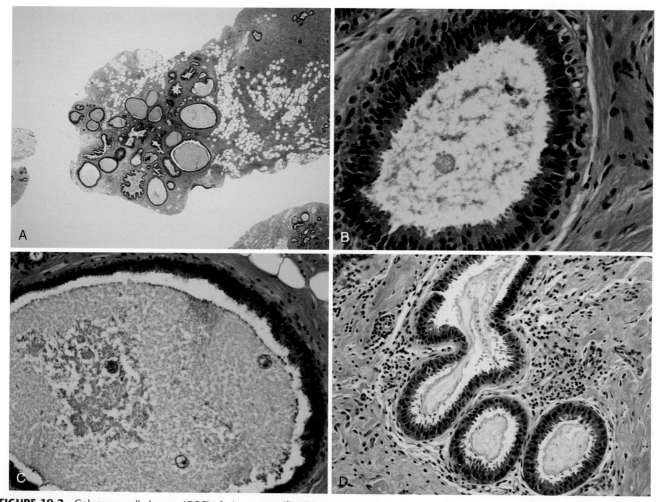

FIGURE 19-2 Columnar cell change (CCC). **A,** Low-magnification appearance of CCC with dilation of terminal duct lobular unit. **B,** CCC with elongated bland nuclei and abundant apical snouts. **C,** Granular calcific debris in the lumen of a terminal duct with CCC. **D,** CCC with dilatation of the lobular unit and prominent apical snouts with luminal content.

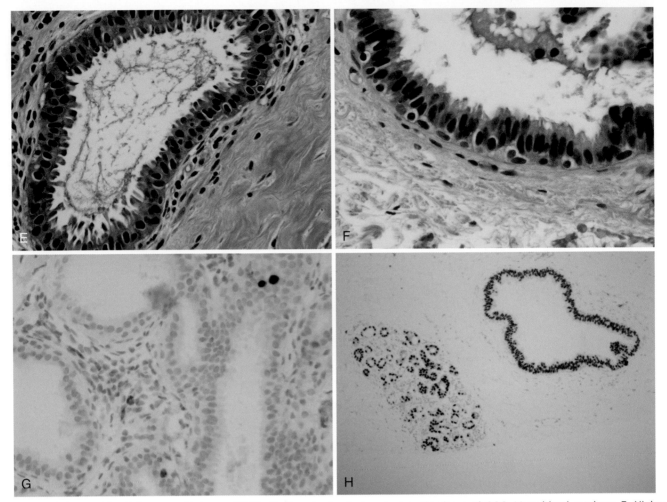

FIGURE 19-2, cont'd Columnar cell change (CCC). **E,** Granular luminal content in this focus of CCC. Note bland cytology. **F,** Higher magnification shows elongated oval bland nuclei, some overlapping, with prominent apical snouts. **G,** Ki-67 index is invariably less than 3%. **H,** Estrogen receptor (ER) in an area of CCC shows diffuse strong immunostaining of nuclei representing ER up-regulation compared with the adjacent lobule where focal nuclear ER expression is usual.

DCIS, and sclerosing adenosis.[21] Mammographic calcifications (Figure 19-1) may appear rounded, branching, amorphous, indistinct, or pleomorphic[5,21,27] and are usually interpreted as "suspicious"; they are assigned a Breast Imaging Reporting and Data System (BIRADS) category 4, which is indication for biopsy.

Gross Pathology

There are no specific gross tissue findings associated with CCC, FEA, or ADH.

Microscopic Pathology

The terminology and names given to the entities of CCC and FEA have changed over the years, and the terminology continues to evolve. Most pathologists currently agree on the terminology of *columnar cell change (CCC), columnar cell hyperplasia (CCH),* and *flat epithelial atypia (FEA).*[28,29] The World Health Organization (WHO) classifies FEA as DIN1a.[9,30]

CCC at low magnification is characterized by dilatation of the TDLU, with replacement of the normal TDLU acinar cells with tall, cytologically bland, columnar cells (Figure 19-2). Such dilatation may be symmetrical or asymmetrical, and the glandular epithelium is lined by one or two layers of columnar epithelium that have uniform, oval or elongated nuclei that are oriented quite regularly, in a perpendicular fashion, to the adjacent basement membrane.[5,25,28,31–33] The nuclei are bland, have a fine chromatin, and no visible nucleoli. The columnar cells have scant apical cytoplasm and apical cytoplasmic blebs or snouts that are extruded into the lumen. The flocculent secretions subsequently formed are invariably calcified to some degree. This lesion, as with all lesions in this classification, is delivered to the pathologist as a result of calcifications discovered on screening mammography. Proliferation is very low in CCC, in the range of 1% to 3%, and most cells show strong estrogen receptor (ER) expression because of up-regulation of ER, compared to adjacent normal breast lobules.

CCH has the same overall appearance at low magnification, with irregularly dilated TDLUs. The cells lining these acini have identical morphologic features, although there is cellular stratification of more than two cell layers (Figure 19-3). There may be cellular crowding or overlapping

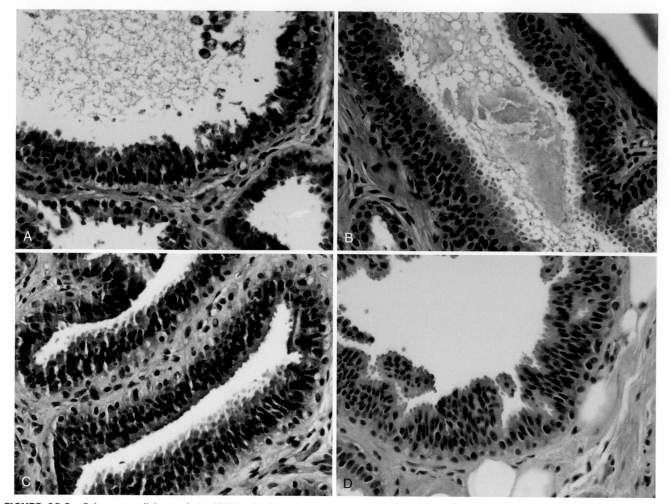

FIGURE 19-3 Columnar cell hyperplasia (CCH). **A,** Crowding and pseudostratification of bland nuclei with prominent apical snouts. **B,** Stratification with bland nuclei and apical cytoplasmic snouts. **C,** Crowding and stratification of bland oval nuclei and luminal apical blebs. **D,** Multiple layers of elongated bland nuclei that maintain polarity.

and, rarely, small tufts or mounds of cells, but no blunt micropapillary projections.[28,31–34] Flocculent secretions and calcifications are universal. Similar to CCC, the Ki-67 is 1% to 3%, and ER expression is up-regulated in most cells, compared with adjacent normal lobules.

FEA also demonstrates variable dilatation of the TDLU, but the cell population is mostly low cuboidal and has columnar configuration. The cytomorphology of these cells is clearly abnormal, manifested as a low-grade monomorphic atypia, in which the nuclei are generally larger, more than twice the size of the nuclei seen in CCC/CCH, rounded, and clearly abnormal in shape, with abnormally shaped nuclear membranes, mild hyperchromasia, occasional small nucleoli, and increased nucleus-to-cytoplasm (N/C) ratios (Figures 19-4 to 19-15).[10,15,25,28,31,33,35–40] The cytomorphologic features of these cells are virtually identical to those of low-grade DCIS. Architecturally, FEA may manifest cellular stratification, but there are no blunt, club-shaped micropapillary projections or Roman bridges. In addition, FEA, including the stratified type, may demonstrate cytoplasmic apocrine features. It is important to recognize that the term "flat" does not exclude cellular stratification, but it does exclude the architectural

manifestations of ADH, namely, Roman arches and blunt micropapillae. Cytoplasmic blebs/snouts are present but, in general, are reduced. Mitotic figures are very uncommon but may be observed. The diagnosis of FEA must not rest on the presence of mitotic figures. The terminology applied to FEA throughout the years is supplied in Table 19-1. An algorithmic approach to aid in the differential diagnosis/morphologic assessment of columnar cell alterations is illustrated in Figure 19-16.

Differential Diagnosis

The CCC, CCH, and FEA all display irregularly dilated TDLUs, often containing secretions and coarse calcium or granular calcific debris. The FEA tends to appear to be "more blue" than CCC/CCH at scanning magnification because the cells are crowded together and have higher N/C ratios. It is important to distinguish CCC and CCH from FEA because FEA will require further patient follow-up whereas CCC/CCH will not.

Apocrine metaplasia is in the differential diagnosis. At times, FEA may have apocrine cytoplasm (see Figure 19-9), and the key here is to recognize the low-grade monomorphic cytology of FEA because apocrine

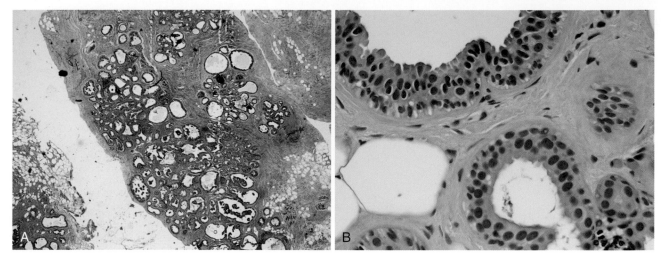

FIGURE 19-4   FEA. **A,** Low magnification demonstrates a more blue appearance due to cellular crowding. Note numerous coarse calcifications. **B,** FEA with rounded, mildly hyperchromatic nuclei and monotonous morphology.

KEY DIAGNOSTIC POINTS

Columnar Cell Change and Hyperplasia versus Flat Epithelial Atypia

	CCC	CCH	FEA
Pattern	Enlarged/di-lated TDLUs Calcifications Lumen secretions	Same	Same
Histology	One or two cell layers	>2 cells/ stratified No complex architecture	Single/stratified No complex architecture May have apocrine cytoplasm
Cytology	Bland oval nuclei No nucleoi Smooth nuclear membranes Apical snouts	Bland nuclei No nucleoli Smooth nuclear membranes Apical snouts	Enlarged, rounded Hyperchromasia Small nucleoli Increased N/C ratio

CCC, columnar cell change; CCH, columnar cell hyperplasia; FEA, flat epithelial atypia; N/C, nucleus-to-cytoplasm; TDLU, terminal duct lobular units.

KEY DIAGNOSTIC POINTS

Differential Diagnosis of Flat Epithelial Atypia/Blunt Duct Adenosis/High-Grade Ductal Carcinoma In Situ Clinging Type

- BDA has curved ducts; mostly nondilated, bland luminal cell cytology; prominent myoepithelial cells; luminal cells variably positive for CK5 or CK5/6 and focally positive for ER.

- FEA has low grade monomorphic (grade 1) cytology, is strongly diffuse ER+, HER2–, very rare mitoses, no atypical mitoses, readily evident myoepithelial cells.

- High-grade DCIS clinging type has high grade 3 cytology; possible luminal necrosis; mitoses, including atypical mitoses, are more likely; mostly ER–; mostly HER2+; Ki-67 index > 20%; myoepithelial cells attenuated; luminal cells may be CK5 or CK5/6 variably positive.

BDA, blunt duct adenosis; CK, cytokeratin; DCIS, ductal carcinoma in situ; ER, estrogen receptor; FEA, flat epithelial atypia.

metaplasia usually has prominent nucleoli, and apical eosinophilic refractile Lendrum's granules, whereas FEA does not. Also, FEA is distinguished from ADH by the presence, in ADH, of club-shaped micropapillary projections and Roman arch formation (Figures 19-17 to 19-26). Micropapillary structures may occur in ductal hyperplasia (DEH), but they are slender, not club-shaped, or part of an obvious bridging area in DEH (see Figures 19-25 and 19-26). Blunt duct adenosis (BDA), described by Azzopardi,[4] is distinguished from FEA by the more rigid, curved, nondilated acinar configuration that is associated with increased stromal cellularity and myoepithelial prominence (see Figure 19-24). Myoepithelial cells are prominent in BDA, and BDA is variably positive for cytokeratin 5 (CK5) or CK5/6 in luminal cells.

High-grade flat DCIS (high-grade flat DIN) is distinguished by the high-grade (grade 3) malignant cytology (Figure 19-27), in contrast to the low-grade monomorphic cytology (grade 1) of FEA.[10] High-grade DCIS is often HER2+, ER– and shows mitotic figures/atypical mitotic figures with Ki-67 indices greater than 20%, whereas FEA is HER2– and strongly positive for ER, with only very rare mitotic figures, no atypical mitotic figures, and Ki-67 indices less than 5%.

IMMUNOHISTOLOGY OF COLUMNAR CELL–RELATED LESIONS

CCCs and FEA are immunoreactive with CAM5.2 and broad-spectrum keratin cocktails such as AE1/ AE3. This immunostaining reflects the presence of

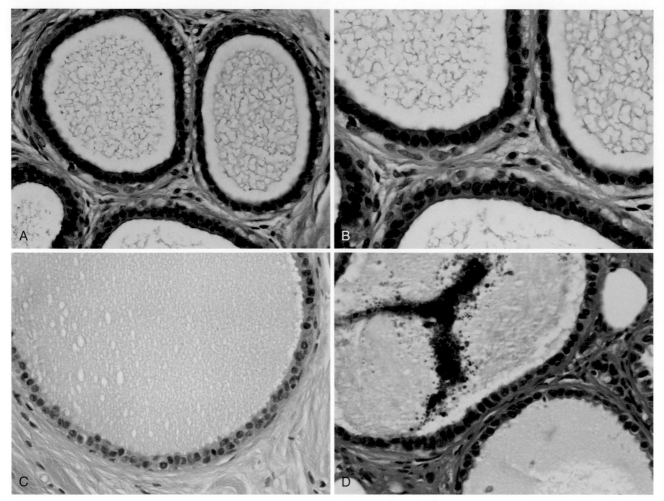

FIGURE 19-5 Slightly dilated FEA. **A,** Attenuated cells have monomorphic rounded nuclei. **B,** Higher magnification of slightly dilated FEA with mildly hyperchromatic rounded nuclei. Loss of apical snouts yields a relative higher nucleus-to-cytoplasm ratio. **C,** Monomorphic atypia and blunting of apical snouts. **D,** Calcific debris and monomorphic rounded atypical cells.

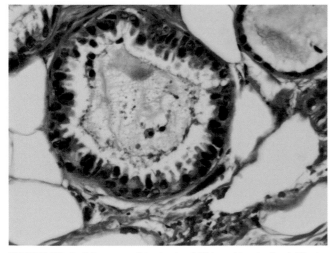

FIGURE 19-6 Monomorphic atypia of FEA and luminal calcific debris and apical blebs.

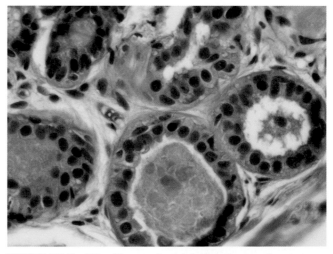

FIGURE 19-7 FEA with granular luminal content and monomorphic atypia. Small nucleoli are evident in some cells.

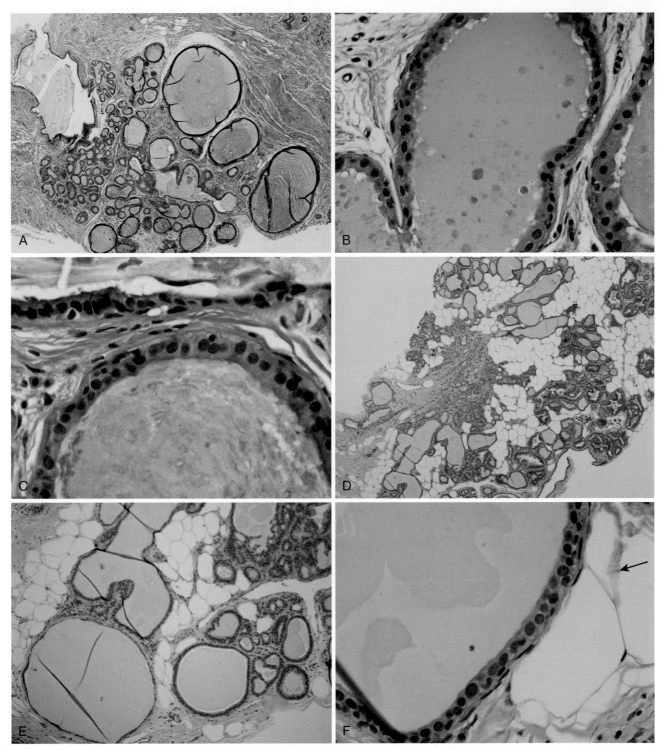

FIGURE 19-8 Colloid-like FEA. **A,** Low magnification of dilated "colloid–like" FEA. **B,** "Colloid-like" FEA in which these cells have apocrine features and monomorphic atypia. **C,** "Colloid-like" FEA shows monomorphic atypia and attenuation of cells with loss of apical snouts. **D,** Low magnification of dilated "colloid-like" FEA. This simulates fibrocystic change. **E,** "Colloid-like" FEA shows dilatation and blue cellular appearance at medium magnification. **F,** Higher magnification shows monomorphic atypia within the area of "colloid-like" FEA.

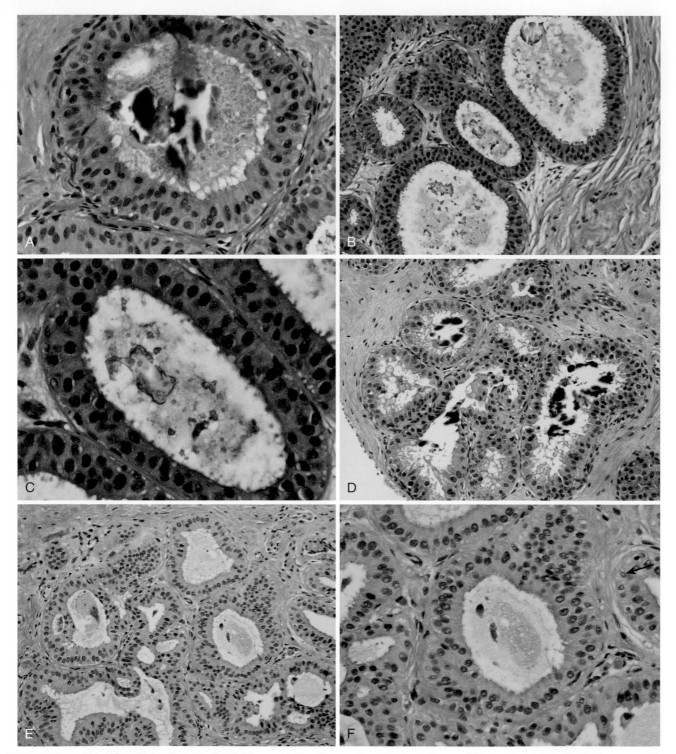

FIGURE 19-9 FEA with apocrine features. **A,** Multilayered FEA with apocrine cytoplasm shows calcific luminal debris. **B,** Medium magnification of FEA with apocrine features. Note multilayered epithelium, prominent apical snouts, and calcific luminal debris. **C,** Higher magnification of FEA with apocrine features and calcific debris. Small nucleoli appear in some nuclei. **D,** This FEA with apocrine features has vacuolated cytoplasm and calcific debris. **E,** This focus of FEA shows architectural abnormality of atypical duct hyperplasia (ADH) on the left side of the image with focal early cribriform architecture. **F,** Apocrine variant of FEA shows monomorphic atypia.

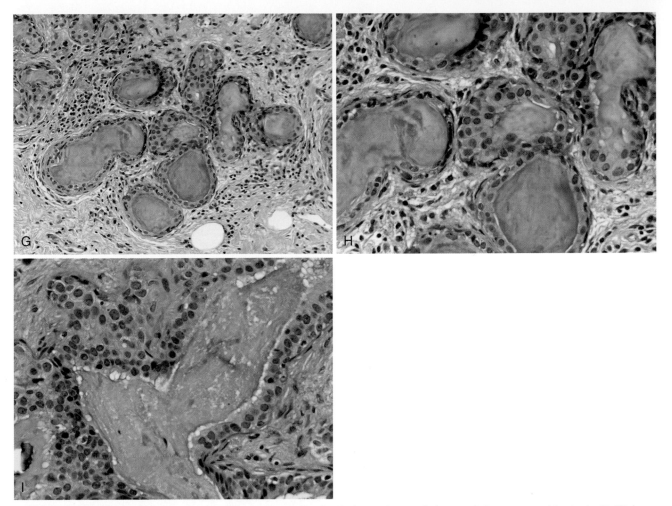

FIGURE 19-9, cont'd **G,** Apocrine variant of FEA with tenacious luminal secretions and characteristic monomorphic atypia. **H,** High magnification shows monomorphic atypia and presence of some nucleoli in focal areas. **I,** Tenacious luminal material in this area of apocrine FEA with characteristic monomorphic cytology.

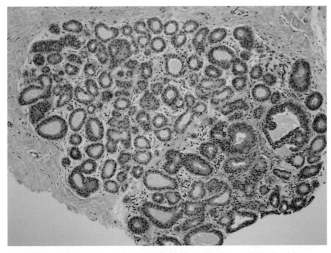

FIGURE 19-10 The *right half* of this lobule shows FEA. At this magnification, the cells appear more blue.

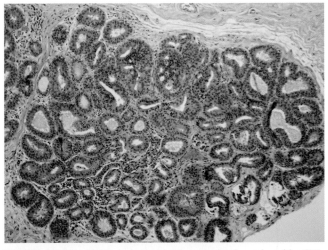

FIGURE 19-11 This lobule is virtually completely replaced by FEA, appears more blue, and shows focal cribriform architecture in the *middle top* of the image.

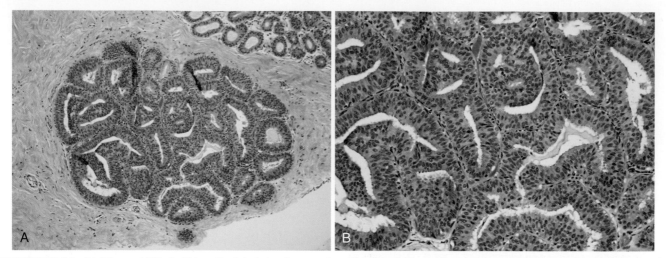

FIGURE 19-12 Multilayered FEA. **A,** This entire lobule has been replaced by FEA of the multilayered type with focal architectural abnormality. Compare with the adjacent normal lobule in the *upper right.* **B,** Higher magnification of the multilayered FEA and focally cribriforming in this lobule.

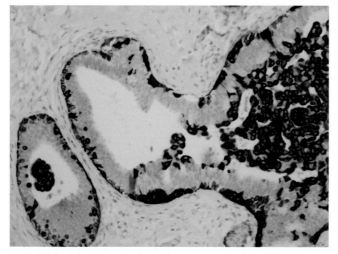

FIGURE 19-13 Cytokeratin (CK) 5 in this lobule of FEA shows no expression in the FEA but strong expression in the luminal area of usual ductal epithelial hyperplasia.

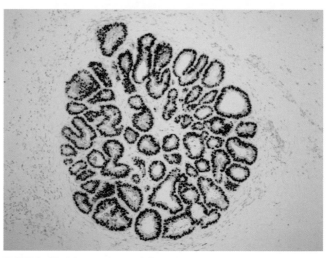

FIGURE 19-14 ER shows diffuse immunostaining because of ER up-regulation, a typical pattern with FEA.

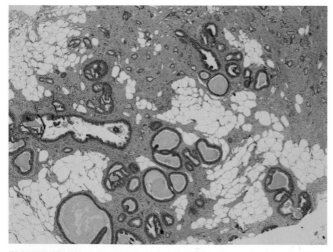

FIGURE 19-15 Low-power magnification shows prominent FEA in dilated acini, foci of ADH with Roman arches, and invasive tubular carcinoma on the *top half* of the image.

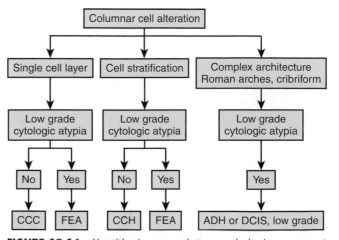

FIGURE 19-16 Algorithmic approach to morphologic assessment of columnar-related lesions. ADH, atypical ductal hyperplasia; CCC, columnar cell change; CCH, columnar cell hyperplasia; DCIS, ductal carcinoma in situ; FEA, flat epithelial atypia.

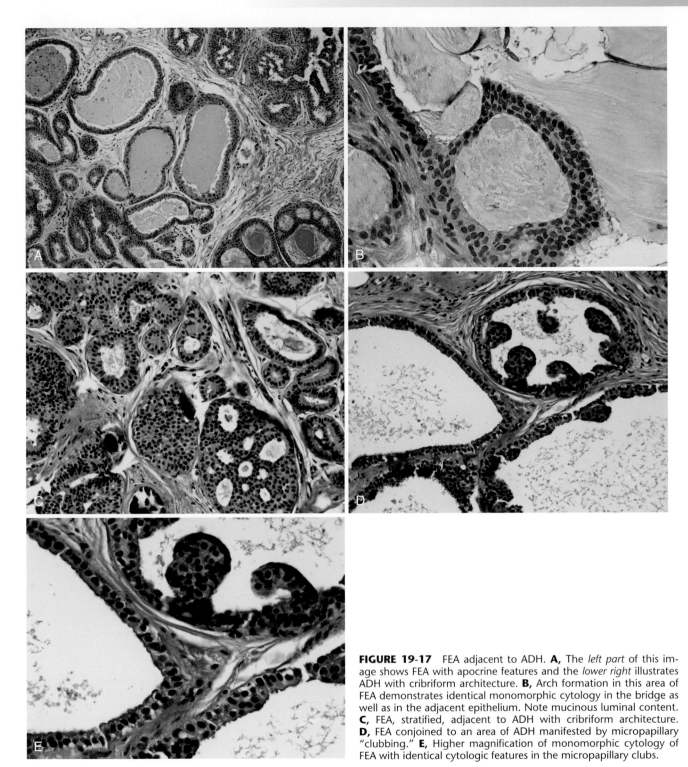

FIGURE 19-17 FEA adjacent to ADH. **A,** The *left part* of this image shows FEA with apocrine features and the *lower right* illustrates ADH with cribriform architecture. **B,** Arch formation in this area of FEA demonstrates identical monomorphic cytology in the bridge as well as in the adjacent epithelium. Note mucinous luminal content. **C,** FEA, stratified, adjacent to ADH with cribriform architecture. **D,** FEA conjoined to an area of ADH manifested by micropapillary "clubbing." **E,** Higher magnification of monomorphic cytology of FEA with identical cytologic features in the micropapillary clubs.

low-molecular-weight keratins such as 8 and 19. There is no immunoreactivity for high-molecular-weight keratins with antibodies 34βE12, CK5, or CK5/6. All forms of columnar alterations show up-regulation of ER compared with adjacent breast lobules, with diffuse strong immunostaining with antibodies directed against ER-α. The cellular constituents also demonstrate increased proliferation rates with Ki-67 compared with adjacent normal breast lobular units. Increasing proliferative

indices are seen with progression from CCH to FEA. Ki-67 indices of proliferation are typically less than 5%. The FEA is commonly positive for bcl-2, an antiapoptotic proto-oncogene, and cyclin D1, a cell cycle regulator.

Abdel-Fatah and coworkers[11] demonstrated the immunohistochemical kinships in FEA and the low-grade neoplasia pathway. The epithelial cells in the putative precursors, FEA, ADH, lobular neoplasia (LN),

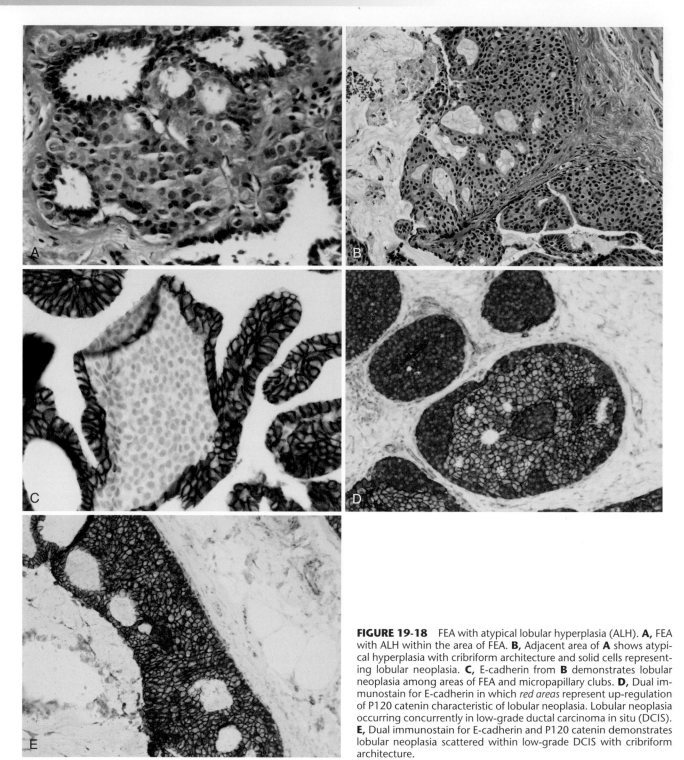

FIGURE 19-18 FEA with atypical lobular hyperplasia (ALH). **A,** FEA with ALH within the area of FEA. **B,** Adjacent area of **A** shows atypical hyperplasia with cribriform architecture and solid cells representing lobular neoplasia. **C,** E-cadherin from **B** demonstrates lobular neoplasia among areas of FEA and micropapillary clubs. **D,** Dual immunostain for E-cadherin in which *red areas* represent up-regulation of P120 catenin characteristic of lobular neoplasia. Lobular neoplasia occurring concurrently in low-grade ductal carcinoma in situ (DCIS). **E,** Dual immunostain for E-cadherin and P120 catenin demonstrates lobular neoplasia scattered within low-grade DCIS with cribriform architecture.

DCIS, and their coexisting invasive low–nuclear grade breast cancers (LNGBCs) were negative for basal and myoepithelial markers, but positive for CK19/18/8, ER-α, bcl-2, and cyclin D1. The ER-α/ER-β expression ratio increased during carcinogenesis, as did expression of cyclin D1 and bcl-2.[11,14]

At the present time, there are no prognostic or predictive factors by immunohistology that can predict progressive behavior of these cellular alterations.

Clinical Relevance, Management, and Risk/Prognosis

There are only a few follow-up studies of patients with columnar cell alterations, and together, they suggest that they may be associated with a very slight increased risk of breast cancer (one- to twofold risk increase).[41]

Boulos and colleagues[42] observed a positive association between CCL and atypical hyperplasia. The

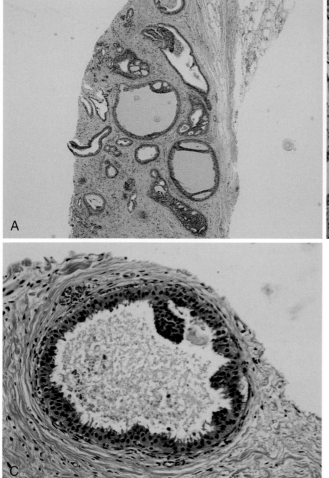

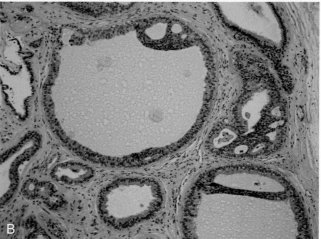

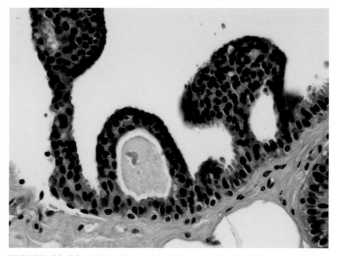

FIGURE 19-19 FEA and ADH. **A,** Low magnification of FEA and concurrent foci of ADH manifested by arches and cribriforming. **B,** Higher magnification demonstrates the stratified FEA and arch and cribriform areas. **C,** FEA with focal areas of micropapillary clubs.

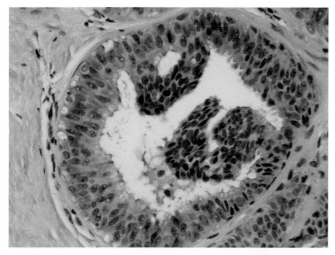

FIGURE 19-20 Stratified FEA with foci of early cribriform architecture.

FIGURE 19-21 FEA with arches. Note similarity of monomorphic cytologic atypia in architectural areas.

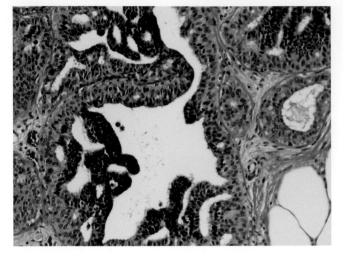

FIGURE 19-22 This area of FEA shows multilayering in continuity with micropapillary clubbing and early arch formation.

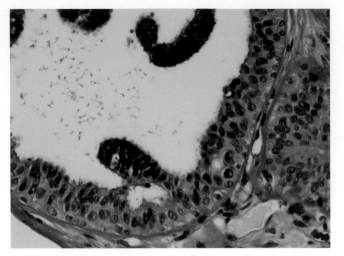

FIGURE 19-23 FEA, multilayered and micropapillary clubs of ADH.

possibility that CCLs by themselves significantly elevate breast cancer risk was not well supported. However, a finding of CCL on a benign breast biopsy may indicate the presence of other, more worrisome lesions.

Aroner and associates,[43] in a nested case control study, provided evidence that CCL may be an important marker of breast cancer risk in women with benign breast disease, but they suggest that CCLs do not increase breast cancer risk independently of concurrent proliferative changes in the breast. These studies indicate that CCL alone probably does not increase risk of breast cancer.

There are only a few studies of patients who have FEA as the only risk lesion on core biopsy, and these patients do have a risk of having a worse lesion on surgical excision, a risk comparable with that of ADH alone on core biopsy. Most of these studies are small, and additional clinical outcome studies are needed to better assess the risk for the individual patient.

In the study by Senetta and coworkers,[44] a total of 41 cases of FEA were available for study. Only 36 (87%) of these cases had follow-up excisional biopsies. Importantly, 14 of these 36 cases were BIRADS 3, and the remaining 22 were BIRADS 4. There was no upstaging to carcinoma in any of these cases.

In the study by Piubello and colleagues,[45] only 20/33 (60%) of patients with pure FEA on core biopsy had surgical re-excision follow-up. Importantly, only 2 of these 20 patients had a BIRADS category 4; the remainder had a BIRADS category 3. None of these 20 patients was upstaged to carcinoma on surgical re-excision.

In the study by Chivukula and associates,[34] there was no statistical difference in upstaging to carcinoma on surgical re-excision for patients who had pure FEA versus those who had FEA plus ADH on 11-gauge vacuum-assisted breast core biopsies. In this study, all patients had BIRADS 4 imaging for calcifications only. Fourteen percent of patients with pure FEA on core biopsy were upstaged to either DCIS or invasive cancer.

In the study by Ingegnoli and coworkers,[46] 15 of 18 (83%) patients with pure FEA on core biopsy had a surgical re-excision, 1 had DCIS, and 2 had invasive carcinoma for an upstaging of 20%. On mammographic

images, all FEA patients had only calcifications and were BIRADS 4 or 3. These results are similar to the studies by Chivukula and associates[34] and Kunju and Kleer,[21] which showed no statistically significant differences for upstaging on surgical biopsies whether pure ADH or pure FEA was present on the core biopsy.

Darvishian and colleagues,[37] in a study of reproducibility of the diagnosis of atypia in breast core biopsies, concluded that upstaging on excisions occurred in 16% of cases of FEA, 15% of ALH, and 20% of ADH, figures that are similar to the studies cited previously.

Guerra-Wallace and associates[47] found upstaging from core biopsies in somewhat more cases when FEA was present than when it was not present, recommending surgical excision.

The degree of upstaging to a worse lesion on surgical excision when FEA is the sole risk lesion on core biopsy of the breast is similar to the degree of upstaging when only ADH is present on core biopsy.[16,20,21,23,34,36,37,41,46,48–57] These findings are consonant with the morphology and molecular kinship of FEA and ADH, as described later.

In summary, the literature suggests that patients with a targeted lesion for calcium with a BIRADS 4 imaging study and pure FEA on core biopsy are at greater risk for

---

KEY CLINICAL FEATURES

Columnar Cell Lesions

- Present as calcifications on mammographic imaging.
- Fourth most common cause of calcifications on mammogram, along with FCC, fibroadenoma, sclerosing adenosis
- CCLs do not independently increase the risk of breast cancer. Concurrent proliferative breast changes are more important in this regard, as is the category of CCL.
- CCL may be a marker for the potential presence of atypia in the breast.

CCLs, columnar cell lesions; FCC, fibrocystic change.

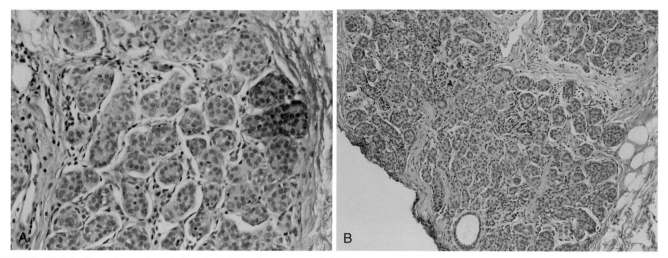

FIGURE 19-24 Blunt duct adenosis (BDA). **A,** BDA demonstrates lobular expansion with cells having benign cytologic features and prominent myoepithelial cells. **B,** Confluent lobules show BDA with lobular architecture.

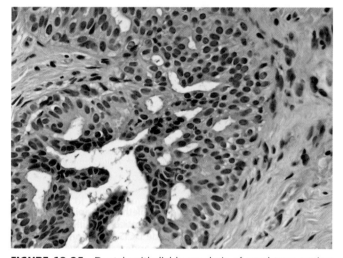

FIGURE 19-25 Ductal epithelial hyperplasia of usual type, noting bland cytology, irregular slitlike spaces, and bridging zones simulating micropapillary clubs.

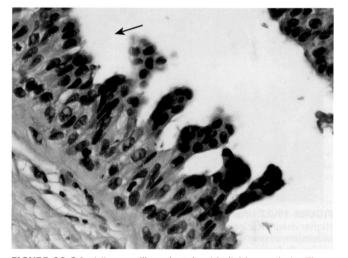

FIGURE 19-26 Micropapillary ductal epithelial hyperplasia. These cells have bland cytology, are multilayered, and lack the club architecture of micropapillary architecture seen in ADH.

upstaging (~20%) to a worse lesion on surgical excision than patients who have a BIRADS 3 image, especially if all calcifications are not removed with core biopsy.

RELATIONSHIPS AMONG FLAT EPITHELIAL ATYPIA, LOBULAR NEOPLASIA, ATYPICAL DUCTAL EPITHELIAL HYPERPLASIA, LOW-GRADE DUCTAL CARCINOMA IN SITU, AND CARCINOMA: A MOLECULAR KINSHIP

Observational studies have demonstrated that FEA commonly coexists on the same microscopic slides as ADH, LN, or low-grade DCIS.[3,5,6,10,28,32,34,38,58–65] ADH in this context is defined by the presence of architectural and cytologic atypia that falls short of the diagnosis of DCIS.[66]

A recent study by Chivukula and associates[34] demonstrated that sequential deeper levels of the paraffin

blocks of core biopsies of the breast that demonstrate FEA revealed transitions from FEA to ADH in 17% of cases on further deeper sectioning of the block.

In addition to ADH, tubular carcinoma (TC) is also a common finding in association with FEA.[62,64,65,67] A noncolumnar associated lesion, LN, has also been described as part of the "Rosen triad" of FEA, LN, and TC.[64] Leibl and coworkers[38] found LN in nearly 87% of cases of FEA in excisional biopsy specimens. Carley and colleagues[68] described the simultaneous occurrence of LN with CCCs without atypia in 54% of core biopsies targeted exclusively for calcification.

A molecular kinship also exists among columnar cell–related alterations. Dabbs and associates[67] investigated, through loss of heterozygosity (LOH) analysis, whether there were molecular aberrations common to CCC, CCH, ADH, and TC that were all present on the same glass slide. The conclusions of this study indicted that there was a low prevalence of molecular alterations, but they were found in very low levels in CCC, with increasing numbers of identical aberrations that (taxane and anthracycline regimen) efficacy with a negative predictive value for pathologic complete response of 97%. Unlike some prior studies, one prominent observation in this study was the significant discordance between clinical receptor status and molecular subtypes. Of the 626 ER+ tumors analyzed in the microarray test set, 73% were luminal (an ER+ molecular subtype), 11% were HER2-enriched (an ER– molecular subtype), 5% were basal-like (an ER– subtype), and 12% were normal-like (also supposed to be ER–). Conversely, the ER– tumors comprised 11% luminal, 32% HER2-enriched, 50% basal-like, and 7% normal-like. There could have been several valid reasons for these discrepancies such as tumor heterogeneity with respect to receptor status; very low degree of hormone receptor positivity, which by defined/accepted criteria are unfortunately labeled as hormone receptor–positive tumors; or admixture of normal or nontumoral tissue resulting in dilution of mRNA used for expression analysis. But instead of examining or providing details, the investigators concluded that ER and HER2 status alone are not accurate surrogates for true intrinsic subtype status.

A recent similar publication also concluded that PAM50 gene expression test for intrinsic biologic subtype can be applied to large series of FFPE breast cancers and gives more prognostic information than clinical factors and immunohistochemistry using standard cutpoints.[23] Once again the key words were "standard cut points," which create artificial categories (such as ER+ and ER– tumors based on 1% cutoff). For example, a tumor expressing ER weakly in 1% of tumor cells is more close to an ER– tumor than to a tumor showing strong expression in nearly every cell. Despite this fact, the tumor showing 1% weak expression is considered an ER+ tumor in the previously mentioned studies and also for statistical analysis in which ER status is considered a categorical variable. This minor deviation then results in a big discrepancy for which details are not provided in the manuscripts or even in supplementary data because semiquantitative results are not always available. There is definitely some truth that ER and HER2 immunohistochemical status has certain limitations in predicting molecular subtype and hence prognosis, but almost none of the previously discussed publications related to molecular subtyping made an attempt to directly compare the prognostic/predictive value of subtype with the combined power of histologic grading, semiquantitative immunohistochemical results, and clinical parameters. A bigger question is whether an expensive nonmorphologic molecular test is required in lieu of immunohistochemistry and histologic grading in all cases. Moreover, concerns about reproducibility of different platforms in predicting the molecular subtype of an individual sample have been recently raised.

Weigelt and coworkers[23a] recently assessed the clinical usefulness of three different SSPs by comparing different methods of breast cancer molecular subtype assignment and to ascertain whether each SSP identifies molecular subtypes with similar associations with outcome. For this purpose, the investigators analyzed 53 microdissected in-house samples and 3 cohorts of breast cancer samples in the public domain. The public domain data sets utilized in this study were NKI-295 (N = 295),[24] Wang and colleagues (N = 286),[25] and TransBig (N = 198)[26] data sets. The three centroid/SSPs used for comparison were described over the last 10 years by Sorlie and associates,[10] Hu and coworkers,[18] and Parker and associates.[22] The results showed a fair to substantial agreement (κ value of 0.238–0.740) between SSPs in each cohort. Only the basal-like class was consistently predicted by each SSPs in all the cohorts. However, the prediction of all other classes varied substantially. Excluding the basal-like and luminal A classes, the significance of associations with outcome of other molecular subtypes varied depending on SSP used. However, different SSPs produced broadly similar survival curves. This study highlighted the lack of stringent standardization of methodologies and definitions for molecular subtypes that led to failure of SSPs to reliably assign the same patients to the same molecular subtypes. As expected, the study was criticized by the original investigators as well as others in the field.[27-31] One reason for discordance was probably the use of publically available data sets with different platforms as pointed out by Perou and colleagues in the letter.[30] In practical terms, an SSP is valid only when a single platform is used for both training and testing predictions because different protocols for the same gene show measurement bias. One way to deal with bias is to use controls that are often unavailable in public data sets. In these cases, normalization estimates or gene centering must be determined from observations of the test cases but it defeats the whole purpose of an SSP because one should not go back to all prior samples in order to determine the subtype for the new sample. Despite the criticism of the Weigelt and coworkers[23a] study by original investigators, it is obvious that variations of the methodology (e.g., probe annotation, choice and averaging of probes, and data centering) exert a substantial effect on the assignment of individual samples to the molecular subtypes. Several issues related to standardization of methodologies need to be addressed before these assays are introduced to routine clinical practice.

KEY PATHOLOGIC FEATURES

Intrinsic Gene Set–Based Classification of Breast Carcinoma

- Reflects intrinsic biologic properties of tumors.

- Currently four distinct classes are recognized: luminal A, luminal B, HER2-enriched, and basal-like.

- Normal breast-like class likely reflects an artificial category created owing to poor tumor sampling.

- Molecular classes broadly reflect steroid HR status; luminal being HR+ and nonluminal classes (HER2-enriched and basal-like) being HR–.

- Luminal B class reflects poor prognosis HR+ tumors.

- Most carcinomas in BRCA1 mutation carriers are of basal-like class.

HR, hormone receptor.

OTHER MOLECULAR SUBTYPES

Claudin-Low Tumors

Claudin-low tumors are a recently identified group of triple-negative tumors that have gene expression profile similar to basal-like breast cancer[32] but also have some distinct differences. These tumors are characterized by enrichment (much more than basal-like cancers) of epithelial to mesenchymal transition markers, immune response genes, and cancer stem cell markers.[33,34] These tumors are named as such owing to low gene expression of tight junction protein claudins 3, 4, and 7. In addition, these tumors also demonstrate low to absent expression of E-cadherin protein but are not lobular carcinomas morphologically. Recently, Prat and associates[35] comprehensively characterized these tumors at the molecular level. Taking tumors from three previously published data sets and 37 new samples (N = 337), hierarchical clustering using approximately 1900 intrinsic genes, the investigators identified the defined intrinsic molecular classes including claudin-low that was placed in close proximity of the basal-like subtype. These tumors showed inconsistent expression of basal keratins such as keratins 5, 14, and 17 and low expression of *HER2*, luminal marker keratins 18 and 19, ER, progesterone (PgR), and ER-related genes. Unlike basal-like tumors, claudin-low tumors as a group did not show high expression of proliferation genes. The prognosis of claudin-low tumors is reported to be significantly worse than luminal A tumors as expected (prognosis of ER– tumors in general is worse than ER+ tumors). It is unclear whether these tumors have a worse or better prognosis than basal-like breast cancers. However, the data on anthracycline/taxane-based neoadjuvant chemotherapy suggest that claudin-low tumors are less responsive to chemotherapy and have significantly lower pathologic complete response rate than basal-like breast cancers.

Molecular Apocrine Class

Subsequent to intrinsic gene set–based molecular classification, Farmer and coworkers[36] reported identification of a "molecular apocrine group." These investigators studied tumor samples from 49 patients with locally advanced breast cancers and, using principal component analysis and hierarchical clustering, defined three tumor groups that they called "luminal," "basal," and "apocrine." The "molecular apocrine" tumors were described to show strong apocrine features on histologic examination and were positive for androgen receptor (AR), but negative for ER and PgR. Further testing also revealed that androgen signaling was most active in molecular apocrine tumors and were commonly *HER2*+. It appears that the "molecular apocrine group" identified by Farmer and coworkers significantly overlap with ERBB2 group (or *HER2*-enriched) of intrinsic gene set–based molecular classification. Through extrapolation of these findings to routine diagnostic and immunohistochemistry analysis, it appears that the molecular apocrine tumors are either ER–/PgR–/*HER2*+/AR+ or ER–/PgR–/*HER2*–/AR+. Both tumor groups demonstrate histologic evidence of apocrine differentiation in a large percentage of cases. The previous assumption is supported by our own study of AR expression in 189 consecutive breast cancers, in which AR was expressed not only in ER+ tumors but also in ER– tumors with apocrine differentiation.[37]

MOLECULAR ANALYSES OF SPECIAL SUBTYPE CARCINOMAS

The molecular classification using "intrinsic" gene set was derived mainly by analyzing invasive ductal carcinomas of no special type. In order to fill this gap on special subtype breast carcinomas, Weigelt and coworkers[38] reported molecular characterization of the various histologic subtypes of breast cancer. Of the 17 known special subtype breast carcinomas, these authors studied 113 tumors belonging to 11 different subtypes using immunohistochemistry and genome-wide gene expression profiling. In this study, the molecular classes (luminal, ERBB2, and basal-like) correlated with immunohistochemical surrogate markers ER, PgR, *HER2* protein expression profile, that is, the "triple-negative" adenoid cystic, medullary, and metaplastic tumors clustered with the usual type of basal-like carcinomas, and the ER+/*HER2*– tumors such as tubular, mucinous, and classic lobular carcinomas clustered together as luminal tumors.[38]

MOLECULAR PROFILING OF METASTATIC DISEASE

Even before gene expression profiling, it was known that any type (low grade, high grade, hormone receptor–positive, hormone receptor–negative) of invasive breast carcinoma can metastasize; however, it was thought that metastatic tumor develops as a result of stepwise progression in a particular cancer type. This concept may still be true for a certain proportion of carcinomas, but it seems like the majority of carcinomas have that potential from the very beginning, and genome-wide expression analyses of primary and metastatic tumors may help unlock these secrets. There are very few molecular studies of matched primary and metastatic tumors, but most suggest that primary and metastatic tumors from one patient are more similar to each other than to metastatic tumors from different patients.[39,40] The concept that "metastatic capability in breast cancer is an inherent feature and is not based on clonal selection" is the basis of a multigene prediction assay now commercially available as MammaPrint. Other investigators have studied metastatic tumor and found site-specific breast cancer metastasis gene signatures, such as bone metastasis,[41] lung metastases,[42,43] and brain metastasis.[44] These signatures may be important if particular targets could be identified and, hence, be treated to prevent metastases. In fact, with respect to bone metastases, Smid and coworkers[45] identified 69 genes that were differentially expressed between patients that developed metastases to bone compared with other sites.

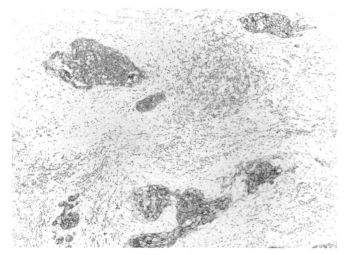

FIGURE 21-36 LCIS and ductal carcinoma in situ (DCIS), E-cadherin immunostaining.

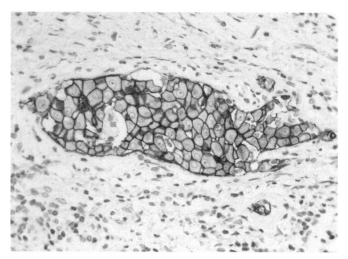

FIGURE 21-38 DCIS, E-cadherin immunostaining, high-power magnification of Figure 21-36.

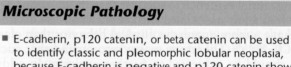

FIGURE 21-37 LCIS, E-cadherin immunostaining, high-power magnification of Figure 21-36.

bona fide ALH/LCIS with E-cadherin expression, cytoplasmic expression of catenin p120 can be used to corroborate a diagnosis of ALH/LCIS.[58,91] Occasionally, lesions show an overlapping range of morphologic features along with variable expression of immunohistochemical markers. This suggests that LCIS and low-grade solid DCIS may truly coexist within the same duct–lobular unit. In these circumstances, differentiation between the two is often not possible and both diagnoses should be given. How a patient should be managed in these unresolved cases remains a challenge, but pragmatically, they will receive treatment as for DCIS.

Likewise, PLCIS must be differentiated from high-grade solid DCIS, given that both lesions display similar features, including high nuclear grade, comedonecrosis, and calcifications. Owing to the massive distention of the TDLUs, PLCIS may not appear so dyscohesive and pose diagnostic problems. In this context, immunohistochemistry plays an essential role because PLCIS must show down-regulation of E-cadherin, β-catenin, and/or catenin p120 (Figures 21-42 to 21-44). Nevertheless, the

same caution as described previously must be exercised when analyzing the immunostains. A small proportion of PLCIS may show focal membranous positivity for E-cadherin.

KEY PATHOLOGIC FEATURES

Microscopic Pathology

- E-cadherin, p120 catenin, or beta catenin can be used to identify classic and pleomorphic lobular neoplasia, because E-cadherin is negative and p120 catenin shows cytoplasmic up-regulation. p120 catenin is currently the only positive marker for lobular neoplasia of all types. Ductal neoplasia shows membranous staining for both E-cadherin and p120 catenin.

- *HER2*/neu is positive by IHC and FISH amplified in up to 5% of cases of classic lobular neoplasia, whereas 15% to 20% of pleomorphic lobular neoplasms have *HER2* amplification.

- ER is present in more than 95% of classic lobular neoplasms.

- In many centers, a core biopsy finding (BIRADS 4) of lobular neoplasia may trigger a surgical re-excision.

- E-cadherin may be present in weak or aberrant patterns in 5% to 15% of cases. In these situations, attention to morphologic features is most helpful.

BIRADS, Breast Imaging Reporting and Data System; ER, estrogen receptor; FISH, fluorescence in situ hybridization; IHC, immunohistochemistry.

INVASIVE LOBULAR CARCINOMA

ILC is defined as an invasive carcinoma usually associated with LCIS and composed of noncohesive cells individually dispersed or arranged in a single-file linear pattern immersed in a fibrous stroma (Figure 21-45).[32] It represents 5% to 15% of all invasive breast cancers.[92–97] Early studies have suggested an incidence around 5%[93,95,96]; however, the use of less restrictive criteria and recognition

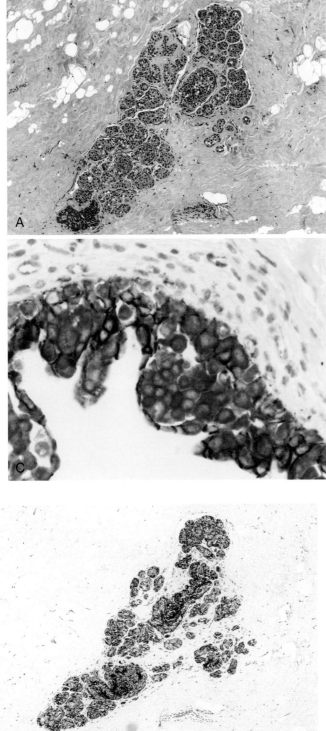

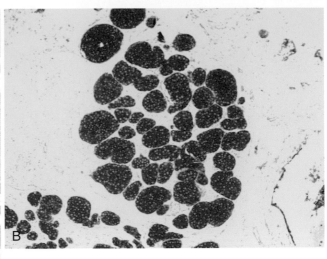

FIGURE 21-39 LCIS. **A,** Lobular distention. **B,** Dual immunostain for p120 catenin *(red)* shows diffuse cytoplasmic stain characteristic of lobular neoplasia. E-cadherin *(brown)* is absent in the cell membranes. **C,** Dual stain in pagetoid spread of LCIS, red cytoplasmic staining of LCIS cells.

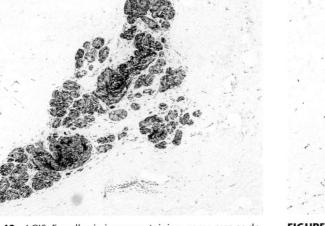

FIGURE 21-40 LCIS, E-cadherin immunostaining, same case as depicted in Figure 21-39. Only myoepithelial cells are decorated.

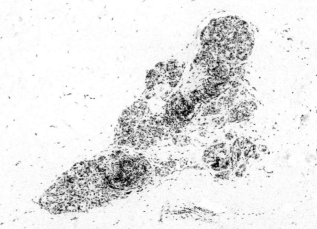

FIGURE 21-41 LCIS, β-catenin immunostaining, same case as depicted in Figure 21-39.

of variants of ILC such as the alveolar, solid, and pleomorphic variants have led to an increase in the percentage of cases diagnosed as ILCs to approximately 10% to 15% of all breast cancers.[20,92,94,98,99] In addition, the incidence of ILCs has increased in the last decades,[16] possibly due to the use of hormone replacement therapy (see earlier).[14,19,20]

Clinical Presentation

In most cases, the presenting symptom is a palpable mass with irregular margins. Not uncommonly, however, the findings are ambiguous and tumors of reasonable size may be clinically reported as a poorly defined thickening or a fine diffuse nodularity without a

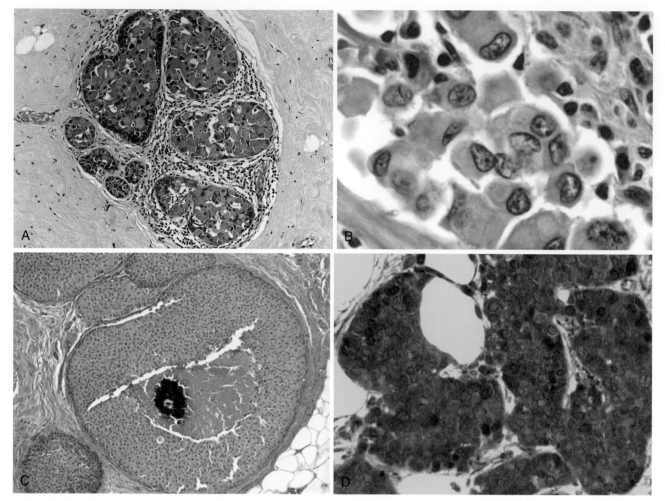

FIGURE 21-42 LCIS. **A,** Pleomorphic type with apocrine differentiation. **B,** Grade 3 nuclei of pleomorphic lobular carcinoma in situ (PLCIS). **C,** Central necrosis and calcification of PLCIS mimics DCIS. **D,** p120 catenin cytoplasmic staining in PLCIS.

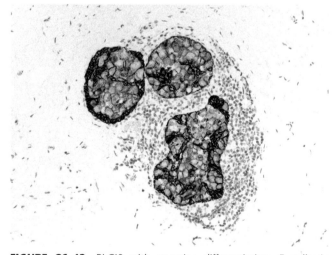

FIGURE 21-43 PLCIS with apocrine differentiation, E-cadherin immunostaining, same case as depicted in Figure 21-41. Note the myoepithelial cell staining.

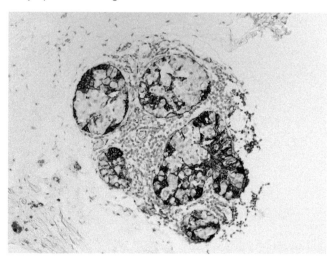

FIGURE 21-44 PLCIS with apocrine differentiation, loss of β-catenin immunostaining, same case as depicted in Figure 21-39.

correlated image at mammograms, resulting in a delay in diagnosis. The age at diagnosis is reported to be similar but slightly higher than that of ductal and mixed carcinomas.[6,97,99] All quadrants may be involved, but when compared with IDCs, ILCs may occur more frequently in the central area.[99] ILCs are traditionally known for being multifocal and bilateral more frequently than other invasive breast tumors. These features seem to be associated (i.e., patients with multicentric disease are more likely to have bilateral disease) and likely to be intrinsic to the biology of lobular proliferations.[100]

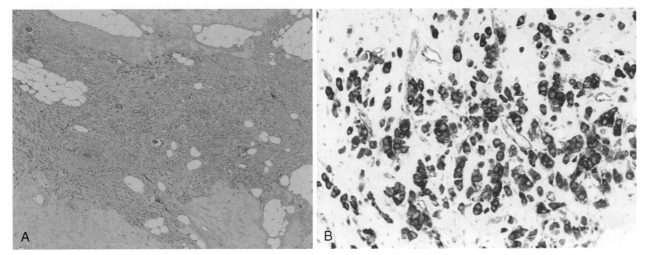

FIGURE 21-45 ILC. **A,** Classic type. **B,** Dual immunostain for p120 catenin (*red,* positive in cytoplasm) and E-cadherin (*brown,* negative).

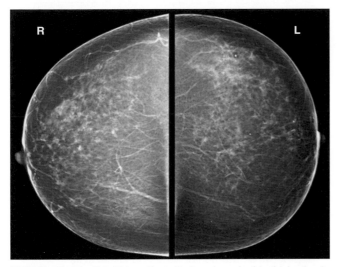

FIGURE 21-46 ILC. This patient displayed a palpable thickening in the upper outer quadrant of the left breast. Mammogram revealed only an architectural distortion in the same region, a common imaging finding with this disease.

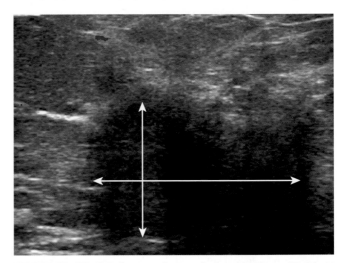

FIGURE 21-47 ILC. Same patient as depicted in Figure 21-46. At ultrasound, an irregular, ill-defined, hypoechoic nodular area with strong posterior acoustic shadowing measuring 2.4 × 2.1 cm was detected.

In addition, multicentricity is more frequently observed in ILCs displaying the classic growth pattern than in those with a variant of ILC.[100]

Clinical Imaging

The most common mammographic manifestations of ILCs are asymmetrical, ill-defined, or irregular masses or densities (24–63%).[101–105] It is not uncommon for ILCs not to result in a mammographic mass, given their typical diffuse growth pattern without well-defined margins, tendency to form multiple nodules throughout the breast parenchyma, and low radiologic opacity. In fact, mammographic examination may detect only indirect signs of malignancy, such as architectural distortion, which has been reported in 10% to 28% of the cases (Figure 21-46).[101–105] Calcifications are uncommonly observed (4–24%).[102–104] The sensitivity of mammograms for detecting ILC is therefore low,[103,106,107] with reported false-negative rates as high as 41%.[103] Even on retrospective analysis, ILCs are often mammographically occult (≤29%).[106,108] Moreover, tumor size estimation by radiographic methods often underestimates the actual tumor size.[103,109] Kepple and associates[103] reported that, in a series of 29 cases, only 4% had measurable abnormalities on mammograms.

Given the low accuracy of mammography, ultrasound is a useful adjunct in the evaluation of ILCs and, in general, it is more sensitive and more accurate than mammography for predicting tumor size and multifocality.[108,110,111] Albayrak and coworkers[108] described that 9 out of 11 mammographically negative ILCs were positive by ultrasonographic examination, leading to a sensitivity of 94.73% when both techniques were applied together. Approximately 60% of ILCs produce on sonography a hypoechoic mass with irregular or indistinct margins and posterior acoustic shadowing (Figure 21-47),[101,108] whereas 15% to 18% of ILCs show shadowing with no appearance of a mass, and 9% to 13% show well-circumscribed mass lesions.[101,108] A significant proportion of cases is ultrasonographically invisible (~10%),[101,108] leading to false-negative rates of up to 36%.[103]

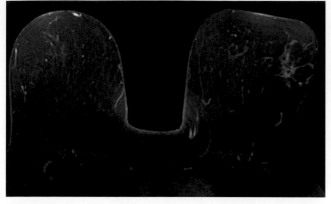

FIGURE 21-48 ILC. Same patient as depicted in Figures 21-46 and 21-47. Magnetic resonance imaging (MRI) showed an architectural distortion with enhancement, with no evidence of a nodule, measuring 6.5 × 2.0 cm.

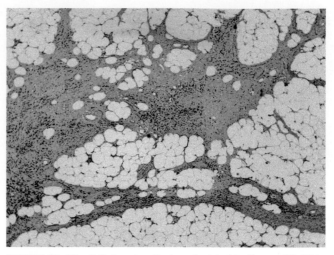

FIGURE 21-49 ILC. Same patient as depicted in Figures 21-46 to 21-48. At gross examination of the surgical specimen, no nodule was visible, only small firm areas were palpable in fat. Histologic examination revealed a classic ILC of 7.0 × 4.0 cm, composed of tumor cells streaming along fibrous septa without a dominant focus, here highlighted with ER immunostaining.

MRI may be useful to estimate disease extent in cases of ILC because it determines tumor size, margins, and multifocality more accurately than ultrasound and mammography (Figure 21-48).[103,112,113] Although one study described that 95% of the cases showed a spiculated enhancing mass,[112] more heterogeneous contrast enhancement patterns might occur[114,115] and, even with the use of MRI, a small proportion of ILCs may remain radiographically occult.[113] It has also been suggested that MRI may be effective in detecting residual tumor after segmental resection,[115] but false-positive rates are yet to be fully determined.

Of note, there is some degree of correlation between histologic subtypes of ILCs and imaging patterns.[101,114] Mirroring its growth pattern, classic ILCs often display only subtle signs of malignancy and absence of a mass lesion is not uncommon. It has been reported that the majority (75%) of ILCs with classic histology are seen as architectural distortion or asymmetrical densities at mammograms and that the ultrasonographic finding of focal acoustic shadowing without a discrete mass is a common presentation of classic ILCs.[101] In contrast, well-circumscribed masses are more frequently observed in cases of ILCs of alveolar, solid, or signet-ring cell variants.[101] Significant correlations between MRI enhancement patterns and histology have also been demonstrated.[114] For instance, classic ILCs with tumor cells streaming along septa are visualised at MRI as enhancing septa without a dominant tumor focus (Figure 21-49).

Gross Pathology

Grossly, ILCs usually form firm to hard tumors with irregular and poorly delimited borders. Tumor size ranges from microscopic lesions to tumors involving the entire breast. In some series, the mean diameters have been reported to be slightly larger than those of IDCs.[6,97,99,116] Sometimes, it may be difficult to determine the tumor edges macroscopically, which may be more accurately defined by palpation than by inspection. In some extreme cases, no tumor is visible and the only findings are small and slightly firm areas in the breast

parenchyma or fat, although microscopic involvement of tissue may be diffuse. These types of cases may be of considerable size, because a diagnostic delay is likely to occur owing to their unusual presentation, and may pose difficulties for assessing margins in intraoperative examination.

Microscopic Pathology

CLASSIC VARIANT

The accepted description of the classic form of ILCs was first provided by Foote and Stewart,[117] 5 years after their seminal paper on LCIS.[2] Classic ILCs are defined by a constellation of architectural and cytologic features. These tumors are hypocellular and composed of small-to-medium-sized dyscohesive cells, which are individually dispersed in a fibroconnective tissue or arranged in single-file linear cords and infiltrate the stroma in a peculiar fashion that is best appreciated at low-power magnification (see Figures 21-45 and 21-49). Classic ILCs invade the breast parenchyma without destruction of residual ductal-lobular structures, often with limited host reaction. Significant desmoplasia and lymphocytic

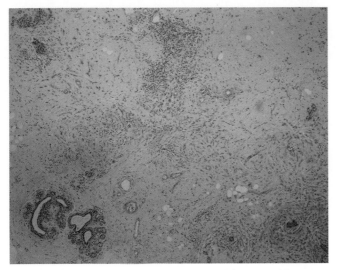

FIGURE 21-50   ILC with little disturbance of the normal breast architecture.

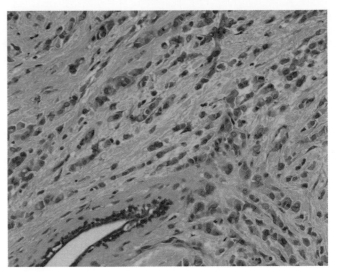

FIGURE 21-52   ILC, classic type. Note the presence of some intracytoplasmic vacuoles.

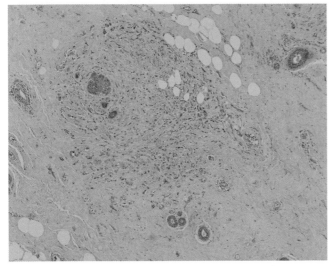

FIGURE 21-51   ILC, targetoid growth pattern.

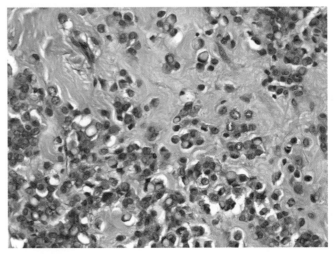

FIGURE 21-53   ILC with numerous signet-ring cells.

reaction are not common features. Moreover, infiltrating cells frequently present a concentric pattern around normal ducts, a feature known as *targetoid* growth pattern (Figures 21-50 and 21-51). Cytologically, the neoplastic cells that compose classic ILCs are similar, if not identical, to those of classic LCIS. These cells have round or notched ovoid nuclei with low-grade nuclear atypia and a thin rim or slightly more abundant cytoplasm (Figure 21-52). As described previously, intracytoplasmic lumina are characteristic of lobular cells, sometimes leading to a signet-ring cell appearance (Figure 21-53). Mitotic figures, albeit present, are not readily found. In the great majority of the cases, this classic form of ILC is associated with LCIS, which is usually of classic morphology, but it can be of the pleomorphic variant.[32] Presence of low-grade DCIS and FEA adjacent to or admixed with the invasive cancer is not uncommon.[12,13]

It is unusual to find an ILC entirely displaying classic histology. In most cases, a mixture of growth patterns is present. To overcome this diagnostic problem, a criterion of at least 70% of the tumor showing classic features has been suggested for a tumor to receive the designation *classic ILC.*[26,96] Moreover, some authors may adopt a very conservative approach and classify as classic only those ILCs with nuclear grade 1.[118] The use of this criterion, however, would limit the clinical usefulness of the subclassification of ILCs because the majority (i.e., those displaying nuclear grade 2) would remain unclassifiable.

HISTOLOGIC VARIANTS

In addition to this common form, ILCs have been traditionally classified according to structural features in histologic subtypes, named *trabecular, alveolar,* and *solid* variants.[119,120] Early studies have suggested that these structural variants would have distinct prognostic implications, with the solid variant indicating a worse prognosis.[119] The trabecular growth pattern is characterized by invasive tumors similar to classic ILCs but composed of broader bands of cells instead of the single-file cell pattern (Figure 21-54).[26,94] In the alveolar pattern, tumor cells are mainly arranged in globular aggregates of at least 20 cells separated by thin bands of fibrous

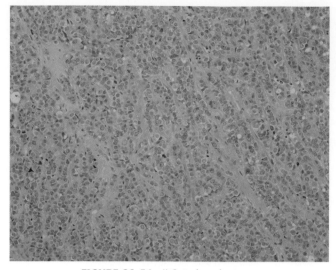

FIGURE 21-54 ILC, trabecular type.

FIGURE 21-56 ILC, solid type.

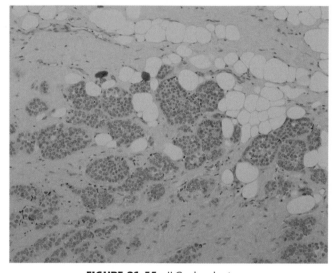

FIGURE 21-55 ILC, alveolar type.

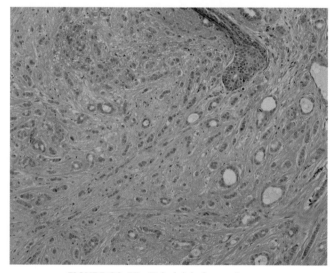

FIGURE 21-57 Tubulolobular carcinoma.

stroma (Figure 21-55).[94] The solid pattern is characterized by large sheets of uniform cells with lobular morphology with little intervening stroma (Figure 21-56).[120] The latter is perhaps the most difficult to recognize. The homogeneity of the tumor cell population, the cellular dyscohesiveness, and the presence of intracytoplasmic lumina are useful diagnostic clues. This variant has been reported as being more pleomorphic and having a higher mitotic rate.[32] Different growth patterns may occur in the same tumor; in this context, the tumor should be classified as an ILC of mixed subtype.

Tubulolobular carcinoma, originally considered to be a lobular variant, is composed of a mixture of low-grade tubular-like glands and dyscohesive lobular-like cells arranged in single-file (Figure 21-57).[121] The tubules are usually smaller and more round than the typically angulated with open lumina of tubular carcinomas. Although recognized as a variant of lobular carcinoma in the last edition of the WHO classification of breast cancer,[32] the majority of these tumors display membranous E-cadherin/β-catenin expression, characteristic of

the ductal lesions.[122–124] These observations have led to the suggestion that most, if not all, tubulolobular carcinomas may be better classified as variants of ductal/tubular rather than lobular carcinomas.

Additional subtypes based on cytologic features have been described, such as the signet-ring cell,[125] apocrine,[126] and histiocytoid[127] variants. Those subtypes, whether structurally or cytologically defined, have not been consistently identified in the literature and are frequently omitted in surgical pathology reports, probably owing to their rarity and the lack of universally accepted criteria for their diagnosis. In addition, there is a paucity of data to support the clinical significance of histologic subtyping of ILCs.

In the last several decades, however, great attention has been given to the pleomorphic variant of ILC, which is reported to be associated with adverse pathologic factors and worse clinical behavior.[32,62,128] It should be noted that these clinical observations are to some extent corroborated by the results of molecular studies of pleomorphic ILCs (see later).[8,129] Pleomorphic ILC is defined as

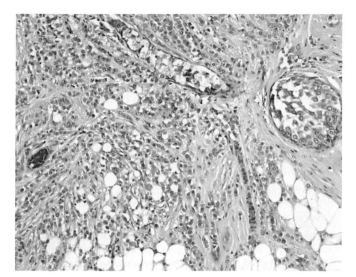

FIGURE 21-58 ILC, pleomorphic type. Note the presence of PLCIS on the right side.

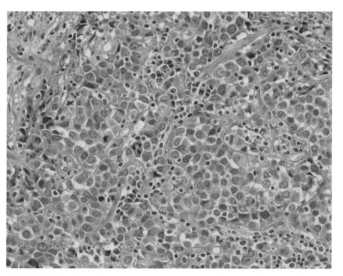

FIGURE 21-60 ILC, pleomorphic type, with a solid growth pattern. Note the presence of atypical mitoses.

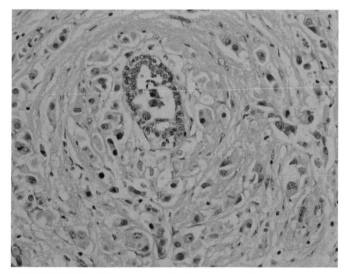

FIGURE 21-59 ILC, pleomorphic type, targetoid growth pattern.

an invasive carcinoma that retains the distinctive growth pattern of classic ILC but exhibits a greater degree of cellular pleomorphism than the classic form (Figures 21-58 and 21-59).[32,62,128] Apocrine differentiation is frequently found[62] but is not required for its diagnosis. Although pleomorphic ILCs tend to display the typical single-file cell and targetoid growth patterns (see Figure 21-58), solid growth pattern is not uncommonly found. In fact, the morphologic features of cases diagnosed in the past as of solid ILC and cases currently diagnosed as pleomorphic ILC overlap (Figure 21-60; see also Figure 21-58). The same is valid for the histiocytoid variant,[32] of which a triple-negative (i.e., ER–, PgR–, and *HER2*–) example is on record.[130] It should be emphasized that the degree of pleomorphism required to warrant a diagnosis of "pleomorphic" ILC is not clear in the literature. A pragmatic solution is to classify ILCs as pleomorphic when the neoplastic cells display grade 3 nuclear morphology, regardless of the structural growth pattern. One of the first studies describing pleomorphic ILC has, however, included cases with nuclear grade 2.[128] Conversely, some

may argue that a nuclear grade 3 morphology is not sufficient for a tumor to receive the "pleomorphic" designation. As discussed previously, Sneige and associates[40] described PLCIS as harboring neoplastic cells with nuclei four times greater than a lymphocyte and mentioned that pleomorphic ILCs displayed similar cytologic features. Adherence to these criteria may be an option to improve the interobserver reproducibility of the diagnosis of pleomorphic ILC, which may have therapeutic implications given that retrospective studies have suggested that pleomorphic ILCs tend to respond to systemic chemotherapy, whereas those with cytologic classic features are chemotherapy-resistant.[131–133] It is unclear, however, whether this is not a mere consequence of the higher histologic grade of pleomorphic ILCs and the fact that patients with low-grade ER+ breast cancers, regardless of histologic type, derive limited benefit from chemotherapy.

In 2008, Orvieto and colleagues[134] directly addressed the issue of whether histopathologic subtyping of ILCs would be clinically useful. Reevaluation of 530 cases of pure ILCs revealed that 301 (57%) were classic, 102 (19%) alveolar, and 59 (11%) solid. Three cases were classified as tubulolobular (owing to the limited number, those cases were considered classic for further analysis) and the remaining 68 (13%) were included in a single group characterized by pleomorphic, signet-ring cell, histiocytoid, or apocrine features. Univariate analysis demonstrated that nonclassic ILCs displayed an increased number of distant metastasis, reduced disease-free survival, and overall survival. On multivariate analysis, the association between histology and survival was no longer significant; however, the association between nonclassic morphology and distant metastasis and breast-related events (locoregional recurrence and distant metastasis) remained significant. The authors, therefore, encouraged pathologists to include in their surgical reports the histologic subtype of ILCs because this information may constitute an independent prognostic factor for patients with ILCs. It should be noted, however, that these observations stem from retrospective analyses and should be interpreted with caution.

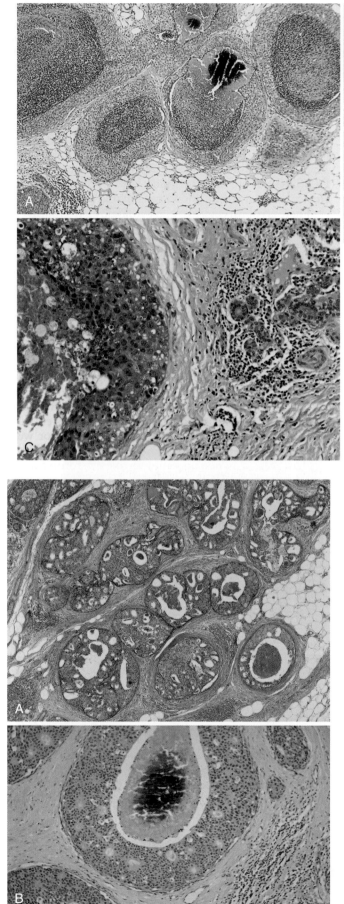

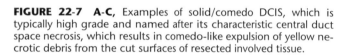

FIGURE 22-7 A-C, Examples of solid/comedo DCIS, which is typically high grade and named after its characteristic central duct space necrosis, which results in comedo-like expulsion of yellow necrotic debris from the cut surfaces of resected involved tissue.

FIGURE 22-8 A and **B,** Examples of cribriform DCIS, which is typically of low or intermediate grade and exhibits a characteristic cribriform architectural growth pattern forming small glandular spaces. Note presence of comedonecrosis.

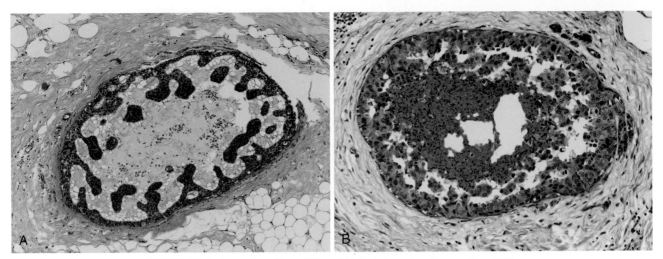

FIGURE 22-9 Examples of low- **(A)** and high- **(B)** grade micropapillary DCIS.

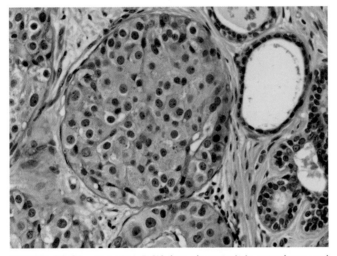

FIGURE 22-10 Apocrine DCIS has characteristic cytoplasm and prominent nucleoli.

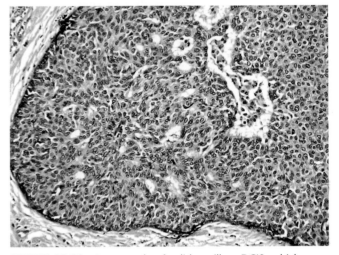

FIGURE 22-11 An example of solid-papillary DCIS, which commonly exhibits neuroendocrine differentiation.

anticipating successful breast conservation.[1,19,31] Grading has also been a component of other classification systems that categorize DCIS based on a combination of nuclear grade and necrosis[18,19] or growth pattern.[32] For example, the Van Nuys system uses a combination of nuclear grade and necrosis.[18] High grade is defined by the nuclear grade. The remainder are divided into non–high grade with necrosis (see Figure 22-8) and non–high grade without necrosis (Figure 22-12). Necrosis, unlike intraductal secretion, is defined by the presence of ghost cells and karyorrhectic debris, is eosinophilic and granular in nature, and does not include single apoptotic cells. Necrosis can be central comedonecrosis within the duct or punctuate nonzonal necrosis.

DCIS Grading

HIGH–NUCLEAR GRADE DCIS

High-grade DCIS (Figure 22-13) is composed of irregularly spaced large pleomorphic cells with irregular nuclear contour and high nucleus-cytoplasm (N/C)

ratio. Cells are typically more than 2.5 times the size of the adjacent normal ductal epithelial cells or greater than three times the size of a red blood cell. The chromatin is typically coarse, and large nucleoli are common. Mitoses are often frequent and may be atypical. If mitoses are prominent, there is a high likelihood that the case is of high grade. Necrosis is often seen. High-grade DCIS may exhibit different growth patterns. A common pattern is central necrosis in a duct distended by a solid pattern of neoplastic cells, previously known as *comedo DCIS* (see Figures 22-3 and 22-7B and C). The necrosis may undergo dystrophic calcification, which mammographically is seen as a branching or linear pattern (see Figures 22-3, 22-6A and B, and 22-7B). High-grade DCIS may also have a cribriform or micropapillary architecture (Figure 22-14; see also Figures 22-3 and 22-9B) frequently associated with central comedo-type necrosis and lacking cell polarization, a feature characteristic of low-grade DCIS. Less commonly, high-grade DCIS exhibits a solid architecture without necrosis (see Figure 22-13B). Periductal fibrosis and adjacent perivascular clusters of inflammatory cells are often present.

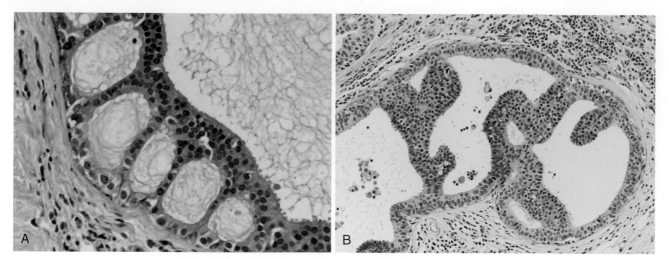

FIGURE 22-12 Low-grade cribriform **(A)** and micropapillary **(B)** DCIS.

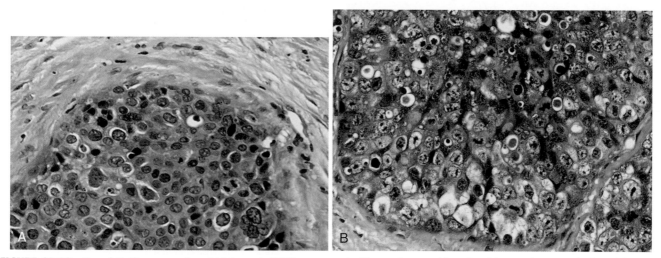

FIGURE 22-13 **A** and **B,** Two examples of high-grade DCIS composed of large pleomorphic cells with prominent nucleoli and frequent mitotic figures.

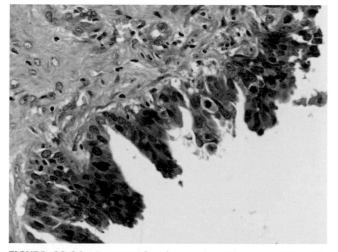

FIGURE 22-14 An example of comedo high-grade DCIS with marked central necrosis of involved duct spaces.

More than 40% of high-grade DCIS are negative for ER, and 70% to 90% of cases are positive for *HER2*,[33–35] which is a strong correlation between larger pleomorphic nuclei and *HER2* positivity.[35] There is also a strong positive correlation between high-grade *HER2*+ DCIS and high proliferation rate.

LOW–NUCLEAR GRADE DCIS

Low-grade DCIS is composed of evenly spaced uniform cells with small regular nuclei (see Figure 22-12). Cells are 1.5 to 2 times the size of a red blood cell or similar in size to the adjacent ductal epithelial cells. Nucleoli, if present, are indistinct. Mitoses are infrequent and necrosis is uncommon. Cribriform and micropapillary architecture are more common than a solid growth pattern. The neoplastic cells form geometric punched-out spaces or bulbous projections around which the cells are polarized. Calcification has a different mechanism from high-grade DCIS. The calcification is found in luminal secretions and has a circumscribed edge and laminated appearance (see Figure 22-1). Mammographically, this is typically seen as clusters of fine granular microcalcification (see Figure 22-2). Low-grade DCIS often coexists with other low–nuclear grade breast lesions such as columnar cell lesion, flat epithelial atypia (Figure 22-15), lobular neoplasia, and low-grade invasive carcinoma such as tubular and lobular carcinomas.[36]

INTERMEDIATE–NUCLEAR GRADE DCIS

These types cannot be assigned readily to the high– or low–nuclear grade categories. The nuclei show moderate pleomorphism, less than in high-grade disease, but lack the uniformity and typically are larger than those seen in the low grade type (two to three times the size of a red blood cell) (Figure 22-16). The N/C ratio is often high; one or two nucleoli may be present but are usually not prominent. Necrosis may be present but is not extensive. There may be some cell polarization. The architectural pattern may be solid, cribriform, or micropapillary. It has been reported that the difference in ipsilateral

recurrence rates between low- and intermediate-grade DCIS is not significant.[37]

DCIS Growth Pattern

Although the growth pattern of DCIS tends to be more heterogeneous than cytologic features in a given case, there is a correlation between growth pattern and nuclear grade; DCIS with comedonecrosis tends to be high grade whereas cribriform and micropapillary DCIS tend to be low to intermediate grade. Cells of DCIS are typically monomorphic; however, not all cells are identical in size and shape. Dimorphic variants of DCIS consisting of two distinctly different populations of cells are unusual. In a case showing an admixture of several architectural patterns, all patterns should be listed in the diagnosis in the order of their relative amount.

CRIBRIFORM DCIS

The proliferating cells of cribriform DCIS form smooth well-delineated regular punched-out microlumina and geometric spaces with cell bridges "rigid," showing

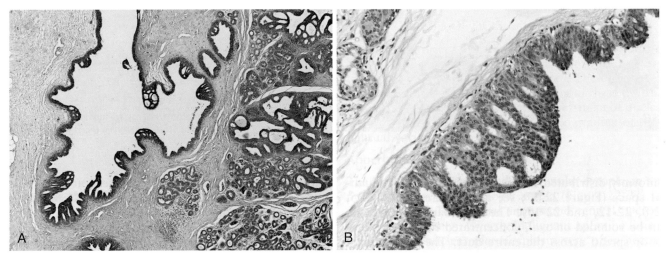

FIGURE 22-15 **A** and **B,** Low-grade cribriform DCIS arising in the background of flat epithelial atypia.

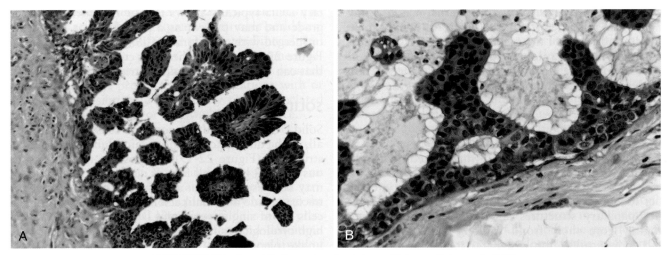

FIGURE 22-16 **A** and **B,** Examples of cytology of intermediate-grade DCIS.

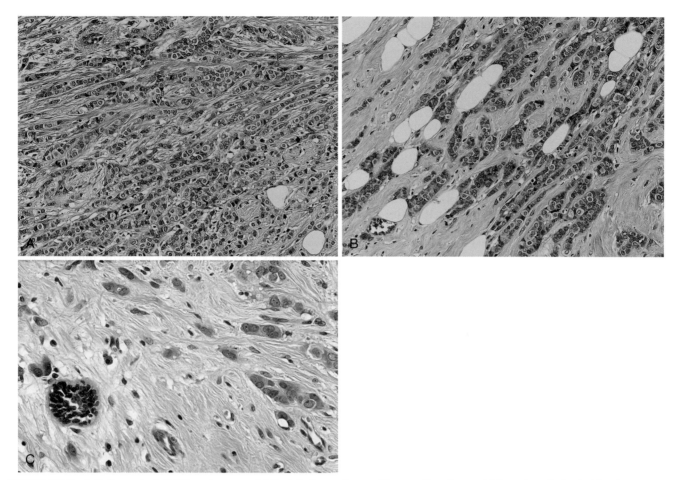

FIGURE 23-2 A-C, Some ductal NST carcinomas exhibit a lobular carcinoma–like growth pattern, which can be admixed with other patterns of growth. These tumors lack the characteristic cytomorphologic features of classic invasive lobular carcinoma and should not be classified as such.

breast cancers invade the skin and involve the dermal-epidermal junction. Although patients with ductal NST carcinoma may have elevated levels of serum β human chorionic gonadotropins (β-hCGs), histologic evidence of choriocarcinomatous differentiation is exceptionally rare.[33] High-grade ductal NST carcinoma may show occasional pleomorphic cells; however, the rare variant pleomorphic carcinoma is characterized by proliferation of pleomorphic and bizarre tumor giant cells comprising more than 50% of the tumor cells (Figure 23-8) in a background of adenocarcinoma or adenocarcinoma with spindle and squamous differentiation.[34]

In most cases (≤80%), foci of associated DCIS are present, and some authorities recognize a subtype with an extensive in situ component.[1,2,30] The growth pattern of a coexisting DCIS component is usually reflected in the structure of the invasive carcinomas, and there is a significant association between grade of DCIS and invasive carcinomas that have both components. Grade 1 ductal NST is usually associated with low-/intermediate-grade DCIS of cribriform and micropapillary pattern, whereas in grade 3 tumors, associated DCIS is often of high-grade type with comedonecrosis, but all other patterns may be seen. Moreover, some invasive ductal tumors mimic solid or cribriform DCIS, which may be of clinical relevance in case of assessment of invasion on NCB and estimation of tumor size in excision specimens. Immunohistochemistry (IHC) for myoepithelial markers may be helpful in such cases.

Immunohistochemistry

Ductal NSTs show reactivity to low-molecular-weight (luminal) cytokeratins (CKs) in the majority of cases and in almost all cases if multiple CKs are used. In our hands, CK18 and CAM5.2 are reliable IHC markers and for ductal NST. Other luminal CKs in use in clinical practice include CK7, CK8, CK19, and AE1/AE3. Ductal NST is usually positive for epithelial membrane antigen (EMA) and E-cadherin, 70% positive for lactalbumin, milk fat globule membrane, and 20% to 50% are positive for gross cystic disease fluid protein-15 (GCDFP-15); the later three markers are more breast specific. Approximately 60% to 80% of ductal NSTs are positive for estrogen receptors (ERs) and androgen receptors (ARs), a slightly lower percentage (55–70%) are positive for progesterone receptors (PgRs), and 12% to 20% are positive for *HER2* or show *HER2* gene amplification. Basal-associated markers such as CK5, CK5/6, CK14, CK17, vimentin, p-cadherin, and laminin are expressed in a small proportion of cases (5–15%). Approximately 5% to 40% of ductal NST tumors are positive for epidermal growth factor receptor

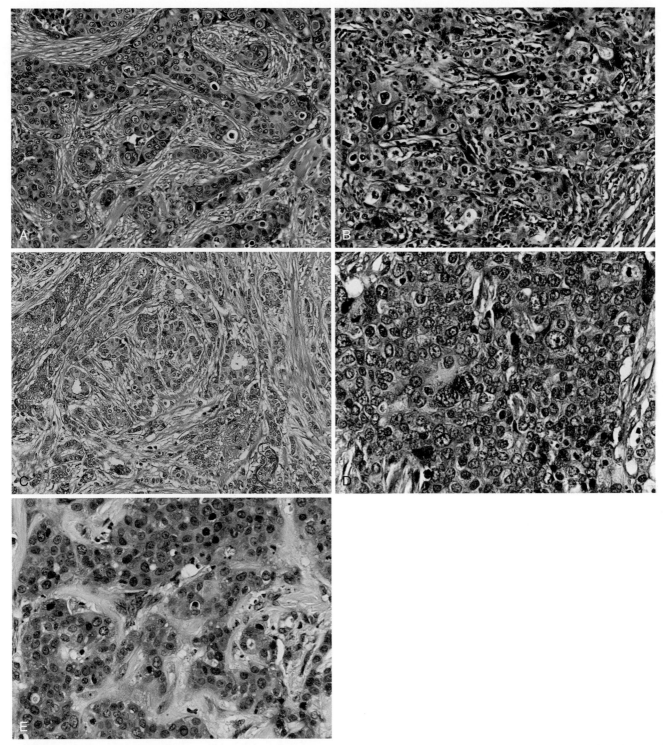

FIGURE 23-3   A-E, The cytomorphology of ductal NST carcinomas is varied in terms of amount and nature of cytoplasm, nuclear shape and size, and the presence of glandular differentiation.

(EGFR; *HER1)* and p53, whereas 80% to 90% are positive for *HER3, HER4,* and FHT protein. Expression of smooth muscle actin (SMA) is reported in 15% of cases. Unlike metaplastic carcinomas, very few cases of ductal NST express p63. Less than 10% of ductal NSTs express neuroendocrine markers (synaptophysin and chromogranin-A). Breast carcinoma of NST is usually negative for WT1, TTF1, CDX2, and CK20, but focal reactivity for WT1 may be seen in mucinous carcinoma,[34a] and focal TTF-1 may occasionally be seen.[34b,34c]

Genetics

The genetic variation seen in breast cancer as a whole is similarly reflected in ductal NST tumors and has, until recently, proved difficult to analyze or explain. The increasing accumulation of genetic alterations seen with increasing grade (decreasing degree of differentiation) has been used to support the hypothesis of a linear progression model in this type and in invasive breast cancer as a whole. However, the observation that specific genetic lesions or regions of alteration are associated with histologic type of cancer or related to grade in the large ductal NST group does not support this view. It implies that breast cancer of ductal NST type includes a number of tumors of unrelated genetic evolutionary pathways[35] and that these tumors show fundamental differences when compared with some special-type tumors including lobular and tubular carcinoma.[36,37] It is now well recognized that ductal NST composes a heterogeneous group of tumors not only at the morphologic level but also at the molecular level. Global gene expression profiling of breast cancer has demonstrated that ductal NST tumors can be classified into subtypes on the basis of expression patterns (see also Chapters 10 and 20).[38,39] At least three main molecular classes have been

identified: luminal/ER+ (60–70%), HER2+ (15–20%), basal-like/triple-negative (ER–, PgR–, and HER2–; 15–20%). Luminal and triple-negative classes have further been subdivided into subclasses based on difference in the expression of other biomarkers. This molecular heterogeneity of ductal NST has also been demonstrated at DNA level and at protein levels. Multiple independent studies have demonstrated an association between these molecular classes of ductal NST and distinct behavior and response to systemic therapy. These observations are consistent with the morphologic spectrum of ductal NST tumors, which, unlike special types, show wide variation in grade and histologic features.

Differential Diagnosis

As mentioned previously, ductal NST has no specific morphologic features and a variety of appearances may be seen; therefore, it is a diagnosis of exclusion. Although ductal NST often shows a variable proportion of tubule formation, distinction must be made between it and pure tubular carcinomas, which have an exceptionally favorable prognosis even compared with grade-matched ductal NST.[24] The diagnosis of pure tubular carcinomas should be restricted to those that exhibit tubule formation in virtually the entire tumor (>90%) with no solid groups of tumor cells in addition to low-grade nuclei. The glands of pure tubular carcinoma are composed of a single layer of cells with relatively uniform calibers. The lumina are often opened and the luminal cell borders may show apocrine-type cytoplasmic tufts or snouts. The cells are usually homogeneous in a given lesion with rounded or oval hyperchromatic nuclei that tend to be basally oriented. Nucleoli are inconspicuous and mitosis is rarely seen. Stromal elastosis is regarded as a hallmark of pure tubular carcinoma, although it is not present in all cases and can be seen in some cases of ductal NST. Tumors showing tubule formation but not fulfilling quantitative criteria described previously can be called *ductal carcinoma with tubular features*. In these tumors, although the pattern of growth is largely tubular, epithelial proliferation tends to be more florid

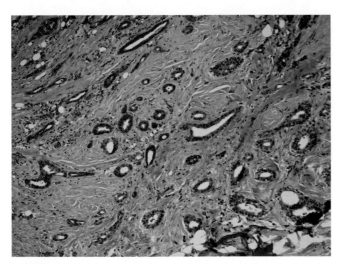

FIGURE 23-4 The stromal component of ductal not otherwise specified (NOS) carcinomas is variable from scant to dense and collagenous and is abundant in this illustration.

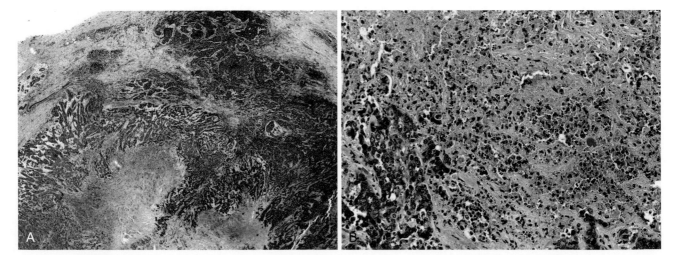

FIGURE 23-5 **A** and **B**, Focal necrosis can be seen in some tumors, particularly those of high histologic grade.

than that observed in pure tubular carcinoma. Epithelial lining of glands may be more than one cell thick. Gland lumina may show micropapillae or transluminal bridging. Cells show a tendency to pleomorphism, and occasional mitotic figures may be seen. The presence of high-grade nuclei or frequent mitotic figures should question the diagnosis of pure tubular carcinoma. In a previous study, we found that, compared with grade 1 ductal NST, pure tubular carcinoma is associated with columnar cell lesions (93%) but the difference in the association with lobular neoplasia or atypical intraductal epithelial proliferation/low-grade DCIS was not significant.[24,40] In routine practice, tumors with tubule formation of 50% to 90% are classified as either ductal NST or tubular mixed or tubular variant carcinoma.[9–12] In the Nottingham series, 55%, 21%, and 24% of ductal NST (tubule formation < 50%) were hormone receptor–positive, *HER2+,* and triple-negative, respectively, compared with 94%, 4%, and 2% for tubular

mixed (tubule formation 50–90%) tumors, respectively. Of ductal NST, 6% was grade 1 compared with 51% of tubular mixed tumors. This emphasizes the good prognostic value of tubular mixed tumors and demonstrates the heterogeneity of tumors with the NST category.

Ductal NST may show areas with cytoarchitecture features of lobular carcinomas. Although the behavior and outcome of both tumor types are significantly different,[41,42] diagnosis of the associated invasive lobular component may have an impact on the use of different imaging modality (i.e., magnetic resonance imaging [MRI]) during preoperative assessment of tumor extent in addition to other features frequently detected with lobular carcinomas such as multifocality and hormone receptor positivity.

There is an overlap between ductal NST, atypical medullary carcinoma, carcinomas arising in *BRCA* germline mutation carriers, and basal-like carcinomas. A proportion of ductal NST carcinomas show features in common with all these subtypes, namely poorly differentiated histology, prominent inflammation, circumscription, syncytial growth pattern, scanty stroma, frequent mitotic and apoptotic figures in addition to absence of hormone receptors, and *HER2* amplification and frequent p53 mutation. Medullary carcinomas are defined by a constellation of histopathologic features; some of them can be found in a proportion of ductal NST carcinoma.[43] The distinction between the two tumor types is often difficult, with low reproducibility. However, medullary carcinomas usually lack fibrosis and gland formation and show well-developed syncytial growth pattern (≥75% of tumor area) in addition to almost complete circumscription. *Atypical medullary carcinoma* is a term given to tumors that show some but not all features of medullary carcinomas.[44] Medullary-like carcinoma is also used to encompass medullary and atypical medullary,[31] and the key features of medullary-like tumors as described in the United Kingdom Royal College of Pathologists (UKRCPath) reporting guidelines are syncytial interconnecting masses of grade 3 tumors that typically

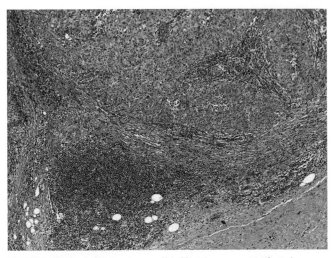

FIGURE 23-6 Inflammatory cell infiltration can vary but, in some tumors, can be intense and comparable with that seen in medullary carcinoma.

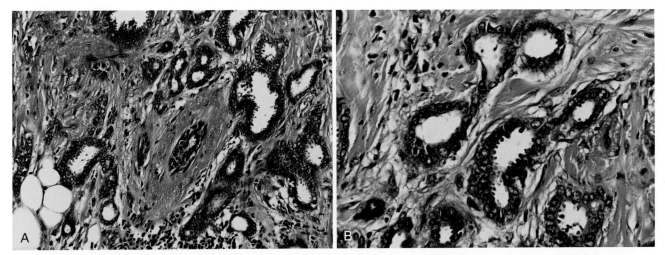

FIGURE 23-7 **A** and **B,** Elements of special type carcinomas can be seen but are disregarded unless they form over 50% of the tumor area, in which case they become "mixed type."

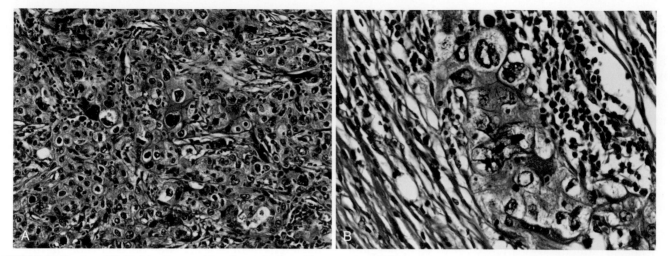

FIGURE 23-8 **A** and **B,** Highly pleomorphic cells can be found in some ductal NOS carcinomas, and if dominant, these tumors have been described as "pleomorphic carcinoma."

have large vesicular nuclei and prominent nuclei and prominent lymphoid inflammatory cell infiltrate in 90% or more of the tumors. It was also mentioned that "if in doubt, the tumor should be classified as being ductal NST."[31] However, owing to difficulties of the diagnosis of medullary carcinomas in routine practice, some cases are included in the NST category, as evident from the observed decline in the diagnosis of medullary carcinoma in routine practice and the low reproducibility of its diagnosis.[45,46] In a previous study of 1597 patients who received no systemic adjuvant treatment, we found that prominent inflammation was associated with high histologic grade and with better survival on multivariate analysis. Medullary carcinoma did not have significantly different prognosis than grade 3 ductal NST carcinoma with prominent inflammation, but both had a better prognosis than grade 3 ductal NST without prominent inflammation, independent of other prognostic factors.[46] In a subsequent study of 165 ductal NSTs that are positive for one of the basal-associated markers (basal-like tumors), we found that anastomosing sheets in at least 30% of the tumor in addition to prominent inflammation were associated with a better prognosis on univariate analysis. The combination of these two features (a simplified definition of medullary-like type that showed good interobserver reproducibility among reporting authors) was an independent prognostic factor on multivariate analysis. These results emphasize the heterogeneity of morphology and behavior of ductal NST tumors.[46] In this series, a fibrotic focus was present in 36% of carcinomas compared with only 3% of medullary-like carcinomas that showed a fibrotic focus. Fibrotic focus of greater than 30% of the tumor was associated with a poor prognosis.

The vast majority (80–94%) of basal-like carcinomas, which account for 10% to 17% of breast cancer, are grade 3 ductal NST and both have shown similar histologic features that are mainly related to hormone receptor negativity.[39,47–50] The diagnosis of basal-like cancer is solely based on assessment of molecular features. In routine practice, basal-like tumors are identified by absence of hormone receptors and *HER2* amplification in addition to positivity of one of the basal-associated markers (e.g., CK5/6, EGFR).[51] Familial breast cancer cases associated with *BRCA1* mutations are commonly of ductal NST type but have basal-like/medullary carcinoma–like features, exhibit solid growth pattern, higher mitotic counts, a greater proportion of the tumor with a continuous pushing margin, and more lymphocytic infiltration, and show triple-negative phenotype than sporadic cancers.[28] Cancers associated with *BRCA2* mutations are also often of ductal NST type but exhibit fewer tubule formation, a higher proportion of the tumor perimeter with a continuous pushing margin, and a lower mitotic count than sporadic cancers.[28]

Duct NST shows focal mucinous differentiation with extracellular and/or intracellular mucin accumulation in 2% to 4% of cases. Tumors are classified as pure mucinous when 90% or greater shows mucinous differentiation; these tumors also show higher mean proportion of extracellular mucin than ductal NST. However, some authors classify tumors as pure mucinous, which is associated with a favorable prognosis,[25,52] when it virtually consists of mucinous pattern, those that have no ductal NST areas, or those in which pools of extracellular mucin make up at least one third of volume throughout.[1,30] In practice, mucinous tumors with greater than 10% of the invasive component as ductal NST or the ductal component is poorly differentiated and should not be classified as pure mucinous. These cases are designated as mixed mucinous/ductal NST or ductal carcinoma with mucinous differentiation.

It is also important to differentiate ductal NST with endocrine differentiation, as revealed by immunohistochemical expression of neuroendocrine markers in scattered cells, which is detected in 10% to 18% of carcinomas. Endocrine breast carcinomas express neuroendocrine markers in more than 50% of the cell population.[53] Focal endocrine differentiation does not seem to carry a special prognostic or therapeutic significance. Similarly, although ductal NST may show variable proportion of oncocytic and apocrine cells, it should be differentiated from oncocytic carcinoma; a breast carcinoma composed of 70% or greater oncocytic cells[54] and apocrine carcinoma; a carcinoma showing cytologic, immunohistochemical, and molecular features of apocrine cells in greater than 90% of the tumor cells.[54]

Finally, it is also important to differentiate ductal NSTs from metastatic carcinomas. The presence of DCIS is indicative of breast origin. Metastatic cancers often surround and displace normal-appearing breast parenchyma and usually exhibit unusual histologic patterns. In addition, the expression of ER and PgR and of the apocrine marker GCDFP-15 is typical of a primary breast carcinoma, whereas other markers may indicate other primary origin such as TTF1 for pulmonary and vimentin for endometrioid carcinomas, WT1 for ovarian serous, and CDX2 for colorectal cancers. In these cases, the constellation of history, clinicoradiologic correlation, histologic appearances, and a panel of biomarkers is helpful.

Prognosis and Predictive Factors

The prognostic characteristics and management of ductal NST carcinoma are similar or slightly worse with 84% and 73% at 5 and 10 years cancer-specific survival, respectively, than breast cancer as a whole, with around 86% and 76% at 5- and 10-year survival. In other nonductal NST breast cancer types, the 5- and 10-year cancer survival are around 93% and 86%.[5,55] Prognosis is influenced profoundly by the classic prognostic variables of histologic grade, tumor size, lymph node status, and vascular invasion and by predictors of therapeutic response such as ER, PgR, and *HER2* status. Approximately 70% to 80% of ductal NST breast cancers are ER+ and between 15% and 25% of cases are *HER2*+. The management of ductal NST carcinomas is also influenced by these prognostic and predictive characteristics of the tumor as well as focality and position in the breast.

KEY PATHOLOGIC FEATURES

Ductal Carcinoma of No Special Type

- Morphologic heterogeneity is the hallmark of these tumors.
- Prognosis is related to the degree of tubule formation, nuclear pleomorphism, and mitotic counts.
- Triple-negative tumors account for 15% of tumors.
- *HER2*-amplified tumors account for 15% to 20% of tumors.
- High-grade tumors need to be differentiated from metastatic tumors to the breast—a DCIS component confirms breast origin.

DCIS, ductal carcinoma in situ.

Histologic Grading

Invasive breast carcinomas are morphologically subdivided according to their growth patterns and degree of differentiation, the latter of which reflects how closely they resemble normal breast epithelial cells. This subdivision is achieved by assessing histologic type and histologic grade, respectively. Histologic grading has become widely accepted as a powerful indicator of prognosis in addition to providing an overview of the intrinsic biologic characteristics of the tumors. Until recently, the most common grading systems used in the United States were the original Scarff-Bloom-Richardson (SBR) system,[56] which combines nuclear grade, tubule formation, and mitotic rate, and the Black method, which emphasizes nuclear grading without assessment of the growth pattern of the tumor.[57] In Europe, the Elston-Ellis modification of the SBR grading system (Nottingham grading system; NGS) is preferred and is becoming increasingly popular in the United States and elsewhere.[2,31,58,59] The prognostic relevance of NGS has be demonstrated in multiple independent studies, and it has been recommended by various professional bodies internationally (WHO, American Joint Commission on Cancer [AJCC], European Union [EU], and UKRCPath).[2,31,58,59] Because NGS has independent but equivalently powerful prognostic value, it has been combined with lymph node stage and tumor size to form prognostic indices—the Nottingham Prognostic Index, which includes NGS and lymph node stage with equal weighting, and the Kalmar Prognostic Index, in which grade is given a higher weighting value.

Although assessment of histologic differentiation will always have a subjective element, NGS provides more objective criteria for the three component elements of grading and specifically addresses mitosis counting in a more rigorous fashion. This grading system is based on semiquantitative evaluation of the morphologic characteristics of the tumor, including how closely the tumor resembles the normal breast TDLU architecture and cell structure (i.e., the degree of differentiation toward normal breast ducts and lobules), the degree of nuclear pleomorphism, and the number of mitotic figures, a measure of proliferation.

Histologic Assessment Methodology

GLANDULAR/TUBULAR DIFFERENTIATION

Tubule/gland (acinar) formation is a histologic feature that reflects degree of tumor differentiation and its resemblance to the normal glandular tissue of the breast. In the assessment of tubule/gland formation, all parts of the tumor are scanned and the proportion occupied by tumor islands showing clear acinar or gland formation or defined tubule structures with a central luminal space is assessed semiquantitatively. This assessment is generally carried out during the initial low-power scan of the tumor sections. Assessment of tubule/gland formation is made on the overall appearances of the tumor and so account is taken of any variation. Only structures in which there are clearly defined central lumens, surrounded by polarized tumor cells, should be counted; the presence of apical snouts within a clear central lumen is useful but not mandatory. Care must be taken not to mistake clefts induced by shrinkage artifact for glands/tubules.

The term *tubule formation* was introduced by Patey and Scarff[59a] for the recapitulation of the acinar structure of the normal lobule. This has subsequently been misinterpreted by some as identification solely of distinct tubular structures reminiscent of those found in tubular carcinoma of the breast, which is an incorrect interpretation. For this reason, we prefer to use the term *glandular/tubular differentiation* rather than just tubular. It is important to emphasize that this refers not only to the tubules seen in pure tubular carcinomas but to any glandular structure, even if it is part of a ductal NST carcinoma or other type. In some rare types of breast cancer, assessment of tubule or gland formation is difficult. For example, the clusters of tumor cells with reversed polarity typically found in micropapillary carcinomas in our opinion do not fulfill the criteria of tubular/glandular formation and tumors composed entirely of this pattern should be scored as 3 for tubule formation.

The cutoff points may appear to be rather arbitrary but they are based on a pilot study that showed them to give the best prognostic separation in life table analyses.

A score of 1 point is given when more than 75% of the area of the tumor cell islands exhibit tubule formation (Figure 23-9). Two points are appropriate for tumors in which between 10% and 75% of the area show tubule formation. Where tubules occupy 10% or less of the tumor, the score is given as 3. These cutoff points may appear to be rather arbitrary but they are based on a study that showed them to give the best prognostic separation in life table analyses.

NUCLEAR PLEOMORPHISM

Nuclear pleomorphism is morphologic measurement of tumor differentiation at the cytologic level, and from a genetic point of view, it can be considered as an indirect measure of levels of aneuploidy, genetic instability, and transcription (i.e., nucleolus). Assessment of nuclear pleomorphism is the most subjective element of histologic grade, and individual pathologists differ markedly in their approach to nuclear grading. It has been reported that breast specialists appear to allocate higher grades than nonspecialists.

In order to introduce a degree of objectivity, we use the size and shape of normal epithelial cells present in breast tissue within or adjacent to the tumor as the reference point. If normal epithelial cells cannot be identified,

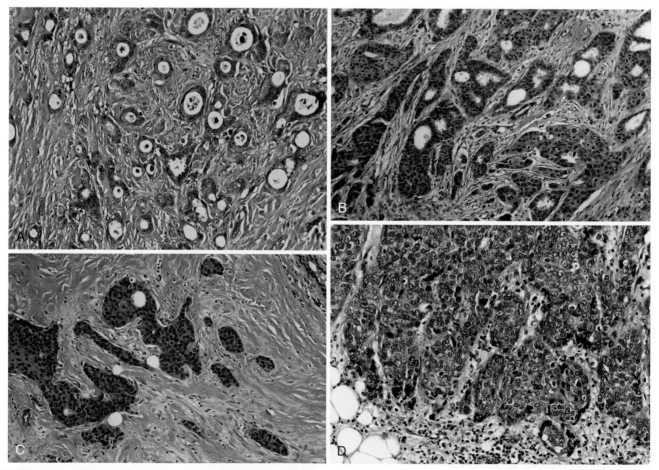

FIGURE 23-9 Examples of glandular/tubular differentiation. **A,** If over 75% of the tumor exhibits glandular/tubular differentiation, a score of 1 point is given. **B,** If this is between 10% and 75%, a score of 2. **C** and **D,** If less than 10%, score 3.

stromal lymphoid cells may be used as a surrogate, with appropriate adjustment for their relatively smaller size. Tumors in which nuclei are small and regular, showing little variation in size and shape compared with normal nuclei, are given 1 point (Figure 23-10). It should be pointed out that most tumors exhibit some degree of nuclear enlargement and pleomorphism, and it is rare to attribute a score of 1 to the common forms of invasive cancer. Two points are given when the nuclei are larger than normal, have a more open vesicular structure, and there is a moderate variation in size and shape. A marked variation in size and shape, particularly when very large and bizarre nuclei are present, scores 3 points. In the latter two categories, nucleoli are often present, and multiple

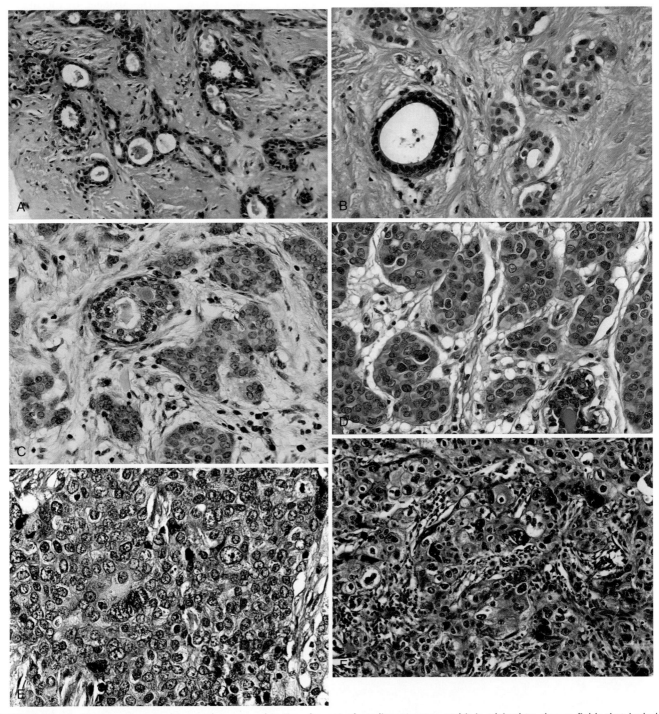

FIGURE 23-10 Nuclear pleomorphism is the most subjective element of grading to score and it is advised to choose fields that include normal parenchymal structures to allow comparison with normal epithelial cells. **A,** It should be noted that it is rare for invasive breast cancer cells to have normal cell characteristics and be allocated a score of 1 for nuclear pleomorphism. **B,** Two points are given when the nuclei are larger than normal, have a more open vesicular structure, and there is a moderate variation in size and shape. **C-F,** A score of 3 is given when there is marked variation in size and shape.

nucleoli in a nucleus favor a score of 3. The finding of an occasional enlarged or bizarre nucleus should not be used to give a score of 3 rather than 2. Relatively regular, single nucleoli do not decide assignment because they may be present in low–nuclear grade cases. Nuclear grading should be evaluated at the periphery and/or at the least differentiated area of the tumor to preclude differences between the growing edge and the less active center.

SCORE

1. Nuclei small with little increase in size in comparison with normal breast epithelial cells, regular outlines, uniform nuclear chromatin, little variation in size.
2. Cells larger than normal with open vesicular nuclei, visible nucleoli, and moderate variability in both size and shape.
3. Vesicular nuclei, often with prominent nucleoli, exhibiting marked variation in size and shape, occasionally with very large and bizarre forms.

MITOTIC COUNTS

Mitotic count reflects the proliferation activity of tumors and is probably the most prognostically significant component of histologic grade. Mitotic count is assessed on routinely prepared hematoxylin and eosin (H&E)–stained sections. Current evidence does not support the use of immunohistochemical stains for routine assessment of proliferative activity in breast cancer. During assessment, only figures that clearly fulfill the morphologic criteria for the various stages of mitosis should be included; application of very strict criteria for prophase figures should eliminate problems caused by apoptotic nuclei and intratumoral lymphocytes. Identification of a mitotic figure is based on the absence of the nuclear membrane and observation of at least one separate chromosome, usually seen as a small protuberance or a clear hairy projection at the outline of the mitotic figure (Figure 23-11). Two parallel clearly separate chromosome clots (metaphase figure) should be counted as one mitosis. Hyperchromatic nuclei, triangular or spiky, rather than the hairy chromosomes of mitosis, favor apoptosis. The surrounding cytoplasm should not be eosinophilic (eosinophilic cytoplasm suggests that the cell is undergoing apoptosis). Structures with empty central zones are often not mitoses. Doubtful structures should be excluded and the fact that pyknotic nuclei and apoptotic bodies are common in most tumors should always be remembered.

Mitosis score depends on the number of mitoses per 10 high-power fields (HPFs). The size of HPFs is very variable, so it is necessary to standardize the mitotic

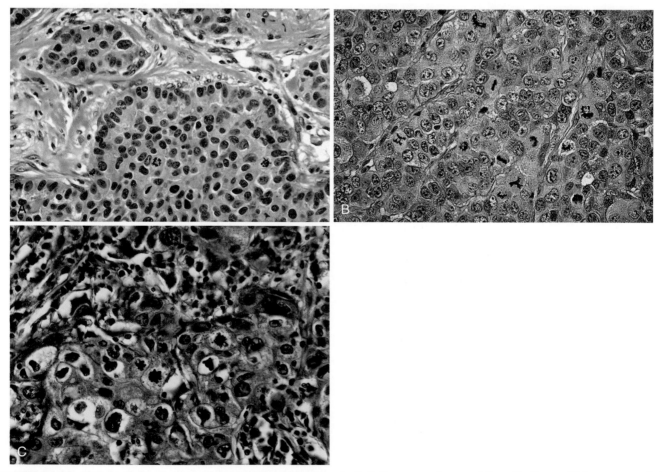

FIGURE 23-11   A-C, Examples of mitotic figures. Good preservation of mitotic figures requires good tissue fixation and it is recommended that tumors within specimens are incised as soon as possible after resection.

count. The size of an HPF may vary up to sixfold from one microscope to another and it has been calculated that the count for the same tumor assessed by different instruments may range from 3 to 20 mitoses/10 HPF. We recommend that the field diameter of the microscope is measured using stage graticule or Vernier scale, and the scoring categories should be determined as previously published.[31] Field diameter is a function of objective and eyepiece, so if either of these is changed, this exercise should be repeated.

A minimum of 10 HPFs should be counted at the periphery of the tumor, where it has been demonstrated that proliferative activity is greatest. If there is variation in the number of mitoses in different areas of the tumor, the least differentiated area (i.e., with the highest mitotic count) should be assessed. If the mitotic frequency score falls very close to a score cut point, one or more further groups of 10 HPFs should be assessed to establish the correct (highest) score. It is recommended that identification of the most mitotically active or least differentiated part of the tumor forms part of the low magnification preliminary assessment of the histologic section. This area should be used for mitotic count scoring. If there is no evidence of heterogeneity, then mitotic scoring should be carried out at a part of the tumor periphery chosen at random. Fields chosen for scoring are selected during a random meander along the peripheral margin of the selected tumor area. We find it helpful to start counting fields when you see at least one mitotic figure and then move the slide and count in 10 consecutive nonoverlapping fields. Only fields with a representative tumor burden should be used. The low-power scan of the tumor can be used to provide an assessment of the typical tumor-to-stroma ratio. Areas of necrosis, inflammation, calcification, and large vessels should be avoided.

OVERALL GRADE

The scores for tubule formation (1–3), nuclear pleomorphism (1–3), and mitoses (1–3) are added together and assigned to grades, as

    Score of 3, 4, or 5 = Grade 1
    Score of 6 or 7 = Grade 2
    Score of 8 or 9 = Grade 3

EXPECTED DISTRIBUTION OF GRADE SCORES

Do not expect equal numbers of cancers to fall in each grade category. Published ratios for grades 1, 2, and 3 are approximately 2:3:5 in symptomatic breast cancer, so about half of all symptomatic cancers are grade 3. If an audit of grade distribution shows substantially fewer grade 3 cases or a majority of grade 2 cases, the grading protocols should be carefully reviewed, although screen-detected cancer series are likely to include a smaller proportion of high-grade cases, approximately 3:4:3.

Misassignments of grade 1 to grade 3 or vice versa are rarely reported; however, grade 2 tumors usually show the lowest degree of concordance. This is an expected phenomenon of scoring of a biologic variable in which scores in the overlap regions are usually most difficult

to be categorized. Attempts have been made to improve biologic and clinical significance of histologic grading by subclassification of grade 2 tumors into two distinct subclasses: a grade 1–like subgroup, which has an excellent outcome, and may not require adjuvant chemotherapy, and a grade 3–like subgroup, which comprises tumors that behave in a way similar to high-grade cancers and need more aggressive systemic treatment. Examples of these studies include application of genomic grade index (GGI) to subclassify histologic grade 2 into two molecular subclasses (GGI1 and GGI3),[60] genetic grade index, or using proliferation biomarkers such as MIB1 expression.[61] However, the clinical usefulness and the cost-benefit ratios of these studies need to be further evaluated.

The relatively wide variation in the proportion of each grade reported in the literature has highlighted the issue of subjectivity and reproducibility of histologic grading.[62] However, current evidence demonstrates an improvement in the consistency and reproducibility of breast cancer grading. Multiple studies have shown an improved interobserver agreement with NGS method compared with other grading systems. Another important point is the introduction of guidelines for the methods for tissue handling, fixation and preparation, and grading of tumors. Differences between centers can, in many cases, be attributed to differences in quality of tissue preparation. Critical evaluation of these issues with recommendations for good practice have been provided by professional organizations (i.e., WHO, EU, UKRCPath, International Union Against Cancer [UICC]).

GRADING OF NEEDLE CORE BIOPSY SPECIMENS

Although no guidelines currently exist for the minimum amount of tissue in NCBs that is needed for sufficient histologic grading, the adequacy of sample for grading is a matter of clinical judgment. Grading is better performed on large, preferably multiple, core biopsies (CBs) of tumor. Current evidence showed that grading on CB can be performed and appears straightforward because formalin fixation is likely to be optimum. Importantly, selection of patients for neoadjuvant therapy requires prognostic information to be available from preoperative diagnostic tumor samples. Amat and coworkers[63] have reported that assessment of grade on CB is a strong predictive factor of response to induction chemotherapy in breast cancer, independent of the type of regimen used. The concordance between grade on CB and that in the definitive excision specimen can be achieved in approximately 75% of cases, varied in different studies from 59% to 91% mainly due to sampling issue.[64] Tubule formation may be overestimated or underestimated and pleomorphism may be underscored. Mitotic counts might be inaccurate because, in tumor grading, the periphery (growing edge) of the tumor is assessed where mitotic figures are more frequent. In addition, the core might have an insufficient amount of tumor to allow 10 HPFs to be counted. For technical reasons, the visibility of mitotic figures on CB may be impaired. As a result, the estimation of mitotic frequency might

Triple-Negative and Basal-like Carcinoma

Magali Lacroix-Triki • Felipe C. Geyer • Britta Weigelt •
Jorge S. Reis-Filho

INTRODUCTION

Breast cancer is a highly heterogeneous disease, encompassing a variety of entities with regards to clinical presentation, biology, response to treatment, and outcome.[1-4] Molecular analyses have now demonstrated that estrogen receptor (ER)–positive and –negative breast cancers are fundamentally different diseases in terms of not only their transcriptomic profiles but also their clinicopathologic features and response to therapy.[1-6] It should be noted, within the ER+ and ER– groups, there is still a great deal of heterogeneity and different tumors display different constellations of genetic and epigenetic aberrations.[7]

Despite the realization of the heterogeneity of breast cancer at the molecular level, breast cancer patient management is still defined based on patients' characteristics (i.e., age, menopausal status, comorbidity), tumor histopathologic features (i.e., tumor size, histologic grade, presence of lymphovascular invasion, lymph node involvement), and tumor biology (in particular, based on predictive factors including hormone receptors and human epidermal growth factor receptor 2 [HER2]). This information is then used in multivariable algorithms to define the modalities of systemic therapies (e.g., hormone therapy, chemotherapy, and targeted therapies) a patient should receive. Adjuvant! Online (www.adjuvantonline. com/), which assigns patients into different risk groups based on a multivariable model combining clinical and pathologic parameters, has become one of the main methods to determine the therapy for breast cancer patients.[8]

The systematic assessment of the ER, progesterone receptor (PgR) and *HER2* status is the cornerstone of current routine clinical management of breast cancer patients, because these markers predict which patients are unlikely to benefit from endocrine and *HER2*-targeted therapies respectively (e.g., ER– breast cancer patients do not derive benefit from endocrine therapy and *HER2–* breast cancer patients are unlikely to derive benefit from anti-*HER2* agents). Based on this limited repertoire of predictive markers, breast cancers are currently divided in ER+ (the vast majority of tumors, accounting for 60–80% of breast cancers) and ER– subgroups.[1-6,9,10]

Although breast cancer patient management based on the assessment of clinicopathologic parameters has been proved successful, given the steady decline in the mortality of breast cancer since the 1980s, it has become blatantly clear that this approach is unable to capture the complexity of breast cancers, and each subgroup has been shown to display a substantial degree of heterogeneity.[4,11] Therefore, it is not surprising that, with the advent of high-throughput molecular methods, several groups endeavored to investigate the molecular heterogeneity of breast cancers.

There is now evidence to suggest that ER+ breast cancers comprise a spectrum of lesions whose outcome can be determined by the assessment of the levels of expression of ER, ER-related genes, and proliferation-related genes.[1-3,6,12,13] In addition, high-grade ER+ breast cancers may originate from low-grade ER+ breast cancers, given that grade 3 ER+ tumors harbor complex karyotypes, yet they do display the hallmark genetic aberrations in low-grade ER+ tumors in approximately 50% of cases. Conversely, ER– breast cancers often present as tumors of high histologic grade and display a constellation of molecular alterations that are responsible for their more aggressive phenotype.[1-6,9,10] Furthermore, there is evidence to suggest that ER– disease comprises multiple molecular entities.

BREAST CANCER MOLECULAR TAXONOMY

Microarray-based gene expression profiling has been extensively used for the characterization of the molecular features of breast cancers. In the early 2000s, the seminal studies performed by Perou and coworkers[14] and Sorlie and colleagues[15] demonstrated that the transcriptomic profiles of ER+ and ER− breast cancers are fundamentally different and that, within each of these subgroups, multiple subtypes exist. Hierarchical cluster analysis of 38 invasive breast cancers using an "intrinsic gene list" (i.e., a list of 496 genes that vary more between tumors from different patients than in paired samples from the same tumor) revealed the existence of four "intrinsic" subtypes: (1) the luminal subgroup, characterized by expression of ER and genes related to the ER pathway, (2) the *HER2* subtype, characterized by overexpression and amplification of the *HER2* gene on 17q12, (3) basal-like cancers, which were reported to lack hormone receptors and *HER2* expression and to express genes normally found in the basal/myoepithelial compartment of normal breast, and (4) the normal breast–like, which displayed an expression profile similar to that observed in normal breast and adipose tissues.[14] Subsequently, a similar approach was applied to additional cohorts of breast cancer patients and revealed that luminal/ER+ tumors could be further divided into at least two subgroups, luminal A and luminal B.[15,16] Additional studies have demonstrated that the differences between luminal A and luminal B cancers were primarily related to the levels of expression of proliferation-related genes.[17,18] For further details on the molecular classes, see Chapter 20.

The "intrinsic" molecular subtype classification has been enthusiastically embraced by the scientific community and clinicians alike. Multiple independent studies have now demonstrated that at least some of these "intrinsic" molecular subtypes (i.e., luminal A and basal-like) are associated with different risk factors, clinicopathologic features, response to therapeutic agents, and outcome (for reviews, see references 1–3). Despite the enthusiasm with this classification system, it has become apparent that it has some important limitations. There is evidence to suggest that the approaches used to identify the "intrinsic" molecular subtypes lack stability[13,19,20] and may be subjective.[21] Furthermore, in a meta-analysis of gene expression profiles of more than 2800 breast cancers from 18 publicly available datasets, Wirapati and associates[10] observed that only three natural clusters (i.e., subgroups stemming from unbiased analyses of microarray data) could be identified, namely ER−/HER2−, HER2+, and ER+/HER2− tumors, which correspond roughly to the intrinsic subtypes of basal-like, HER2, and luminal A/B, respectively.[10] In fact, the luminal ER+/HER2− subtype was shown to constitute a continuum of tumors rather than a subgroup comprising two biologically distinct subgroups.[1,6,10] Conversely, ER−/HER2− cancers were shown to form a discrete transcriptomic entity. These observations were further confirmed by independent studies, which have demonstrated that the identification of luminal A, luminal B, normal breast–like and *HER2* "intrinsic" subtypes is strongly dependent on the bioinformatic methods employed.[13,20] Conversely, the basal-like subtype appears to comprise a group of tumors fundamentally different from ER+ and *HER2*+ cancers.[1–3,6] Taken together, these observations indicate that out of all "intrinsic" molecular subtypes, basal-like breast cancer is the only class that can be reliably identified across different data sets, platforms, and methodologies, providing additional evidence in support of the concept that this subtype represents a discrete spectrum of lesions.[13,20,21]

BASAL-LIKE BREAST CANCER

Although the existence of breast cancers harboring ultrastructural features of, or expressing proteins usually found in, basal/myoepithelial cells of the normal breast was recorded many decades ago,[22–31] it was the gene expression profiling studies by Perou and coworkers[14] and Sorlie and associates[15] that brought the existence of this subgroup of breast cancers to the forefront of breast cancer research and clinical practice. Basal-like breast cancer constitutes the first entity in breast cancer pathology primarily defined by its expression profile and not histopathologic features.[32,33] Basal-like breast cancers were so named because their common denominator is a transcriptomic profile characterized by the lack or low levels of expression of ER and *HER2*, and expression of genes that are found in basal/myoepithelial cells of the normal breast (e.g., cytokeratins [CKs] 5/6 and 17, epidermal growth factor receptor [EGFR]).[14–18,31–34]

Basal-like cancers are also characterized by a high expression of a constellation of genes (Table 24-1) pertaining to different gene ontology categories (e.g., extracellular matrix, receptors, or oncogenes), such as P-cadherin, fatty acid–binding protein 7, c-kit, matrix metalloproteinase 7, caveolin 1 and 2, metallothionein IX, transforming growth factor–beta (TGF-β) receptor II, and hepatocyte growth factor.[14–18,31–34] Moreover, these tumors display increased expression of cell growth- and cell proliferation–related genes (e.g. topoisomerase IIα, CDC2, and PCNA),[15,34] confirming the observations that these cancers display remarkably high proliferation rates.[9,10,17,34] The fact that the large majority of basal-like cancers do display high levels of expression of proliferation-related genes constitutes one of the reasons why gene signatures based on proliferation are not necessarily important in this subgroup of breast cancer patients.[1,9,10]

Despite the interest in the biologic and clinical characteristics of these cancers, it should be noted that there is still no internationally accepted definition for basal-like breast cancers.[3,31–33] Although these tumors can be robustly identified by gene expression profiling,[1–3,13,21] there is no agreement as to how these tumors would be best defined in clinical practice.[32] Although microarray-based expression profiling has been used by some groups to define basal-like breast cancers,[18,35] others have employed panels of immunohistochemical markers as surrogates for basal-like breast cancers.[32,33] It should be noted, however, that direct comparisons between the proposed immunohistochemical markers and the microarray-defined molecular subtypes are scarce.[13,32,35–37] The most commonly used immunohistochemical

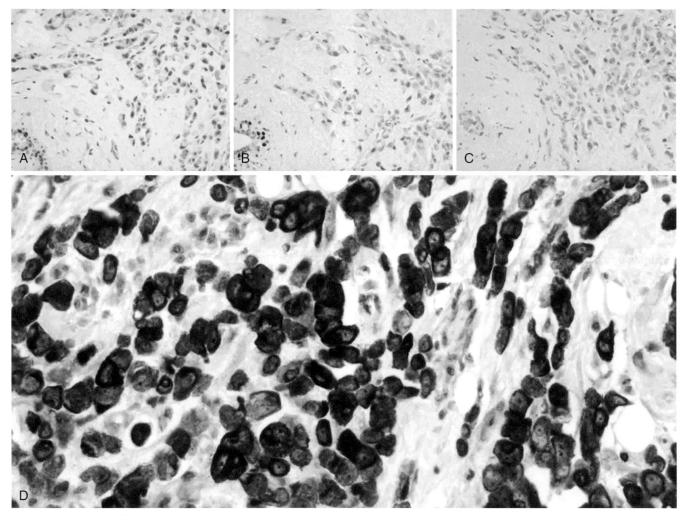

FIGURE 24-42   Basal-like carcinoma. Pleomorphic lobular carcinoma (same case as Figures 24-38 to 24-41) is negative for ER **(A)**, PgR **(B)**, and *HER2* **(C)**, and express CK8/18 **(D).**

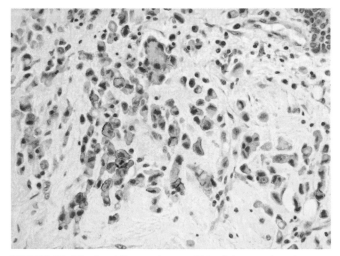

FIGURE 24-43   Basal-like carcinoma. This triple-negative pleomorphic lobular carcinoma (same case as Figures 24-38 to 24-42) displays a membranous EGFR expression.

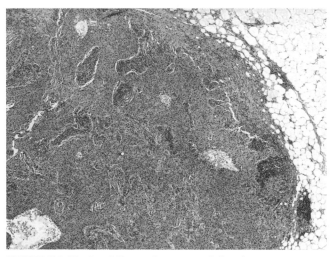

FIGURE 24-44   Basal-like carcinoma. Medullary breast carcinomas belong to the basal-like subtype. They display pushing margins.

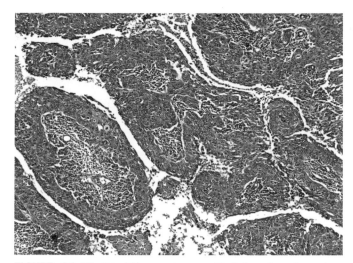

FIGURE 24-45 Basal-like carcinoma. Medullary breast carcinoma shows prominent lymphocytic infiltrate and syncytial growth pattern.

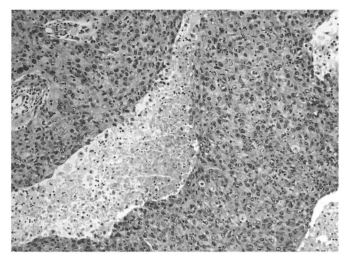

FIGURE 24-46 Basal-like carcinoma. Medullary breast carcinoma is composed of solid sheets of neoplastic cells with extensive necrosis.

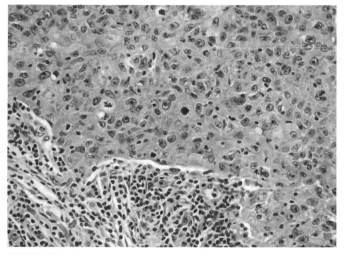

FIGURE 24-47 Basal-like carcinoma. Medullary breast carcinomas display high-grade features with pleomorphic nuclei and high mitotic activity. The syncytial growth pattern is characteristic.

to the *ETV6-NTRK3* chimeric fusion gene.[73,96] This fusion gene has been shown to have oncogenic properties and to be a defining feature of secretory carcinomas of the breast, because it has not been identified in other types of breast cancer.[97–99]

Taken together, these findings illustrate the heterogeneity of the basal-like subgroup and the overlapping phenotypes of entities that have completely distinct histologic features and clinical outcome.[32] These observations highlight the fact that a clinically relevant definition of basal-like carcinomas ought to also be based on morphology and should not solely rely on immunophenotypic or gene expression criteria.

Immunoprofile

Despite meritorious efforts made by the medical and scientific community to characterize basal-like breast cancers, there is still no internationally accepted definition for these cancers (see Table 24-2). Gene expression

profiling–based methods are yet to be implemented in routine clinical practice; however, with the development of PAM50,[18,35] a quantitative reverse-transcriptase polymerase chain reaction (qRT-PCR) or nanostring-based method that can be readily applied to formalin-fixed paraffin-embedded tissue sections, it is possible that in the near future the identification of basal-like breast cancers will be made based on transcriptomic analyses. Given that the use of this methodology is still restricted, attempts have been made to develop surrogate markers for basal-like breast cancers based on their transcriptomic definition. Several limitations, however, have been encountered in the current development of an immunohistochemical definition of basal-like breast cancers. Apart from the known caveats of immunohistochemical surrogates (e.g., lack of standardization of the technical protocol, variability in the interpretation criteria and cutoffs used),[100] the major criticism for the immunohistochemical surrogates developed for basal-like cancers is that only a few immunohistochemical surrogates have been established using gene expression profiling as a gold standard (see Table 24-2).

Out of all surrogates put forward for basal-like breast cancers, the most commonly used definition for these tumors is the triple-negative phenotype (i.e., lack of ER, PgR, and *HER2*).[33] It should be noted that this definition was based more on convenience than on scientific merit, given that, even in the initial transcriptomic studies of basal-like cancers, it was apparent that not all basal-like breast cancers display a triple-negative phenotype and not all triple-negative breast cancers are classified as basal-like tumors by gene expression profiling.[14–18,33] Bertucci and colleagues[101] demonstrated that only 71% of triple-negative cancers as defined by immunohistochemical analysis are of basal-like subtype by gene expression profiling and that only 77% of basal-like tumors as defined by gene expression profiling are of triple-negative subtype by immunohistochemical analysis. Similar observations have also been made by de Ronde and associates[102] and Parker and coworkers[18] who reported that 8% to 29%

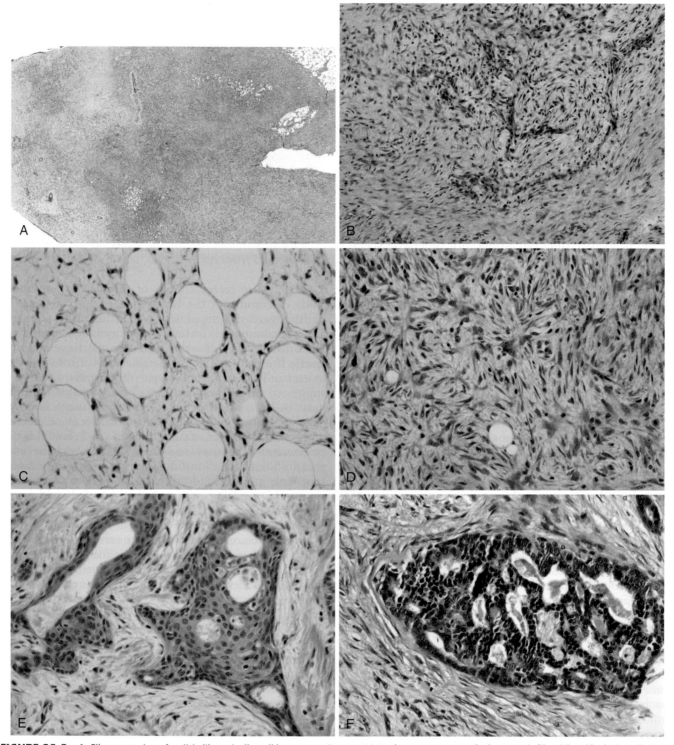

FIGURE 25-5 **A,** Fibromatosis or fasciitis-like spindle cell breast carcinoma. Note the appearance of a low-grade fibroblast-like lesion. **B,** Note the fibroblast-like cells and angiectoid treachery mimicking branching capillary vessels. **C,** Note subtle fibroblast-like invasion of adipose tissue by the bland fibroblast-like spindled tumor cells. **D,** Higher magnification shows the low-grade cytologic features. **E,** Note the islands of bland squamous carcinoma from which the spindle cells appear to arise. **F,** Sometimes, only areas of atypical duct hyperplasia or low-grade duct carcinoma in situ can be found and represent evidence of spindle cell carcinoma.

20 cases in which axillary nodes were biopsied, definitive nodal metastases were identified in only 1 (5%), and this was in a case with a significant component of invasive ductal carcinoma. Three patients developed local recurrences. Extranodal metastases occurred in 11 of 24 patients (46%), most commonly to the lungs. Ten of 24 patients (42%) died of disease at a median interval of 11.5 months (range 1–46 mo), and 3 patients were alive with metastatic disease. Eight patients were alive with no evidence of recurrent or metastatic disease (median 29.5 mo). Based on this series, spindle cell/sarcomatoid carcinoma of the breast is a highly aggressive neoplasm with a high

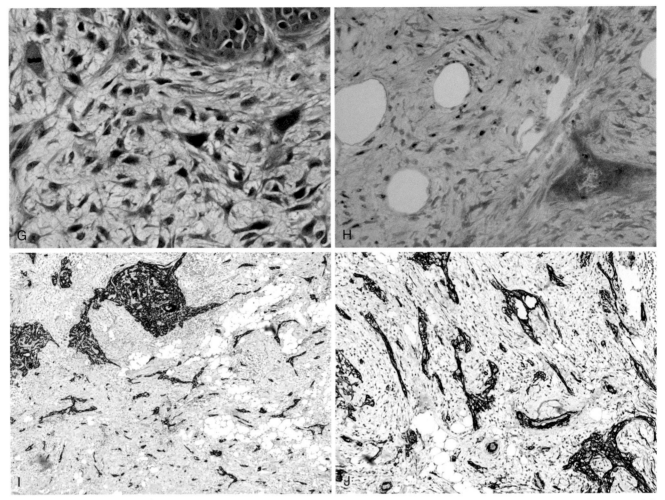

FIGURE 25-5, cont'd G, Careful search can sometimes reveal evidence of malignancy such as nuclear atypia or mitotic figures. **H,** Other evidence of malignancy may be found such as necrosis. **I,** Keratin stain shows that the angiectoid treachery is actually invasive strands of carcinoma, which are arising from islands of low-grade squamous carcinoma. **J,** Higher magnification of the keratin-positive treachery.

rate of extranodal metastases. Purely spindled/sarcomatoid tumors have a significantly lower rate of nodal metastases than conventional ductal and lobular breast carcinomas. Not surprisingly, large tumors with high nuclear grade and frequent mitoses were generally (but not always) aggressive. They also found, somewhat surprisingly, that even low-grade tumors were capable of aggressive behavior with metastases and subsequent mortality. Of the 6 low-grade tumors with follow-up information, 33% (2 of 6) died of metastatic disease, 1 patient was alive with widespread metastases, and 1 patient was alive with chest wall involvement and metastases to the axilla. They further observed that this group of tumors appeared to be more aggressive than conventional ductal carcinomas of similar size, with an apparent tendency for somewhat earlier systemic metastasis and that there appear to be no histologic features that reliably predict good prognosis in this group of tumors.

Treatment and Prognosis

Some early reports indicated that metaplastic breast carcinomas had a poor survival, possibly in the range of 35% at 5 years follow-up; and this poor survival

---

KEY PATHOLOGIC FEATURES
Metaplastic Breast Carcinoma

- Usually biphasic epithelial and spindle components.

- Spindle cell component may be dominant, epithelial component inconspicuous.

- Grade varies from low to high grade.

- Spindle cell component may be very bland and fasciitis-like.

- Differential diagnosis includes many spindle cell lesions, benign and malignant.

- Immunohistology panels with CAM5.2, AE1/AE3, CK7, CK5, CK14, CK17, will demonstrate at least one keratin-positive profile. In the absence of any keratin, another diagnosis should be entertained.

- Vimentin, p63, SMA are other immunostains that may be positive, in decreasing order of staining frequency.

CAM, cell adhesion molecule; CK, cytokeratin; SMA, smooth muscle actin.

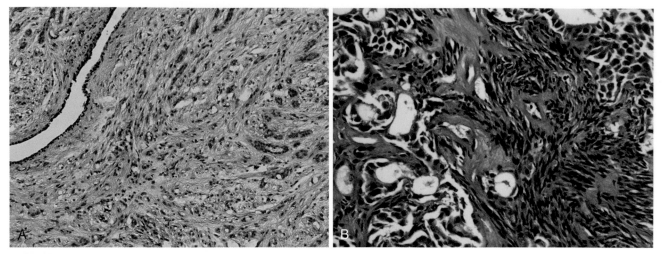

FIGURE 25-8 **A,** Sclerosing adenosis with spindle cell myoepithelial cells, which can be confused with spindle cell breast carcinoma. **B,** Note abundant spindle cells in this example of sclerosing adenosis.

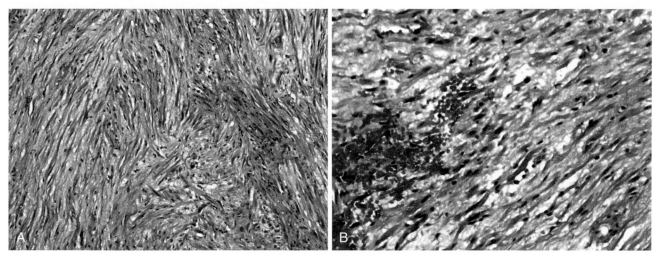

FIGURE 25-9 **A,** Inflammatory myofibroblastic tumor of the breast. **B,** Note myxoid and low-grade myofibroblastic (desmoplasia) features of inflammatory myofibroblastic tumor.

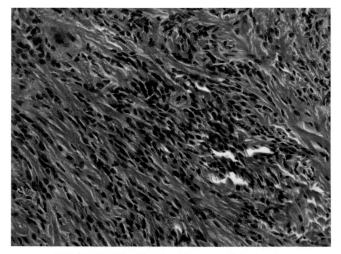

FIGURE 25-10 Myofibroblastoma of the breast.

sarcomas (also called stromal sarcoma) (Figure 25-16), and angiosarcoma (Figure 25-17). We begin our discussion with benign lesions.

Benign Spindle Cell Breast Lesions

Desmoid or aggressive fibromatosis of the breast is a rare benign mesenchymal transformation of connective tissue origin, usually associated with the fascia of the pectoral muscles or the Cooper ligaments.[44–49] Occasional cases are associated clinically with Gardner's syndrome or familial multicentric fibromatosis.[44] (Early recognition of Gardner's syndrome allows prophylactic colectomy to prevent colon carcinoma.) After clinical and radiologic examination, it can be difficult to differentiate fibromatosis from mammary carcinoma or other malignant tumors of the breast. Only histologic examination can lead to the final diagnosis.

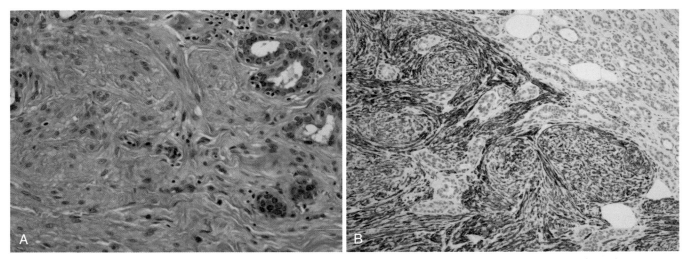

FIGURE 25-11 **A,** Breast containing leiomyoma. **B,** Positive smooth muscle actin in the spindled leiomyoma cells.

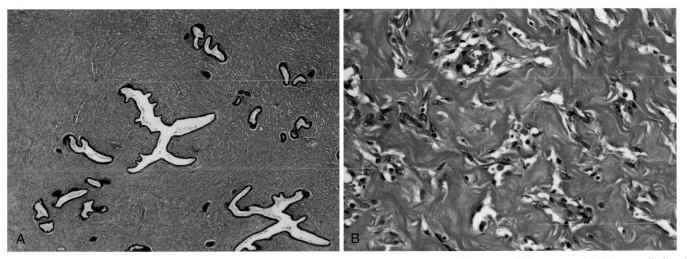

FIGURE 25-12 **A,** Pseudoangiomatous stromal hyperplasia (PASH). **B,** Higher magnification shows vessel-like spaces of PASH, actually lined by fibroblasts.

In the breast, desmoid or aggressive fibromatosis behaves the same as when it arises in other soft tissue sites—an aggressive infiltrative lesion with a proclivity for local recurrence after inadequate excision but without potential for distant metastases.[44–50] The therapy of choice is excision with margins clear of the fibromatosis.[44–50] Mastectomy is not necessarily indicated, but inadequate excision can lead to multiple recurrences, chest wall invasion, and eventual death due to pulmonary complications.[46]

Of interest, Pettinato and associates[51] reported two cases of a peculiar "fibromatosis" of the breast characterized by a proliferation of spindle cells containing intracytoplasmic, spherical, eosinophilic inclusion bodies. Both patients were free of disease 16 and 18 months after surgery described as "simple excision" and "excision biopsy." The light and electron microscopic features, as well as the immunohistochemical features, are indistinguishable from those found in infantile digital fibromatosis. The proliferating spindle cells are characterized as myofibroblasts, whereas the inclusion bodies showed a nonreactive, hollow-like pattern with peripheral reactivity for actin filaments. These lesions, observed for the first time in the breast, expanded the number of extradigital inclusion body fibromatoses. Exactly how this form relates clinicopathologically to desmoid fibromatosis is unclear. Other cases of inclusion body–like fibromatosis arising in other extradigital sites in adults have not recurred after surgical excision.[51] Electron microscopy shows the cells of desmoid fibromatosis to have fibroblastic or myofibroblastic differentiation.[47] They also often immunoreact with antibodies to muscle actins and desmin, but they are negative with antikeratin antibodies.[51]

Sclerosing lymphocytic lobulitis is an inflammatory breast lesion that can mimic carcinoma. It is of probable autoimmune cause.[52,53] Moreover, many reports emphasized the association of sclerosing lymphocytic lobulitis with diabetes, especially type 1, less commonly type 2 (also called diabetic mastopathy).[54–56] But essentially identical lesions occur in nondiabetic patients, often with other evidence of autoimmune disease (e.g., Hashimoto's thyroiditis or circulating autoantibodies).[52,57] Diabetic patients with sclerosing lymphocytic lobulitis usually have early-onset, longstanding, insulin-dependent diabetes, which developed premenopausally.

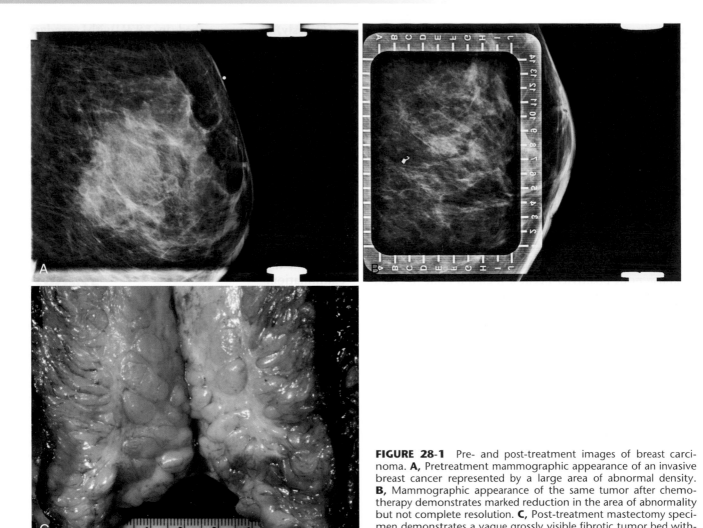

FIGURE 28-1 Pre- and post-treatment images of breast carcinoma. **A,** Pretreatment mammographic appearance of an invasive breast cancer represented by a large area of abnormal density. **B,** Mammographic appearance of the same tumor after chemotherapy demonstrates marked reduction in the area of abnormality but not complete resolution. **C,** Post-treatment mastectomy specimen demonstrates a vague grossly visible fibrotic tumor bed without grossly identifiable residual tumor.

typically well defined and the cells tend to shrink away from the stroma (see Figure 28-6). This feature should not be misinterpreted as lymphatic or vascular invasion. In cases of near-pCR, scattered single tumor cells may show multinucleation, hyperchromasia, and nuclear smudging, making them difficult to detect on routine stain (Figure 28-7). In certain cases, IHC stains are helpful in distinguishing between epithelial cells (cytokeratins [CKs] AE1/AE3 or CK7) and macrophages (CD68). Residual ductal carcinoma in situ (DCIS) may or may not show morphologic alteration after treatment (Figure 28-8). However, residual DCIS in lobules (cancerized lobules) may pose a diagnostic dilemma leading to misinterpretation as residual invasive carcinoma (see Figure 28-8). IHC stains for myoepithelial cells (p63 or myosin heavy chain) would resolve the diagnostic dilemma in those instances. For reasons not completely clear, in situ carcinoma and vascular tumor emboli are relatively resistant to chemotherapy when compared with invasive carcinoma.[44] Although immeasurable, if residual tumor is identified only in vascular spaces, it should be considered as incomplete pathologic response (Figure 28-9). However, this is an extremely rare phenomenon, and if thorough examination of the

breast is performed, an invasive component is usually identified.

EVALUATION OF MARGINS The significance of tumor bed changes at a margin is unclear in cases in which no residual carcinoma is identified (Figure 28-10). However, cases in which residual invasive or in situ carcinoma is scattered throughout the tumor bed, tumor bed changes at a margin may be predictive of residual carcinoma in the breast (Figure 28-11). In rare instances, CK stain may help to delineate the extent of residual tumor cells and assessment of margin if single tumor cells are scattered throughout the tumor bed (see Figure 28-11).

CHANGES IN NON-NEOPLASTIC BREAST Cytotoxic effect of either chemotherapy or radiation therapy can affect the non–tumor-bearing breast parenchyma. Scattered epithelial cells of the terminal duct lobular unit demonstrating cytoplasmic and nuclear enlargement and sclerosis of basement membranes may be seen outside the tumor bed area (Figure 28-12). These changes should not be misinterpreted as residual in situ carcinoma, especially when present near a margin.

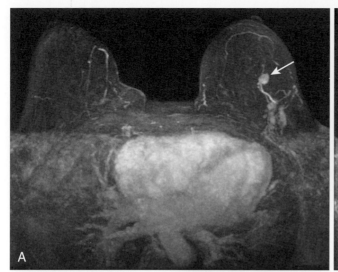

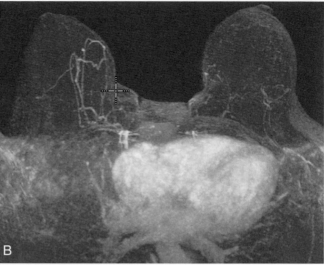

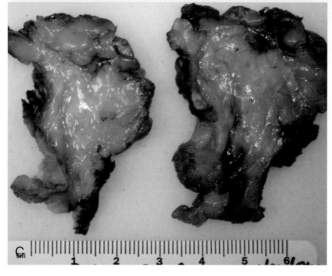

FIGURE 28-2 Pre- and post-treatment contrast-enhanced magnetic resonance imaging (MRI). **A,** Pretreatment maximum intensity projection (MIP) image of a patient presented with a 1.5-cm "triple-negative," node-positive breast carcinoma correlating with a 1.2-cm area of intensity on MRI. **B,** The patient received four cycles of chemotherapy. Post-therapy MIP image shows complete resolution of the abnormality. **C,** Post-treatment partial mastectomy was localized for excision using a clip that had been placed before treatment. Partial mastectomy specimen was differentially inked. The cut surface demonstrating no grossly visible tumor bed but a small area showing characteristic changes of tumor bed was found on microscopic examination.

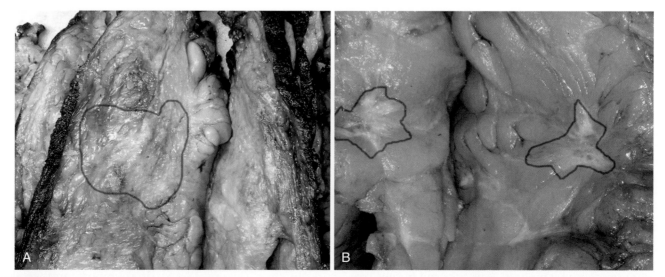

FIGURE 28-3 **A,** Post-treatment mastectomy specimen with a vague grossly visible fibrotic tumor bed without grossly identifiable residual tumor. On pathologic examination, this patient had small foci of residual tumor. **B,** Partial mastectomy specimen with small tan nodules of residual tumor in an irregular fibrotic tumor bed.

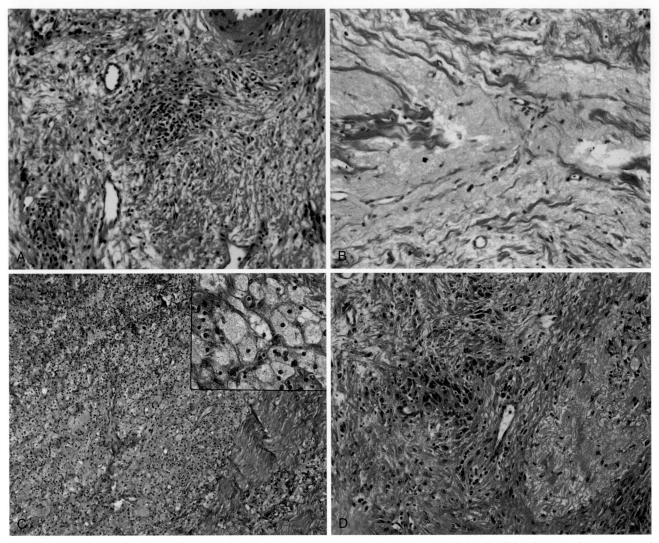

FIGURE 28-4 Tumor bed with complete pathologic response. **A,** Hyalinized vascular stroma without glandular elements demonstrates edema, elastosis, and chronic inflammatory cells. **B,** Tumor bed with prominent myxoid change. **C,** Tumor bed with large sheets of macrophages. Inset: high power. **D,** Tumor bed with hemosiderin-laden macrophages.

POST-TREATMENT LYMPH NODE EVALUATION

Gross Examination

Axillary fat should be carefully searched for lymph nodes and all nodes thinly sectioned along the long axis and completely submitted. In general, after chemotherapy, lymph nodes are difficult to recognize because of atrophy and fibrosis.[45] Whereas one study reported low axillary lymph node counts after neoadjuvant chemotherapy,[46] others have shown not much difference.[47,48] In cases in which it is difficult to identify lymph nodes, submitting fibrotic areas in the axillary fat and tissue around the vessels may reveal small atrophic nodes on microscopic examination.

Microscopic Examination

Not all of a patient's lymph node metastases will respond equally to chemotherapy. Some nodes may show pronounced lymphoid depletion and fibrous scarring with little or no residual carcinoma, whereas other nodes may have large metastases after treatment.

In general, the degree of response to therapy in the lymph nodes corresponds to that observed in the breast. Lymph node metastases that show CR to therapy are often replaced by hyaline sclerosis, mucin pools, or aggregates of macrophages without any viable tumor cells (Figure 28-13). pCR to prior metastatic involvement in some cases cannot be determined with certainty because small metastasis can resolve without a scar or may leave small fibrous scars. However, it is unusual to see large fibrous scars in lymph nodes of patients who undergo surgery first.[45] Therefore, the presence of a large scar in lymph nodes without tumor cells most likely represents CR to therapy.

Metastatic nodes with PR to therapy are characterized by isolated or clusters of tumor cells often surrounded by thin or thick hyaline fibrosis (Figure 28-14). IHC stain for CK is helpful to identify tumor cells that are difficult to delineate on routine hematoxylin and eosin stain (Figure 28-15). It is important to make note of any treatment effect in the residual metastatic nodes.

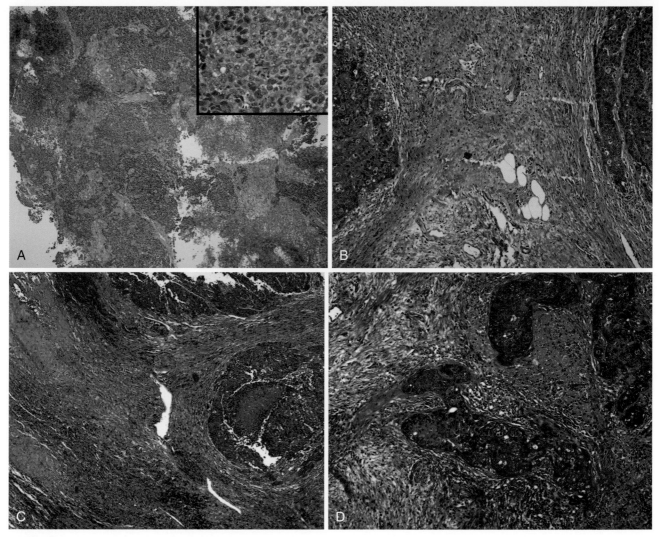

FIGURE 28-5 Loss of tumor cellularity after therapy. **A,** Pretreatment core biopsy of a high-grade invasive ductal carcinoma. Inset: high power. **B-D,** Foci of residual tumor nodules separated by fibrous stroma.

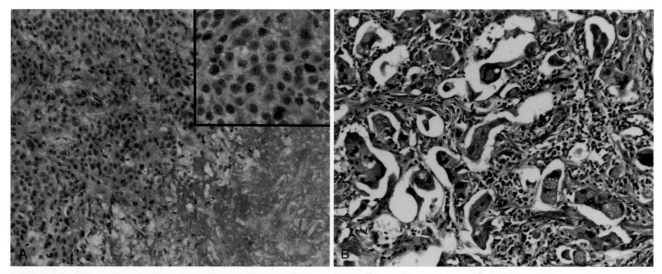

FIGURE 28-6 Pre- and post-treatment tumor. **A,** Pretreatment core biopsy of a high-grade invasive ductal carcinoma. Inset: high power. **B,** Nests of residual tumor cells with marked therapy effect. Note the prominent retraction artifact.

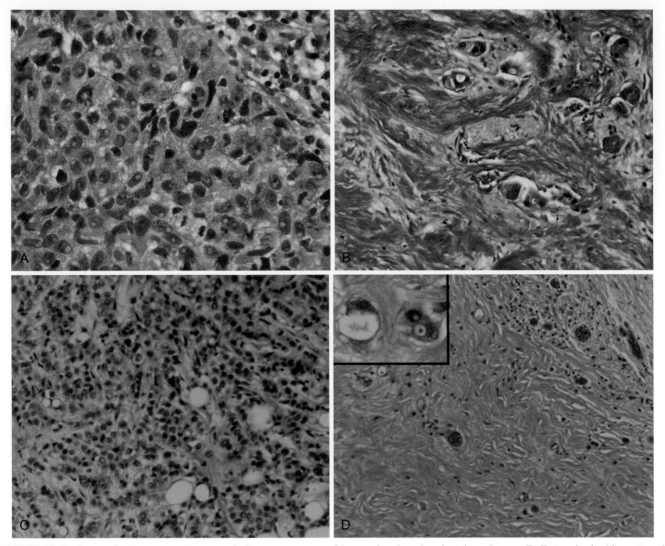

FIGURE 28-7 Pre- and post-treatment tumor. **A,** Pretreatment core biopsy of an invasive ductal carcinoma. **B,** Tumor bed with scattered single tumor cells with therapy effect. **C,** Pretreatment core biopsy of an invasive lobular carcinoma. **D,** Tumor bed with marked loss of cellularity with scattered single cells showing therapy effect *(inset).*

POST-TREATMENT PROGNOSTIC AND PREDICTIVE FACTORS

Postneoadjuvant Prognostic Factors

The prognosis of breast cancer patients treated with neoadjuvant systemic agents before surgery is determined by both the pretreatment clinical stage and the post-treatment pathologic stage.[49] Patients who obtain the greatest survival advantage from neoadjuvant chemotherapy are those who experience complete abolition of their tumor.[14,15,17,19,50] Following are the post-treatment tumor characteristics that are commonly associated with prognosis.

TUMOR SIZE

In most patients, NAT reduces the size of the primary tumor. Size is relatively easy to determine in patients with a minimal response to treatment. However, it is difficult to measure residual tumor that has undergone a marked response, because multiple small foci of invasive carcinoma or scattered tumor cells are present throughout the tumor bed. Nonetheless, smaller tumor size remains as a good prognostic factor after chemotherapy.[17,51,52] In a study, Chen and associates[53] reported pathologic residual tumor larger than 2 cm was associated with higher rates of locoregional tumor recurrence in patients who underwent breast-conserving surgery and radiation therapy after NAT.

TUMOR CELLULARITY

Carcinomas often become less cellular after treatment. The loss of cellularity is not always reflected by a decrease in tumor size due to chemotherapy-induced fibrous stromal involution, which can result in clinical and macroscopic overestimation of residual tumor size.[33] For tumors that remain as a contiguous mass, cellularity can be estimated over the entire carcinoma. Estimation of cellularity is problematic in cases with marked

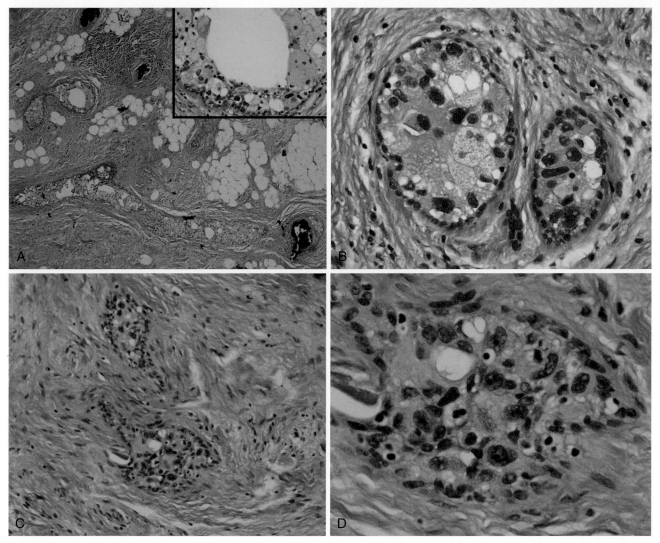

FIGURE 28-8 Ductal carcinoma in situ (DCIS) with treatment effect. **A,** Some of the ducts are replaced by histiocytes with microcalcification. Inset: high power. **B,** The residual DCIS with large cells with enlarged nuclei. **C** and **D,** Scattered foci of DCIS within the tumor bed simulate residual invasive carcinoma.

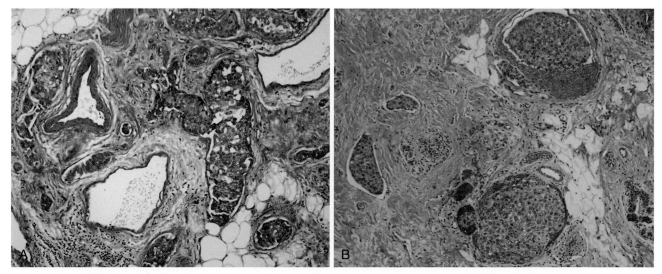

FIGURE 28-9 **A** and **B,** Tumor bed changes with prominent vascular tumor emboli after chemotherapy.

response, because islands of highly cellular carcinoma may be interspersed within a large, difficult-to-delineate tumor bed. Because carcinomas may vary greatly in cellularity before treatment, a change in cellularity can be determined with certainty only if the pretreatment carcinoma is available for comparison.

Loss of cellularity has been shown to correlate with better prognosis and clinical outcome.[15,54] Ideally, a combination of residual tumor size and changes in tumor cellularity is useful in documenting treatment response and outcome. In one study, the authors reported an inverse relationship between tumor HR content and percentage of tumor volume reduction using a formula that requires pre- and post-treatment tumor size and tumor cellularity.[23]

TUMOR GRADE

In the majority of cases, the microscopic appearance of carcinoma does not change after treatment. However, some carcinomas may appear to be higher grade and, in

rare instances, may be of lower grade owing to changes in mitosis and histologic appearance of the tumor cells.[4,35,44] The pretreatment assessment of histologic grade remains an independent prognostic factor for DFS and OS in patients treated with neoadjuvant chemotherapy.[24] The cytotoxic effects of treatment resulting in a change in the grade of cancers have not been clearly correlated with clinical outcome.

LYMPH NODE

Post-treatment lymph node status is the most important prognostic factor in patients who receive NAT.[2,11,55] In fact, patients with no residual tumor in the breast but who have residual tumor in the lymph nodes have worse prognosis than patients who have negative nodes but residual tumor in the breast.[11,16,55] Most studies have shown that patients with an increasing number of residual positive nodes had progressively worse distant DFS and OS than patients with negative nodes.[56,57]

The significance of the size of a metastatic deposit in a lymph node depends on whether or not the patient has been treated with chemotherapy before surgery. In the National Surgical Adjuvant Breast and Bowel Project (NSABP) B-18, at 9 years of follow-up, patients in the adjuvant arm with negative nodes or micrometastases had identical survival, whereas those patients with macrometastases had a significantly worse prognosis. In contrast, survival rates of patients in the NAT arm with minimetastases (<1.0 mm) and micrometastases (<2.0 mm) in nodes were similar to patients with macrometastases but significantly worse than those with negative nodes.[4] Similar results were reported by other studies.[56] This is attributed to the fact that micrometastases in lymph nodes in patients who receive NAT probably represent macrometastases that have responded to therapy. Furthermore, patients who have residual metastatic tumor with evidence of treatment effect have better DFS and lower relapse rates than patients who have metastatic nodes without evidence of treatment effect.[58] However, the significance of isolated tumor cells in the lymph nodes after NAT is somewhat conflicting. In a

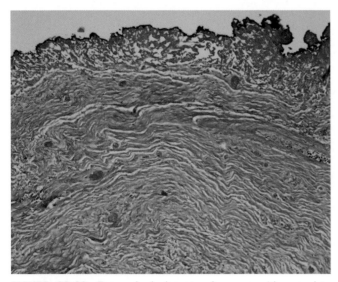

FIGURE 28-10 Tumor bed changes of a case with complete pathologic response seen at a cauterized inked margin.

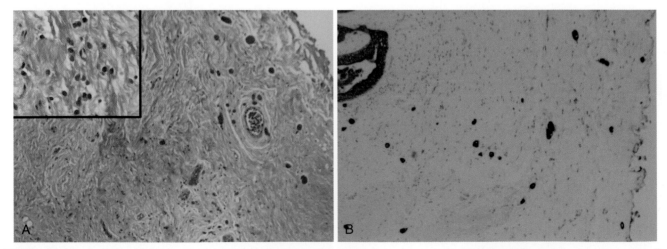

FIGURE 28-11 **A,** Tumor bed changes of a case with pronounced response seen at a cauterized inked margin. Inset: scattered tumor cells. **B,** Cytokeratin stain highlights single tumor cells very close to the margin.

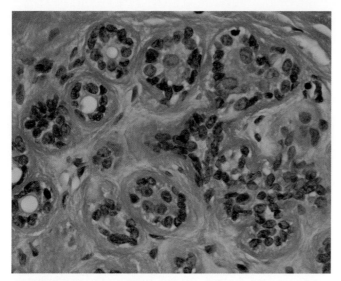

FIGURE 28-12 Normal terminal duct lobular unit with therapy effect.

study by Loya and coworkers,[57] no statistically significant difference was found in DFS or OS between patients with and without occult metastases (isolated tumor cells found on IHC stain for CK) after a median follow-up of 63 months.

Postneoadjuvant Predictive Factors

In general, patients who achieve pCR have better long-term DFS and OS regardless of the tumor subtypes. Despite higher pCR rate in "triple-negative" and *HER2*+/ER– tumors, patients who failed to achieve pCR with these tumors have a worse outcome (frequent relapse and worse OS) when compared with patients with residual ER+ tumors. This phenomenon has been described as the "triple-negative paradox" or rather "HR– paradox."[18,19]

In patients with substantial residual disease, questions regarding the stability of HR and *HER2*/neu expression in residual tumor after therapy are raised in order to optimize additional targeted therapy. Little discordance

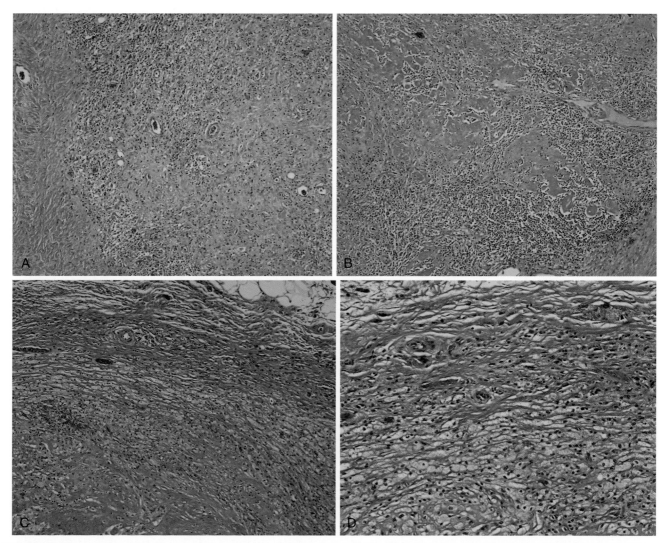

FIGURE 28-13 Lymph node with complete response to therapy. **A** and **B,** Lymph node with marked depletion of lymphocytes and fibrous scar without viable tumor cells. **C** and **D,** Lymph node with sheets of foamy macrophages and hemosiderin without viable tumor cells.

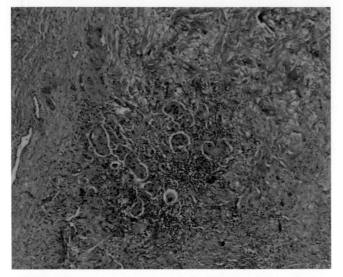

FIGURE 28-14   Lymph node with partial response to therapy. Tumor cells are surrounded by fibrosis.

between core needle biopsy and excisional biopsy for ER (discordance 1.8%), PgR (discordance 15%), and *HER2*/neu (discordance 1.2%) overexpression has been reported in untreated tumors.[59] However, with NAT, the discordance rate between pre- and post-treatment samples for HR have been reported to be as high as 8% to 33%, particularly in studies in which endocrine agents were used.[60] Unlike HRs, *HER2*/neu overexpression seems to be more stable during chemotherapy. Discordance was reported in only one of the seven trials that tested *HER2* using fluorescence in situ hybridization (FISH).[61] However, diminished *HER2*/neu expression was reported in up to 32% of the carcinomas when trastuzumab was combined with neoadjuvant chemotherapy.[62] Similarly, down-regulation of *HER2*/neu was reported in as many as 41% of *HER2*+ tumors treated with an aromatase inhibitor without a *HER2*-blocking agent.[63]

In cases of discrepancy of tumor markers between pre- and post-treatment tumor, one must consider the confounding factors such as variability in tissue

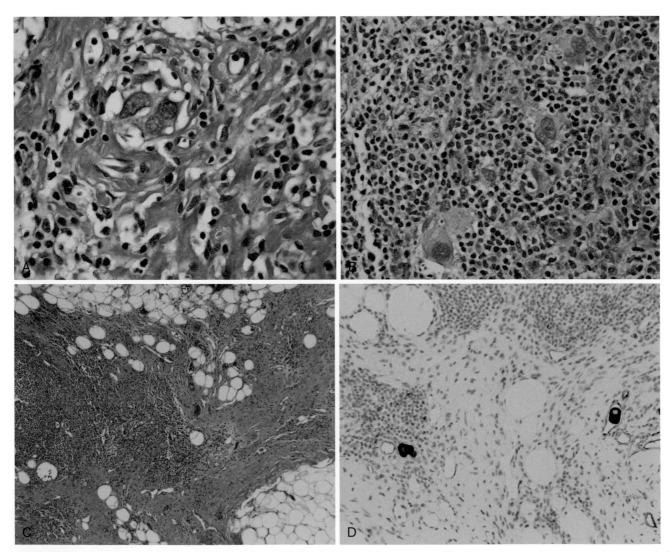

FIGURE 28-15   **A-C,** Postchemotherapy lymph node with isolated enlarged single tumor cells with large hyperchromatic nuclei surrounded by fibrosis. **D,** Cytokeratin AE1/3 stain highlights single tumor cells.

processing and fixation, laboratory error in testing, variability in interpretation of the stains, tumor sampling, tumor multiplicity, and intratumoral heterogeneity before attributing the results to therapy. Possible mechanisms of change in tumor marker expression related to therapeutic agents include change in tumor biology (down-regulation of markers) or selection of resistant tumor cells in the residual disease.

When there has been a change in tumor markers after treatment, little is known whether the pre- or post-treatment expression profile will be more predictive of the pattern in future recurrences or distant metastases. Nonetheless, a positive switch of the HR status could be an indicator for a better outcome and, indeed, was significantly correlated with better OS and DFS in patients who were treated with adjuvant endocrine therapy compared with those who were not treated.[64] In a small study population of *HER2*+ tumors treated with neoadjuvant trastuzumab, a diminished *HER2*/neu expression in the post-treatment tumor sample was associated with poor recurrence-free survival (RFS).[62]

Changes in proliferation index as determined by Ki-67 (MIB-1) stain have been suggested as a means to measure response to therapy, particularly in patients with HR+ tumors receiving hormonal agents, because inhibition of proliferation is the primary goal of treatment.[65] The significance of change in proliferation index after treatment has been linked to survival benefit.[66–68] Most studies have demonstrated low post-treatment Ki-67 to be an independent predictor of RFS and OS and suggest using Ki-67 in residual tumors as surrogate biomarkers to personalize additional adjuvant treatment.[68]

The prognostic significance of detecting circulating tumor cell has been shown in patients with metastatic breast cancer.[69] Pierga and colleagues[70] reported that persistence of circulating tumor cells at the end of neoadjuvant chemotherapy did not correlate with treatment response. However, after a short median follow-up of 18 months, the presence of circulating tumor cells, HR negativity, and large tumor size were shown to be independent prognostic factors for shorter distant metastasis-free survival.

SYSTEMS FOR EVALUATING DEGREE OF RESPONSE

Many pathologic classification systems have been developed to correlate treatment response with survival outcomes. All of the systems recognize a category of pCR and a category of NR. In most systems, a pCR requires the absence of invasive carcinoma in the breast. In systems that include lymph nodes, the nodes must also be free of carcinoma for a pCR. The number of categories of PR varies from study to study including systems in which response is expressed as a continuous variable. No single method of assessing response has been shown to be superior in predicting clinical outcome.

Listed later are some of the systems with a brief description on the classification and category of responses (Table 28-1).

American Joint Committee on Cancer System (7th Edition)

Carcinomas are assigned a post-treatment T and N category indicated by the prefix "y." The AJCC (American Joint Committee on Cancer) stage does not recommend using pretreatment clinical stage to calculate post-treatment tumor stage. Post-treatment AJCC stage relies predominantly on information about tumor size and lymph node status in the post-treatment specimen, unless the patient was M1 prior to NAT, in which case, the M status remains unchanged regardless of response to therapy (and, therefore, stage IV). The postneoadjuvant pathologic tumor size (ypT) is based on the largest contiguous focus of invasive tumor unless there were clearly defined multiple scattered foci of tumor, which is designated with a modifier "m." Measurement of the largest tumor focus should not include areas of fibrosis within the tumor bed. Although the system does not include changes in cellularity in the classification, it is recommended that additional information regarding extent of residual disease and overall tumor cellularity be included in the report to assist clinicians in the assessment of treatment response.

The post-treatment yp "N" categories are the same as those used for untreated tumors (pN). For example,

TABLE 28-1	Different Systems of Categorizing Response to Neoadjuvant Treatment
NSABP B-18[4]	
pCR: No recognizable invasive tumor cells present.	
pPR: The presence of scattered individual or small clusters of tumor cells in a desmoplastic or hyaline stroma.	
pNR: Tumors not exhibiting the changes listed previously.	
Miller-Payne Grading System[13]	
Grade 1: No change or some alteration to individual malignant cells, but no reduction in overall cellularity (pNR)	
Grade 2: A minor loss of tumor cells, but overall cellularity still high; up to 30% loss (pPR).	
Grade 3: Between an estimated 30% and 90% reduction in tumor cells (pPR).	
Grade 4: A marked disappearance of tumor cells such that only small clusters or widely dispersed individual cells remain; more than 90% loss of tumor cells (almost pCR).	
Grade 5: No malignant cells identifiable in sections from the site of the tumor; only vascular fibroelastotic stroma remains, often containing macrophages; however, ductal carcinoma in situ may be present (pCR).	
Residual Cancer Burden System[15]	
RCB-0: No carcinoma in breast or lymph nodes (pCR).	
RCB-I: Minimal residual disease (marked response).	
RCB-II: Moderate response.	
RCB-III: Minimal or No response (chemoresistant).	

NSABP, National Surgical Adjuvant Breast and Bowel protocol; pCR, pathologic complete response; pNR, pathologic no response; pPR, pathologic partial response.

presence of isolated tumor cells or metastases no greater than 0.2 mm is classified as ypN0 (i+). However, patients with this finding are excluded from being classified as pCR.

The Miller-Payne Grading System

Response was divided into five grades based on a comparison of tumor cellularity before and after treatment and was correlated with DFS and OS.[15] This study showed that a grade 4 response (almost CR) had a worse prognosis than a pCR (grade 5), providing evidence that this type of response should be kept as a separate group. However, this system did not include the response in lymph nodes for classification of pCR. Thus, it is possible that the patients with a grade 4 response who did poorly could have had residual tumor in the lymph nodes.

Residual Cancer Burden System

This system was developed to calculate residual cancer burden (RCB) in 382 patients in two different treatment cohorts for prediction of distant relapse-free survival.[17] The system used residual invasive carcinoma cellularity distributed over the tumor bed, the number of lymph nodes with metastases, and the size of the largest metastasis combined mathematically to provide a continuous parameter of response (RCB index) and devised four classes of RCB (RCB-0 through RCB-III). Based on the RCB classes, patients with minimal residual disease (RCB-I) had the same 5-year survival as those with pCR (RCB-0), irrespective of the type of neoadjuvant chemotherapy administered. Conversely, extensive residual disease (RCB-III) had poor prognosis, in particular, patients who did not receive adjuvant hormone therapy. Interestingly, patients who had a moderate response to chemotherapy (RCB-II) appeared to have survival benefit from subsequent hormone therapy.

Although this system requires the use of a formula, a Web-based calculation script (http://www.mdanderson.org/breastcancer_RCB) is freely available to calculate the scores and the RCB class. The Web site also provides a stepwise guide for the pathologic evaluation of post-treatment breast specimens along with links to illustrative examples.

Magee Method

At Magee-Womens Hospital of University of Pittsburgh Medical Center (UPMC), we follow a simple, objective method for assessing tumor volume reduction secondary to NAT. The process starts with examination of the gross specimen. In this method, the largest dimension of the gross tumor bed/fibrotic area identified on gross examination should be noted in the gross description of the pathology report. This area should be either entirely submitted (if small, i.e., ≤3 cm) or sampled extensively (if large, i.e., >3 cm), with sections serially submitted at 0.5-cm intervals along the largest dimension. The entire region should be submitted regardless of the size if no tumor is detected on initial sections. The tumor

TABLE 28-2	Magee Method of Estimating Tumor Volume Reduction
Pre-therapy Tumor Size	
A1	Maximum tumor dimension (use following in preferential order: MRI; ultrasound; mammogram; physical exam): _____cm.
Post-therapy Tumor Size	
B1	Maximum dimension of tumor bed/fibrotic area by gross exam: _____cm.
B2	Percentage cellularity of tumor bed (in comparison to pre-therapy biopsy): _____%.
B3	Revised tumor size after correcting for cellularity (B1 × B2): _____cm.
Estimated Tumor Volume Reduction	

$$\frac{\text{pre-therapy size (A1)} - \text{revised tumor size (B3)}}{\text{pre-therapy size (A1)}} \times 100$$

cellularity of the resection specimen should be compared with the pretherapy biopsy. Specifically, the pretherapy biopsy should be screened for de novo sclerosis and necrosis. If these areas are present in pretherapy biopsy, similar areas in post-therapy resection specimens should not be counted toward therapy-related changes. After excluding these de novo changes, the resection specimen showing treatment-related fibrosis should be compared with the cellularity of pretherapy biopsy and the residual cellularity of the tumor bed is estimated. The revised tumor size is calculated by multiplying the largest dimension of gross tumor bed/fibrotic area with the tumor cellularity (compared with pretherapy biopsy) of the resection specimen. The percentage tumor size/volume reduction is calculated by subtracting revised tumor size from pretherapy size, divided by pretherapy size times 100 (Table 28-2). Although this method may also be used for determining response within the lymph nodes, it is generally not possible because it requires pretherapy size and core biopsy of the lymph node, which is not always available. Only the presence or absence of tumor within lymph nodes should be noted at the post-therapy resection specimen to judge whether pathologic response is complete or incomplete. Although not measurable, if residual tumor is identified only in vascular spaces, it should be considered as incomplete pathologic response. However, this is an extremely rare phenomenon and, if thorough examination of the breast is performed, generally an intraparenchymal component is also identified. In a few cases of inflammatory carcinoma in which pretherapy size is not available, the size of the tumor bed/fibrotic area on gross examination can be used to estimate the pretherapy size.

REPORTING OF POST-TREATMENT SPECIMEN

Pathology reports on treated tumors should include the following information.

Breast Specimen

1. Identification and measurement of tumor bed: important for documentation, especially in cases with pCR.
2. Size and extent of residual tumor:
   - Two-dimensional measurements of the largest area of invasive cancer.
   - Number of foci or number of blocks with foci of invasion.
3. Average tumor cellularity of the residual tumor (compare with pretreatment carcinoma).
4. Appearance of the residual tumor and grade, if applicable: compare with pretreatment carcinoma, if possible.
5. Viability (necrosis, mitotic figures); proliferation index by MIB-1 (Ki-67) may be requested for some protocols.
6. Lymphovascular invasion.
7. Presence and extent of DCIS (percentage of in situ carcinoma when using the RCB system).
8. Margins with respect to tumor bed, invasive, and in situ carcinoma.
9. A comment on the overall response to treatment.

Lymph Nodes

1. Number of lymph nodes.
2. Number of lymph nodes with metastases.

KEY PATHOLOGIC FEATURES
Neoadjuvant Therapy

- Identification of the tumor bed is important for documentation of therapy response.
- Obtain specimen x-ray in excisional biopsy specimen to confirm presence of tumor bed.
- In mastectomy specimens, complete clinical information of the tumor (e.g., size, clock position, and distance from nipple) is invaluable for handling of the specimen.
- Thorough sampling and microscopic documentation of tumor bed is essential, particularly in cases of complete or near-complete response.
- Failure to find the tumor bed can result in an erroneous conclusion that there has been a complete response.
- Tumor bed at the margin should be reported, especially in specimens where residual invasive carcinoma or DCIS is identified.
- Extent, largest contiguous focus, cellularity, and treatment effect of any residual tumor should be analyzed carefully to grade the extent of response in both the breast and the lymph nodes.
- In certain cases, use of IHC stain to characterize residual in situ and invasive carcinoma to evaluate margins and lymph nodes is helpful for accurate staging.
- Treatment-related changes can be mistaken for carcinoma if careful attention is not paid to the history of prior therapy.

DCIS, ductal carcinoma in situ; IHC, immunohistochemistry.

3. Size of the largest metastasis.
4. Presence of extranodal extension (measurement of largest extent of extranodal spread).
5. Number of metastases with evidence of treatment response.
6. Number of lymph nodes with evidence of treatment response but without tumor cells (i.e., fibrosis, necrosis, mucin pools, aggregates of macrophages).

Classification of Response

1. By AJCC staging, pT category and pN category are assigned a prefix "y" for post-treatment ("p" refers to pathologic classification).
2. Response category according to one of the classification systems as used by specific institutions or for clinical protocols.

SUMMARY

Proper handling of the NAT specimen centers around ensuring the status of neoadjuvant chemotherapy response. The key item is proving or disproving a pCR, which can be ensured only if the entire sample is examined microscopically or sampled very generously according to the previously discussed guidelines.

REFERENCES

1. Dawood S, Ueno NT, Valero V, et al. Differences in survival among women with stage III inflammatory and noninflammatory locally advanced breast cancer appear early: a large population-based study. Cancer 2011;117:1819-1826.
2. Kuerer HM, Newman LA, Smith TL, et al. Clinical course of breast cancer patients with complete pathologic primary tumor and axillary lymph node response to doxorubicin-based neoadjuvant chemotherapy. J Clin Oncol 1999;17:460-469.
3. van der Hage JA, van de Velde CJ, Julien JP, et al. Preoperative chemotherapy in primary operable breast cancer: results from the European Organization for Research and Treatment of Cancer trial 10902. J Clin Oncol 2001;19:4224-4237.
4. Fisher ER, Wang J, Bryant J, et al. Pathobiology of preoperative chemotherapy: findings from the National Surgical Adjuvant Breast and Bowel (NSABP) protocol B-18. Cancer 2002;95:681-695.
5. Mauri D, Pavlidis N, Ioannidis JP. Neoadjuvant versus adjuvant systemic treatment in breast cancer: a meta-analysis. J Natl Cancer Inst 2005;97:188-194.
6. Makris A, Powles TJ, Ashley SE, et al. A reduction in the requirements for mastectomy in a randomized trial of neoadjuvant chemoendocrine therapy in primary breast cancer. Ann Oncol 1998;9:1179-1184.
7. Mieog JS, van der Hage JA, van de Velde CJ. Preoperative chemotherapy for women with operable breast cancer. Cochrane Database Syst Rev. 2007;2:CD005002.
8. Chen AM, Meric-Bernstam F, Hunt KK, et al. Breast conservation after neoadjuvant chemotherapy. Cancer 2005;103:689-695.
9. Jones RL, Lakhani SR, Ring AE, et al. Pathological complete response and residual DCIS following neoadjuvant chemotherapy for breast carcinoma. Br J Cancer 2006;94:358-362.
10. Mazouni C, Peintinger F, Wan-Kau S, et al. Residual ductal carcinoma in situ in patients with complete eradication of invasive breast cancer after neoadjuvant chemotherapy does not adversely affect patient outcome. J Clin Oncol 2007;25:2650-2655.
11. Rouzier R, Extra JM, Klijanienko J, et al. Incidence and prognostic significance of complete axillary downstaging after primary chemotherapy in breast cancer patients with T1 to T3 tumors and cytologically proven axillary metastatic lymph nodes. J Clin Oncol 2002;20:1304-1310.

- **Definition:** An extremely well differentiated type of invasive mammary carcinoma characterized by well-formed tubules in over 90% of the lesion.

- **Incidence/location:** Accounts for less than 2% of all breast carcinomas and 7% to 27% of carcinomas in the mammographically screened population.

- **Clinical features:** Most patients present with a nonpalpable mass and are diagnosed on routine imaging studies.

- **Imaging features:** Irregular spiculated lesion with central densities on mammography; and hypoechoic mass with ill-defined margins and posterior acoustic shadowing on ultrasonography.

- **Prognosis/treatment:** Excellent prognosis with a 10-year survival of over 81%. Lymph node metastases occur in approximately 10% of patients with pure tubular carcinoma. Most patients are eligible for breast-conserving surgery.

are relatively larger are most likely examples of mixed tumors (invasive ductal carcinoma [IDC] with tubular features) or coalescence of multifocal tubular carcinomas.

Grossly, tubular carcinomas are gray-white, ill-defined firm, stellate or spiculated lesions that often retract from the cut surface and are not distinguishable from invasive duct carcinomas. The cut surface of tumors that have extensive elastosis may appear tan or pale yellow.

Microscopic Pathology

Tubular carcinoma is characterized by a haphazard proliferation of well-formed glands or tubules distributed in a stellate configuration (Figure 29-2). The neoplastic tubules are round to ovoid in shape and have sharply angular contours with tapering ends and open lumina. The tubules are formed by a single layer of monotonous cuboidal to low columnar epithelial cells with basally oriented low-grade nuclei and inconspicuous nucleoli (Figure 29-3). Mitoses, when present, are rare. The

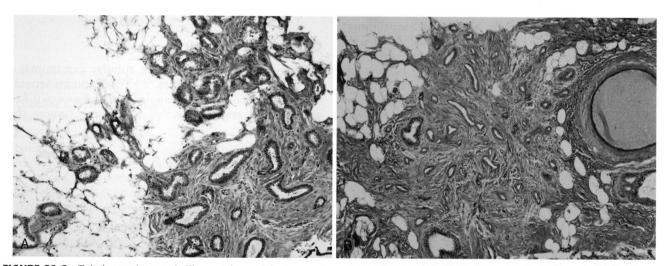

FIGURE 29-2 Tubular carcinoma. **A,** The periphery of the tumor shows infiltrative margins. **B,** A microscopic focus (2 mm) of tubular carcinoma with characteristic stellate appearance and altered stroma from a case with multifocal tubular carcinoma.

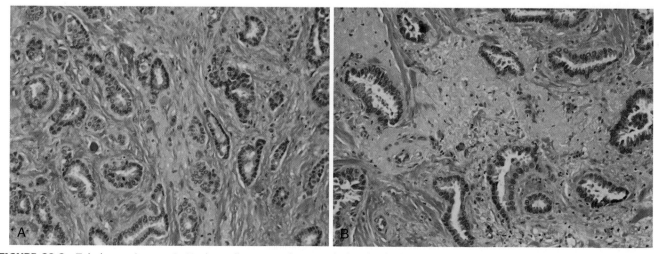

FIGURE 29-3 Tubular carcinoma. **A,** Haphazardly arranged open tubular glands distributed in a desmoplastic stroma. **B,** The glands are mostly angulated and surrounded by stroma with elastosis. Note apical snouts.

cytoplasm is usually eosinophilic to amphophilic, often exhibiting prominent apical "snouts" (Figure 29-4).

The stroma of tubular carcinomas often appears different from the surrounding normal breast tissue, rendering it easily recognizable on low-power magnification. The alteration of normal stroma is usually due to desmoplasia or fibroelastosis (Figure 29-5). Some consider stromal elastosis as a characteristic finding in tubular carcinoma, but it may not be present in every tumor.[31] In addition, stromal elastosis can be observed in other nontubular invasive carcinomas and in benign lesions, particularly in radial scar. Approximately half of tubular carcinomas have calcifications identified microscopically. The calcifications can be seen in the stroma, in the intraductal component, or within the neoplastic tubules (Figure 29-6). Lymphatic and vascular invasion is extremely rare in tubular carcinoma.

The proportion of tubule formation required for the diagnosis of tubular carcinoma varies from 75% to 100% according to published studies. There is now general agreement that a diagnosis of "pure" tubular carcinoma should be reserved for cases in which more than 90% of the tumor exhibits this characteristic morphology.[32,33] Tumors comprising less than 90% tubular elements should be classified as "mixed" tubular carcinomas or well-differentiated ductal carcinoma. Tubular carcinomas should not be confused with IDCs with glandlike structures in which the glands are more complex in architecture and the cells are typically less well differentiated.

The majority of tubular carcinomas are associated with a range of atypical epithelial hyperplasia including atypical ductal and lobular hyperplasia, ductal and lobular carcinoma in situ (DCIS and LCIS), and columnar cell change with or without atypia (flat epithelial atypia). DCIS associated with tubular carcinoma typically has cribriform, micropapillary, papillary, or mixed patterns, usually of low nuclear grade, and overall, constitutes a minor component of the tumor mass (Figure 29-7).

The coexistence of columnar cell change and hyperplasia with or without atypia, including flat epithelial atypia, lobular neoplasia, and tubular carcinoma has

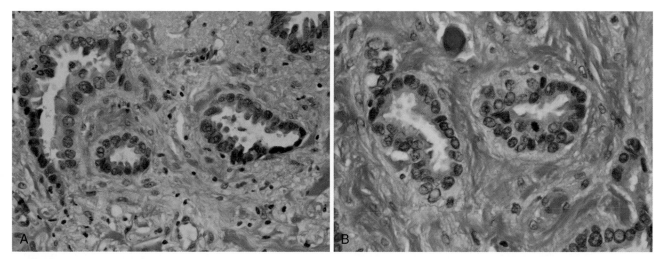

FIGURE 29-4 Tubular carcinoma. **A,** Angulated open glands with basally oriented nuclei and prominent "apical snouts." **B,** The glands have low-grade nuclei and a single mitosis, a rare finding in tubular carcinoma.

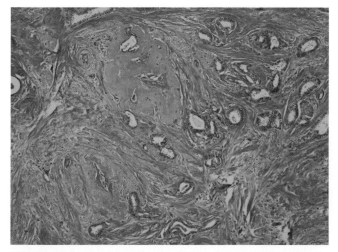

FIGURE 29-5 Tubular carcinoma shows extensive stromal elastosis.

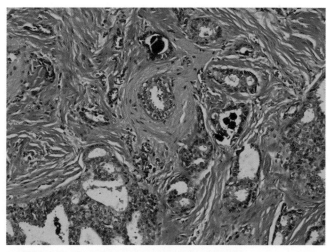

FIGURE 29-6 Tubular carcinoma with invasive and intraductal components. The neoplastic glands contain calcification.

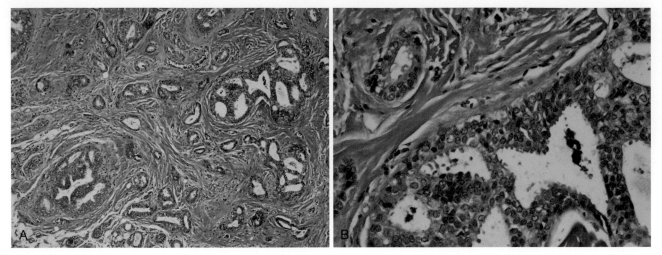

FIGURE 29-7 Tubular carcinoma. **A,** Micropapillary intraductal carcinoma admixed with invasive glands. **B,** High-power magnification reveals cells with similar appearance in both in situ and invasive components.

led some to use these lesions as a "triad" of pathologic changes.[34–37] In fact, some of the incidental tubular carcinomas are detected in breast biopsies performed for microcalcifications associated with columnar cell change (Figure 29-8). Columnar cell lesions are reported in 93% to almost 100%, whereas coexistent lobular neoplasia is found in approximately 50% of tubular carcinoma cases.[36,38,39]

In lymph node metastases, tubular carcinoma retains its well-formed tubular architecture (Figure 29-9). Interestingly, some of the metastases involve the lymph node capsule, which may be mistaken for benign glandular inclusions.

Prognosis and Treatment

The biologic behavior of tubular carcinoma is very favorable. The reported local recurrence rate in patients with tubular carcinoma is 4% to 7%.[10,11,13,38] Rakha and colleagues[38] reported a 6.9% local recurrence rate among 102 patients with tubular carcinomas compared with 25% for those with invasive grade 1 ductal carcinoma. All 7 patients with tubular carcinoma who experienced local recurrence were treated with wide local excision, 5 patients did not receive postoperative radiotherapy, and none of the 7 patients received adjuvant systemic therapy.

The reported incidence of axillary lymph node metastases in patients with tubular carcinomas varies widely, mostly owing to variation in the pathologic criteria used in the past for the diagnosis. Some of the studies have shown a direct relationship between the degree of differentiation of the tumor and the incidence of lymph node metastases.[16,19,40–45] In most studies of "pure" tubular carcinoma, the incidence of lymph node metastases is less than 15%.[10,11,18,19,21,29,38] In cases in which tubular carcinoma metastasizes to axillary lymph nodes, usually only one to three level 1 lymph nodes are involved.[1,3,9,18,19,30,38] Furthermore, the presence of nodal disease does not appear to affect disease-free or overall survival.[9,10,38] In view of the low frequency of nodal disease, most patients undergoing sentinel lymph node (SLN) biopsy are spared an axillary lymph node dissection.

Most studies suggest that patients with tubular carcinoma have a longer disease-free survival.[3,5,9,16–19,29,30,33,40–48] In the randomized prospective National Surgical Adjuvant Breast and Bowel Project (NSABP) B06 trial, 1090 node-negative and 651 node-positive patients in the "favorable" histology category included 120 patients with tubular carcinoma.[48] In an univariate analysis, both node-negative and node-positive patients in the "favorable" category experienced significantly greater overall survival at 10 years compared with other patients, and "favorable" histology proved to be an independent predictor of survival in node-negative patients by multivariate analysis.[48] In a recent study by Rakha and colleagues,[38] longer disease-free survival and breast cancer–specific survival were reported in 102 patients with pure tubular carcinoma when compared with 212 patients with grade 1 IDC with a median follow-up of 127 months. There was no cancer-specific death in patients with pure tubular carcinoma diagnosis compared with 9% cancer-specific deaths in patients with grade 1 ductal carcinoma. Other studies have reported significantly lower rates of distant recurrences in patients with tubular carcinoma compared with patients with IDC.[46,47] In two large studies, the overall survival rates (94.1% 5-yr and 81.7% 10-yr) of patients with tubular carcinoma were not significantly different from those of rates of the aged-matched set of women (91.3% 5-yr and 77.6% 10-yr)[13] or in the general population.[1]

Most patients with unifocal tubular carcinoma are excellent candidates for breast-conserving surgery. SLN biopsy should be performed at the time of definitive surgery in patients who have prior diagnosis on a needle core biopsy. If an incidental small tubular carcinoma is found in a breast biopsy performed for an unrelated reason, the need for subsequent SLN biopsy is questionable, considering the infrequency of lymph node metastases.

One of the earlier studies reported no breast recurrences in 17 of 38 patients with tubular carcinoma who did not receive postoperative radiotherapy after lumpectomy. However, most recent studies have found no significant differences in local recurrence rates

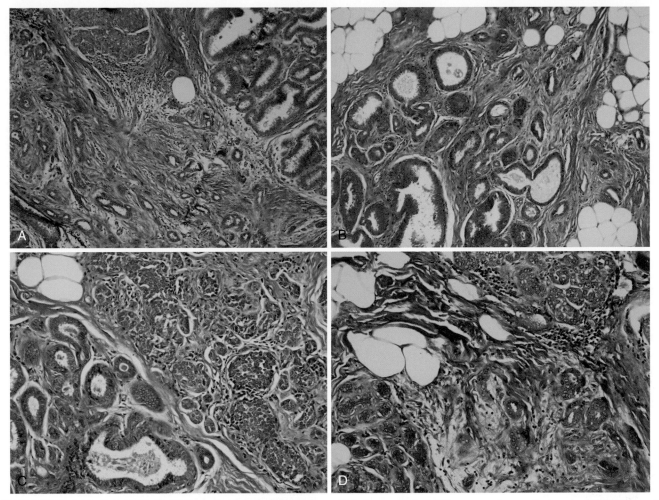

FIGURE 29-8 The triad of "tubular carcinoma, columnar cell change, and lobular neoplasia." All images are from a single case. **A,** Tubular carcinoma *(lower half),* lobular carcinoma in situ (LCIS; *upper left),* and columnar cell change *(upper right).* **B,** A different focus of tubular carcinoma intermingled with columnar cell change. **C,** Columnar cell change and LCIS. **D,** Normal lobule, tubular carcinoma, and LCIS (higher magnification).

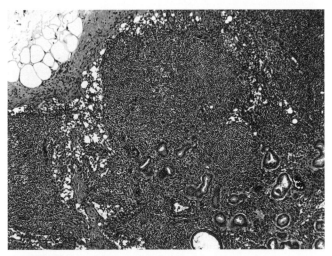

FIGURE 29-9 Axillary lymph node with metastatic tubular carcinoma recapitulating the well-formed glands of the primary site.

between patients with tubular carcinomas and those with IDC.[47,49–51] One may speculate that at least some patients with tubular carcinoma may be adequately treated with local excision alone if the margins are widely clear (i.e., without postoperative radiation therapy); however, currently, insufficient data prevent lumpectomy alone to be widely considered as a standard treatment option.

Because almost all tubular carcinomas express hormone receptors, some form of adjuvant hormonal treatment is offered to most patients.

Prognostic and Predictive Factors

The various biologic markers expressed in tubular carcinomas generally reflect the well-differentiated nature and good prognosis of these tumors. Estrogen receptor (ER) positivity has been reported in more than 80% to 98% of tubular carcinomas, and progesterone receptor (PgR) positivity in 72% to 92%.[1,9,13,38] The pattern of ER immunoreactivity is usually diffuse (>90% of the tumor) and strong in most cases (Figure 29-10). Tubular carcinomas are almost always diploid, have a low proliferation rate, and are negative for *HER2*/neu overexpression or p53 protein accumulation.[1,38,52–54]

Molecular and genetic studies have demonstrated tubular carcinomas to be associated with a low frequency of cytogenetic abnormalities compared with the complex abnormalities exhibited by most breast cancers of

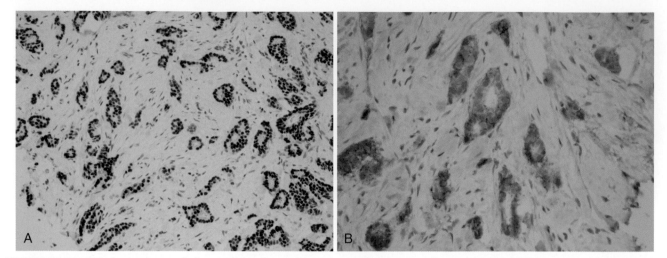

FIGURE 29-10 Tubular carcinoma. **A,** Immunohistochemical stain for estrogen receptor shows strong and diffuse staining of tumor nuclei. **B,** Immunostain for *HER2*/neu often shows partial membrane staining (1+ reactivity).

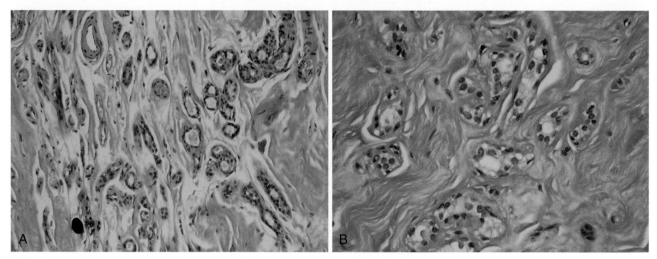

FIGURE 29-11 Sclerosing adenosis. **A** and **B,** Small open distorted acini with somewhat edematous and sclerotic stroma, but myoepithelial cells and basement membrane are evident.

no special type.[55] Tubular carcinomas show higher frequency of 16q loss and 1q gain and lower frequency of 17p loss,[56] an abnormality more commonly found in most low-grade, luminal-type breast carcinomas. Tubular carcinoma also shares transcriptome and immunohistochemical expression profiles similar to other low-grade luminal-type breast carcinoma, including classic invasive lobular carcinoma.[57,58]

Differential Diagnosis

Benign entities such as sclerosing adenosis, complex sclerosing lesions/radial scar, tubular adenosis, and microglandular adenosis may mimic tubular carcinoma and vice versa. Small tubular carcinoma with relatively uniform round to oval glands may mimic microglandular adenosis. However, microglandular adenosis is a diffuse lesion whereas tubular carcinoma is often localized. Both lesions lack myoepithelial cells, but glands in microglandular adenosis retain basement membrane, which can be easily seen on routine hematoxylin and

eosin (H&E) stain and further demonstrated by reticulin or periodic acid–Schiff (PAS) stains, or collagen IV immunohistochemistry.

Because angulated glands are commonly encountered in sclerosing adenosis, tubular adenosis, and radial scars, these entities are often considered in the differential diagnosis for tubular carcinoma, particularly in core biopsy specimens. Tubular adenosis is more diffuse and not associated with a desmoplastic reaction. Examination on higher magnification reveals investment of glands by myoepithelium (Figure 29-11). Because the proliferation pattern in sclerosing adenosis is lobulocentric, it is almost always helpful to examine these lesions at low magnification to avoid misinterpretation (Figure 29-12). In difficult cases, immunohistochemical stains for myoepithelial cells such as p63 or smooth muscle myosin–heavy chain are helpful. Smooth muscle actin is not recommended owing to its concomitant staining of adjacent myofibroblasts, which can be misinterpreted as myoepithelial staining of an invasive lesion. The center of a radial scar exhibits not only angulated glands seen in

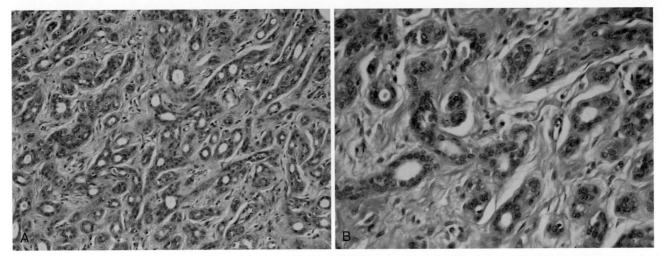

FIGURE 29-12 Tubular adenosis. **A,** Extensive adenosis with tubular architecture, mimics tubular carcinoma. **B,** Higher magnification clearly demonstrates myoepithelial cells and basement membrane around the tubules.

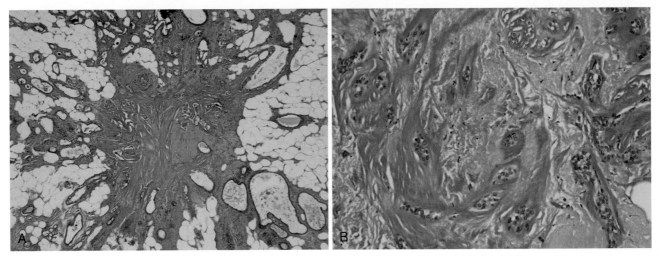

FIGURE 29-13 Radial sclerosing lesion. **A,** On low power, characteristic central sclerosis from which dilated ducts radiate. **B,** Higher magnification of the center reveals marked stromal elastosis and entrapped tubular glands.

tubular carcinoma but also stromal changes such as elastosis, sometimes making the distinction between the two very difficult. In excisional biopsy specimens, radial sclerosing lesions are easy to recognize owing to the characteristic appearance of a sclerotic and distorted nidus from which dilated ducts admixed with ductal hyperplasia and papillomas radiate (Figure 29-13). Complex sclerosing lesions/radial scar are the most problematic if the center of the lesion is sampled in a core biopsy (Figure 29-14). In most cases, immunostains for myoepithelial cells will demonstrate immunoreactivity in a radial scar. However, in highly sclerotic lesions of radial scar, immunoreactivity of myoepithelial cells may be focally attenuated or inapparent in some of the glands. Therefore, one must be cautious of relying heavily on immunohistochemical staining pattern to distinguish between these two entities, especially in needle core biopsy.

Tubulolobular carcinomas are invasive tumors that are now classified as ductal phenotype.[59] Some tumors that are mixed ductal and lobular carcinomas have been referred to by some as "tubulolobular" (Figure 29-15) whereas other tumors may have cytologic features that are more typical of IDCs but invade the stroma in a single-file pattern or have cytologic features of invasive lobular carcinoma but form well-formed ducts (Figure 29-16). This has led some to consider these tumors to be a variant of tubular carcinoma whereas others regard this as a form of lobular carcinoma. Although DCIS is an integral part of the tubular carcinoma, tubulolobular carcinomas are more likely to be associated with LCIS. Tubulolobular carcinomas are also more likely to be multifocal and metastasize to axillary lymph nodes than pure tubular carcinomas.[21,59] Immunohistochemical staining for E-cadherin may be useful in making the distinction between ductal and lobular carcinomas in problematic or indeterminate cases. The fact that it may be difficult for the pathologist to categorize a given lesion as ductal or lobular in some cases should not be surprising in view of reports suggesting that some low-grade invasive duct carcinomas share similar chromosomal abnormalities with invasive lobular carcinomas.[60–62]

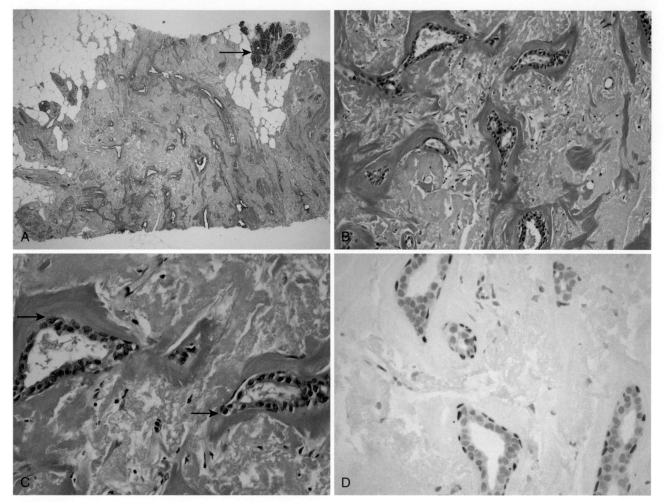

FIGURE 29-14 Core biopsy of radial sclerosing lesion. **A,** On low power, the center of a radial scar with extensive elastosis mimics tubular carcinoma. A focus of atypical lobular hyperplasia *(arrow)* is also seen. **B,** High power reveals open angulated glands, making the diagnosis difficult. **C,** Careful examination reveals myoepithelial cells *(arrows)*. **D,** Immunostain for p63 decorates the myoepithelial cells around the tubules.

KEY PATHOLOGIC FEATURES

Tubular Carcinoma

■ **Gross:** Most tumors are approximately 1 cm in diameter and appear as an ill-defined firm to hard tumor with a stellate to spiculated margin that retracts from the cut surface.

■ **Microscopic:** An irregular haphazard collection of well-formed neoplastic tubules (>90% of the lesions) with angulated margin and apical "snouts" embedded in a fibroelastotic and desmoplastic stroma. Coexistent columnar cell lesions including flat epithelial atypia and lobular neoplasia are common in the vicinity of tubular carcinoma.

■ **Immunohistochemistry:** The neoplastic glands lack myoepithelial cells and well-formed basement membrane around the glands.

■ **Other special studies:** Almost all tumors express strong ER and PgR and do not overexpress *HER2* oncoprotein. Very low proliferation index (<10% Ki-67 labeling).

■ **Differential diagnosis:** Radial scar, sclerosing adenosis, microglandular adenosis, and tubular adenosis.

ER, estrogen receptor; PgR, progesterone receptor.

Finally, the distinction of grade 1 invasive duct carcinoma from tubular carcinoma is somewhat arbitrary and can be challenging in some cases (Figure 29-17). However, if one adheres to the criteria of tubular carcinomas as tumors showing more than 90% tubule formation of mostly single-layered cells of low nuclear grade, the distinction between the two should be more apparent.

MUCINOUS CARCINOMA

Mucinous carcinoma (also known as *colloid carcinoma*) is a special type of invasive breast carcinoma characterized by the presence of extracellular mucin and is associated with a better prognosis than infiltrating ductal carcinoma of no special type. The reported incidence of mucinous carcinoma varies, depending on the percentage of the mucinous component used to define mucinous carcinoma. Depending on the study, the mucinous component of mucinous carcinomas range from as low as 33% to 50% to 90% to 100% of the tumor.[33,63–67] Although an exact percentage necessary to diagnose mucinous carcinoma

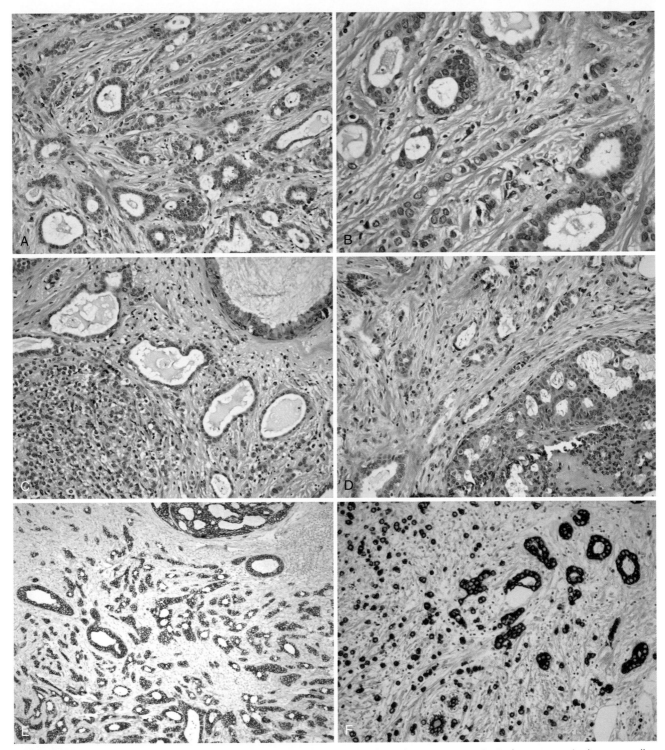

FIGURE 29-15 Mixed tubular and invasive lobular carcinoma. All images are from the same tumor. **A,** On low power, single tumor cells are scattered between well-formed tubules. **B,** Higher magnification reveals classic invasive lobular carcinoma and neoplastic tubules. **C,** Columnar cell change, tubular carcinoma, and invasive lobular carcinoma in the same field. **D,** Intraductal carcinoma is identified at the periphery of the tumor. **E,** Immunostain for E-cadherin highlights positive membranous staining in the tubules; invasive lobular carcinoma is negative for E-cadherin. **F,** Cytokeratin AE1/3 highlights both the single neoplastic cells and the tubules.

is not clearly established, currently, most agree that a diagnosis of a pure mucinous carcinoma should be reserved for tumors in which at least 90% is mucinous. Pure mucinous carcinomas are uncommon and account for approximately 2% of all primary breast carcinomas.[1,68–70] It is important to recognize pure mucinous carcinomas from "mixed" mucinous carcinomas, the latter containing a mixture of mucinous and nonmucinous components because the prognosis of pure mucinous carcinoma is better.[66,71,72]

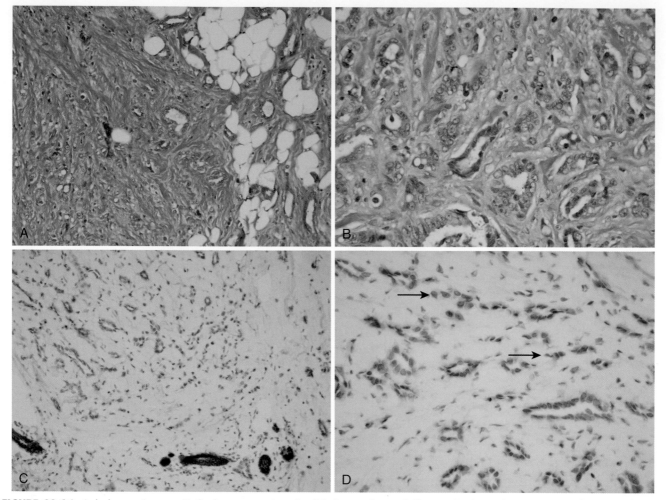

FIGURE 29-16 Lobular carcinoma. **A,** On low power, invasive lobular carcinoma infiltrates the fat and stroma. **B,** Higher magnification reveals intimate association of pseudotubules and single tumor cells. **C,** E-cadherin immunostain demonstrates no reactivity in the single cells and in the pseudotubules (normal tubules stain positive). **D,** Higher magnification of E-cadherin.

Clinical Presentation

Mucinous carcinoma has been reported to occur over a wide age range (age range 21–94 yr), but the mean age at presentation for patients with this tumor is older than those with breast cancers of no special type.[63,64,66,67,71–77] A retrospective analysis of SEER (Surveillance Epidemiology and End Results) database between 1973 and 2002 revealed 11,422 patients with pure mucinous carcinoma of the breast.[74] Although no difference was seen in the distribution of gender and race between patients with pure mucinous carcinoma and those with IDC, the median age at diagnosis of patients with the former was 71 years compared with 61 years for IDC patients. Fifty-six of the 11,422 pure mucinous carcinoma patients were males. The majority of mucinous carcinomas (44%) occur in the upper outer quadrant, and the remaining (56%) tumors are evenly divided in the other quadrants and central breast, a distribution pattern not significantly different from that of IDC.[74]

In the past, most patients with mucinous carcinoma presented with a palpable breast mass. However, with the widespread use of screening mammography, a large

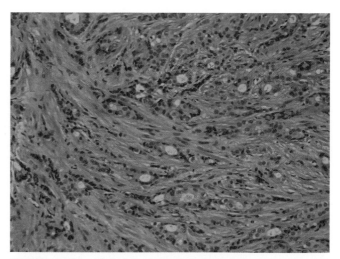

FIGURE 29-17 Well-differentiated invasive duct carcinoma with complex fused glands and solid nests of cells with intermediate nuclear grade.

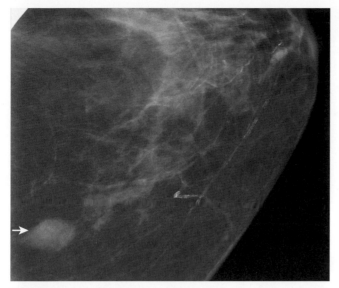

FIGURE 29-18 Mucinous carcinoma, gross appearance. A well-circumscribed lobulated tumor with a bulging gelatinous cut surface *(arrow).*

proportion of patients (30–70%) with mucinous carcinoma are diagnosed with nonpalpable mammographic abnormality.[78,79] Fixation to skin or chest wall is rare but can occur with large lesions.

Clinical Imaging

On mammographic examination, mucinous carcinoma tends to present as an oval or lobulated mass, rarely associated with calcification.[78–81] Tumors with a large mucinous component (pure mucinous carcinomas) tend to be well circumscribed on mammography (Figure 29-18) and sonography in contrast to the irregular borders of mixed mucinous tumors.[78,80,82,83] In addition, mammographically occult mucinous carcinomas have been reported to account for 17% to 21% of cases in two different studies.[80,82] On ultrasonographic examination, some mucinous carcinomas exhibit well-defined borders and isoechogenic echo texture relative to that of the fat,[82,83] whereas others are hypoechogenic with microlobulated margins.[81] For these reasons, a number of pure mucinous tumors could be misinterpreted as benign tumors on routine imaging studies.

Magnetic resonance imaging (MRI) findings such as lobular shape, rim or heterogeneous enhancement, gradually enhancing contrast pattern, and homogeneous strongly high signal intensity on T2-weighted images may be useful in diagnosing pure mucinous carcinoma.[84,85]

Gross Pathology

Mucinous carcinomas are generally slow-growing tumors. Although a wide range of size ranging from nonpalpable tumors to tumors as large as 25 cm have been reported in the literature,[63,65,86–88] most mucinous carcinomas measure approximately 3 cm on average.[89] Based on a study using the SEER database, 83% of 11,422 patients with pure mucinous carcinoma had

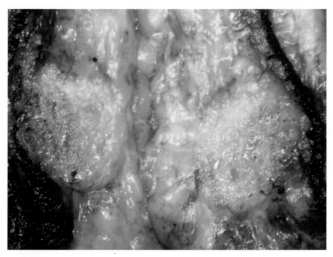

FIGURE 29-19 Mucinous carcinoma, mammographic appearance. A 1.3-cm oval density with well-defined border resembles a benign tumor.

tumors measuring 3 cm or less, the mean and the median tumor size was 2.2 cm and 1.6 cm, respectively.[74] Other studies have also reported pure mucinous tumors to be smaller, on average, than mixed tumors.[72,78]

Pure mucinous carcinomas have a distinctive gross appearance. These tumors are generally well circumscribed and bosselated and have a relatively soft consistency due to sparse fibrous stroma (Figure 29-19). However, lesions with a greater amount of fibrous stroma may have a firmer consistency. Presence of abundant extracellular mucin imparts a characteristic gelatinous and glistening appearance to the cut surface.

Microscopic Pathology

The characteristic feature of mucinous carcinomas is the presence of extracellular mucin around the tumor cells. Although the relative proportion of extracellular

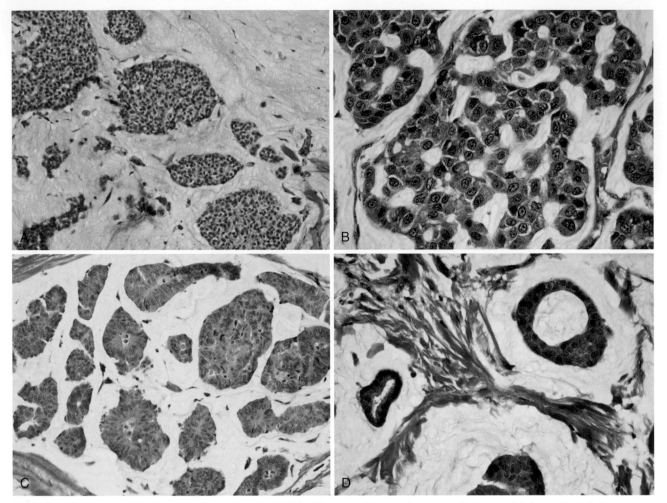

FIGURE 29-20 Mucinous carcinoma. Cellular component with different architectural patterns. **A,** Large solid sheets. **B,** Cribriform appearance. **C,** Micropapillary pattern. **D,** Tubular pattern.

mucin and neoplastic cells vary from tumor to tumor, the distribution of each component is fairly uniform in any given case. Typically, the neoplastic cells are dispersed in small clusters, large sheets, or papillary or cribriform configurations within pools of extracellular mucin (Figure 29-20). This characteristic histology should be present in at least 90% of the tumor to qualify for the diagnosis of mucinous carcinoma. A tumor should be classified as "mixed" mucinous carcinoma if more than 10% of the invasive component is of nonmucinous morphology. Because mucinous carcinomas are slow-growing tumors, the periphery of most tumors is characterized by a pushing border (Figure 29-21).[80] The cellularity in mucinous carcinomas varies among individual cases (Figure 29-22). In paucicellular tumors, multiple sections may be required to detect the neoplastic cells to establish the diagnosis (Figure 29-23). The cells in most mucinous carcinomas are usually of low or intermediate nuclear grade (Figure 29-24). Occasionally, mucinous carcinomas may harbor cells with high nuclear grade (Figure 29-25).[74] Some authors recommend excluding such high-grade tumors from the classification of mucinous carcinoma.[90] Nonetheless, all mucinous carcinomas should be graded using the Nottingham histologic grading system. Calcifications can be found in mucinous carcinomas (Figure 29-26). Rarely, psammomatous-type calcification in mucinous carcinomas of the breast have been reported.[91]

Mucinous carcinomas with micropapillary pattern have been described.[92,93] In a study of pure mucinous carcinoma, cells forming a focal to diffuse micropapillary pattern were observed in 20% of tumors studied.[93] The average age of patients with the micropapillary variant of mucinous carcinomas was lower (47 yr) than of those with mucinous carcinoma of all variants (60 yr). The average tumor size was, however, similar in the micropapillary variant (1.7 cm). Although in this study, mucinous carcinoma with a micropapillary pattern was more frequently associated with nodal disease,[93] this finding has not been observed by others.[92]

A subset of mucinous carcinomas show endocrine differentiation as defined by cytoplasmic argyrophilia or immunoreactivity to markers such as synaptophysin or chromogranin.[94-96] Although in one study endocrine differentiation was associated with favorable histology,[95] others did not find this association.[97,98]

In 60% to 75% of cases, mucinous carcinomas are accompanied by an intraductal component, noted generally at the periphery of the lesion (Figure 29-27). The in situ component may have a papillary, micropapillary,

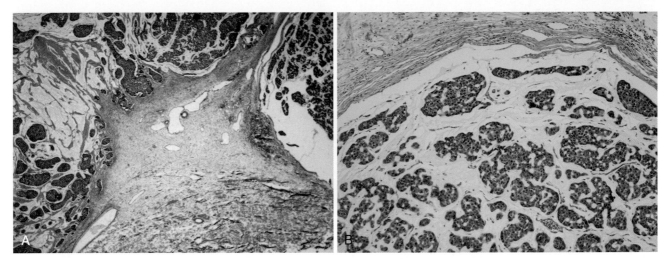

FIGURE 29-21 **A** and **B,** Mucinous carcinoma. A scanning view demonstrates pushing border in two different tumors.

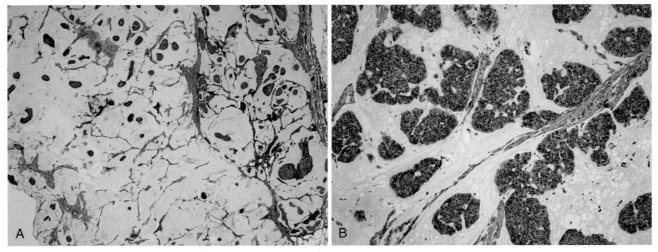

FIGURE 29-22 Mucinous carcinoma. **A,** A moderately cellular tumor. **B,** A rather cellular variant of mucinous carcinoma.

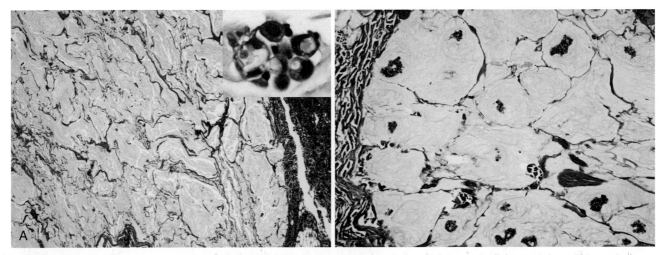

FIGURE 29-23 Mucinous carcinoma. **A,** A paucicellular type mucinous carcinoma. **B,** Another paucicellular carcinoma. This particular case was treated with neoadjuvant chemotherapy before surgery.

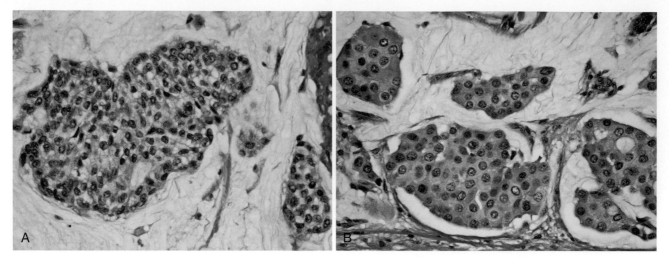

FIGURE 29-24 **A** and **B,** Mucinous carcinoma. Monotonous-appearing tumor cells with low nuclear grade.

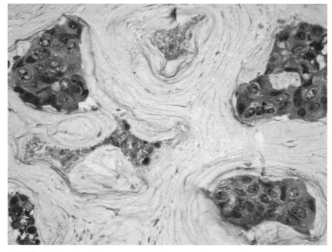

FIGURE 29-25 Mucinous carcinoma. Pleomorphic-appearing tumor cells with higher nuclear grade and prominent nucleoli.

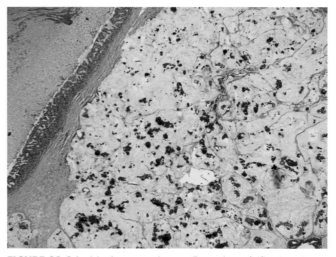

FIGURE 29-26 Mucinous carcinoma. Extensive calcifications in extracellular mucin.

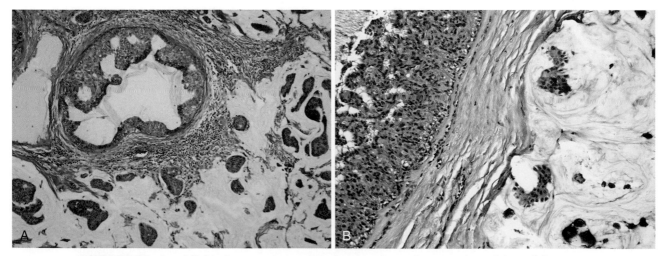

FIGURE 29-27 **A** and **B,** Mucinous carcinoma. Intraductal carcinoma is seen at the periphery of the tumor.

or cribriform pattern. In some cases, the in situ carcinoma may exhibit prominent extracellular mucin production (Figure 29-28).[89] Determination of vascular or lymphatic tumor emboli can be challenging in mucinous carcinoma. Clusters of tumor cells suspended in clear spaces with little mucin may mimic lymphatic vascular invasion (Figure 29-29). Special stain for mucin or immunohistochemical stain for endothelial markers such as CD31, Factor VIII, or D2-40 may help in uncertain cases. When assessing the margins of excision in mucinous carcinomas, the presence of extracellular mucin without epithelial cells at a margin should be considered positive (Figure 29-30). Lymph node metastases often contain abundant mucin with neoplastic cells floating in it (Figure 29-31).

Prognosis and Treatment

Although mucinous carcinomas are uncommon and the definition of mucinous carcinoma varies from study to study, the favorable prognosis of pure mucinous carcinoma has been supported by numerous studies. The prognostic significance of tumor size in mucinous carcinomas is particularly interesting. Some studies and reports have found tumor size not to be a significant prognostic factor and may not affect survival because the majority of the tumor volume consists of mucin.[65] Indeed, lymph node metastasis was not found in two isolated reports of pure mucinous carcinoma patients with 17-cm tumors.[86,87] However, in a multivariate analysis of 11,422 patients with pure mucinous carcinoma, tumor size was found to be an independent prognostic indicator, although less significant than nodal status.[74]

Patients with pure mucinous carcinomas have a lower rate of axillary lymph node metastases. The frequency of node involvement in large series varies from 12% to 14%,[1,65,67,72,74] although rates as low as 0% to 2% have been reported.[80,94,99] This range, however, is significantly less than the rate of node positivity seen in mixed mucinous tumors or breast cancers of no special type (36–64%).[63,66,71-74]

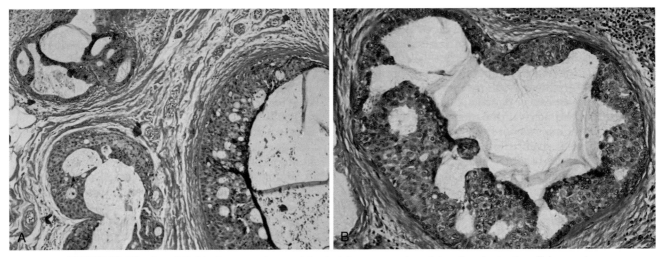

FIGURE 29-28 **A** and **B,** Mucinous carcinoma. Intraductal component contains abundant extracellular mucin.

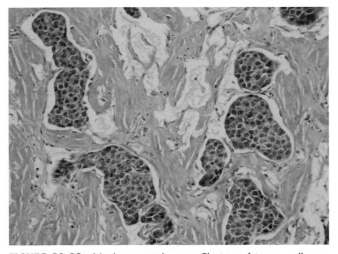

FIGURE 29-29 Mucinous carcinoma. Clusters of tumor cells suspended in clear spaces with little mucin, mimicking lymphatic invasion. Note this focus is in the middle of the tumor.

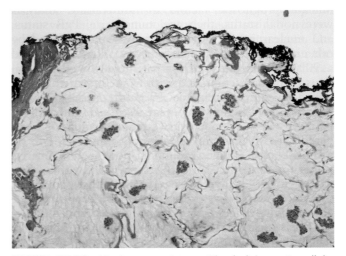

FIGURE 29-30 Mucinous carcinoma. The bulging extracellular mucin with tumor cells is present at an inked margin.

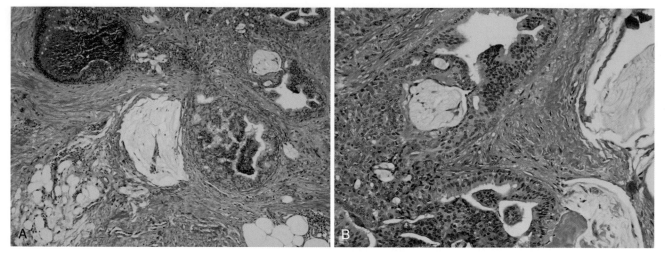

FIGURE 29-33 Benign mucocele-like lesion with atypia. **A,** Low-power view of a small radial sclerosing lesion with extravasation of mucin and scarring from a prior core biopsy. **B,** Higher-power view reveals sclerosis, extravagated mucin, and atypical ductal hyperplasia with mucin in it.

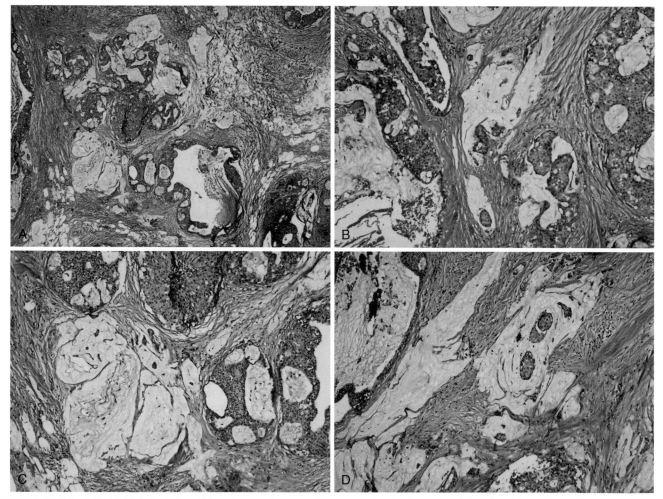

FIGURE 29-34 **A-D,** Multiple foci of small invasive mucinous carcinoma arise in a background of ductal carcinoma in situ (DCIS) containing abundant extracellular mucin. All the pictures are from the same case.

extracellular mucin. In addition, micropapillary carcinomas express MUC1 instead of MUC2 and MUC6, often described in mucinous carcinoma.[107–109,118] MUC1 is a glycoprotein usually found on apical surfaces of glandular epithelial cells, facing and maintaining the lumen. In micropapillary carcinomas, MUC1 is expressed in the stroma-facing surface of epithelial cell clusters.[118] Mucinous carcinoma exhibiting a micropapillary-like growth pattern has been described.[92,93] It is debatable whether mucinous carcinomas with micropapillary architecture

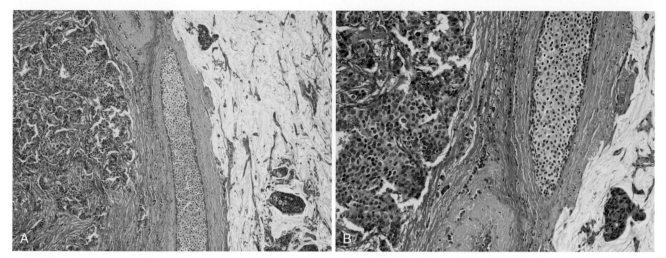

FIGURE 29-35 Mixed mucinous and ductal carcinoma. **A,** A scanning power view of a mixed ductal *(left)* and mucinous carcinoma *(right).* **B,** Higher-power view of the invasive ductal carcinoma and invasive mucinous carcinoma. These tumors should not be classified as mucinous carcinoma.

are associated with frequent nodal metastases and less favorable prognosis.[92,93]

Finally, accurate diagnoses of mucinous lesions on core biopsies or needle aspiration biopsies can be challenging owing to limited sampling. Whereas some recommend that all MLLs on core biopsy should prompt further excision of the lesion in order to exclude mucinous DCIS or invasive mucinous carcinoma,[114] others have questioned whether, because most benign MLLs can be reliably diagnosed on a core biopsy, all such lesions require excision.[116] Nonetheless, it is prudent to adopt a cautious approach if MLLs or extracellular mucin pools are found on a core biopsy, particularly if a mass is apparent radiologically or by palpation or if the sample exhibits atypical hyperplasia.[90]

KEY PATHOLOGIC FEATURES

Mucinous Carcinoma

- **Gross:** Most tumors are less than 3 cm in diameter and appear as a well-circumscribed, soft, gelatinous lobulated mass with a glistening cut surface.

- **Microscopic:** Most tumors have a pushing border; in over 90% of the lesions, the low–nuclear grade tumor cell nests are dispersed in abundant extracellular mucin. Coexistent low-grade intraductal carcinoma is often present, mostly at the periphery of the lesion, sometimes filled with extracellular mucin.

- **Immunohistochemistry:** Although not clinically significant, the neoplastic cells in most tumors demonstrate endocrine differentiation, MUC2 and MUC6 and sometimes WT1.

- **Other special studies:** Almost all tumors express strong ER and PgR, rarely overexpress *HER2*/neu oncoprotein.

- **Differential diagnosis:** Mucocele-like lesions, "mixed" mucinous carcinomas, and invasive micropapillary carcinomas.

ER, estrogen receptor; PgR, progesterone receptor; WT1, Wilms' tumor antigen-1.

INVASIVE CRIBRIFORM CARCINOMA

Invasive cribriform carcinoma is a well-differentiated carcinoma that exhibits a cribriform growth pattern similar to that of cribriform intraductal carcinoma. Morphologic features of invasive tubular carcinoma can be admixed as a minor component in some cases.

Clinical Presentation

Most patients are females in the fifth decade, but a wide age range exists (19–91 yr).[119–122] A rare example occurring in a male patient has been reported.[123] These patients may present with a breast mass that is radiologically occult.[121] The mean tumor size is 3.1 cm; however, it can be up to 20 cm in rare cases.[119,120] Multifocality is uncommon.[119,120]

Clinical Imaging

By one report, a significant proportion of invasive cribriform carcinomas can be mammographically occult.[121] If apparent, these tumors usually appear as spiculated masses with or without associated microcalcifications, but they can also show nonspecific features.[121,123,124] Examples with extensive calcifications are rare.[123,124]

Gross Pathology

When apparent, the gross findings are similar to that of mass-forming invasive duct carcinoma, not otherwise specified. No unique features specific to this carcinoma have been described.

Microscopic Pathology

Pure examples have cribriform pattern constituting greater than 90% of the invasive carcinoma or an admixture of cribriform and tubular patterns in which the former composes the majority (>50%) of the tumor.[120] Noncribriform histologic patterns can be seen

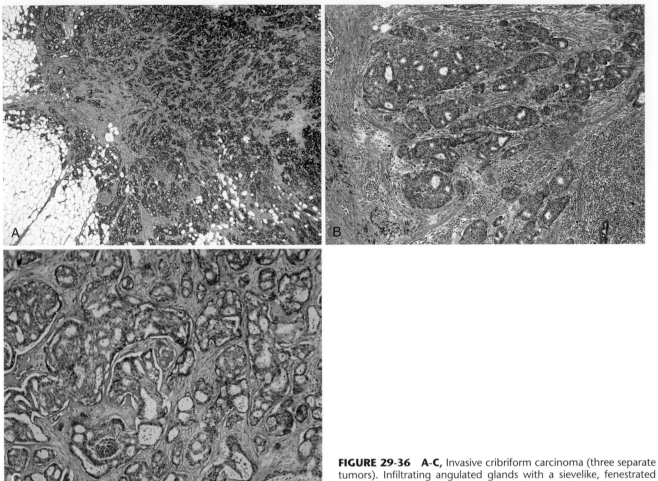

FIGURE 29-36 **A-C,** Invasive cribriform carcinoma (three separate tumors). Infiltrating angulated glands with a sievelike, fenestrated pattern.

KEY CLINICAL FEATURES

Invasive Cribriform Carcinoma

- **Definition:** A well-differentiated invasive duct carcinoma with cribriform pattern similar to that of cribriform intraductal carcinoma. In pure examples, the cribriform pattern comprises greater than 90% of the lesion.

- **Incidence:** Unknown.

- **Clinical features:** Typically affects female patients in their 50s who present with a breast mass.

- **Imaging features:** Can be radiologically occult but, if apparent, a spiculated mass with or without calcifications is appreciated.

- **Prognosis/treatment:** The biologic behavior is similar to that of invasive tubular carcinoma. The prognosis is favorable compared with that associated with invasive duct carcinoma of no special type. Treatment is the same as it is for invasive mammary carcinoma of other histologic types.

in 17% to 23% of cases and are commonly tubular in type. Conversely, approximately 5% to 6% of invasive breast cancers show at least a partial invasive cribriform component.[120,122] "Mixed" examples of invasive cribriform carcinoma are those that either do not fit the

morphologic criteria of pure invasive cribriform carcinoma or do not have any component that is nontubular in type.[120,122]

Individual glands are often angulated and fenestrated (Figure 29-36). Tumor cells show low or intermediate nuclear grade and apical snouts can be appreciated (Figure 29-37). Mitoses are rare. Calcifications can be seen associated with neoplastic glands. The surrounding stroma is often fibroblastic (reactive-appearing) with or without inflammatory infiltrates (Figure 29-38), and in some cases, associated osteoclast-like giant cells of histiocytic origin have been described.[125–127] Concomitant intraductal carcinoma, typically cribriform type, can be seen in up to 80% of cases[120] (Figure 29-39). As true for other well-differentiated invasive duct carcinomas, these tumors are consistently ER+ (100%) and many are also PgR+ (69%).[122] Moreover, none has been found to have *HER2*/neu oncoprotein overexpression.[52,128] Other biomarkers have not been well studied in this variant of invasive duct carcinoma.

Prognosis and Treatment

The biologic behavior of invasive cribriform carcinoma is very similar to that of tubular carcinoma.[120] A favorable prognosis has been reported in these patients

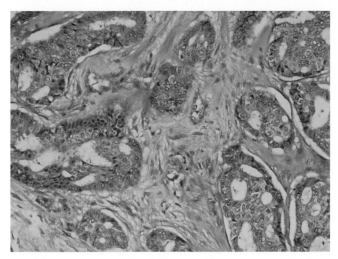

FIGURE 29-37 Invasive cribriform carcinoma. Individual glands exhibit low– or intermediate–nuclear grade, and some also show apical snouts.

compared with patients with invasive carcinoma of no special type in which the former had a 10-year survival of 91% in 13 patients versus 47% in the latter.[33] Other studies have reported a 100% 5-year survival in these patients.[122] In addition, patients with pure invasive cribriform carcinoma experienced a better overall survival than those with mixed type.[120,122]

Axillary lymph node metastases have been seen in 14% and 37% of pure examples in two studies, respectively.[120,122] No examples showed lymphovascular invasion.[120] This is unlike patients with mixed types who had a greater frequency of lymph node involvement (16%, 48–50%) and lymphovascular invasion (19%).[120,122] Similarly, no cancer-related deaths were observed in any patients with pure tumors (up to median follow-up of 14.5 yr) compared with those with mixed type (7%, 38%).[120,122] An exceptional case of macrometastasis to one ipsilateral internal mammary lymph node with two SLNs free of metastatic carcinoma has been described.[128]

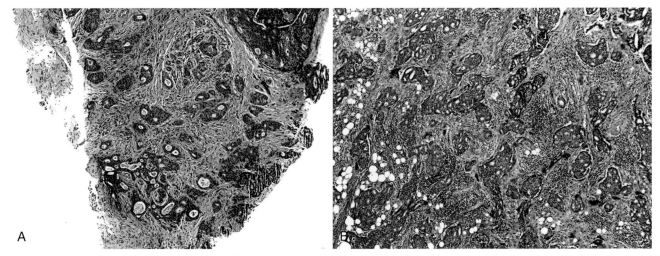

FIGURE 29-38 Invasive cribriform carcinoma. **A,** Intervening stroma characteristically appear desmoplastic or "reactive." **B,** Stroma with scattered chronic inflammatory cell infiltrates.

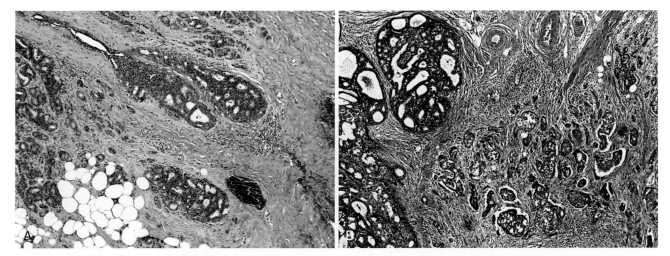

FIGURE 29-39 **A** and **B,** DCIS associated with invasive cribriform carcinoma. DCIS is often cribriform in type.

Differential Diagnosis

Two lesions that invasive cribriform carcinoma must be distinguished from are cribriform DCIS and invasive mammary carcinoma with osteoclast-like giant cells. Adenoid cystic carcinoma is a consideration in some examples that may have a superficial resemblance.

Discrimination from cribriform DCIS is clinically important, not only because one is invasive and the other is in situ but also because precise proportions of invasive and in situ components in a given tumor are necessary to accurately measure the pathologic tumor size as well as identify cases of invasive tumor with an extensive intraductal component. Invasive cribriform carcinoma is characteristically composed of irregular or angulated glands infiltrating between duct and lobules without regard for normal breast architecture. In addition, the stroma through which it invades tends to show a desmoplastic reaction. Similar to other invasive carcinomas, neoplastic glands lack myoepithelium, which can be demonstrated by absence of staining with myoepithelial-specific immunostains. In contrast, cribriform DCIS has smooth, rounded contours and respects the normal breast architecture. Also, cribriform DCIS is invested by intact myoepithelium, which can be confirmed by immunohistochemistry.

Invasive mammary carcinoma with osteoclast-like giant cells is an uncommon type of carcinoma characterized by invasive duct carcinoma associated with osteoclast-like giant cells. The invasive duct carcinoma is commonly moderately or poorly differentiated and more commonly exhibits cribriform pattern but can show other patterns such as tubular, lobular, squamous, papillary, apocrine, mucinous, and metaplastic carcinomas. The extent of cribriform pattern in any given case is highly variable. However, unlike invasive cribriform carcinomas, several to numerous osteoclast-like giant cells can be seen in the intervening stroma or juxtaposed to ("hugging") neoplastic glands (Figure 29-40). Reactive-appearing stroma can be seen in both entities, but in cases of invasive mammary carcinoma with osteoclast-like giant cells, the stroma also contains numerous erythrocytes or hemosiderin, both of which are indicative of recent or past hemorrhage (see Figure 29-40). The presence of stromal red blood cells directly relates to the typical red-brown color of the tumor grossly.

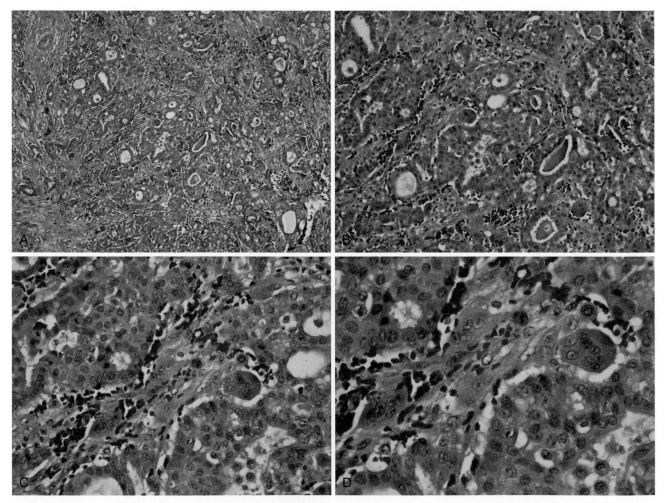

FIGURE 29-40 Invasive mammary carcinoma with osteoclast-like giant cells. **A** and **B,** There is evidence of recent and past hemorrhage in the stroma, as evidenced by extravagated erythrocytes and abundant hemosiderin pigments. **C** and **D,** Unlike invasive cribriform carcinoma, the tumor has significant numbers of giant cells in the intervening stroma, juxtaposed to neoplastic glands.

INVASIVE MICROPAPILLARY CARCINOMA

Invasive micropapillary carcinoma of the breast is a morphologically distinct and clinically aggressive variant of ductal carcinoma that resembles micropapillary carcinoma of other primary sites. In the 2003 World Health Organization (WHO) classification of breast tumors, invasive micropapillary carcinoma was listed as a subtype of invasive carcinoma; however, no percentage of the micropapillary component was proposed as a criterion for diagnosis.[128a] Pure micropapillary carcinomas are rare and accounted for 1.7% of all breast carcinomas in one study[129] and 2.3% in another.[130] However, a higher incidence (3–6%) of micropapillary carcinoma has been reported in studies that have included carcinomas with focal areas of micropapillary differentiation.[131–133] Unlike other special type carcinomas, the poor prognosis associated with this entity appears to be the same whether the micropapillary component is present focally or diffusely within a tumor.[132,134]

Clinical Presentation

The age range (26–92 yr) and the mean age (52–61 yr) at presentation for patients with invasive micropapillary carcinoma are not significantly different from ductal carcinoma of no special type.[130,132,135–138] The majority of patients present with a palpable mass; however, in some, the tumor is detected during routine imaging studies.[130,135,138] As with carcinomas of no special type, these tumors most frequently occur in the upper outer quadrant of the breast.[131,136,139]

Clinical Imaging

The imaging characteristics of invasive micropapillary carcinoma are highly suggestive of malignancy.[131,136,140] Mammography typically shows a high-density irregular mass with spiculated margins that is often associated with microcalcifications. In a study of 28 patients with 29 invasive micropapillary carcinomas, mammographic mass with microcalcifications was visible in 13 tumors

(45%), mass only in 7 (24%), microcalcifications only in 5 (17%), focal asymmetry with microcalcifications in 1 (3%), density in 1 (3%), and architectural distortion in 1 (3%). One tumor was mammographically occult and was detected on MRI. On sonographic examination, most tumors present as a homogenously hypoechoic, irregular mass with posterior acoustic shadowing or normal sound transmission.[131,136] The ultrasonographic appearance of 27 micropapillary carcinomas revealed solid mass in 23 tumors (21 hypoechoic and 2 with mixed echogenicity), most were irregular with indistinct or spiculated margins, and architectural distortion in one. Three tumors were sonographically occult. In this study, sonography helped to determine the extent of disease in some cases. Of the 23 masses, 8 (35%) were multifocal and 1 (4%) was multicentric.[136] In two different studies, ultrasonography revealed frequent involvement of axillary nodes.[131,136] Adrada and colleagues[136] found suspicious axillary lymphadenopathy in 48% of cases and supraclavicular nodes in 11% of cases with ultrasonography.

MRI performed in four patients with invasive micropapillary carcinoma who had equivocal mammographic and ultrasonographic findings revealed an irregular mass with spiculated margins in four and a non-mass-like enhancement in two. The kinetics of all lesions suggested the presence of malignancy with a rapid initial increase and washout or plateau on dynamic contrast-enhanced studies.[136]

Gross Pathology

Tumors ranging from a few millimeters to as large as 11 cm have been reported.[129,132,133,135,141] The median size of the tumor was 2.8 cm in one study[133] and 4.9 cm in another study.[134] Overall, these tumors are significantly larger than ductal carcinoma of no special type.

The gross appearance of invasive micropapillary carcinoma is not different from IDC of no special type.

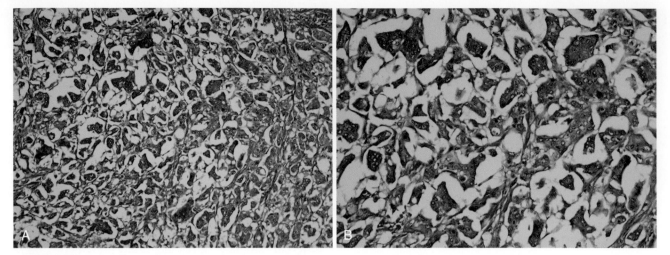

FIGURE 29-41 **A** and **B,** Invasive micropapillary carcinoma. The characteristic spongelike appearance is due to the tumor cell clusters surrounded by clear spaces.

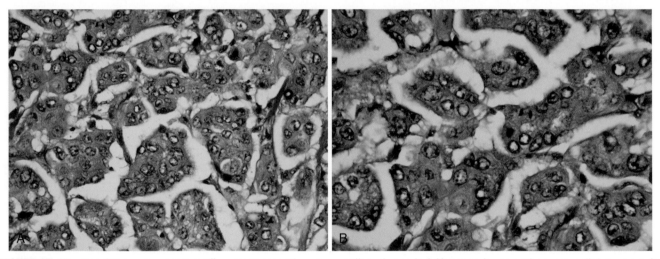

FIGURE 29-42 **A** and **B,** Invasive micropapillary carcinoma. The micropapillary clusters lack fibrovascular core. The tumor cells have granular pink cytoplasm, high nuclear grade, and mitosis.

However, a high percentage of patients have metastases to multiple axillary lymph nodes.

Microscopic Pathology

In most cases, invasive micropapillary carcinoma is admixed to a variable degree with IDCs of no special type. The micropapillary component in both pure and mixed forms has a characteristic morphologic appearance. The tumor cells are arranged in micropapillary, tubuloalveolar, or morular clusters and appear to be suspended in clear spaces, imparting a sponge-like appearance on low magnification (Figure 29-41). On rare occasions, the spaces may contain clear aqueous fluid or extracellular mucin. The micropapillary clusters, unlike "true" papillary carcinomas, lack fibrovascular cores (Figure 29-42). In the tubuloalveolar structures, a central lumen may be present. The tumor cells have finely granular or dense eosinophilic cytoplasm and intermediate- to high-grade nuclei with frequent mitoses (Figure 29-43; see also Figure 29-42). In a study

of 80 invasive micropapillary carcinomas, Walsh and Bleiweiss[135] reported high nuclear grade in 67.5% of cases and intermediate nuclear grade in the remaining 32.5% of cases. None of the tumors in their series were well-differentiated. No well-differentiated tumor was identified in three large studies that examined a total of 136 cases of micropapillary carcinomas.[129,130,133] The cells in micropapillary carcinoma have reversed polarity with the apical surface polarized to the outside, which some have referred to as an "inside-out" growth pattern. This morphologic observation has been supported by the presence of microvilli on electron microscopy as well as the characteristic staining of the cell membranes facing toward the stroma with epithelial membrane antigen (EMA) (Figure 29-44).[134] Others have demonstrated a similar reverse-staining pattern of the tumor cell clusters with MUC1, a glycoprotein localized to the apical surface of glandular cells. It is postulated that the role of MUC1 in lumen formation may be linked to detachment of cells from the stroma resulting in the characteristic histologic appearance of invasive

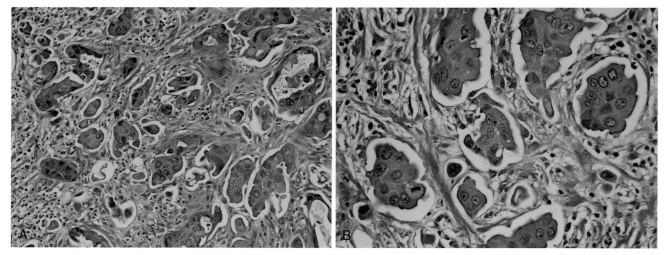

FIGURE 29-43 **A** and **B**, Invasive micropapillary carcinoma, apocrine type. The tumor cells have abundant cytoplasm and high nuclear grade and are surrounded by clear spaces.

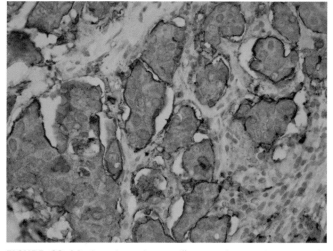

FIGURE 29-44 Invasive micropapillary carcinoma. Immunostain for epithelial membrane antigen shows the characteristic reverse membranous staining at the outer border of the cells, facing the stroma.

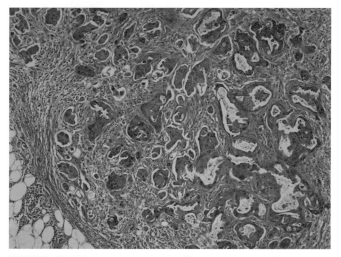

FIGURE 29-45 Invasive micropapillary carcinoma. The stroma contains marked lymphocytic infiltrates.

micropapillary carcinoma as well as the more aggressive biology of this tumor.[118]

The intervening stroma between the tumor cell nests can be loose delicate reticular to dense collagenous stroma. In some cases, the stroma may show myxoid change or infiltration by lymphoid cells (Figure 29-45). The overall morphologic appearance of invasive micropapillary carcinoma of breast is similar to that described in other primary sites such as urinary bladder, lung, pancreas, and ovary. Indeed, the micropapillary architecture is preserved in lymphatic tumor emboli, lymph nodes, and distant metastatic sites (Figure 29-46).

The prominent clear spaces around the cell nest may simulate lymphatic/vascular space invasion. However, true lymphatic/vascular space invasion has been reported in many studies to be as high as 33% to 67% of cases. In some cases, it can be extensive.[133–135,139] This may be due to increased lymphangiogenesis and increased lymphatic density as demonstrated by overexpression of vascular endothelial growth factor-C (VEGF-C) in these

tumors.[142] VEGF-C induces lymphangiogenesis and that, in turn, promotes lymphatic invasion and lymph node metastases.

The majority of tumors (67–70%) are associated with an intraductal component of micropapillary and cribriform patterns.[134,139] The intraductal carcinoma, including the micropapillary architecture type, exhibits higher nuclear grade (Figure 29-47). Microscopic evidence of calcifications have been identified in up to 33% of cases.[139] Two studies have reported the frequent presence of psammoma bodies (42% and 67%).[142,143]

Prognosis and Treatment

Patients with invasive micropapillary breast carcinoma experience a high relapse rate and short disease-free survival. Most series with follow-up have reported early skin or chest wall recurrence. Pettinato and associates[133] reported 29 of 41 (71%) of their patients developed local recurrence in the skin and chest wall. The time to local recurrence was from 3 to 60 months (mean

be seen. This invariably produces a microscopic invasive tumor edge. The lymphoplasmacytic infiltrate is found not only at the periphery of but also admixed within the invasive tumor (Figure 29-51). Formation of germinal centers can be seen in some examples. There has been an attempt to better define the lymphocytic infiltrate associated with medullary carcinoma, and one study found that these lymphocytes were proportionately more CD3–, CD8–, and TIA-1 and granzyme-B–positive than those in usual breast cancer. The authors surmised that such an increase in infiltrating cytotoxic lymphocytes in medullary carcinoma may be, in part, related to its known association with a favorable prognosis.[177] The invasive carcinoma cells are high grade and exhibit pleomorphic nuclei, a coarse chromatin pattern, and prominent nucleoli (Figure 29-52). Scattered pyknotic nuclei are common. Not surprisingly, a brisk mitotic rate is reliably present in all cases. Some examples of medullary carcinoma can show metaplastic changes, most commonly squamous metaplasia.[89] Necrosis can be associated with the invasive carcinoma and tends to be more extensive in larger tumors. Extensive necrosis can lead to cystic degeneration and is often found concomitantly with squamous metaplasia.

Coexisting in situ carcinoma is not uncommon in cases of medullary carcinoma. Typically, the lymphoplasmacytic infiltrate evident in and around the invasive tumor also surrounds ducts and lobules that are involved by in situ carcinoma. Moreover, similar infiltrates can be seen in more distantly located ducts and lobules uninvolved by carcinoma. The in situ carcinoma associated with medullary carcinoma is usually solid type with or without central necrosis and high nuclear grade (Figure 29-53). Lobular extension by in situ carcinoma can be appreciated in some cases. At times, particularly expansile foci of in situ carcinoma with surrounding lymphoplasmacytic infiltration can, themselves, form smaller nodules of tumor. These should not be mistaken for peripheral foci of invasive carcinoma (Figure 29-54).

Medullary carcinomas possess a biomarker profile similar to that of other tumors with aggressive histologic features, which is not considered to be specific for

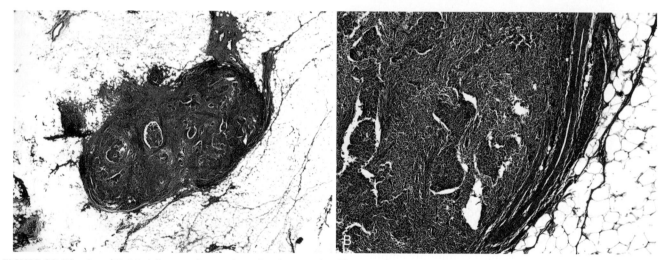

FIGURE 29-51 A and **B,** Medullary carcinoma. Lymphoplasmacytic infiltrate is characteristically abundant and found not only at the periphery of but also admixed within the tumor.

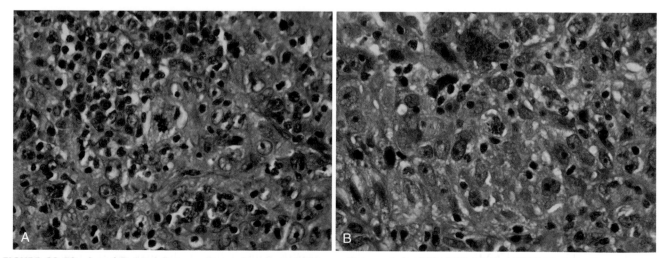

FIGURE 29-52 A and **B,** Medullary carcinoma. Invasive carcinoma cells are poorly differentiated with high nuclear grade and frequent mitoses.

this tumor type but rather a function of its high-grade morphology.[151–154,156,158,178] ER and PgR positivity is relatively infrequent in these tumors (ranges 0–33% and 0–36%, respectively).[103,104,106,153,179] *HER2*/neu overexpression is also relatively uncommon (0–14%).[52,53]

Prognosis and Treatment

As previously mentioned, correctly classifying medullary carcinoma is fraught with difficulties including determining which classification system is "best" in terms of diagnostic accuracy and high consensus and reproducibility rates among pathologists. One study directly compared all three classification schemes (Ridolfi, Wargotz, and Pedersen) and found the one of Pedersen and associates[153] to be the most reproducible; however, none was found to correlate with axillary lymph node status or overall survival in these patients.[172] A recent study proposed a simplified definition of "medullary-like" type of

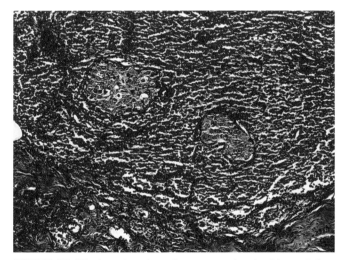

FIGURE 29-53 Intraductal carcinoma associated with medullary carcinoma. Intraductal carcinoma is typically solid type with high nuclear grade. A prominent lymphoplasmacytic infiltrate surrounds foci of in situ carcinoma.

breast carcinoma that was based on the presence of two histologic findings: the presence of prominent inflammation and anastomosing sheets in at least 30% of the tumor.[180] The investigators found significant overlap between tumors that were "medullary-like" and medullary carcinoma classified by conventional histologic criteria; however, some atypical medullary carcinomas did not meet the simplified definition. Tumors that fulfilled this highly reproducible (90% agreement) histologic definition were found to be associated with a better prognosis on univariate analysis. Survival at 10-year follow-up was 80% to 90% in patients with "medullary-like" type compared with 50% to 60% in those that were "nonmedullary" type.[180] Additional studies of larger cohorts will be needed to validate the accuracy of this simplified version of classification.

With that said, most published studies have reported a lower incidence of axillary lymph node involvement in patients with medullary carcinoma (19–46%) than those with atypical medullary carcinomas (30–52%) or invasive duct carcinomas (29–65%).[151,153,156,157,174]

Reported survival differences between those with medullary carcinoma and those with other histologic types including atypical medullary carcinomas are conflicting. Whereas some studies[156,174] have reported significantly better 10-year and 5-year survival rates in patients with medullary carcinoma (84–94.9% and 95%, respectively) compared with 77.5% of invasive duct carcinomas,[155] others have found no difference (51%, 79%) compared with those with atypical medullary carcinoma (55%) and patients with carcinoma of no special type (47%, 77%).[33,51] However, when compared with patients with grade 3 tumors of no special type, patients with medullary carcinoma experienced a more favorable survival rate.[33,181] Another large study showed only a modestly improved survival rate in patients with node-negative medullary carcinomas and no improved survival rate in node-positive patients with this tumor type.[179]

Treatment is no different from what is prescribed in patients with other types of invasive breast carcinoma;

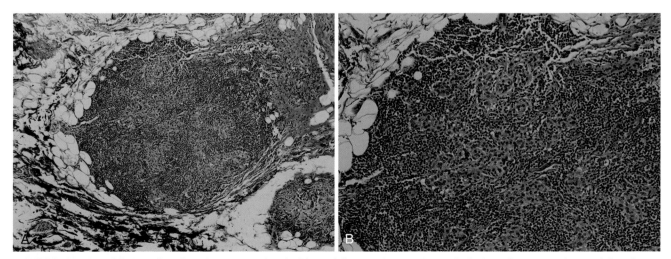

FIGURE 29-54 **A** and **B**, Intraductal carcinoma associated with medullary carcinoma. Expansile foci can form secondary nodules of tumor, which should not be mistaken for peripheral foci of invasive carcinoma.

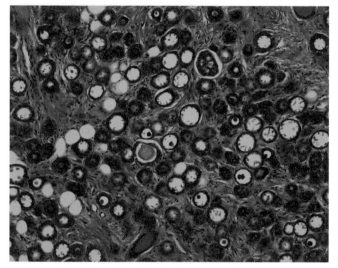

FIGURE 30-5 AdCC, tubular growth pattern.

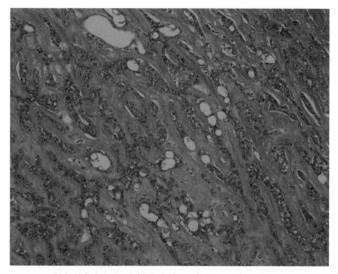

FIGURE 30-6 AdCC, trabecular growth pattern.

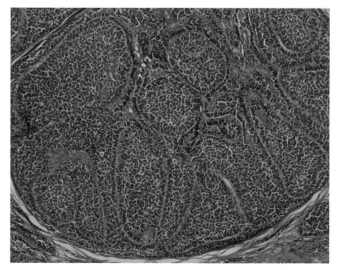

FIGURE 30-7 AdCC, solid growth pattern.

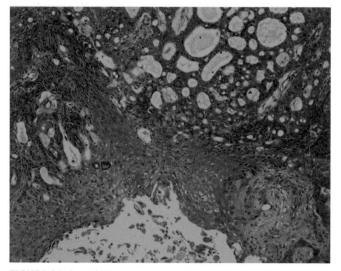

FIGURE 30-8 AdCC, squamous metaplasia. Same case as depicted in Figure 30-2 exhibits overt squamous metaplasia lining the central cystic area.

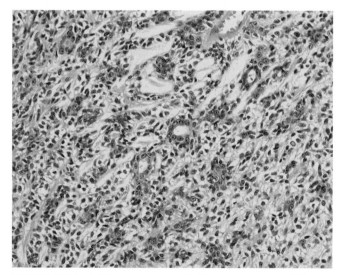

FIGURE 30-9 AdCC, adenomyoepitheliomatous pattern. This case displays areas indistinguishable from an adenomyoepithelioma.

for AdCC of the salivary glands can also be applied. This system, based on the proportion of solid growth pattern, qualifies as G1 tumors with a cribriform or tubular pattern, as G2 tumors with 30% of solid areas, and as G3 tumors with greater than 30% of solid elements. Although Ro and associates[19] suggested that this grading system was prognostic in breast AdCC, Kleer and Oberman[13] reported a lack of association between tumor grade and prognosis.

Immunoprofile

Breast AdCCs are generally negative for estrogen receptor (ER), progesterone receptor (PgR), and *HER2* expression.[7,23–28,33] Whereas rare cases morphologically reviewed to confirm the diagnosis of AdCC showed focal positivity for ER and less frequently for PgR,[24,28] *HER2* overexpression and/or *HER2* gene amplification has not been described.[7,24,25,27,28,33] Taken together, it is reasonable to conclude that the vast majority of breast AdCCs display a triple-negative phenotype. Moreover, AdCCs frequently, if not always, express basal-like markers such as c-kit,[7,12,27,28] epidermal growth factor receptor (EGFR),[24] and high-molecular-weight cytokeratins (CKs),[25] being therefore classified as part of the basal-like molecular phenotype according to a validated immunohistochemical surrogate panel.[36] Proliferative ratios as defined by Ki-67 index are variable, with levels ranging from 4% to 70% in one series,[28] and may not be associated with prognosis.[13]

The two distinct cell populations of AdCCs are best appreciated by immunohistochemistry. The basaloid cells express basal CKs, such as CK14 and CK17, vimentin, S100 protein, actin, calponin, p63, and maspin, whereas the epithelial cuboidal cells lining the true glandular lumina show strong positivity for luminal CKs, including CK7 and CK8/18, carcinoembryonia antigen (CEA), epithelial membrane antigen (EMA) and c-kit.[1] Furthermore, the stromal hyaline material can be highlighted by staining for collagen IV and laminin.[1]

Molecular Pathology

Although microarray has been extensively applied to the study of breast cancer, most analyses, including the seminal studies by Perou and Sorlie and coworkers,[37–39] have not included representative numbers of special histologic types of breast cancer. Therefore, the so-called molecular taxonomy of breast cancer (i.e., luminal A, luminal B, *HER2*, basal-like, and normal breast–like molecular subtypes) has been derived from analysis of only IDC-NSTs and few invasive lobular carcinomas. Weigelt and colleagues[33] directly investigated the transcriptome of 11 histologic special types of breast cancer, including AdCCs. Unsupervised hierarchical cluster analysis revealed that AdCCs clustered together with metaplastic and medullary carcinomas and that these tumors displayed a basal-like phenotype, corroborating the basal-like immunohistochemical profile of these tumors (i.e., lack of ER, PgR, and *HER2* expression; low levels of CK19, androgen receptor [AR], and CK8/18; and high levels of c-kit, vimentin, S100, CK14, and CK5/6 expression). In addition, molecular subtype analysis using a single sample predictor showed that two AdCCs were of basal-like phenotype, whereas two AdCCs were of normal breast–like phenotype, a molecular subtype that is currently considered to be an artifact of sample representation (i.e., high content of normal tissue contamination).[40] These data also illustrate the heterogeneity of the basal-like phenotype, which is predominantly composed of high-grade IDC-NSTs and metaplastic carcinomas but also includes a subgroup of breast cancers with low-grade histology and an indolent behavior such as AdCCs and secretory carcinomas (see later).[41,42] Importantly, however, there is evidence to suggest that, in contrast with high-grade IDC-NSTs of basal-like phenotype,[43] AdCCs do not display *BRCA1* down-regulation,[25] which may in part explain the differences in prognosis.

These observations highlight the importance of histologic subtyping of breast cancer, given that, although a subgroup of IDC-NSTs and AdCCs display triple-negative/basal-like phenotype, the management of patients with IDC-NSTs is fundamentally different from those with AdCCs (see later).

At the genomic level, AdCCs rarely display aneuploidy[4,44] and often harbor simple genomes,[25] indicating low levels of genetic instability. Frequent copy number alterations detected by microarray comparative genomic hybridization include focal gains of 1p, 11p, 12p, 16p, 19p, and focal losses on 6q and 9p. Of note, AdCCs do not harbor concurrent gains of 1q and 16p and losses of 16q as typically do low-grade IDC-NSTs.[45] Moreover, breast AdCCs significantly differ at the genomic level from other basal-like IDC-NSTs.

In a way akin to secretory carcinomas, another form of indolent triple-negative and basal-like disease, AdCCs are also characterized by a recurrent specific translocation. Although the existence of t(6;9)(q22–23;p23–24) as characteristic of salivary gland tumors was known for many years,[46] it was only in 2010 that Persson and associates[17] reported that this translocation was found in all AdCCs analyzed (breast, salivary, ceruminal, and lachrymal glands) and that it leads to the fusion of the oncogene *MYB* (6q22-q23) with the transcription factor *NFIB* (9p23-p24). Although distinct breakpoints and fusion transcripts were reported, the common denominator of these rearrangements is the deletion of a microRNA target site of *MYB*, ultimately resulting in *MYB* overexpression. Subsequent analyses have confirmed that the translocation t(6;9)(q22–23;p23–24) is specific of AdCCs in the context of salivary gland tumors,[30,31] but the prevalence seems to be lower than initially suggested.[25,30,31] The *MYB-NFIB* fusion has been found in about a third to a half of salivary gland AdCCs tested; however, *MYB* overexpression as defined by immunohistochemistry or quantitative reverse-transcriptase polymerase chain reaction (qRT-PCR) was far more prevalent. Wetterskog and coworkers[25] studied by fluorescence in situ hybridization (FISH) 13 breast AdCCs, of which 1 did not harbor the *MYB-NFIB* fusion gene. Nevertheless, qRT-PCR analysis revealed that all cases, including the fusion-negative, displayed *MYB* overexpression as compared with histologic grade–matched IDC-NSTs and basal-like IDC-NSTs. Those results provide strong circumstantial evidence to suggest that *MYB* overexpression is a molecular driver of AdCCs, is often, but not always, underpinned by t(6;9)(q22–23;p23–24), and may be a novel specific therapeutic target.

Additional potential targets have been reported based on the analysis of an AdCC metastatic to the kidney. *PTEN* and *PIK3CA* mutations were found in both primary and metastatic lesions, possibly explaining the more aggressive behavior displayed by this case.[47] Although *PIK3CA* and *PTEN* mutations may be more prevalent in breast cancers of the basal-like subtype, such as metaplastic breast cancers,[48] additional studies with large cohorts are needed to determine the prevalence of PI3K/AKT pathway mutations in breast AdCCs.

neuroendocrine carcinomas of all variants must be differentiated from metastasis of neuroendocrine tumors of other anatomic sites. The presence of an in situ component, ideally displaying similar cytologic features, may be considered the best evidence in favor of a breast primary. Immunohistochemistry should be evaluated with caution because hormone receptor expression may occur in nonmammary neuroendocrine tumors, in particular PgR expression. Likewise, antibodies for site-specific transcription factors, such as TTF-1 and CDX2, are of limited use in tumors with neuroendocrine differentiation. For instance, TTF-1 has been shown to be expressed in 20% of mammary small cell carcinomas,[68] whereas the entire spectrum of lung neuroendocrine neoplasms may display focal to diffuse ER and PgR expression.[62] In this context, the expression of gross cystic disease fluid protein-15 (GCDFP-15) and/or mammaglobin may indicate a breast primary, because nonmammary neuroendocrine tumors failed to express both markers in one study.[70] Finally, before rendering a diagnosis of a breast neuroendocrine carcinoma without an in situ component, one may best rule out any evidence of a neuroendocrine neoplasm in another anatomic site.

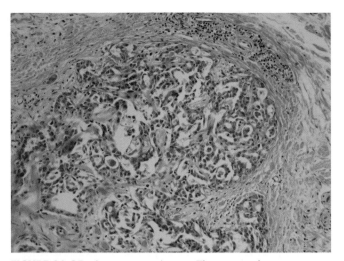

FIGURE 30-15 Secretory carcinoma. The tumor often presents as a well-circumscribed nodule with margin stromal invasion.

KEY PATHOLOGIC FEATURES

Neuroendocrine Carcinoma

- WHO recognizes three variant growth patterns: solid, large cell, and small cell.

- Nottingham scoring is the best method to grade these tumors.

- Well-differentiated solid types are 95% ER+, >90% *HER2*–.

- Differential diagnosis is to exclude metastatic neuroendocrine carcinoma to breast: ER positivity and an in situ component are the best ways to prove a primary breast carcinoma. TTF-1 CDX2 and neuroendocrine markers (chromogranin, synaptophysin, CD56) have limited usefulness.

- Neuroendocrine carcinomas are in the luminal molecular subtype.

ER, estrogen receptor; WHO, World Health Organization.

SECRETORY CARCINOMA

Secretory breast carcinoma (SBC) is a rare histologic special type of breast cancer, accounting for less than 0.1% of all breast cancers.[51,71–73] This tumor, defined by a pattern of clinical, pathologic, phenotypic, and specific molecular features, exemplifies the concept of genotypic-phenotypic correlation in breast cancer. SBC was first described by McDivitt and Stewart in 1966[74] under the term "juvenile breast carcinoma," because the average age of the seven patients included in their study was 9 years (range 3–15 yr). Subsequently, over 100 cases have been reported, leading to the observation that only a third of all SBCs affect children. Therefore, the term "juvenile breast carcinoma" was replaced by the descriptive term *secretory breast carcinoma*.[75]

Clinical Presentation

This entity occurs preferentially during the third decade, with a median age at presentation of 25 years and a range from 3 to 87 years.[51,72,74–80] SBC occurs more frequently in females, with approximately 20 reported cases in males,[81] and a male-to-female ratio of 1:6.[82,83] The tumor usually presents as a solitary, well-circumscribed mobile nodule in the subareolar region, but it may also be located anywhere in the breast (Figure 30-15). Multifocal lesions are infrequently described.[75,76] An associated bloody nipple discharge may rarely occur.[84]

Clinical Imaging

Ultrasound examination usually shows an ovoid hypoechogenic formation with regular margins, concordant with an opaque, dense, and homogeneous mass showing rather well-delineated outlines on mammography.[85–88] Taken together, the clinical presentation may, therefore, prove misleading, especially in young women in whom it may be misdiagnosed as a fibroadenoma.

KEY CLINICAL FEATURES

Secretory Carcinoma

- Tumors tend to be circumscribed on imaging.

- Generally good prognosis, despite lymph node spread in up to a third of cases. Death is rare from this entity.

Gross Pathology

Reported dimensions of tumors range from 0.3 to 16 cm.[73,75,76] The lesion is often lobulated, nonencapsulated, firm and fibrous, with a gray to yellow-tan cut surface.[75,88] Infiltrating margins may sometimes be seen on gross examination.[75]

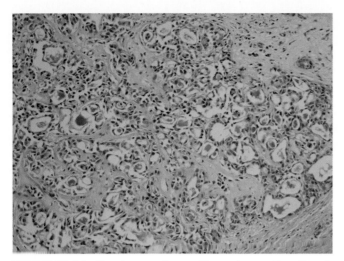

FIGURE 30-16 Secretory carcinoma. The main growth pattern is microcystic with sclerotic or myxoid stroma.

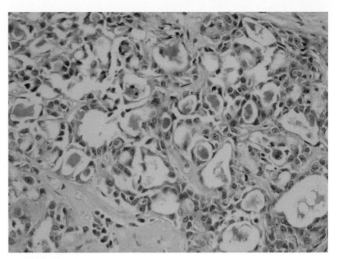

FIGURE 30-17 Secretory carcinoma. An abundant eosinophilic secretory material is seen in extracellular lumina.

Microscopic Pathology

At optical microscopy, SBCs are characterized by partially circumscribed nodules composed of cells arranged in three main histologic patterns—solid, microcystic (so-called honeycomb pattern, composed of multiple small cysts simulating thyroid follicles), and tubular.[75,80,89] Some papillary central areas may also be observed.[75] The three main patterns are often associated in variable proportions within a given case.[75,76,80,89] Neoplastic cells are uniform, round to polygonal, and display a finely granular or vacuolated cytoplasm containing dense, eosinophilic secretion in the center of the vacuole. Some signet-ring cells may be observed. Extracellular secretory material positive for PAS, diastase-PAS, and alcian blue (i.e., corresponding to acid mucopolysaccharides, mainly in sulfated groups), similar to that found in the intracellular compartment, is a characteristic feature of these tumors, thus the preferred term *secretory*.[75,80]

Albeit apparently well delimited on gross examination, microscopically, SBCs often have irregular margins with foci of infiltration of tumor cells in the surrounding stroma.[75] Within the tumor, the stroma separating the nests and cords of neoplastic cells is either sclerotic, fibroblastic, or myxoid (Figures 30-16 to 30-18).[75] Lymphocytic infiltration is usually sparse and focal.[75] Of note, a component of in situ carcinoma, usually harboring the same secretory features, is observed within or at the margins of the tumor in 46% to 100% of the cases, rendering the complete surgical excision of these lesions challenging.[72,75,76]

The vast majority of SBCs are low-grade neoplasms, with mild nuclear atypia and low mitotic activity.[72,75,76] The nuclei are round to oval, occasionally with vesicular chromatin and discrete nucleoli. Necrosis is rarely observed. The presence of lymphovascular invasion is infrequently reported.[72]

Immunoprofile

SBCs display a distinct and characteristic immunoprofile. Most SBCs lack expression of ER and PgR and do not overexpress *HER2;* therefore, these tumors

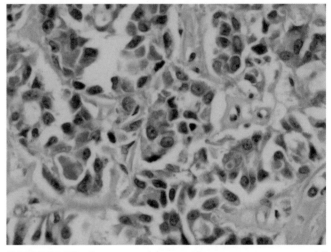

FIGURE 30-18 Secretory carcinoma. The same secretory material is found in intracellular vacuoles. Nuclear atypia are mild with discrete nucleoli and low mitotic activity.

display a "triple-negative" phenotype (Figures 30-19 to 30-21).[72,73,76,82,85,90,91] In rare cases, low reactivity for ER, often in the absence of PgR expression, has been reported.[72,76,92] *HER2* overexpression was described in one case.[76] SBCs express the CKs 8/18 and 19 at least focally and E-cadherin.[72,91] Furthermore, recent studies have demonstrated that SBCs often express at least in a minority of the tumor cells high-molecular-weight CKs (e.g., CK5/6, CK14, CK17, 34βE12), EGFR, vimentin, and c-kit (Figures 30-22 to 30-25).[72,88,91] Thus, despite being low-grade neoplasms, the vast majority of SBCs display a basal-like phenotype, if the surrogate described by Nielsen and coworkers[36] is employed.

Other markers consistently expressed include S100 protein (strong and diffuse cytoplasmic and nuclear staining), smooth muscle actin (focal expression), EMA, α-lactalbumin, and less frequently, polyclonal CEA (Figures 30-26 and 30-27).[72,73,88,91] Positivity for amylase, lysozyme, α_1-antitrypsin, Leu-M1, immunoglobulin A (IgA), and GCDFP-15 has also been reported.[92] In addition, in contrast to other histologic subtypes,

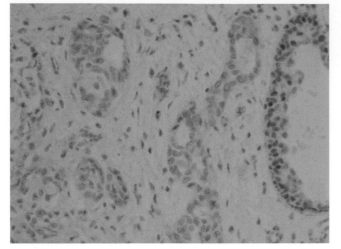

FIGURE 30-19 Secretory carcinoma. These tumors are usually estrogen receptor (ER)–negative. Note the presence of positive internal controls.

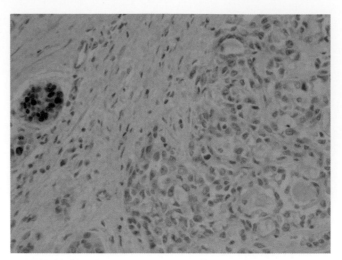

FIGURE 30-20 Secretory carcinoma. Absence of progesterone receptor (PgR) expression, in the presence of positive internal controls.

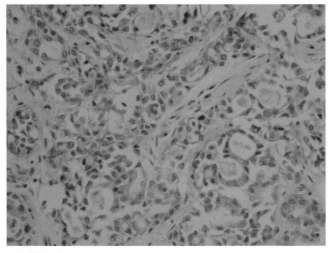

FIGURE 30-21 Secretory carcinoma. Absence of *HER2* overexpression is a rule.

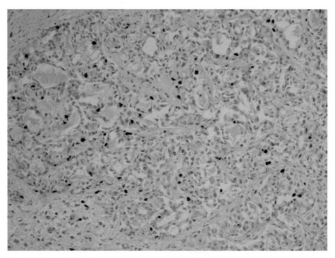

FIGURE 30-22 Secretory carcinoma. These tumors are low proliferative with a Ki-67 labeling index less than 15%.

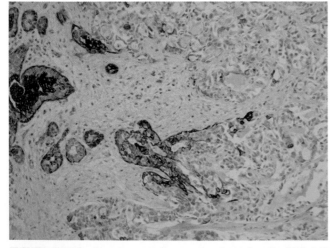

FIGURE 30-23 Secretory carcinoma. Focal cytokeratin (CK) 5/6 expression is often observed at the periphery of the tumor.

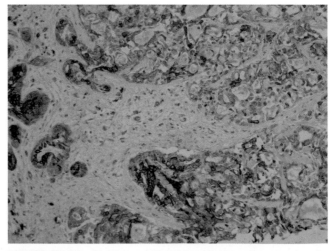

FIGURE 30-24 Secretory carcinoma. c-kit expression may be observed.

presence of an *ETV6* gene rearrangement may be useful to rule out an apocrine carcinoma, lipid- or glycogen-rich carcinoma, mucinous carcinoma, or lactating adenoma.

CARCINOMA WITH OSTEOCLAST-LIKE GIANT CELLS

Osteoclast-like multinucleated giant cells can occur in association with carcinomas of many organs, including the breast, lung,[105] gastrointestinal tract,[106] kidney,[107] as well in the context of nonepithelial tumors such as mesothelioma[108] and leiomyosarcoma.[109] This histologic type of breast carcinoma was first described in 1979 by Agnantis and Rosen,[110] and its features further catalogued in multiple publications.[111–120] Its incidence is estimated to be between 0.5% and 1.2% of breast carcinomas.[113,115]

Despite the unusual morphologic features of breast carcinomas with osteoclast-like giant cells, it was not included as a distinct special histologic type in the last edition of the WHO classification of breast cancer.[51] According to this classification, the presence of osteoclast-like giant cells in association with an epithelial breast invasive lesion would be better viewed as a morphologic pattern that can occur within any type of breast carcinoma, instead of a diagnostic criterion for a discrete pathologic entity. In fact, osteoclast-like giant cells have been reported in association with tubular/cribriform,[115] lobular,[114,118] squamous,[111] papillary,[110] mucinous,[116] and metaplastic[112] carcinomas.

Clinical Presentation

The clinical features of carcinomas with osteoclast-like giant cells are similar to those of breast cancer generally. A palpable or imaging-detected mass in the upper outer quadrant is the main finding, but the lesion can occur in any quadrant and may be multifocal[117] and, rarely, bilateral.[114] The average age at diagnosis is 50 years, ranging from 28 to 88 years.

Clinical Imaging

At imaging analysis, carcinomas with osteoclast-like giant cells are usually round well-circumscribed masses, which may contain calcifications.[113,119,121] Less frequently, architectural distortion, heterogeneous density, or tumors with marginal spikes may occur. The frequent well-defined contours of the tumors may suggest benign lesions, such as cysts or fibroadenomas, and delay the diagnosis of malignancy.[113,118]

KEY CLINICAL FEATURES

Carcinoma with Osteoclast Giant Cells

- Imaging mimics benign tumors because they are usually circumscribed.

- Similar prognosis to IDC-NST.

IDC-NST, invasive ductal carcinoma, no specific type.

Gross Pathology

Carcinomas with osteoclast-like giant cells display rather characteristic gross features. The tumors are typically well circumscribed, spongy and firm, and display a red to dark-brown color. The striking color is due to hemorrhage and hemosiderin-laden macrophages and may suggest a heavily pigmented metastatic melanoma. The latter, however, tends to be black rather than reddish/brownish, which is the typical presentation of carcinomas with osteoclast-like giant cells. Although typical, it should be noted that this gross appearance is not specific of carcinomas with osteoclast-like giant cells because other tumors, in particular papillary carcinomas, may display similar features due to conspicuous hemorrhage. Moreover, tan or white tumors, which correspond to lesions with less osteoclast-like giant cells and less hemorrhage at microscopic examination as well as lesions with ill-defined margins, have also been recorded.[34]

Microscopic Pathology

The defining histologic feature of this type of breast cancer is the presence of a stromal reaction with varying amounts of non-neoplastic multinucleated osteoclast-like giant cells, whereas the carcinomatous component may display a panoply of morphologic patterns. The majority of the lesions are well- to moderately differentiated IDC-NSTs, frequently with a cribriform growth pattern (Figure 30-29); however, osteoclast-like giant cells can also be found in association with several special histologic types of breast cancer as previously described, including metaplastic carcinomas (Figure 30-30).[110–112,114–116,118] If present, the intraductal component is usually of conventional ductal type, with solid, cribriform, or papillary architectural patterns, and is sometimes intimately admixed with the giant cells as the invasive counterpart. Nevertheless, it is uncommon to find osteoclast-like giant cells in pure in situ lesions.

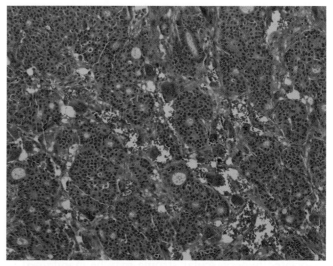

FIGURE 30-29 Carcinomas with osteoclast-like giant cells. A grade 1 invasive ductal carcinoma with a cribriform growth pattern and neoplastic cell immersed in a hypervascular stroma with multinucleated giant cells and red blood cell extravasation.

Gross Pathology

Lipid-rich carcinoma has been described at gross examination as a white to yellow firm mass with well-defined and lobulated contours[132] or ill-defined margins.[133] Tumor size has been reported to range from 1.2 to 15 cm.[128,132,133,137]

Microscopic Pathology

Lipid-rich tumors are usually poorly differentiated lesions, with high nuclear grade, few or no gland formation, and high mitotic indices. They are composed of nests, sheets, or anastomosing cords of large cells, with ill-defined borders. The neoplastic cell population comprises a mixture of cells with finely granular eosinophilic cytoplasm, which merge with large, clear cells showing univacuolated, multivacuolated, or foamy cytoplasm. The nuclei are irregular, hyperchromatic, and pleomorphic, frequently containing one or more prominent nucleoli of varying size. The nuclei can be eccentric or peripherically located and often scalloped, somewhat resembling the nuclei of lipoblasts. As a rule, neoplastic cells stain strongly for neutral lipid. Mucin and glycogen can be found but are far less conspicuous and unevenly distributed.[134–137] The intraductal component can be of ductal or lobular type. When performing histologic analysis of lymph nodes from patients with lipid-rich carcinomas, one must be aware that neoplastic cells may resemble vacuolated histiocytes or a malignant histiocytic lesion instead of a metastatic carcinoma.[127,138]

Immunoprofile

Lipid-rich carcinomas usually lack or express low levels of hormone receptors.[128,132,133] Shi and coworkers[128] described 0% and 10% of positivity rates for ER and PgR expression, respectively. In the same study, 31 out of 49 (71%) cases displayed 2+/3+ levels of *HER2* expression, whereas another study failed to detect a higher prevalence of *HER2* overexpression and *HER2* gene amplification in lipid-rich carcinomas than in breast cancer in general.[139] Russo and colleagues[133] described a case of lipid-rich carcinoma that was negative for ER, PgR, and *HER2* (i.e., triple-negative phenotype) and displayed diffuse and strong positivity for basal-like markers, such as high-molecular-weight CKs, EGFR, and c-kit. High proliferation rates as defined by Ki-67 staining have also been reported, with 55% of the samples showing nuclear staining in more than 30% of the tumor cells.[128]

Treatment and Prognosis

Patients with lipid-rich carcinomas must be treated accordingly to routine guidelines for breast invasive carcinoma. In the largest series,[128] all patients received surgery, from lumpectomy plus axillary dissection to radical mastectomy. Axillary dissection was performed in nearly all patients and lymph nodes were involved in 79% of them, 65% with more than three positive nodes. Considering its aggressiveness, chemotherapy was given to all patients, with different regimens. The reported 2- and 5-year overall survival rates were 64.6% and 33.2%, respectively. Most lipid-rich tumors appear to be sensitive to paclitaxel, carboplatin, cisplatin, teniposide, and vincristine but resistant to adriamycin, rubidomycin, cytarabine, methopterin, and 5-fluorouracil.[128] The clinical validity of the assays employed by Shi and coworkers[128] is, however, yet to be demonstrated.

It has been suggested that lipid-rich carcinomas display a more aggressive clinical behavior, due to the frequent association with adverse prognostic factors, such as high-grade histology, low levels of hormone receptors expression, and high rates of lymph node metastasis. However, this is yet to be systematically demonstrated in a stage- and grade-matched basis.

Differential Diagnosis

All tumors that may display vacuolated or clear cells must be included in the differential diagnosis of lipid-rich carcinoma, such as glycogen-rich carcinoma, secretory carcinoma, apocrine carcinoma, myoepithelial carcinoma, and epithelioid liposarcoma.[132] Diffuse and strong positivity for neutral lipid is highly suggestive of lipid-rich carcinomas; in addition, other features may help in the differentiation of lipid-rich carcinoma from its mimics. Secretory carcinomas typically affect younger women, display lower-grade histology and consistently harbor the chromosomal translocation t(12;15) (p13;q25). Glycogen-rich carcinomas display PAS-positive diastase-sensitive glycogen in the cytoplasm of neoplastic cells. Apocrine carcinomas express GCDFP-15 strongly and diffusely, whereas lipid-rich carcinomas show focal, if any, GCDFP-15 expression. Myoepithelial carcinomas composed entirely of clear cells may be identified on the basis of immunoreactivity of neoplastic cells for myoepithelial markers, including p63 and smooth muscle markers. Epithelioid liposarcoma must display at least focal adipocytic differentiation, and scattered areas with spindle cells may also be found.

KEY PATHOLOGIC FEATURES

Lipid-rich Carcinoma

- High-grade, clear cell components mimic metastatic tumors.
- Vacuolated or foamy tumor cells mimic histiocytes.
- Tend to be hormone receptor–negative or weak, and *HER2*–.

GLYCOGEN-RICH CLEAR CELL CARCINOMA

Glycogen-rich clear cell carcinomas are tumors in which more than 90% of the neoplastic cells display abundant clear cytoplasm containing glycogen. First described in 1981 by Hull and associates,[140] its incidence varies depending on the series and set criteria (50% or 90%

of neoplastic cells with clear appearance) from less than 1% to 3% of all invasive breast carcinomas.[141–144] Ultrastructural analysis has demonstrated that the neoplastic cells contain massive quantities of non–membrane-bound particulate glycogen in the cytoplasm.[140]

Clinical Presentation

No specific feature characterizes glycogen-rich clear cell carcinomas at clinical presentation. In a series reporting on 20 cases, the patients' age ranged from 33 to 68 years (mean 52 yr).[143]

Clinical Imaging

The imaging findings of glycogen-rich carcinomas are similar to those of breast carcinomas generally.

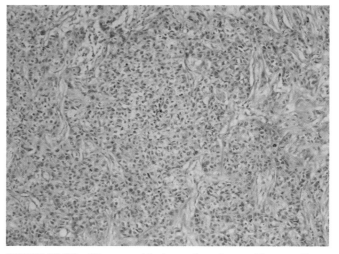

FIGURE 30-33 Glycogen-rich clear cell carcinoma. Tumor cells are organized in solid sheets with few intervening stroma.

KEY CLINICAL FEATURES

Glycogen-rich Clear Cell Carcinoma

- No distinct imaging or clinical presentation compared with IDC-NST.
- Prognosis similar to that of high-grade IDC-NST variant.

IDC-NST, invasive ductal carcinoma, no specific type.

Gross Pathology

No specific gross feature has been identified.[143] Reported tumor size ranges from 1 to 15 cm.[143,145] When present, an intraductal/intracystic papillary carcinoma may be noted grossly.[142,146]

Microscopic Pathology

Cytologic features are the defining criteria for glycogen-rich carcinomas. The tumor cells range in shape from polygonal to tall columnar, with sharply defined borders, large clear cytoplasm, and hyperchromatic irregular nuclei, which is often centrally located (Figures 30-33 and 30-34). Nuclear atypia may be significant, with clumped chromatin and conspicuous nucleoli. To establish a diagnosis of glycogen-rich carcinoma, high content of PAS-positive, diastase-labile glycogen must be demonstrated. It should be noted, however, that up to 58% of breast carcinomas without significant clear cell features may display intracytoplasmic glycogen.[141] Neoplastic cells of glycogen-rich carcinomas may also display mucin content, but this tends to be sparsely distributed.[145]

Glycogen-rich clear cell carcinomas may be purely intraductal or composed of intraductal and invasive components. Intraductal lesions may have solid, comedo, cribriform, or papillary growth patterns. Of note, glycogen-rich intracystic papillary lesions have been recurrently described.[146,147] In most cases, the predominant pattern of the invasive component is that of solid growth with sheets and nests of clear cells; less frequently, tubular or papillary formations may be found.[143]

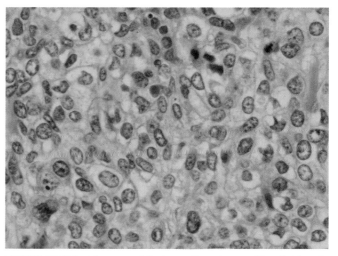

FIGURE 30-34 Glycogen-rich clear cell carcinoma. Neoplastic cells display an optically clear cytoplasm, with well-defined boundaries. Nuclei show moderate pleomorphism and are mostly centrally located. Mitotic activity is promptly observed.

Immunoprofile

The immunophenotype of glycogen-rich clear cell carcinomas has been described as similar to that of IDC-NSTs[51]; however, in the study by Kuroda and coworkers,[143] glycogen-rich clear cell carcinomas less frequently expressed ER (35%) and PgR (30%) than consecutive IDC-NSTs. The prevalence of *HER2* overexpression and *HER2* gene amplification seems indeed to be similar in glycogen-rich carcinomas as in breast cancer in general.[139,143]

Molecular Pathology

Flow cytometric analysis of six cases revealed that glycogen-rich clear cell carcinomas display a high DNA index. All cases analyzed to date were shown to be nondiploid and to display high S-phase fractions.[144]

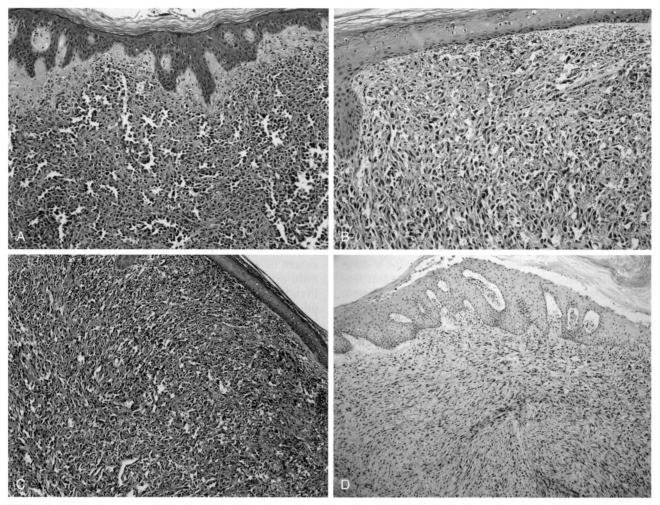

FIGURE 31-12 Angiosarcoma. Hobnail pattern **(A)** and vasoformative patterns **(B)** indicate the tumor is vascular. Spindled **(C)** and solid **(D)** growth patterns may make vascular differentiation less obvious.

and the infiltrative distribution is important to separate this tumor from a benign entity. Better-defined pattern areas of angiosarcoma are usually found nearby, further assisting in recognition.

Papillary endothelial growth is a feature of intermediate- and high-grade angiosarcoma. This pattern refers to a spectrum of endothelial proliferation ranging from small mounds and tufts of endothelium protruding into the vascular lumen to complex papillary branching that may fill and expand the vascular lumen. Whereas a rare focus of mild endothelial tufting may be seen in what is otherwise the vasoformative pattern of a low-grade angiosarcoma, these findings, particularly papillary growth, are generally indicative of a higher-grade tumor. Exuberant papillary endothelial growth may result in a complex pattern that appears nearly solid. Nuclear atypia may be subtle and mitoses may be rare in these papillary endothelial proliferations, resulting in a deceptively bland appearance. Endothelial cell shape may become more plump or spindled with increasing complexity of growth and with transition to more cellular solid growth.

Solid pattern of tumor growth typically presents as one or more foci within a background of vasoforma-tive growth. Occasionally, the tumor may present as

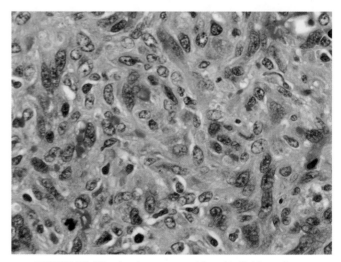

FIGURE 31-13 Angiosarcoma with epithelioid cytology.

multiple scattered cellular nodules that appear to arise from adjacent vessels. Endothelial cell shape is usually spindled in solid foci and arranged in a concentric or swirling pattern (Figure 31-21).

Epithelioid features in the tumor cells may be pronounced enough to result in an appearance equivalent

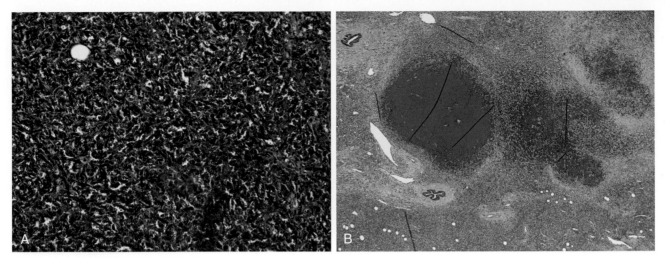

FIGURE 31-14 Angiosarcoma, high grade, with intratumoral hemorrhage **(A)** and large blood lakes **(B)**.

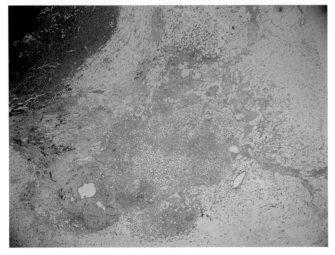

FIGURE 31-15 Angiosarcoma. High-grade tumors may be admixed with larger zones of intermediate- and low-grade tumor; therefore, a core biopsy may significantly underestimate the true tumor grade.

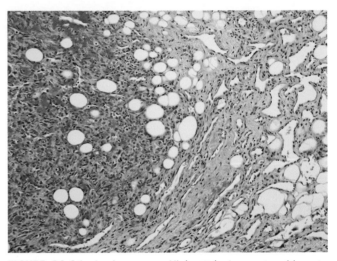

FIGURE 31-16 Angiosarcoma. High-grade tumor transitions to lower-grade architecture and cytology.

to that of epithelioid angiosarcoma seen in other anatomic sites. Few cases of epithelioid angiosarcoma or angiosarcoma with areas of epithelioid growth have been reported in the breast (Figure 31-22).[42,56–59] The growth pattern is predominantly solid. This morphology should raise the differential diagnosis of relatively more common entities such as metaplastic breast cancer or high-grade ductal carcinoma. Given the rarity of this entity, confirmatory immunohistochemistry with markers of vascular differentiation should be considered before diagnosing epithelioid angiosarcoma if there are no foci of well-developed vasoformative growth adjacent to the solid epithelioid areas.

A mixture of morphologic patterns and nuclear atypia may be found in some angiosarcomas. In tumors with mixed morphology, low-grade patterns may be common at the borders of the tumor or may form the bulk of the tumor. This poses several potential

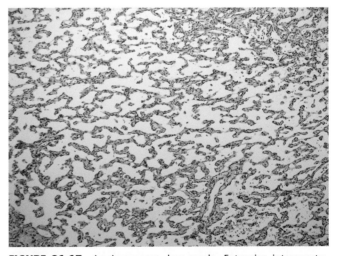

FIGURE 31-17 Angiosarcoma, low grade. Extensive interanastomoses of vascular channels.

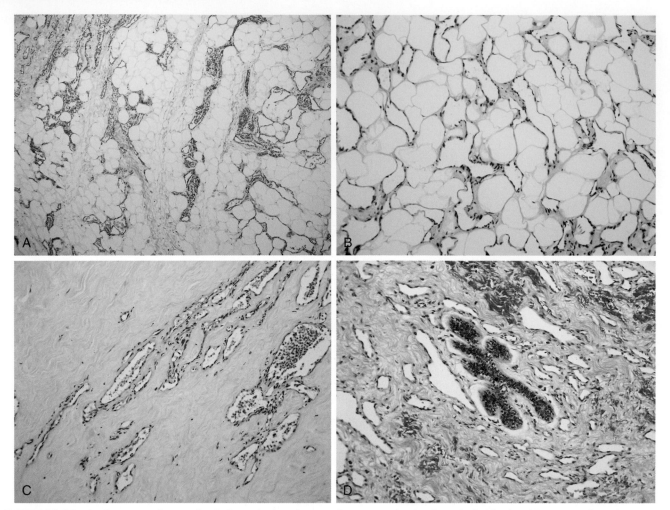

FIGURE 31-18 Angiosarcoma, low grade. **A,** Extensive invasion may be present despite deceptively bland architecture and cytology. Neoplastic vascular spaces may mimic adipocytes **(B),** native vascular structures within stroma **(C)** or around lobules **(D).**

diagnostic pitfalls. First, an angiosarcoma detected by core biopsy or incisional biopsy may be undergraded if the biopsy represents only the low-grade component of a tumor that has heterogeneous areas of lower- and higher-grade morphology. Designation of an angiosarcoma as low grade should be done only on evaluation of a complete excision. Second, a low-grade angiosarcoma may be misinterpreted as a hemangioma or angiolipoma in a core biopsy if the nuclear features are bland and if the density of neoplastic vascular spaces is low in the sampled tissue. A low threshold for excision is prudent when a vascular proliferation is identified at core biopsy, even when cytologically bland. Third, tumor size and margin status may be underestimated in cases in which the low-grade morphology at the tumor borders blends imperceptibly with the adjacent fat.

Immunohistochemistry is generally not required to confirm vascular differentiation for tumors in which convincing infiltrating vasoformative growth is identified. In cases of solid growth without obvious vascular differentiation, the distinction of angiosarcoma from carcinoma may be challenging on routine hematoxylin and eosin (H&E)–stained slides alone. In general, most vascular markers used in other anatomic sites, such as CD31, CD34, and Factor VIII, will also work in the breast.[42] It should be noted, though, that the sensitivity and staining intensity among vascular markers are variable and so a panel approach may be advisable. Keratins and epithelial membrane antigen (EMA) should be negative in most angiosarcoma, although some expression has been reported in areas of epithelioid growth pattern.[42,57,60] A diagnosis of angiosarcoma is supported by expression of vascular markers and by absence of EMA and absence, or limited focal expression, of keratins. Estrogen receptor (ER) and progesterone receptor (PgR) are absent in most angiosarcomas.[43,61,62] The role of immunohistochemistry in separating benign vascular lesions from low-grade angiosarcoma is not well defined, but at least one study suggests that Ki-67 can be useful. A Ki-67 index of 175 positive tumor cells per 1000 tumor cells correlates with the morphology of low-grade angiosarcoma whereas hemangiomas, with or without atypical features (e.g., mitoses or nuclear atypia without endothelial proliferation) exhibit lower Ki-67 indices.[63] High Ki-67 index in a vascular proliferation in a core biopsy should prompt excision; a low index should not be used to preclude excision if the morphologic features are at all suspicious.

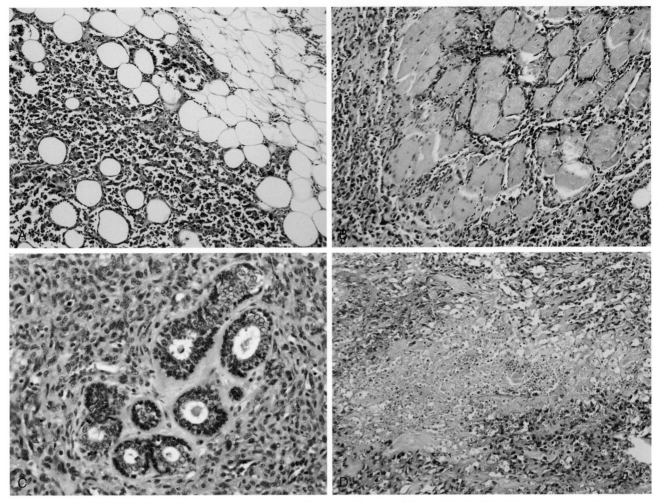

FIGURE 31-19 Angiosarcoma, high grade. Invasion into fat **(A)**, skeletal muscle **(B)**, and lobules **(C). D,** Tumor necrosis is common.

TREATMENT AND PROGNOSIS

The prognosis of primary breast angiosarcoma is poor. Although nodal metastasis is not common, these tumors have a predilection for local recurrence, distant metastasis, disease-related death, and short survival time.[40,42,43,45,46,50,55] Recent studies confirm the aggressive nature of this disease: the median time to recurrence has been reported to be as low as 5 months.[64] More than half of patients develop metastases.[40,42] The median time from diagnosis to metastasis was 2.8 years in one recent study.[42] Median disease-free survival is reported to be 2 to 3 years.[42,46,50,65] The median time from diagnosis to death is reported to be just over 2 years.[45,55] Overall survival at 5 years is reported to be 46% to 59%.[45,65] Among patients presenting with recurrence or subsequent metastasis, the median survival was under 1.2 years.[46] Bone, lung, liver, and skin are the most common sites of metastasis; metastasis is also reported in the contralateral breast.[40,42,45] Axillary lymph node involvement occurs in fewer than 10% of patients.[40,43,45]

Prognostic variables for primary breast angiosarcoma have been evaluated by various authors. Findings in these studies are difficult to compare because most studies are limited in sample size and some studies combine primary angiosarcomas with treatment-associated angiosarcoma. Most studies are too small to draw meaningful conclusions about prognostic variables. Tumor grade and tumor size are the best-studied variables. The literature contains conflicting conclusions for both. Two studies demonstrate that tumor grade predicts outcome: 5 year disease-free survival was 76% and 70% for low- and intermediate-grade angiosarcoma, compared with 15% for high-grade angiosarcoma in one study.[40] A smaller study showed a similar relationship between tumor grade and outcome.[55] In contrast, several more contemporary studies do not demonstrate any association between grade and outcome.[42,43,45,46] It is unclear why there are conflicting findings but it is notable that, for statistical analysis, some studies lump intermediate-grade tumors with high-grade tumors and others lump intermediate-grade tumors with low-grade tumors. The variables used in multivariate models also differ across these studies. The prognostic value of tumor size is similarly controversial. Some studies do not demonstrate any association between tumor size and outcome.[40,42,45,46] However, at least one study demonstrated in multivariate analysis that tumor size was the only prognostic factor.[43] One study demonstrated that tumor recurrence was the only predictor of outcome in a multivariate analysis model; median overall survival dropped from

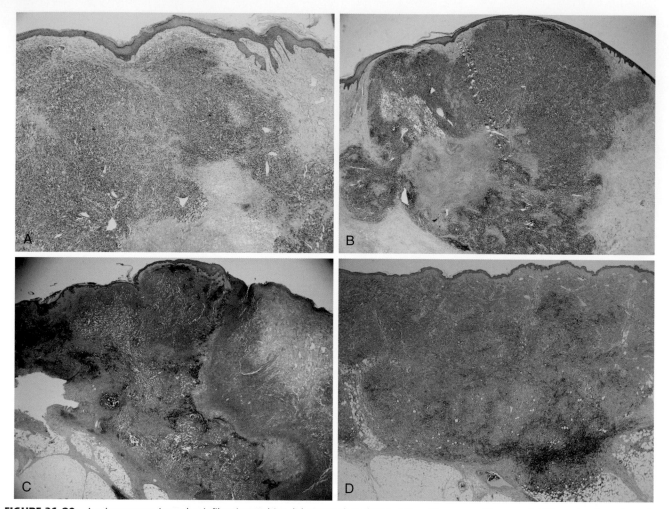

FIGURE 31-20   Angiosarcoma. Irregular, infiltrative multinodular growth in dermis **(A)**, with geographic necrosis **(B)**, and surface ulceration **(C)**. **D**, Tumor growth may also be diffuse without forming a discrete mass.

6.7 years to 1.2 years among patients with recurrent disease.[46]

Mastectomy is the main treatment reported in most studies.[40,42,43,45,46,64,65] Axillary lymph node sampling or dissection is variable; many studies report mastectomy without node sampling whereas some report node dissection in up to about half of patients. As mentioned earlier, nodal involvement by angiosarcoma is uncommon. Adjuvant treatment has not been well studied in breast angiosarcoma. The use of adjuvant chemotherapy and/or radiotherapy varies across studies, most of which have limited sample size and lack systematic approach to treatment, making it challenging to evaluate. Overall, adjuvant therapy is not currently viewed as a proven mainstay of treatment, although its potential role for local control is of interest.[65]

DIFFERENTIAL DIAGNOSIS

There are two major settings that raise a differential diagnosis with primary breast angiosarcoma: benign mimics of low-grade angiosarcoma and malignant mimics of high-grade angiosarcoma.

Benign mimics of angiosarcoma include hemangioma, angiolipoma and PASH.

Because most hemangiomas exhibit well-circumscribed borders, do not infiltrate intralobular stroma, or grow larger than 2 cm, the presence of ill-defined borders, infiltrative growth, or size greater than 2 cm favors low-grade angiosarcoma. The presence of a paired thick-walled artery and vein is often noted in hemangioma, as well as mural smooth muscle cells in venous hemangioma, but neither finding is observed in angiosarcoma.[40] Endothelial proliferation, piling up, tufting, or papillary growth is not a feature of hemangioma and should raise concern for low-grade angiosarcoma.

Malignant mimics of high-grade or epithelioid angiosarcoma include metaplastic breast carcinoma, invasive ductal carcinoma, metastatic carcinoma to the breast, acantholytic variant of squamous cell carcinoma, and melanoma. Metaplastic breast cancer, especially spindle cell/sarcomatoid variants, may contain foci of pseudovascular spaces resulting in an overall appearance that mimics angiosarcoma.[66] A similar pseudovascular pattern is produced in rare variants of squamous cell carcinoma with acantholytic growth.[67,68] Poorly differentiated invasive ductal carcinoma should be excluded before diagnosing epithelioid angiosarcoma, as should poorly differentiated tumors of metastatic origin, including melanoma,

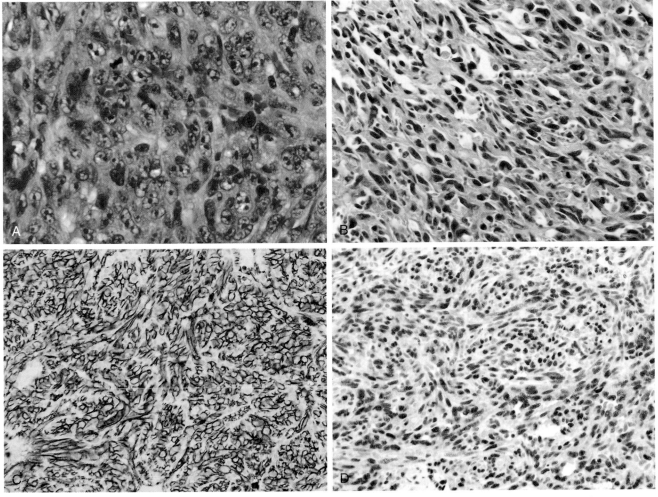

FIGURE 31-21 Angiosarcoma, high grade. Solid growth may mimic adenocarcinoma **(A)**. Spindled growth may mimic other sarcomas or metaplastic carcinoma **(B)**, necessitating confirmatory immunohistochemical staining: CD31 **(C)** or FLI-1 **(D)**.

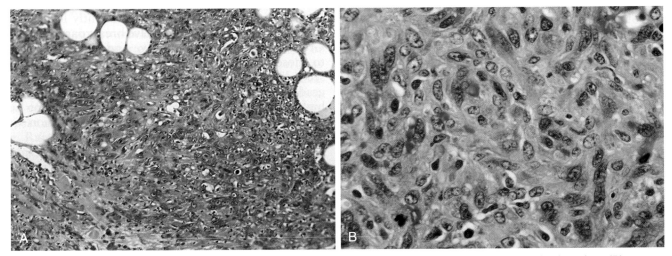

FIGURE 31-22 Angiosarcoma, epithelioid variant. Solid growth mimics carcinoma **(A)** as does epithelioid cytology **(B)**.

although these latter entities are uncommon.[69] Ductal carcinoma in situ is not typically reported in cases of primary angiosarcoma and so its presence weighs more in favor of a carcinoma; immunohistochemistry should be considered in this setting, as discussed earlier.

Secondary (Postradiation) Angiosarcoma

A spectrum of vascular pathology, from benign to malignant, may occur after radiation treatment of breast cancer. Benign vascular lesions include entities

TREATMENT AND PROGNOSIS

Local recurrence, distant spread, and death due to disease occurs in approximately one quarter of patients, generally within a few years of diagnosis. Mastectomy is the main treatment.

Although the number of cases in the literature is small, it appears that there is a prognostic difference between pure liposarcoma of the breast and liposarcoma arising as a component of phyllodes tumor. In the case of the latter setting, the behavior appears to follow that of the phyllodes tumor component in contrast to the more aggressive behavior of pure liposarcoma.[219–224]

OTHER SARCOMAS

Sarcomas arising in the breast make up a heterogeneous group of neoplasms and account for less than 1% of all breast neoplasms.[225,226] After excluding malignant phyllodes tumors, which account for the majority (and the only biphasic) of these neoplasms, primary and metastatic sarcomas remain.[227] The former consists of those arising from the specialized, hormonally responsive periductal stroma as well as from the fibroconnective tissue and adipose tissue. Tumors arising from the specialized, hormonally responsive periductal stroma are collectively termed "stromal sarcomas,"[202] whereas others are further subtyped by cell of origin and represent in order of frequency: angiosarcoma, malignant fibrous histiocytomas, fibrosarcoma, liposarcomas, and leiomyosarcoma.[204,227–229] Mammary osteosarcoma or chondrosarcoma that is not fundamentally a metaplastic carcinoma is exceedingly rare. Compared with other anatomic sites, the breast appears to give rise to a relatively higher proportion of angiosarcomas, some of which are secondary to radiation therapy.[202] Also, sarcomas are not uncommonly seen arising within malignant phyllodes tumor. Other sarcomas are more commonly metastatic tumors originating from other sites such as rhabdomyosarcoma and alveolar soft part sarcoma. Stromal sarcoma is discussed here, and select histogenetically and immunohistochemically well-defined subtypes such as angiosarcoma, leiomyosarcoma, and liposarcoma are discussed elsewhere in this chapter. Malignant phyllodes tumors and lymphomas are discussed in Chapters 12 and 35, respectively.

Clinical Presentation

Most commonly, patients complain of a progressively enlarging breast mass/lump for a number of months. Associated pain or skin changes occur in some cases.[228] The vast majority affects women, but these tumors can also occur in men. Although the average age at presentation is in the sixth decade of life,[214,239] adolescents and the elderly can also be affected.[204,227–229] Clinically, the tumor sizes span a broad range (1–20 cm) but most are 3 to 5 cm.[202,229] There is no predisposition in laterality or quadrant, and they are typically solitary and unilateral. Coexisting lymphadenopathy can occur in up to one third of patients; however, virtually

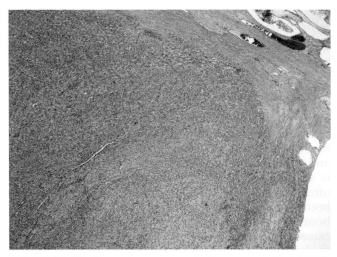

FIGURE 31-52 Stromal sarcoma, not otherwise specified (NOS). Grossly circumscribed tumor shows invasive microscopic tumor borders.

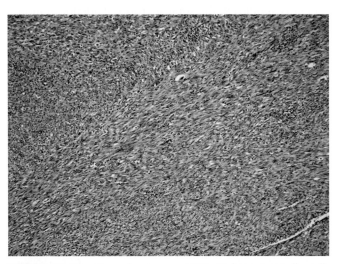

FIGURE 31-53 Stromal sarcoma, NOS. Malignant spindle cells grow in sheets or fascicles.

all have shown only reactive lymph nodes at histologic examination.[204]

Gross Pathology

Tumors are firm, fleshy, and pale to gray. Soft, cystic areas, and necrotic and/or hemorrhagic components can be seen. Typically, the tumors are unencapsulated. Tumor borders are grossly well circumscribed despite being microscopically invasive.

Microscopic Pathology

Pure stromal sarcomas are composed of malignant spindle cells with or without associated hemorrhage and necrosis in interlacing fascicles (Figures 31-52 to 31-54). However, the growth pattern can show considerable intratumoral heterogeneity (Figures 31-55 to 31-57). The degree of nuclear atypia can be low, intermediate, or high (Figure 31-58). Mitoses are variably present and heterogeneously distributed. The histologic or tumor

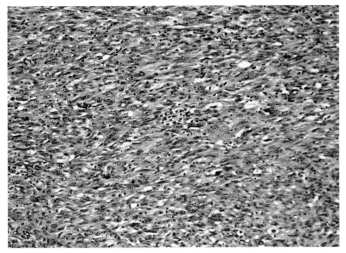

FIGURE 31-54 Stromal sarcoma, NOS. Higher magnification of Figure 31-53 shows malignant spindle cells and frequent mitoses.

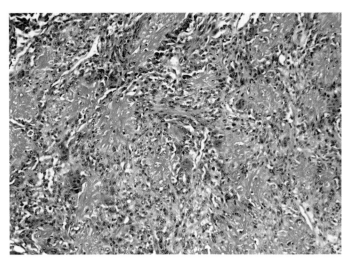

FIGURE 31-57 Stromal sarcoma, NOS. However, focal areas showed osseous differentiation.

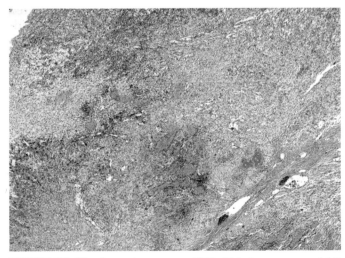

FIGURE 31-55 Stromal sarcoma, NOS. This tumor can exhibit morphologic heterogeneity including heterologous components. All immunostains were negative for metaplastic carcinoma in this case.

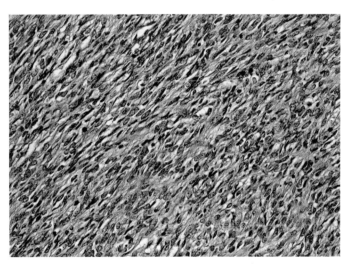

FIGURE 31-58 Stromal sarcoma, NOS. Example of high nuclear grade.

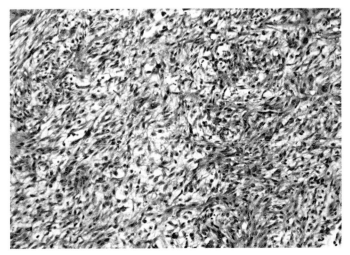

FIGURE 31-56 Stromal sarcoma, NOS. Case in Figure 31-55 showed a predominantly spindle cell pattern.

grade is based on prognostically significant features such as nuclear grade, mitotic index, and tumor border characteristics (invasive vs. pushing).[225] Others have used the presence of necrosis in place of tumor border.[227]

Treatment and Prognosis

Primary treatment should consist of at least simple mastectomy. Breast conservation with postoperative radiotherapy with or without chemotherapy should be reserved for only low-grade and/or smaller-sized sarcomas. Because tumor spread is rarely via lymphatics, involvement of axillary lymph nodes is rare and usually indicative of end-stage disease.[229–231] As such, axillary lymph node evaluation is not indicated in these patients unless they are clinically involved, in which case removal ensures local clearance of tumor.[232,233] Adjuvant treatment is controversial. Postoperative radiation therapy was found to achieve good locoregional

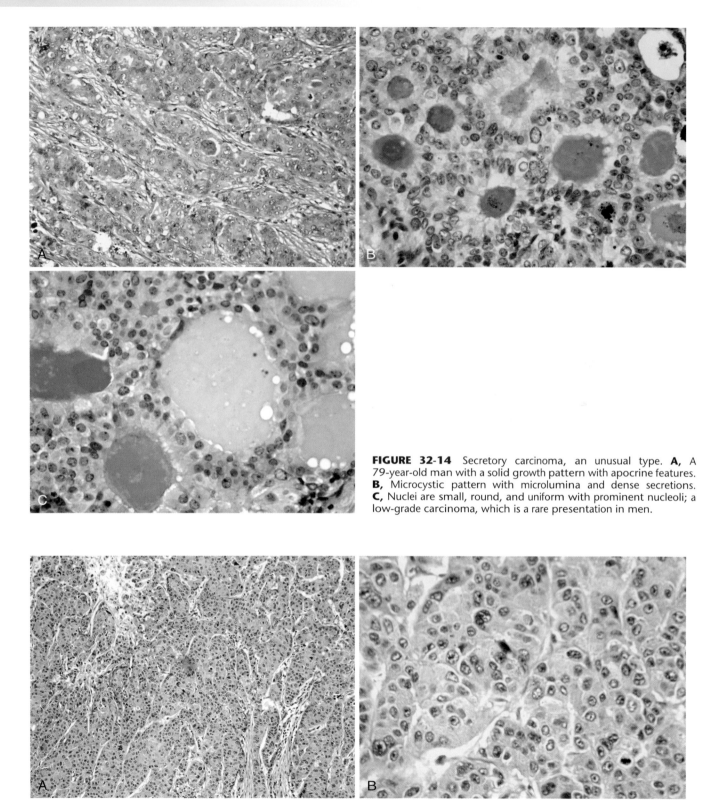

FIGURE 32-14 Secretory carcinoma, an unusual type. **A,** A 79-year-old man with a solid growth pattern with apocrine features. **B,** Microcystic pattern with microlumina and dense secretions. **C,** Nuclei are small, round, and uniform with prominent nucleoli; a low-grade carcinoma, which is a rare presentation in men.

FIGURE 32-15 Apocrine carcinoma. **A,** Solid pattern with apocrine features mimics metastatic prostatic carcinoma. **B,** Poor–nuclear grade features resembles a metastatic prostatic carcinoma.

by immunohistochemistry. Several studies have evaluated the incidence of *p53* mutations in breast cancer in men.[96-102] A large review of male breast carcinomas revealed *p53* mutation in up to 30% by immunohistochemistry.[98] These results are comparable with data reported for breast cancer in women. However, the prognostic significance of *p53* mutations in breast cancer in men has not been clearly established, but most studies have found *p53* mutations to be associated with decreased survival.[99]

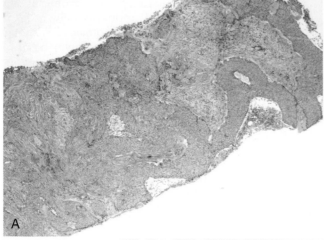

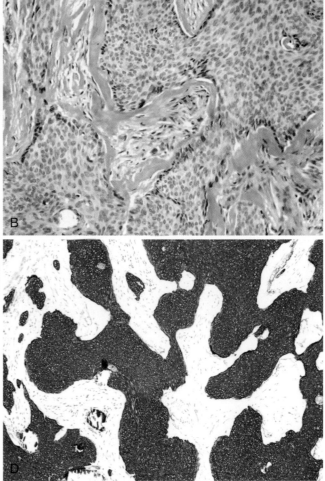

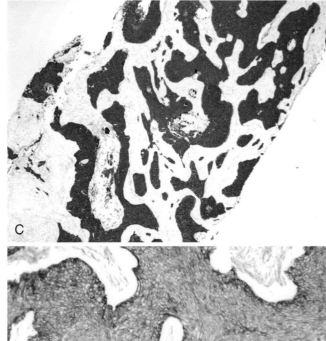

FIGURE 32-16 Basal cytokeratins and epidermal growth factor receptor (EGFR) expression in male breast tumors. Whereas the basal-like variant of carcinoma has been described in males, this case represents a pitfall—a squamous cell carcinoma of the skin of the breast. **A,** The invasive carcinoma on core needle biopsy shows a spindle growth pattern. **B,** Spindle squamous cell carcinoma. **C,** Basal cytokeratins (CK)—CK5 shows a diffuse strong staining. **D,** CK14 and CK17 show similar diffuse strong staining. **E,** EGFR shows strong and diffuse staining. An identical keratin pattern is seen in the basal-like carcinoma of breast.

BCL-2

bcl-2 is a proto-oncogene that inhibits apoptosis and thereby promotes cell growth. In women with breast cancer, expression of *bcl-2* has been associated with favorable prognosis.[103,104] Overall, *bcl-2* expression in male breast carcinoma is reported to be positive in 79%.[104] Men tend to have significantly higher *bcl-2* expression than women[103]; however, the expression has not been shown to have prognostic significance in men.[104] The high rates of expression of *bcl-2* in male breast cancer suggest that apoptotic mechanisms may be important in the etiology of the carcinoma in men.

CYCLIN D1

Cyclin D1 is involved in cell cycle regulation and helps to control the cell's entry into S-phase. In women with breast carcinomas, this gene is oncogenic but appears to be associated with a favorable prognosis. In a study of 111 of male breast carcinomas tested for cyclin D1 overexpression, 60 (58%) were immunoreactive.[100] The study results are similar to women who have shown about 50% overexpression for cyclin D1.[105] Rayson and coworkers[100] have found that cyclin D1 negativity was associated with significantly decreased progression-free survival, indicating that overexpression of this gene may be a favorable prognostic factor in men with carcinoma of the breast.

BASAL CYTOKERATINS AND EPIDERMAL GROWTH FACTOR RECEPTOR

The expression of distinct basal cytokeratins (CKs) such as CK5/6, 14, 17 and EGFR or *HER1* have been utilized to identify a subset of tumors with basal-like differentiation in female breast cancers.[88,106,107] Basal-like carcinomas show a typical immunoprofile of estrogen receptor (ER)–/progesterone receptor (PgR)–, *HER2*–, CK5/6+, or EGFR+.[88,89] In a few studies that aimed to classify the molecular subtypes of male breast cancers based on the expression profile of immunomarkers, CK5/6 expression was seen in 28% of ER+ carcinomas.[108-110] However, in this study, no basal-like carcinomas were seen.

Another study that evaluated the CK profiles in male breast cancer have reported approximately a 12.5% (4/32) prevalence of basal-like carcinomas.[110] Although, at present, the existence of (triple-negative) basal-like phenotype in male breast carcinomas is uncommon, it is also plausible that a subset of luminal B type of aggressive high-grade carcinomas may show patchy basal keratin expression.[110]

In male breast cancers, the reported expression of EGFR ranges from 20% to 76%.[111,112] Luminal B subtype of cancers tend to have high nuclear grade and more frequent expression of EGFR, probably attributing to their aggressive biology. No association was found with either ER status or with prognosis, although conclusions are limited by the small study size.

Hormone Receptors in Male Breast Cancer

Carcinomas of the male breast have a slightly higher rate of hormone receptor positivity than female breast carcinomas when matched for tumor stage, grade, and patient age (48–50 yr).[108-110] The literature indicates that 81% of breast cancers in men express ER, and

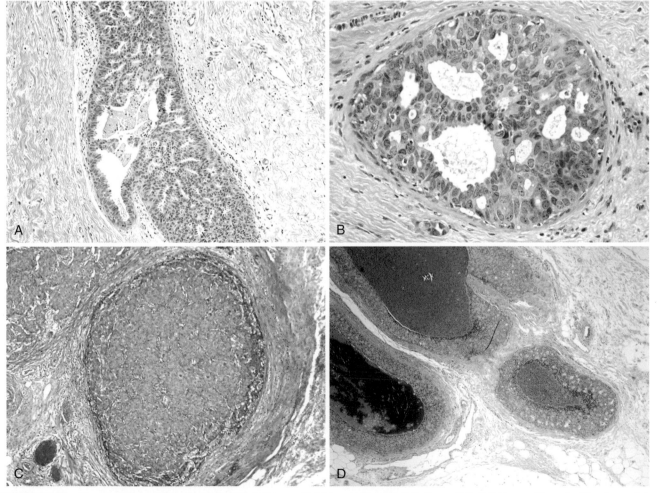

FIGURE 32-17   Morphologic variants of intraductal carcinoma. **A,** Micropapillary. **B,** Cribriform. **C-E,** Solid type with and without associated comedo necrosis.

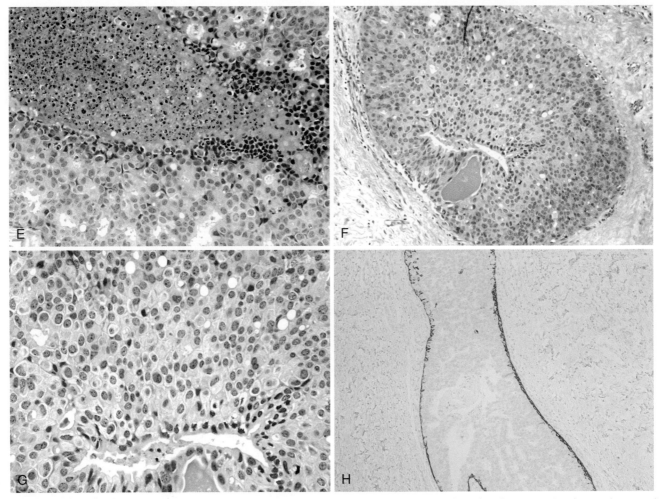

FIGURE 32-17, cont'd Morphologic variants of intraductal carcinoma. **C-E,** Solid type with and without associated comedo necrosis. **F** and **G,** Apocrine type with high nuclear grade. The morphologic variants seen in male breast cancer are similar to those seen in females. **H,** SMM-HC demonstrates the presence of myoepithelial cells in a continuous membrane staining pattern in this ductal carcinoma in situ (DCIS).

74% express PgR. In contrast to women, men do not have a higher incidence of ER+ tumors with advancing age.[108-111]

HER2/Neu

Studies of HER2 expression in male breast carcinoma are limited, and with conflicting results. Recent studies indicate that HER overexpression occurs in about 15% of cases,[112] no different than the prevalence of HER2 overexpression in women. HER2 overexpression predicts far poorer outcome, and with limited outcome data, men are treated analogous to women (Figure 32-18).[112-115]

Management

SURGERY AND RADIOTHERAPY

The optimal recommended treatment includes modified radical mastectomy. Breast-conserving therapies are more successful in women than men owing to the abundant amount of breast tissue. Conversely, because

DCIS in the male breast carries a good prognosis, total mastectomy without axillary dissection has been the standard therapy.[99]

ROLE OF SENTINEL NODE BIOPSY AND AXILLARY LYMPH NODE DISSECTION

The morbidity due to axillary lymph node dissection is similar for men and women. The role of sentinel lymph node (SLN) biopsy in males with breast cancer is evolving owing to lack of experience and lack of large randomized trials. In a large retrospective review of SLN biopsies in men, the procedure was successful in 97% of patients.[116] Negative SLNs were found in 51% of patients and positive SLNs were found in 49% of patients. In 59% of the men, node positivity was determined intraoperatively, prompting immediate axillary lymph node dissection. At a median follow-up of 28 months (range 5–96 mo), there were no axillary recurrences. In comparison with their female counterparts, men with breast cancer had larger tumors and were more likely to have positive nodes. SLN biopsy is successful and accurate in male breast cancer patients. Although a

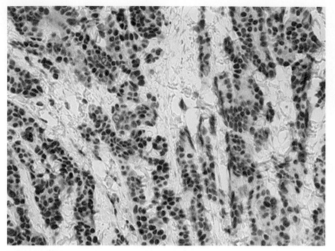

ER pos 270

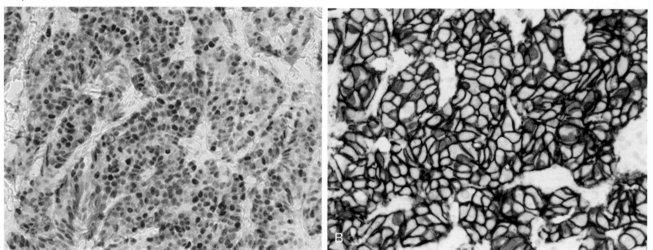

PR pos 210

A

FIGURE 32-18   Hormone receptor expression. The majority of male breast cancers express estrogen (ER) and progesterone (PgR) receptor. **A,** Nuclear expression of ER (H score 270) and PgR (H score 210) in male breast carcinomas. **B,** *HER2* 3+ (clone 4B5; Ventana, Tucson, AZ) by IHC is seen in about 15% of male breast carcinomas.

larger proportion of men have positive nodes, for men with negative nodes, SLN biopsy may potentially reduce morbidity related to axillary lymph node dissection.

The role of adjuvant radiation therapy is still evolving and is unclear in male breast carcinomas. Radiation has shown to reduce the risk of locoregional relapse but does not change the overall survival.[40] The reported 5-year locoregional recurrence rates range from 3% to 20%.[40] Radiation is considered in patients with risk factors of local relapse such as nodal capsular extension, large tumors, and cutaneous or muscle involvement. Further locoregional failure carries an unfavorable prognosis.[115,117]

SYSTEMIC THERAPY

Hormonal Therapy

Hormonal therapy with tamoxifen in ER+ breast cancers in women has shown significantly improved survival rates.[117–121] Because the hormone receptor expression

is prevalent in men, adjuvant hormonal therapy seems undeniably promising. Although large randomized trials have not been performed to demonstrate the efficacy of hormonal therapy, large retrospective studies have addressed and demonstrated the benefit of using tamoxifen as first-line adjuvant treatment in hormone receptor–positive men.[39,40] In a study by Ribeiro and colleagues,[125] the overall 5-year survival rates were found to be superior in patients treated with tamoxifen (61% vs. 44%) particularly in stage II or III. Hormonal therapy for a 5-year period has been recommended for patients who are hormone receptor–positive.[121,122]

Chemotherapy

The role of adjuvant chemotherapy in men is less well established and data are limited. In a National Cancer Institute (NCI) case-control study of 24 male patients with stage II breast cancer, the overall 5-year survival rates among treated patients was 80%.[123]

In another study, male patients who were node-positive and treated with anthracycline therapy had a better overall 5-year survival rate of up to 85% compared with the control study group. Although there are no data to determine which group of men benefit from chemotherapy, in routine practice, chemotherapy is offered to men with node-positive disease and tumors larger than 1.0 cm.[123,124]

Prognosis

Axillary lymph node status, tumor size, histologic grade, and hormone receptor status have shown to be significant prognostic factors in men. In a large retrospective study reported by Guinee and associates,[115] the reported 5-year survival rates in node-negative versus node-positive patients were 90% versus 65%. In the same study, the authors reported that the number of positive lymph nodes were predictive of survival as well. The 10-year reported survival in patients who were node negative was 84% in comparison with patients with one to three lymph nodes involvement was 44% and 14% for four or more positive nodes.[115] In a retrospective French study of 397 patients, the 5-year survival rates for tumors less than 5 cm in size were better than tumors larger than 5 cm.[120]

Poor histologic grade was similarly associated with decreased survival rates.[119,125,126] Ribeiro and colleagues[118] found a statistically significant difference in 5-year survival based on histologic grade of tumor (grade I: 76%; grade II: 66%; grade III: 43%).

Hormonal status in men as a prognostic factor is debatable owing to limited number of studies. In a retrospective study of 229 patients from Princess Margaret Hospital in Toronto, after adjustment for patient age, tumor size, lymph node status, and type of therapy, hormone receptor positivity was not significant.[123] However, in a similarly designed study of 215 patients from Wisconsin, it was demonstrated that men with hormone receptor–positive tumors had improved overall survival, even after adjustment for tumor stage and axillary lymph node status.[124]

Clinical outcome for men with breast cancer is similar to that for women. The overall 5-year survival rates for all stages of breast cancer in men have been reported to range from 36% to 66%, and 10-year overall survival rates range from 17% to 52%.[125-134] Disease-specific survival rates are somewhat higher; 52% to 74% of patients are alive at 5 years and 26% to 51% are alive at 10 years.[121-124] Overall 5-year survival rates are greater than 90% for stage I, 41% to 78% for stage II, 16% to 57% for stage III, and 0% to 14% for stage IV disease.[125,128]

Although prior studies have reported poorer survival rates in men than in women, most recent studies show that men and women have fairly equivalent prognoses when matched for age and stage of disease.[125-134] Men do have lower overall survival rates, but this is probably due to later stage at presentation, more advanced age, and high rates of death from intercurrent illness. The cause of these high death rates in men with breast cancer remains unclear; however, it may in part be due to the older age of presentation in these men.

Metastatic Disease

The reported prevalence of metastatic disease in males is in the range of 7% to 15%.[39,132] The pattern of metastasis is similar to that in females, and rare sites such as the choroid have been reported as well.[129] Hormonal therapy has been the mainstay of treatment for metastatic carcinoma of the male breast since the 1960s.[133] Prior to tamoxifen, ablative orchiectomy, adrenalectomy, and hypophysectomy were the initial hormonal therapies. ER positivity appears to predict response to hormonal therapy. Jaiyesimi and coworkers reported that 69% of men with ER+ tumors responded to hormonal manipulation compared with 0% of men with ER– tumors.[134] Chemotherapy, however, can offer significant palliation to men in whom hormonal therapy has failed, or those with hormone receptor–negative disease.[117,118] Radiotherapy is effective as a palliative treatment for choroidal metastases.[133]

SUMMARY

The incidence of breast carcinomas in males is approximately 1% and has been slowly increasing. Male breast carcinomas tend to express ER and tend to have similar rates of *HER2* expression as seen in female breast carcinomas. Male breast carcinomas have been shown to be associated with *BRCA2* rather than *BRCA1*. Although similarities exist between breast carcinomas in males and females, it is not appropriate to extrapolate data from female disease for the treatment of males. Future studies are in need, particularly specific multi-institutional trials, to better understand the clinicopathologic features and establish optimal therapy.

REFERENCES

1. Vorherr H. Fibrocystic breast disease: pathophysiology, pathomorphology. Clinical picture and management. Am J Obstet Gynecol 1986;154:161-179.
2. Banik S, Hale R. Fibrocystic disease in the male breast. Histopathology 1988;12:214-216.
3. Robertson KE, Kazmi SA, Jordan LB. Female-type fibrocystic disease with papillary hyperplasia in a male breast. J Clin Pathol 2010;63:88-89.
4. McClure J, Banerjee SS, Sandilands DGD. Female type cystic hyperplasia in a male beast. Postgrad Med J 1985;61:441-443.
5. Rosen PP, Cantrell B, Mullen DL, DePalo A. Juvenile papillomatosis (Swiss cheese disease) of the breast. Am J Surg Pathol 1980;4:3-12.
6. Ståle Sund B, Kåre Topstad T, Nesland JM. A case of juvenile papillomatosis of the male breast. Cancer 1992;70:126-128.
7. Rosen PP, Lyngholm B, Kinne DW, Beattie EJ Jr. Juvenile papillomatosis of the breast and family history of breast carcinoma. Cancer 1982;49:2591-2595.
8. Rosen PP, Holmes G, Lesser ML, et al. Juvenile papillomatosis and breast carcinoma. Cancer 1985;55:1345-1352.
8a. Rice HE, Acosta A, Brown RL, et al. Juvenile papillomatosis of the male breast in infants: two case reports. Pediatr Surg Int 2000;16:104-106.
8b. Pacilli M, Sebire NJ, Thambapillai E, Pierro A. Juvenile papillomatosis in a male infant with Noonan syndrome, café au lait spots, and family history of breast carcinoma. Pediatr Blood Cancer 2005;95:991–993.

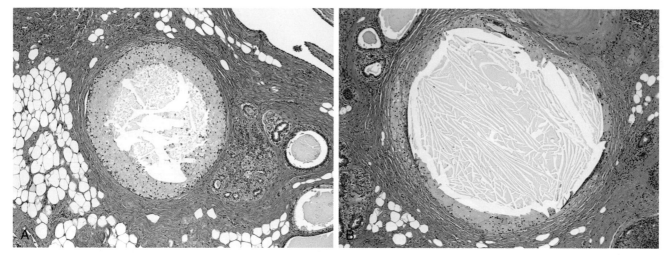

FIGURE 33-4 JP. **A** and **B,** Some cysts are filled with foamy histiocytes, which can rupture with spillage of histiocytes into the adjacent stroma, causing an inflammatory response.

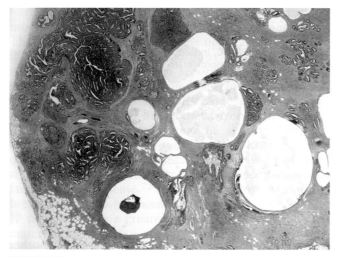

FIGURE 33-5 JP. Papillomas can represent a dominant component in some cases.

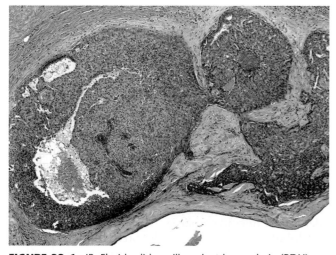

FIGURE 33-6 JP. Florid solid papillary duct hyperplasia (PDH) can contain central necrosis and occasional mitoses, neither of which should be considered atypical findings.

Rarely, atypical duct hyperplasia (ADH) and carcinoma arise in JP. ADHs of the cribriform and micropapillary patterns are most common (Figure 33-11). Coexisting carcinoma is rare at the time of diagnosis but has been found in up to 15% of studied patients.[8,13,15] Ductal carcinoma in situ, lobular carcinoma in situ, invasive duct carcinoma, and secretory carcinoma in association with JP have been described.[7,8,13,14,22–24] Thus far, *BRCA1* or *BRCA2* mutations has not been reported to play a role in these patients.

Treatment and Prognosis

Wide local excision is curative. Although recurrence can occur if incompletely excised, further excision for lesions that have been grossly excised is not recommended.[7,8,13,15,20] Re-excision should be considered in incompletely excised JP cases with atypical hyperplasia or instances of recurrent disease. The risk of developing breast carcinoma in patients previously diagnosed with unilateral JP without recurrence has not been adequately assessed because published studies have insufficiently long follow-up to draw such prognostic conclusions. Nonetheless, 10% of patients with JP developed carcinoma in one study of 41 patients with a median follow-up period of 14 years.[15] The long-term prognosis of these patients remains undefined, and hence, postoperative close clinical surveillance is recommended. Furthermore, the studies suggest that JP may be a marker for breast carcinoma in the patient's female relatives, and consequently, screening of these family members is advisable.

Differential Diagnosis

Because individual components of JP represent the spectrum of fibrocystic disease, the distinction from fibrocystic changes must be made. Histologic findings of a localized arrangement of proliferative components, the presence of multiple cysts, some filled with foamy macrophages, and the histologic transition of duct hyperplasia to apocrine metaplasia/hyperplasia are more affirming of JP than other features. Correlation with clinical features,

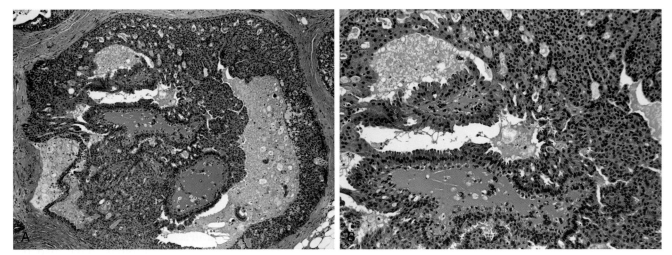

FIGURE 33-7 JP. **A** and **B,** Histologic merging of duct hyperplasia and apocrine metaplasia/hyperplasia is an uncommon finding outside the context of this entity.

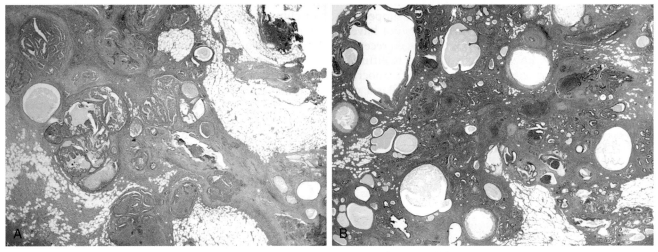

FIGURE 33-8 JP. **A** and **B,** Sclerosis can involve parts of this entity.

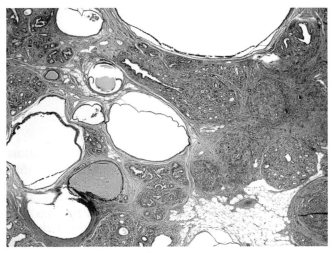

FIGURE 33-9 JP. Nodular sclerosing adenosis is a prominent component in this example and the source of microcalcifications.

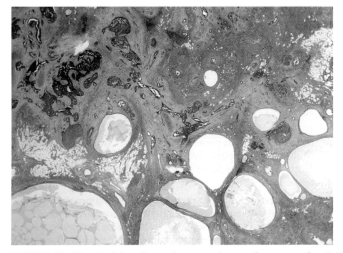

FIGURE 33-10 JP. Sclerosis can be extensive, to the extent that it obscures the fundamental lesion.

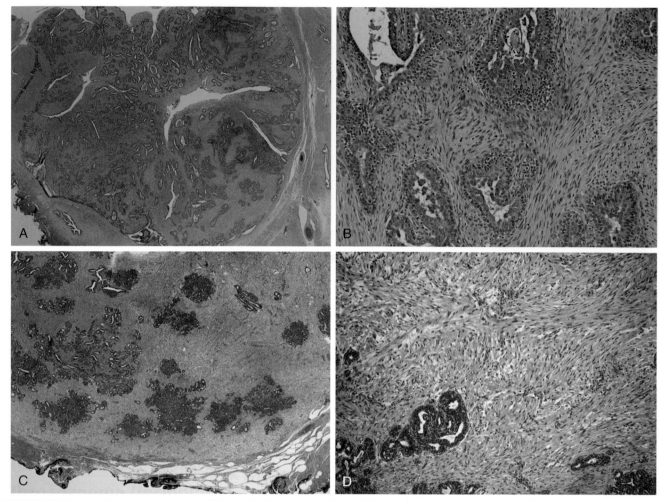

FIGURE 33-16 Juvenile fibroadenomas in 19-year-old females. **A-D,** Each of these two examples show hypercellular but cytologically bland stroma, and one (**C** and **D**) also shows diffuse micropapillary duct hyperplasia. Note the sharply circumscribed tumor border in both cases.

appreciably higher in this clinical context, managing patients similarly to those with conventional fibroadenomas is reasonable.[39]

Phyllodes Tumor

Phyllodes tumor (historically known as *cystosarcoma phyllodes*) is a biphasic tumor that constitutes 0.3% to 0.9% of all breast neoplasms.[48] At least 45 cases of phyllodes tumor arising in this age group have been described[49–62] and together account for 5% to 8% of phyllodes tumors across all ages.[35]

CLINICAL PRESENTATION

Similar to those with juvenile fibroadenoma, a patient's chief complaint is a rapidly growing but painless breast mass. The mass is usually present for several months. Physical examination reveals a mobile, rubbery breast mass that ranges in size from 2 to 13 cm (average 6 cm).[49-61] Tense skin or distended veins can be seen in some cases, features also mimicking that of juvenile fibroadenoma.[5] Less common signs include skin ulceration or erythema, nipple retraction, nipple discharge, and axillary lymphadenopathy (reactive).[35]

CLINICAL IMAGING

Regardless of the age of the patient, distinguishing phyllodes tumor from other fibroepithelial lesions is difficult if not impossible by mammography, sonography and MRI due to significant overlap in features.[5] The sonographic features of phyllodes tumor and fibroadenoma are the same. Anechoic cysts or clefts can be seen in both phyllodes tumors and juvenile fibroadenomas. By some, the presence of peripheral cysts is the only indication by imaging that could suggest the diagnosis of phyllodes tumor.[36,43] There are no particular features of phyllodes tumors arising in this age group that are unique. Furthermore, there are no distinguishing features by imaging which can discern benign from malignant phyllodes tumors.[5] Like fibroadenomas, sonography is the imaging modality of choice in these patients for diagnosis and follow-up.

GROSS PATHOLOGY

As with phyllodes tumors in adults, these tumors appear unencapsulated but well-circumscribed, the latter even if microscopically found to have invasive tumor borders. Multinodularity, if present, is characteristic of phyllodes

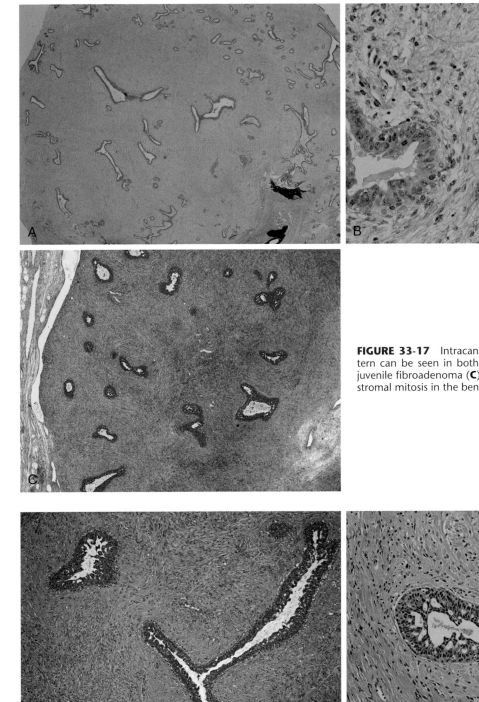

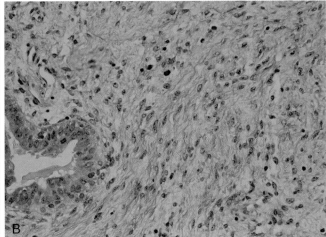

FIGURE 33-17 Intracanalicular growth pattern. This growth pattern can be seen in both benign phyllodes tumor (**A** and **B**) and juvenile fibroadenoma (**C**), both from 14-year-old females. **B**, Note stromal mitosis in the benign phyllodes tumor.

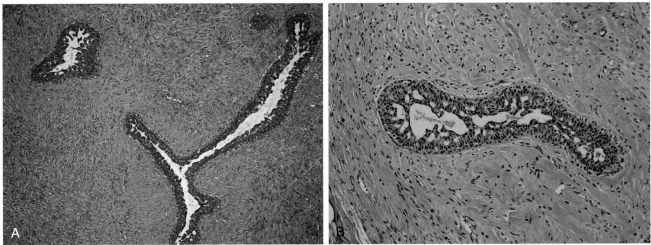

FIGURE 33-18 Micropapillary duct hyperplasia. **A** and **B**, Micropapillary duct hyperplasia can be seen in both juvenile fibroadenoma and benign phyllodes tumor. Note tapering of cells toward the tips of individual micropapillary fronds.

tumor, which can also be appreciated microscopically. More often, however, the mass is solitary. The cut surface of the tumor is usually bulging and firm like fibroadenomas; the color is similarly tan or white-gray. A cystic appearance can occur in some examples that have a particularly exaggerated intracanalicular growth pattern. Necrosis or hemorrhage is more likely to be found in malignant forms.

MICROSCOPIC PATHOLOGY

In general, the morphologic features used to diagnose phyllodes tumors are the same as those applied to ones of older patients. Phyllodes tumors are biphasic tumors with varying degrees of stromal cellularity and epithelial hyperplasia as well as variable number of stromal mitoses. The tumor borders can be well-circumscribed

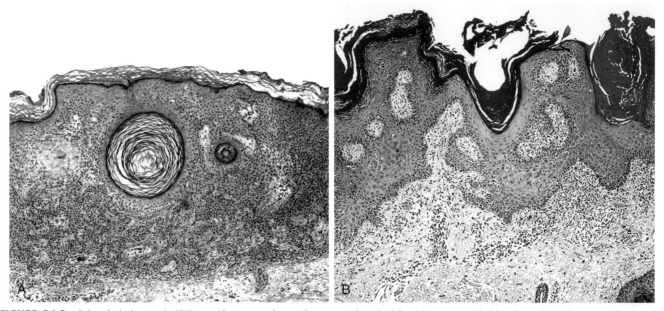

FIGURE 34-3 Seborrheic keratosis (SK) manifests cross-bars of compact basaloid keratinocytes with bland cytologic features. **A,** Circular intraepithelial deposits of lamellated keratin ("horn cysts") are typical. **B,** When SK becomes inflamed or irritated, it may acquire moderate nuclear atypia and advanced squamous differentiation, potentially simulating squamous carcinoma.

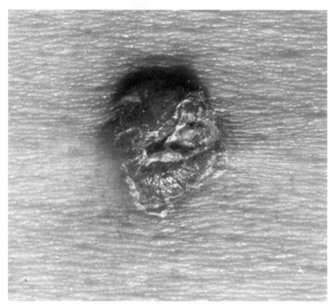

FIGURE 34-4 Clear cell acanthoma is a crusted, red-brown papule, which is clinically nondescript.

squamous cell carcinoma in situ. The microscopic findings include irregular acanthosis, focal hypergranulosis, hyperkeratosis, and lichenoid lymphocytic inflammation that tend to obscure the dermoepidermal junction. There is also vacuolar change in the basal layer keratinocytes, and numerous densely eosinophlic Civatte bodies are present (Figures 34-6 and 34-7).[9] Although there are microscopic differences between LPLK and lichen planus,[10] the most pragmatic way of separating the two entities is to obtain a clinical history. If a lesion in question is solitary, it is likely an LPLK.

SURFACE CARCINOMAS OF THE MAMMARY SKIN

Basal cell carcinoma (BCC) is the most common cutaneous malignancy.[11,12] The overwhelming majority of BCCs appear as a papule or nodule, often with a pearly surface or edge, as well as erythematous plaques or ulcerated areas of induration (Figure 34-8).

Despite the existence of numerous morphologic subtypes, BCCs have several constant morphologic features. The typical appearance is that of a multinodular dermal proliferation of basaloid cells with hyperchromatic nuclei and scant amphophilic cytoplasm. Palisading of columnar cells is common around the periphery of the nodules. In formalin-fixed specimens, the adjacent fibromyxoid stroma tends to retract from the edges of the tumor cell nests (Figure 34-9). Small collections of stromal mucin are often present among or around the cell groups. Internal cystic change and brisk apoptosis are also common in BCC. Nuclear features are usually rather bland, but a variant with marked nuclear atypia does exist. Surprisingly, its clinical behavior is similar to that of "ordinary" BCCs.[13] Mitotic activity is variable but is usually not brisk.

Some histologic subtypes of BCC are associated with a more aggressive clinical behavior. The *infiltrative* or *morpheaform* pattern shows small angular nests, short cords, and single cells in a desmoplastic stroma (Figure 34-10). The term *metatypical* BCC has been used for those tumors having intermixed areas of squamous differentiation. *Superficial* BCC is not clinically aggressive but may be difficult to eradicate because of its broad growth over a rather large skin area.

Other histologic variants that have an indolent clinical evolution are *nodulocystic* BCC, in which the cell islands are arranged as dermal nodules with limited or no epidermal attachment; *adenoid* BCC, forming pseudoglandular structures that often contain stromal mucin (Figure 34-11); *pigmented* BCC, which contain melanin and may clinically simulate malignant melanoma; and *fibroepitheliomatous* BCC (of Pinkus), which manifests thin, interconnected strands of basaloid cells in a background of fibrous stroma (Figure 34-12). A misdiagnosis of BCC as an adnexal neoplasm may be made when necrosis or mitotic activity is unusually notable. The basaloid nature of both BCC and Merkel cell carcinoma (see later) may also cause a striking histologic similarity between those two tumor types.

BCC is most commonly treated successfully by surgical excision. Local recurrence may be encountered, but metastases are extraordinarily rare. Imiquimod, a topical immune modulator, has also been used effectively in the treatment of superficial BCC.[14]

Mammary cutaneous *squamous cell carcinoma in situ* is known in the clinical lexicon as *Bowen's disease (BD)*. It presents as a circumscribed erythematous, slightly scaly patch (Figure 34-13). This lesion becomes invasive in only a small percentage of cases.[15] BD exhibits panepidermal keratinocytic atypia with disordered maturation, mitotic figures at all levels of the epidermis, acanthosis, and elongation of rete ridges (Figure 34-14). Multinucleation and dyskeratosis are common as well.[16]

The pagetoid (clonal) variant of BD is particularly important to recognize in the mammary skin because it can simulate true mammary Paget's disease (MPD; see later). Clonal BD comprises atypical keratinocytes with pale to clear cytoplasm, arranged as nests and single cells throughout the epidermis (Figure 34-15). Immunostains are helpful in distinguishing pagetoid BD from

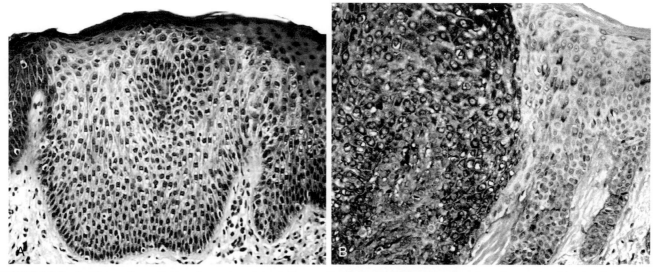

FIGURE 34-5   A, Clear cell acanthoma shows sharp lateral demarcation from the adjacent epidermis and comprises bland polygonal cells with clear cytoplasm. **B,** The lesion stains with periodic acid–Schiff (PAS) without diastase digestion, indicating the presence of glycogen.

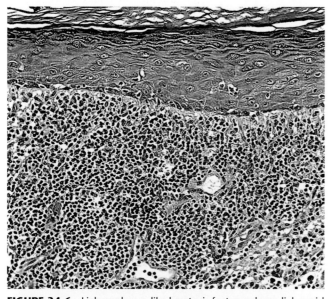

FIGURE 34-6   Lichen planus–like keratosis features dense lichenoid lymphoplasmacytic inflammation, basal epidermal vacuolization, and pigment incontinence. It is a solitary lesion, unlike the process it simulates, namely, lichen planus.

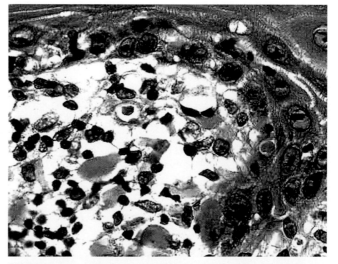

FIGURE 34-7   Globular eosinophilic "cytoid" bodies are prominent in this lichen planus–like keratosis beneath the epidermis. They represent effete keratinocytes.

MPD or superficial-spreading melanoma. Melanomas express S100 protein, whereas BD does not. MPD is almost always positive for cytokeratin-7 (CK7), but BD usually lacks that marker and stains for high-molecular-weight CKs (with antibodies 34BE12 or anti-CK 5/6) instead.[17]

Merkel Cell (Primary Cutaneous Neuroendocrine) Carcinoma

Primary cutaneous neuroendocrine tumors have been thought to show differentiation toward the Merkel cell, a neurotactile element in normal skin. However, that conceptual linkage is probably not altogether valid. *Merkel cell carcinoma* (MCC) appears as an erythematous or violaceous nodule (Figure 34-16), which is ulcerated in 20% of cases.[18]

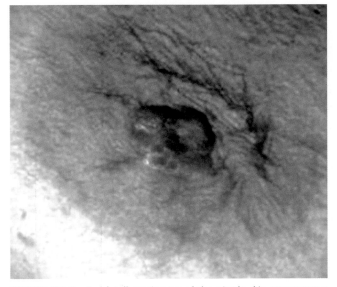

FIGURE 34-8 Basal cell carcinoma of the nipple skin represents a reddish, crusted, discrete lesion.

The original examples of MCC had a trabecular growth pattern (*trabecular* carcinoma), but growth in solid sheets or nests of cells is more common (Figure 34-17). Focal epidermal involvement is seen in approximately 10% of cases.[19-21] Subcuticular infiltration is frequent and adipocytes are entrapped by MCC cells, as seen in lymphoproliferative disorders. Cytologic features of MCC include finely stippled chromatin, high nuclear-to-cytoplasmic ratios, inconspicuous nucleoli, and extremely numerous mitoses (Figure 34-18). As many as 15 division figures may be seen in each high-power (×400) field, along with apoptosis and necrosis. The stroma may be sclerotic or delicately fibrovascular, and a lymphoplasmacytic infiltrate is present in many examples of MCC.[22] A distinction from metastatic small cell carcinoma of the lung may be difficult in selected cases. However, if one observes DNA encrustation around intratumoral blood vessels (the Azzopardi phenomenon), metastasis *to* the skin from a visceral neoplasm must be strongly considered.[23]

Immunoreactivity of MCCs for CK may be diffuse in the cytoplasm or take the form of paranuclear "dots." CK20 is present in approximately 90% of cases[24,25]; chromogranin-A has been reported in 33% to 100% of cases.[26] Synaptophysin is demonstrable in 40%.[27] Other markers that are helpful in diagnosis include CD56 (probably the best screening determinant for neuroendocrine lesions), CD57, and PAX5. CD99 and FLI-1 (friend leukemia virus–related nuclear antigen) expression is potentially shared by both MCC and primitive neuroectodermal tumors (PNETs) of the subcutis,[28] but only the latter lesions contain vimentin.

MCC is an aggressive cutaneous neoplasm, second in that regard only to melanoma. It is prone to local recurrence and has a high incidence (~50% of cases) of lymph node metastasis.[29] Complete surgical excision provides the best chance of cure; irradiation and chemotherapy are largely palliative, producing only rare instances of long-term remission.

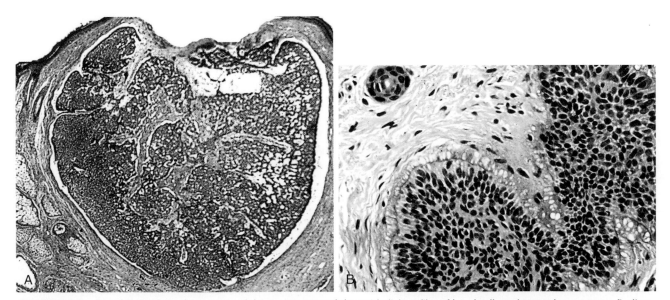

FIGURE 34-9 **A** and **B,** Artifactual retraction of the stroma around the epithelial profiles of basal cell carcinomas is a common finding.

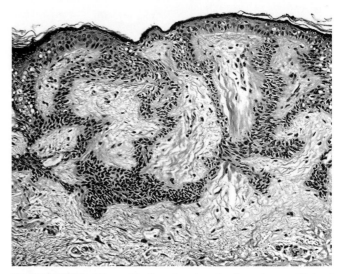

FIGURE 34-12 Fibroepitheliomatous basal cell carcinoma (Pinkus' tumor) comprises a meshwork of basaloid tumor cell cords, which enclose collagenized stroma.

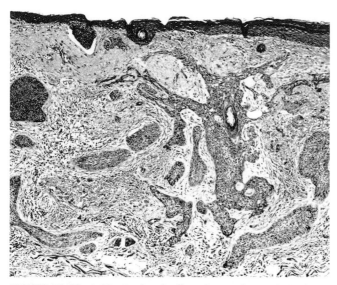

FIGURE 34-10 Infiltrative basal cell carcinoma demonstrates irregular, "spiky" cords of tumor cells that tend to blend with surrounding stroma. This variant shows an increased level of local recurrence.

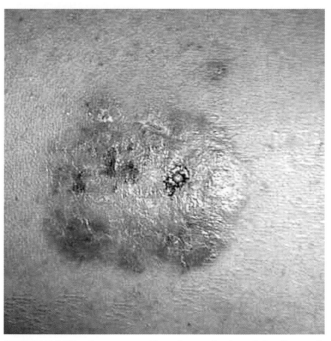

FIGURE 34-13 Squamous cell carcinoma in situ of the "Bowen's disease" type is represented by a velvety and scaly reddish patch.

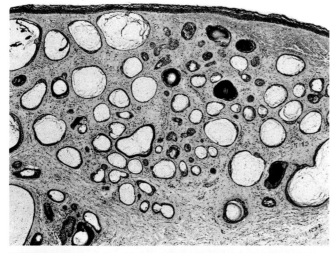

FIGURE 34-11 Adenoid (pseudoglandular) basal cell carcinoma forms spaces within tumor cell nests that contain stromal mucin. As a consequence, it may be mistaken for a glandular tumor.

Benign Adnexal Tumors of the Mammary Skin

PILOMATRIXOMA (CALCIFYING EPITHELIOMA OF MALHERBE)

Pilomatrixoma (PMX) is a relatively common dermal tumor that presents in children and young adults as a solitary, deeply seated nodule.[30] It is sharply circumscribed and centered in the dermis, often extending into the subcutis as well. Microscopically, one sees a biphasic cell population comprising basaloid cells and eosinophilic cells with "ghost" or "shadow" nuclei (Figure 34-19). The basaloid cells have scant cytoplasm,

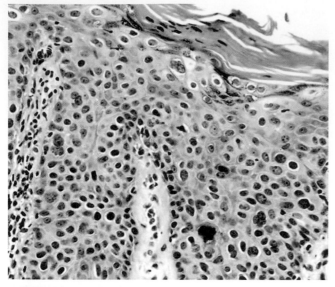

FIGURE 34-14 Conventional squamous carcinoma in situ manifests transepidermal cytologic atypia, often with numerous mitotic figures and multinucleated cells.

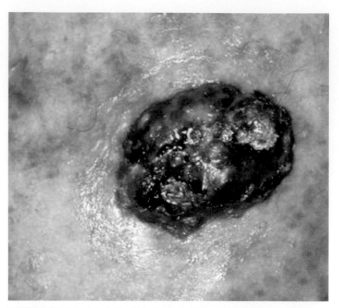

FIGURE 34-16 Merkel cell (primary cutaneous neuroendocrine) carcinoma usually presents as a reddish-violet, variably ulcerated nodule.

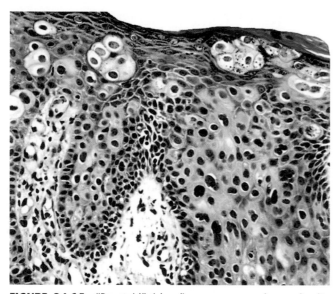

FIGURE 34-15 "Pagetoid" (clonal) squamous carcinoma in situ shows intraepidermal nesting of the tumor cells, potentially imitating Paget's disease or pagetoid melanoma.

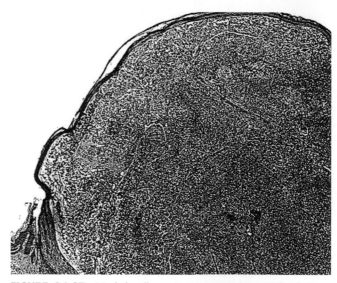

FIGURE 34-17 Merkel cell carcinoma most commonly demonstrates a confluent sheetlike growth pattern and is composed of uniform small cells.

hyperchromatic nuclei, easily seen nucleoli, and numerous mitotic figures. In contrast, the shadow cells contain abundant eosinophilic cytoplasm and are often calcified. Other findings include foreign body granulomas and hemosiderin deposits.[31,32] Typical PMX rarely recurs, even if marginally excised.

CYLINDROMA

Cylindroma is a basaloid dermal neoplasm, composed of small cell nests and forming a pattern that resembles pieces of a jigsaw puzzle (Figure 34-20). Within the cell nests, peripheral cells are more polygonal; between the tumor cells, one finds eosinophilic, hyalinized stroma.[33,34]

Similar material is often deposited as globules inside cell nests. Spiradenoma may sometimes be mimicked by cylindroma; however, the latter tumor lacks the presence of intratumoral lymphocytes, as routinely observed in spiradenomas.

MIXED TUMOR

Formerly called *chondroid syringomas*, mixed tumors of the mammary skin are identical morphologically to their deeper counterparts in the breast parenchyma (Figure 34-21).[35] In contrast to their analogues in salivary glands, mammary cutaneous and intramammary mixed tumors rarely recur and virtually never metastasize.

SPIRADENOMA

Spiradenoma is a variably colored nodule that is centered in the dermis and may be painful on palpation.[36,37] This tumor morphologically resembles cylindroma in many respects, as just noted previously. Mature lymphocytes are consistently seen throughout spiradenomas; moreover, dilated blood vessels and lymphatics are typically seen in or around spiradenomas (Figure 34-22).

ACROSPIROMA

Acrospiroma (nodular hidradenoma) takes the form of a nondescript, tan-pink, dermal-based nodule. It is often misinterpreted clinically as a cutaneous cyst. Microscopically, the lesion demonstrates a circumscribed, partially cystic, multinodular proliferation of polygonal cells in the dermis, with possible focal attachments to the epidermis (Figure 34-23).[38,39] The cell population is variable in its cytologic appearance, potentially comprising

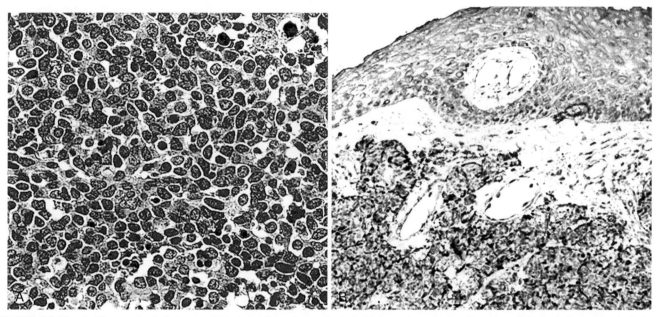

FIGURE 34-18   A, The cytologic features of Merkel cell carcinoma include high nucleocytoplasmic ratios, dispersed chromatin, indistinct nucleoli, and an extremely high mitotic rate with brisk apoptosis. **B,** Paranuclear "dots" of keratin are present in immunohistochemical staining of Merkel cell carcinoma.

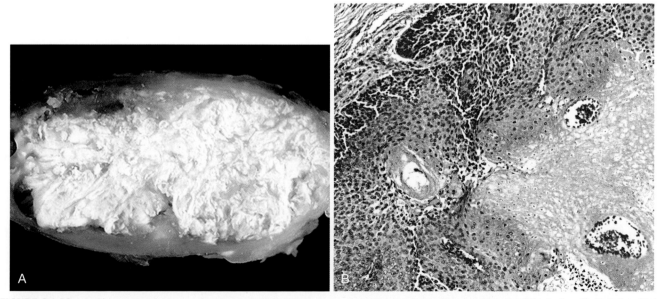

FIGURE 34-19   A, This gross specimen of excised pilomatrixoma shows the abundantly keratinous contents of the lesion. **B,** Peripheral lobules of basaloid cells with numerous mitotic figures surround zones of "ghost-cell" keratinization in pilomatrixoma.

banal polygonal cells with amphophilic cytoplasm, clear cells, or squamoid elements. In fact, mixtures of those cell types are common.

EROSIVE ADENOMATOSIS OF THE NIPPLE

Strictly speaking, *erosive adenomatosis of the nipple* (papillary subareolar adenoma; nipple adenoma) is a proliferative lesion of the subareolar mammary ducts rather than the skin appendages. However, it presents as an eczematoid reddish lesion of the areola and nipple, often with clear discharge, in women of reproductive age.[40,41] The clinical diagnosis in such cases is often that of mammary Paget's disease.

Histologically, one sees a papillary epithelial proliferation in subareolar ducts immediately beneath the nipple-skin surface. Constituent cells are cytologically bland, resembling those of "usual" intraductal epithelial hyperplasia of the breast (Figure 34-24). A chronic inflammatory infiltrate may accompany the proliferation in the dermis.[40]

Wedge excision of the nipple complex is curative. Erosive adenomatosis does not predispose to carcinoma of the breast.

Borderline and Malignant Sweat Gland–type Tumors of the Breast

In contradistinction to the views of other authors,[42] this author does not recognize the existence of sweat gland carcinomas in the skin of the breast. That opinion may

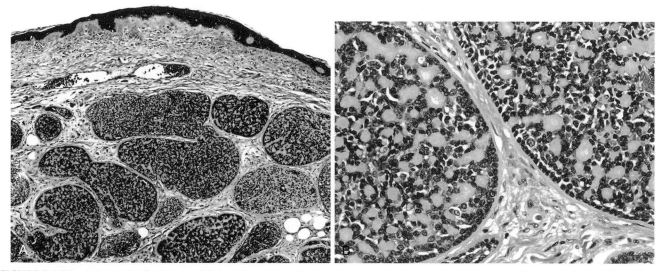

FIGURE 34-20   A, Dermal cylindroma exhibits a "jigsaw puzzle piece" appearance on scanning microscopy, because its basaloid tumor cell nests appear to fit into one another. **B,** Prominent eosinophilic deposits of basement membrane material are present in and around the tumor cell clusters in dermal cylindroma.

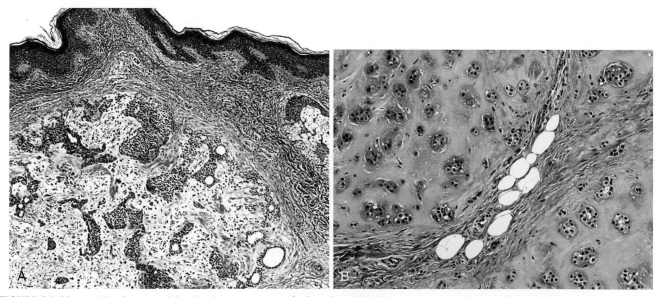

FIGURE 34-21   A, Mixed tumor of the skin shows a variety of adnexal epithelial lineages, potentially including eccrine, apocrine, sebaceous, and pilar. **B,** Its stroma likewise may comprise cartilage-like, lipomatous, or myoid tissue.

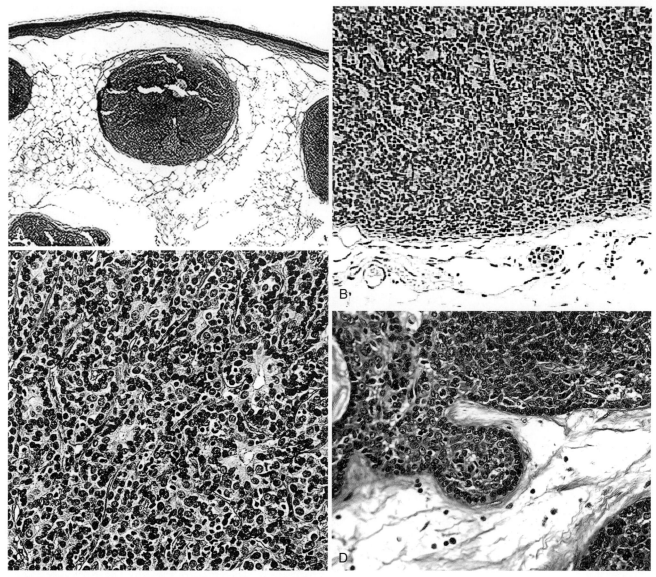

FIGURE 34-22   A, Eccrine spiradenoma is typified by multiple, sometimes discontinuous, compact nests of basaloid epithelioid cells in the dermis. **B-D,** Prominent intratumoral lymphatic spaces and intralesional lymphocytosis are typical findings.

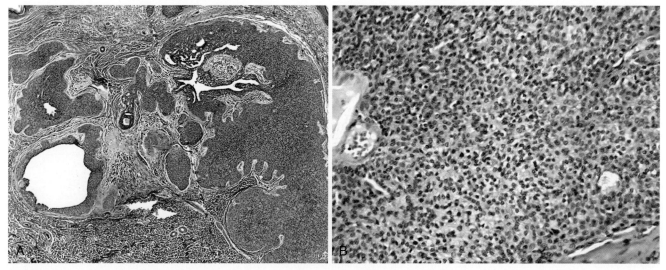

FIGURE 34-23   A and **B,** Eccrine acrospiroma (solid and cystic nodular hidradenoma) comprises a variably cystic nodule of polygonal or squamoid cells in the dermis. It is well circumscribed but may show focal attachment to the epidermis.

seem to be a strange and dogmatic idiosyncracy, but it is based on the concept that the breasts have great similarities to sweat glands. Thus, literally all of the pathologic characteristics of breast cancers are recapitulated in sweat gland carcinomas, and one is, therefore, completely unable to separate superficial parenchymal mammary carcinomas from tumors that may theoretically have arisen in the dermis.

As a consequence, when faced with an obviously malignant glandular neoplasm in the mammary skin, the author uses a descriptive and generic diagnosis, such as "poorly differentiated adenocarcinoma." A note in the accompanying surgical pathology report discusses the points just made previously and recommends that the lesion be treated as a primary *breast* tumor.

Related concepts pertain to other special skin tumors of the breast that also may be seen as primary cutaneous lesions in nonmammary sites. These are discussed later.

SYRINGOMATOUS ADENOMA OF THE NIPPLE/ MICROCYSTIC ADNEXAL CARCINOMA

Microcystic adnexal carcinoma (MAC) is an appendageal skin tumor of "borderline" malignant potential that almost always arises on the face or scalp.[43–46] It demonstrates frequent perineural and perivascular extension along with deep infiltration, even though it is cytologically banal. Small, tubular or angulated cell cords are widely scattered throughout the dermis and subcutis in MAC, and interspersed microcysts may contain pilar-type

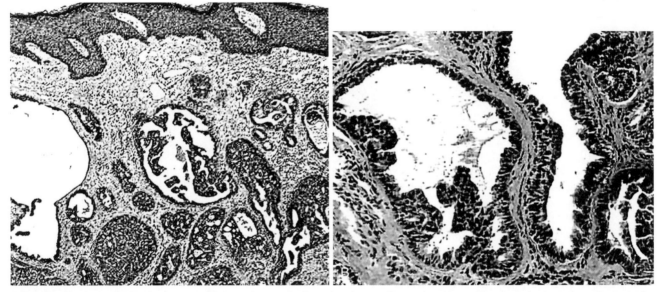

FIGURE 34-24 **A** and **B**, Erosive adenomatosis of the nipple ("nipple adenoma") represents a proliferation of subareolar mammary ducts that may cause ulceration of the overlying skin. The lesional ducts contain micropapillary epithelial profiles.

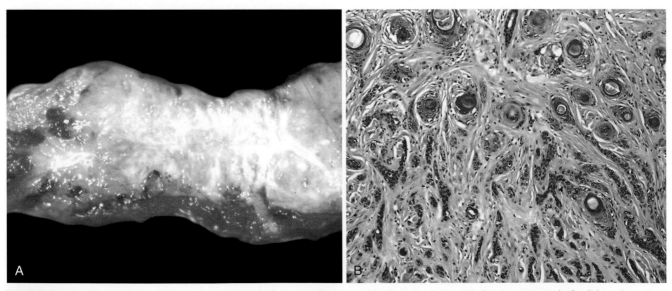

FIGURE 34-25 "Syringomatous adenoma" of the nipple is an infiltrative and sclerosing lesion (**A**) that is composed of solid cords and microcystic arrays (**B**). The tumor cells are cytologically bland. In the author's opinion, this lesion is analogous to microcystic adnexal carcinoma of the extramammary skin.

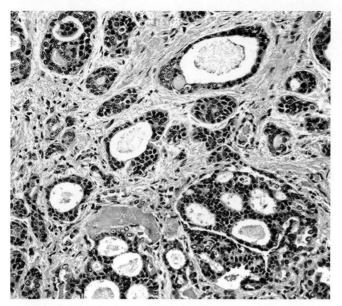

FIGURE 34-26 Adenoid cystic carcinoma of the mammary skin is identical histologically to its deeper counterpart in the breast parenchyma.

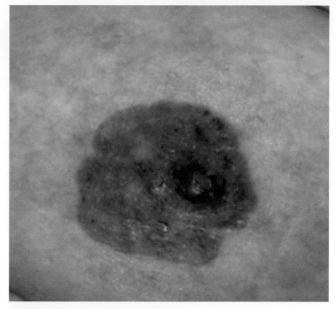

FIGURE 34-27 Paget's disease of the nipple and areola, manifesting as a scaly, erythematous, eczematoid patch.

keratin (Figure 34-25). Ward and coworkers[47] have concluded—and the author concurs—that the lesion known as *syringomatous adenoma of the nipple (SAN)* is actually a MAC-like tumor in the mammary skin. Like facial MAC, SAN also may recur locally but does not metastasize.

ADENOID CYSTIC CARCINOMA

Adenoid cystic carcinomas in the skin of the breast have morphologic features that are identical to their counterparts in the deep mammary parenchyma (Figure 34-26).[48] Thus, the same comments made previously, in reference to "sweat gland carcinomas" of the breast in general, pertain here as well.

MAMMARY PAGET'S DISEASE

An erythematous or eczematous plaque in the mammary skin of the areola, or around it, suggests the possibility of *mammary Paget's disease* (Figure 34-27). This condition is associated with an underlying carcinoma of the breast in 85% to 90% of cases.[49–51] Large, pale, epithelioid tumor cells are scattered haphazardly throughout the epidermis in MPD. They have pleomorphic nuclei that, along with cytoplasmic clearing and vacuoles, help to distinguish them from surrounding keratinocytes (Figure 34-28). Epidermal hyperplasia or "pseudobullous" acantholysis may be present, and when the second of those changes is prominent, confusion with pemphigus may eventuate (Figure 34-29).[52,53]

In comparison with pagetoid BD and pagetoid melanoma, mucin is much more often demonstrable in MPD with several histochemical stains. Those include alcian blue at pH 2.5, the periodic acid-Schiff (PAS) method, Best's mucicarmine stain, and Hale's colloidal iron.[50] Immunohistochemistry is also helpful, as discussed earlier (Figure 34-30).

The author's conceptual synthesis of MPD differs from that of doctrinaire writings on this disease. The usual explanation for the presence of glandular-type cells in the epidermis is that an underlying carcinoma has "migrated" upward, through the mammary ducts, and into the skin of the breast. That premise is illogical on biologic grounds. Instead, the author believes that the cells of MPD originate in the epidermis, as they clearly do in *extramammary Paget's disease* (EPD).[50] In other words, MPD and EPD are one and the same process, but with differing values as biomarkers. MPD is an indicator of an associated breast carcinoma in a high proportion of cases (>85%), whereas EPD has a similar marker value of no more than 20% in other sites, such as the perineum.

In support of its intraepidermal origin, the author has seen examples of MPD that invaded through the epidermal basement membrane into the dermis and superficial subareolar tissue, in the *absence* of a deeper breast cancer. In parallel with comments made previously, the author would still recommend that the patient be treated as if she had a primary mammary-parenchymal carcinoma. That approach is chosen because invasive MPD has all of the histopathologic attributes of infiltrating apocrine carcinoma of the breast.[54] Further details on this subject are found in Chapter 27 on MPD.

NONVASCULAR CUTANEOUS MESENCHYMAL LESIONS OF THE MAMMARY SKIN

Hypertrophic scar and *keloid* are two terms for the same morphologic continuum of reparative fibroblastic and myofibroblastic proliferation in the skin.[55] Keloids arise *from* tumefactive hypertrophic scars, showing broad, brightly eosinophilic bands of hyalinized collagen in the dermis.

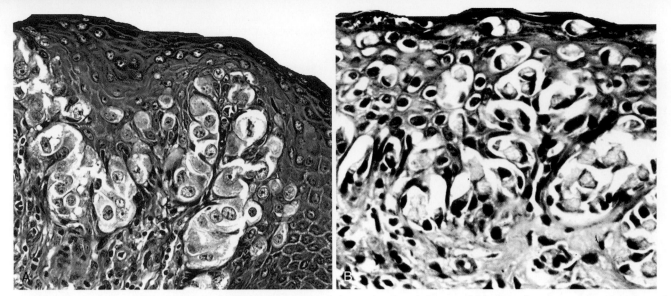

FIGURE 34-28 A, Tumor cells in mammary Paget's disease are usually larger than keratinocytes, with increased nucleocytoplasmic ratios and pale cytoplasm. **B,** They may be distributed singly or in groups throughout the epidermis.

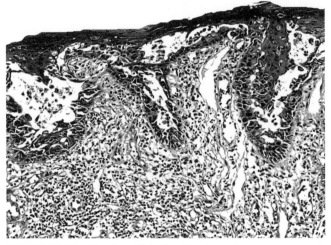

FIGURE 34-29 The "pseudobullous" variant of mammary Paget's disease may be mistaken for an immunobullous dermatosis because of extensive intralesional acantholysis.

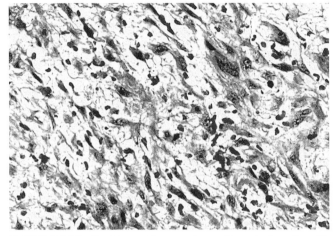

FIGURE 34-31 Post-traumatic or postoperative spindle cell proliferations of the skin are the dermal analogues of nodular fasciitis in deeper tissues. Accordingly, one sees a "tissue-culture" appearance in which spindle cells are separated from one another by myxoedematous material. Nuclear features are bland, despite brisk mitotic activity, and extravasated stromal erythrocytes are common.

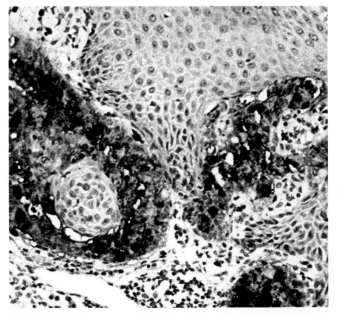

FIGURE 34-30 Immunoreactivity for keratin-7 separates mammary Paget's disease from its microscopic imitators.

Post-traumatic spindle cell nodules (PSCNs) are the dermal counterparts of nodular fasciitis in deeper tissues. They may follow injury to the mammary skin or arise in and around surgical incision scars as rapidly enlarging tan-pink nodules and plaques. Microscopic examination shows a very loosely aggregated ("tissue culture") appearance of proliferating, bland spindle and stellate cells in a myxoedematous stroma, with evenly distributed chromatin, ample amphophilic cytoplasm, numerous mitotic figures, complex capillary-sized stromal blood vessels, and extravasated erythrocytes (Figure 34-31). Focal deposition of keloid-type collagen may be observed as well, along with hemosiderin.[56,57]

Dermatofibromas (DFs) are the most common mesenchymal tumors of the skin. The synonymous term *fibrous histiocytoma* is sometimes used in reference to these lesions. Usually, they measure less than 1 cm in diameter and are often pigmented. "Dimpling" of the skin upon centripetal compression of the lesion is seen with DF and any other tumor with a deep dermal

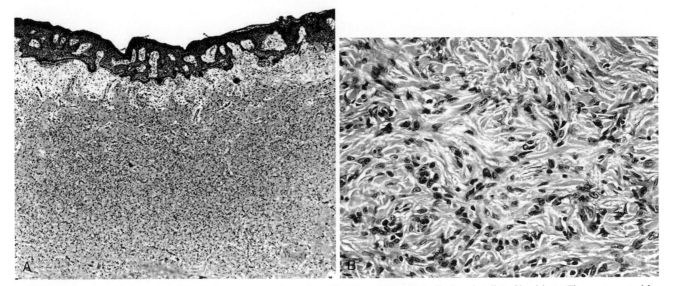

FIGURE 34-32 **A** and **B,** Dermatofibroma is a common dermal proliferation of bland spindled and stellate fibroblasts. They entrap and fragment collagen in the corium.

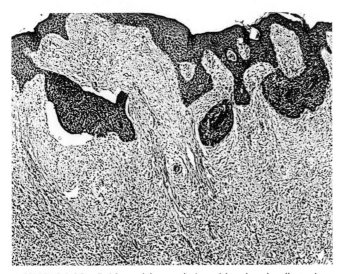

FIGURE 34-33 Epidermal hyperplasia—either basal cell carcinoma–like (shown here) or pseudoepitheliomatous—often overlies dermatofibromas.

or subcutaneous attachment.[58,59] Recurrence of DFs after simple excision is uncommon. The dermis in DFs contains a haphazard and cytologically bland spindle cell proliferation with possible storiform areas (Figure 34-32). An admixture of foamy histiocytes and multinucleated or floret-type giant cells is very common.[60,61] "Encircled" collagen fibers at the periphery of the lesion are another characteristic finding in DF. Associated epidermal changes include acanthosis, sometimes with basal cell hyperplasia that resembles superficial BCC (Figure 34-33), as well as hyperpigmentation. Mitotic activity is variable but has no clinical significance.

Dermatomyofibroma is distinct from DF, in that the former lesion has a platelike configuration and comprises spindle cells with more eosinophilic cytoplasm.[62,63] Markers of smooth muscle differentiation (muscle-specific actin, caldesmon, calponin) or Factor XIIIa, or both, may be present in dermatomyofibromas. Their treatment and behavior overlap with those of DF.

Granular cell tumor (GCT) may be seen either within the breast parenchyma or on the mammary skin.[64,65] It is represented by sheets and nests of large, polygonal, oxyphilic cells, which permeate through the dermal collagen. They have a distinctively granular cytoplasm, in which small targetoid inclusions are often present as well (Figure 34-34). Nuclei are bland, oval, and peripherally located; mitoses are rare. The granules in GCT can be highlighted with a PAS stain after diastase digestion. Immunohistologically, GCT is reactive for S100 protein in 80% of cases; most of the remaining examples express CD57, calretinin, or inhibin.[66]

Neurofibroma can be either single or multiple in the skin of the breast (Figure 34-35). Multifocality suggests the possibility of syndromic neurofibromatosis, especially if several café au lait spots are also apparent on the breasts or in other skin fields.[67,68] Microscopically, neurofibroma can be either "diffuse" or "plexiform." In the first instance, sheets of bland spindle cells with serpiginous contours replace the dermis and are accompanied by fibromyxoid stroma (Figure 34-36). Plexiform neurofibroma resembles a caricature of a nerve trunk, comprising several intermingled fascicular arrays, each of which comprises tissue similar to that of diffuse neurofibroma (Figure 34-37).[69] Virtually all neurofibromas are immunoreactive for S100 protein, CD56, CD57, Factor XIIIa, or combinations thereof.

Neurilemmoma (schwannoma) usually presents clinically as a single, nondescript, flesh-colored papule or nodule in the skin.[69,70] Histologically, it has a biphasic appearance; one portion of the tumor comprises closely apposed elongated spindle cells (Antoni A areas); whereas the other shows loosely arranged fusiform or polygonal cell elements in a myxoedematous stroma

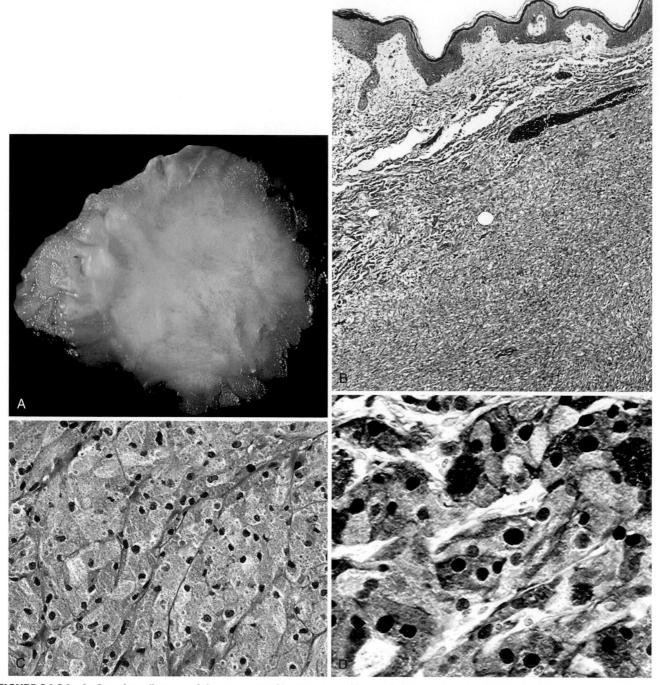

FIGURE 34-34 **A,** Granular cell tumor of the mammary skin, represented by an ill-defined dermal and subcuticular mass that may be mistaken grossly for a carcinoma. The tumor is composed of uniform, polygonal, eosinophilic cells with bland ovoid nuclei and numerous cytoplasmic granules. **B** and **C,** Intracellular "targetoid" bodies are also common. **D,** Immunoreactivity for S100 protein, calretinin, inhibin, and CD57 may be seen in granular cell tumors.

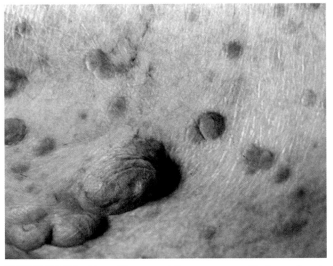

FIGURE 34-35 Neurofibromas of the mammary skin in syndromic neurofibromatosis (von Recklinghausen's disease) are multifocal. They may be papular, nodular, plaquelike, or pedunculated.

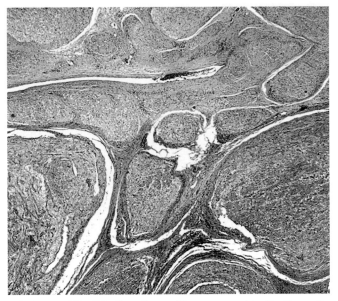

FIGURE 34-37 "Plexiform" neurofibromas are virtually diagnostic of neurofibromatosis and resemble miniature nerve trunks on scanning microscopy.

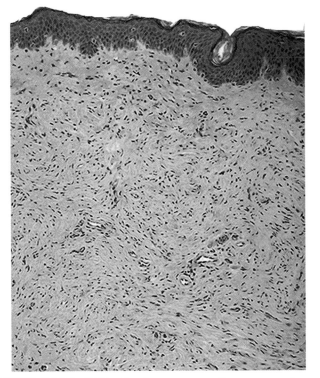

FIGURE 34-36 "Diffuse" cutaneous neurofibroma comprises a disorganized but circumscribed proliferation of bland spindle cells whose nuclei often show serpiginous contours.

(Antoni B foci) (Figure 34-38). Zones of Antoni A tissue may furthermore manifest a peculiar alignment of tumor cell nuclei in register with one another, yielding structures called *verocay bodies*. Immunostains for S100 protein are virtually always strongly reactive in neurilemmoma.[70]

Lipoma variants in the skin of the breast parallel those seen in other cutaneous fields. Pleomorphic, spindle cell, and angiolipomas may all be potentially

encountered. These respectively feature large, multinucleated, "floret"-type giant cells; variably dense zones of spindle cells that are immunoreactive for CD34; and congeries of small capillary-sized blood vessels at the periphery of adipocytic lobules in the lesions (Figures 34-39 and 34-40).[71]

Leiomyoma cutis tends to occur in or around the nipple-areolar complex, and it may be represented by a solitary plaque or multiple, grouped nodules that are tan-pink (Figure 34-41).[72–74] They are sometimes tender on palpation. Microscopically, leiomyoma of the skin is a relatively superficial and circumscribed dermal lesion, composed of fusiform cells with bluntly tapered nuclear contours and eosinophilic fibrillar cytoplasm (Figure 34-42). Mitoses are extremely rare. Some leiomyomas may have a neuroid histologic image, and in those cases, immunohistochemical confirmation of smooth muscle differentiation is helpful. Potentially positive immunostains include desmin, muscle-specific actin, alpha-isoform actin, caldesmon, and calponin.[75] In cases of multifocal leiomyoma cutis, a possible syndromic association with renal cell carcinoma and uterine leiomyomas may pertain. This finding is related to heterozygous germline mutations in the fumarate hydratase gene on chromosome 1.[76]

Dermatofibrosarcoma protuberans (DFSP) is a cutaneous tumor of borderline malignancy. It is usually seen in adults, but uncommon examples in childhood may include morphologic foci, known as *giant cell fibroblastoma*, that imitate the lesion. DFSP may recur in up to 50% of cases after simple excision but very rarely metastasizes.[77,78] The lesion usually takes the form of a violaceous nodule or a plaque (Figure 34-43). A tendency for protrusion above the skin surface gives DFSP its name. Deep intradermal involvement is the norm, but that finding is not invariable.[79,80] Storiform (pinwheel-like) growth is virtually always present in DFSP, with the constituent elements

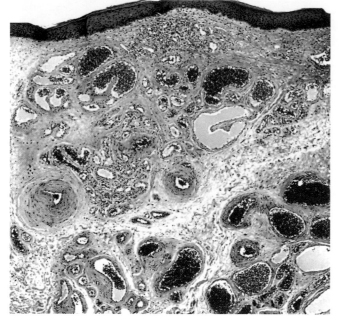

FIGURE 34-51 Arteriovenous hemangioma ("acral arteriovenous tumor") features at least partial composition by small vessels with muscularized walls. Areas resembling lobular capillary hemangioma may be admixed.

surround small vessels (Figure 34-54). The individual cells are uniform with eosinophilic cytoplasm and oval nuclei; the background stroma may be fibrous or myxoid. A lack of cellular pleomorphism and mitotic activity is characteristic. Glomus cells are immunoreactive for vimentin, muscle-specific actin, and alpha-isoform ("smooth muscle") actin.[103] Endothelial cell markers are absent.[104]

Biologically Borderline Vascular Tumors of the Mammary Skin

Epithelioid hemangioendothelioma (EHE) is a distinctive vascular neoplasm, first described by Weiss and Enzinger in 1982.[105] It only extraordinarily arises in the skin of the breast, where it takes the form of a red-violet plaque. Microscopically, one sees nests, cords, or sheets of polygonal cells with modest nuclear atypia, irregularly permeating the dermis and subcutis (Figure 34-55). Tumor cell groups may be closely apposed to the adventitia of large blood vessels. On close examination, at least some of the cellular elements show cytoplasmic vacuolization (Figure 34-56), and erythrocytes may be demonstrable in those spaces as well. A peculiar myxochondroid stroma is common to many EHEs.[106] Differential diagnosis with signet-ring-cell carcinomas or adipocytic neoplasms is sometimes difficult, but among those possibilities, only EHE is immunoreactive for endothelial determinants such as CD31, CD34, FLI-1, and thrombomodulin.[107]

EHE of the skin is a borderline malignancy, characterized by potential recurrence (~30% of cases) but a low risk of metastasis (<10%).[105,108] Complete excision is the treatment of choice.

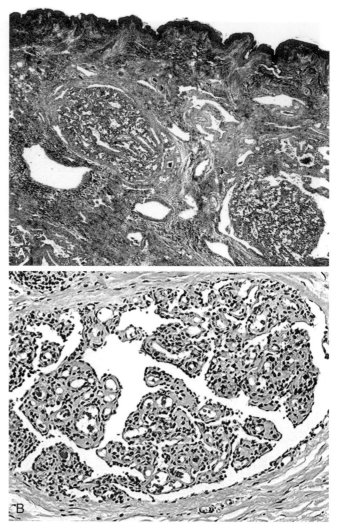

FIGURE 34-52 **A** and **B,** Glomeruloid hemangioma show dermal vascular profiles that strongly resemble renal glomeruli. It is usually a marker of the POEMS (polyneuropathy, organomegaly, endocrinopathy, M-protein production, and skin changes) syndrome.

Malignant Vascular Tumors of the Mammary Skin

Kaposi's sarcoma (KS) is a locally aggressive endothelial tumor that is reproducibly associated with infection by human herpesvirus type 8 (HHV-8). With regard to involvement of the mammary skin, KS of the Mediterranean (classic) and African types is virtually never encountered. The breast is affected only in iatrogenic and immunosuppressive forms of KS, which are interrelated (Figure 34-57).[109]

Iatrogenic KS is a rare complication of long-term immunomodulatory therapy for solid organ transplantation or prolonged corticosteroid use. Tumor regression may sometimes eventuate if immunosuppressive treatment is discontinued.[110] *Acquired immunodeficiency syndrome (AIDS)–associated KS* is the most aggressive form. The anatomic distribution of lesions in that variant is broad, often involving the skin of the trunk as well as mucosal surfaces and viscera. Most patients with this form of the disease die

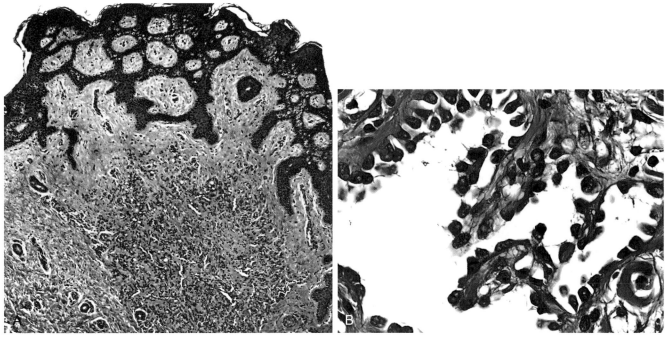

FIGURE 34-53 **A** and **B**, Hobnail hemangioma comprises small, interconnecting vascular channels that are lined by endothelial cells whose nuclei protrude into the lumina—resembling the bottom of a hobnail boot.

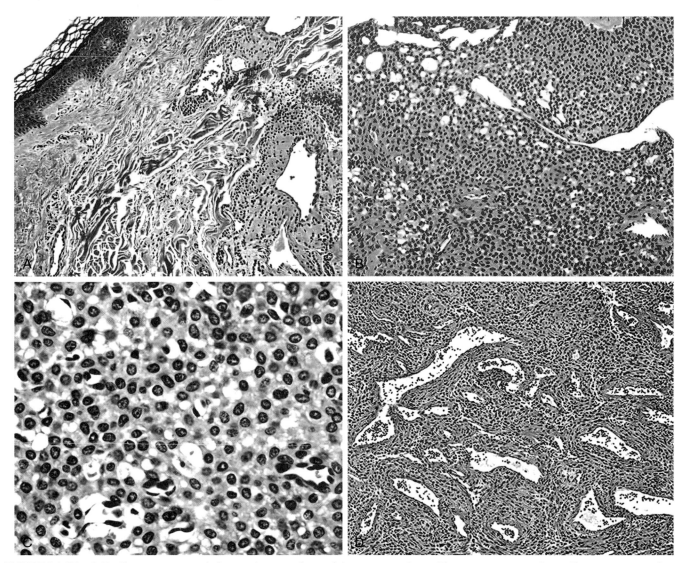

FIGURE 34-54 **A-D**, Glomus tumor and glomangioma are faces of the same neoplasm. Glomus tumor comprises uniform compact polygonal cells in groups, usually with small blood vessels in their centers. In turn, those vessels may be dilated in some lesions, producing the image of glomangioma.

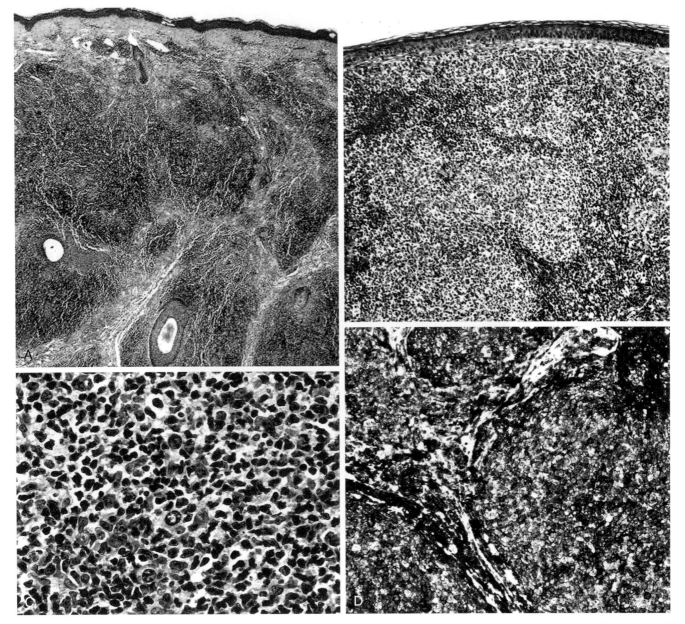

FIGURE 34-90 A and **B,** Nodular aggregates of atypical lymphocytes are seen throughout the superficial and deep dermis in cutaneous follicular lymphoma. The tumor cells exhibit folded nuclear contours (**C**) and show diffuse nuclear immunoreactivity for *bcl-6* (**D**).

mantle zones, and a lack of intrafollicular tingible-body macrophages.

Extranodal marginal zone lymphoma of mucosa-associated lymphoid tissue type (MALToma) is the most common primary low-grade cutaneous B-cell malignancy.[216] This form of lymphoma was formerly called "immunocytoma." In the skin of the breast, it presents as multiple red or purple nodules or plaques. Although the long-term prognosis is generally good, subsequent involvement of lymph nodes and visceral organs has been reported.[217]

Histologically, the dermis in MALToma is infiltrated by neoplastic lymphocytes that show a spectrum of cytologic images including centrocyte-like, monocytoid

B-cell–like and small lymphocyte-like cells (Figure 34-91). Aggregates of plasma cells and plasmacytoid cells may also be present, with or without Dutcher's bodies.[216] The overall pattern of tissue infiltration may be nodular or diffuse, and reactive lymphoid follicles can be scattered throughout infiltrate. Although MALTomas in other anatomic locations (e.g., stomach; salivary glands) show prominent infiltration of glandular epithelium by the tumor cells,[217] that feature is only rarely seen in adnexal structures of the skin.

Immunohistologically, MALTomas express CD20, CD79a, and *bcl-2*.[218] An absence of CD5 and cyclin-D1 helps to distinguish this tumor respectively from mantle cell and small lymphocytic lymphomas that may

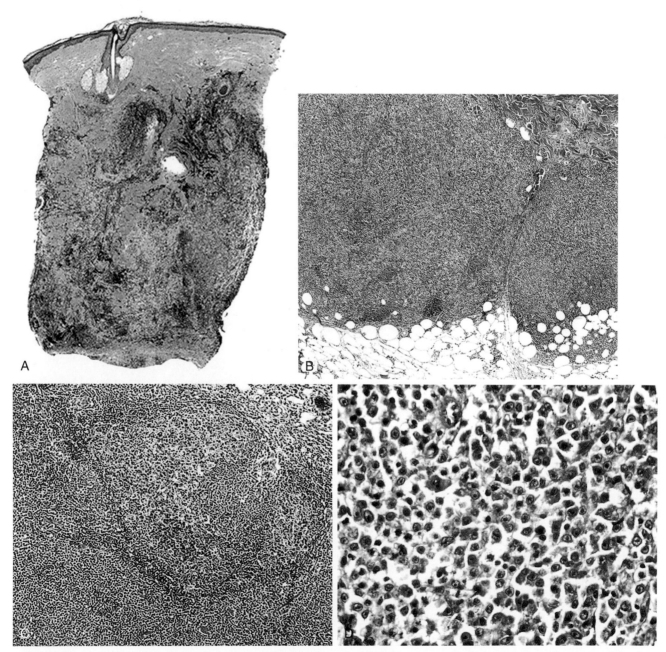

FIGURE 34-91 **A** and **B**, Marginal zone lymphoma of the skin (formerly called "immunocytoma") demonstrates effacement of the dermis and involvement of the subcutis. Germinal centers are focally present (**C**), and the lesion contains a substantial number of plasma cells (**D**).

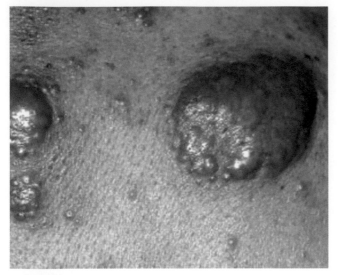

FIGURE 34-92 Cutaneous large cell lymphoma, manifesting as several reddish plaques and nodules in the skin of the breast.

secondarily involve the skin.[216] A lack of CD10 in cutaneous extranodal marginal zone lymphoma separates it from follicular lymphomas.

Primary cutaneous diffuse large B-cell lymphoma (PCDLBL) is a proliferation of large neoplastic B cells with nuclear sizes two or more times that of a normal lymphocyte.[219] Although PCDLBL may arise de novo in the skin, some cases represent diffuse variants of grade 3 cutaneous follicular lymphomas or transformed marginal zone lymphomas of the MALT type.[218,220–223] The course of PCDLBL is usually indolent, but visceralization has been reported. In the skin, the lesions tend to be single violaceous nodules or grouped papules (Figure 34-92). The cytologic appearance of the neoplastic cells is variable. Usually, they resemble centroblasts, with large round nuclei and peripheral nucleoli (Figure 34-93). However, large cells with prominent macronucleoli, cleaved nuclear contours, or overt anaplasia may also be seen. Biopsies of early lesions may show a periadnexal and perivascular distribution for the tumor in the corium. Later, diffuse effacement of the dermis and subcutis is common.[220,223] The epidermis is uninvolved. Immunophenotyping demonstrates

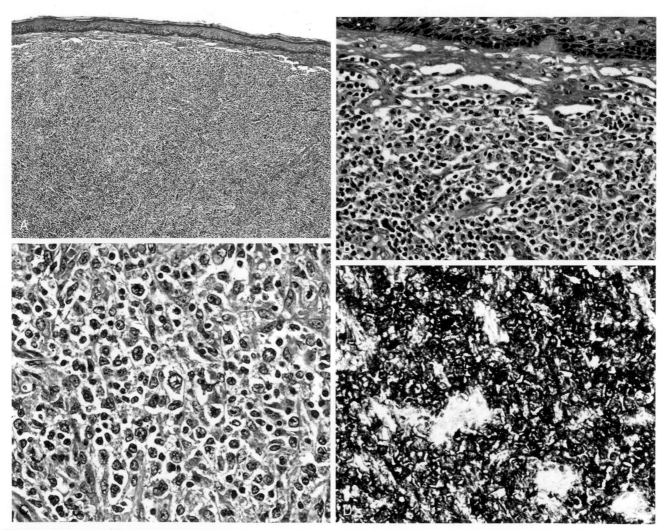

FIGURE 34-93 **A** and **B,** Large cell lymphoma of the skin, replacing the dermis. **C,** The tumor cells have high nucleocytoplasmic ratios, open chromatin, and discernible nucleoli. **D,** They are immunoreactive for CD20, reflecting B-cell differentiation.

the presence of CD20 and CD79a, and many cases also express PAX-5, CD10, and *bcl-2*.[224]

A highly unusual variant of cutaneous large B-cell lymphoma is represented by the lesion known as *intravascular lymphomatosis* (IVL). In that tumor type, neoplastic large lymphoid cells are almost totally confined to the lumina of blood vessels in the dermis and subcutis, with little or no involvement of the interstitial connective tissue or epidermis (Figure 34-94).[223,225] In contrast to PCDLBL, IVL in the skin is usually part of a systemic process that involves several visceral organs. The neoplastic elements in IVL almost always have a B-cell immunophenotype.[225]

T-cell lymphomas of the mammary skin comprise a bifid group, including peripheral T-cell lymphomas (PTCLs)[226] and variants of mycosis fungoides (MF).[227–229] PTCLs are clinically indistinguishable from B-cell lymphomas, as described previously. Histologically, they encompass a spectrum of specific lesions, such as PTCL, not otherwise specified (NOS); anaplastic large cell lymphoma (ALCL); extranodal NK/T-cell lymphoma; angioimmunoblastic T-cell lymphoma; gamma/delta T-cell lymphoma; and subcutaneous panniculitis–like T-cell lymphoma (SPTCL).[230–232] All of these tumors, except perhaps for ALCL, generally feature a greater cytologic spectrum of neoplastic lymphoid cells and non-neoplastic elements than that associated with B-cell tumors. Neutrophils and eosinophils are the nontumoral hematopoietic cells that are common in PTCL. A high level of stromal vascularity is another aspect of PTCLs that is usually not seen in B-cell neoplasms.[233]

The author will give particular attention here only to the ALCL and SPTCL forms of PTCL, because they most commonly pose particular problems in differential diagnosis. The first of these two entities comprises sheets of large polygonal cells that efface the dermis. They have markedly pleomorphic cytologic features, often with large nucleoli, numerous mitoses, and multinucleate cells (Figure 34-95). A tendency for the tumor cells to cluster together may be responsible for potential confusion of ALCL with melanoma or carcinoma diagnostically.[234] Immunohistochemically, the elements of ALCL are variably reactive for CD45, with up to 30% of cases being nonreactive for that marker.[234,235] By mandate of current classification systems, all ALCLs must express CD30 (Figure 34-96) in order to be so categorized; most also label for at least one pan-T-lymphocyte marker for paraffin sections (e.g., CD2, CD3, CD5, CD7, CD43, and CD45RO). CK and S100 protein are absent. Primary cutaneous ALCL lacks the t(2;5) chromosomal translocation that is seen in its lymph nodal counterpart; accordingly, the first form of the tumor is also negative for *ALK-1* (anaplastic lymphoma kinase-1), which is encoded on chromosome 2.[236,237]

The distinction between primary and secondary ALCL in the skin is prognostically important. Despite its aggressive histologic appearance, primary ALCL often remains confined to the skin for a prolonged period, and individual lesions may spontaneously involute. In contrast, secondary cutaneous ALCL is associated with a rapidly deteriorating clinical course.[234,237]

Another odd lesion that is microscopically interchangeable with ALCL is *lymphomatoid papulosis* (LYP) (Figure 34-97). It is manifested by grouped, variably sized red-violet papules that spontaneous resolve, only to be replaced by others.[238,239] At virtually every level of pathologic evaluation, there is no certain recipe for diagnostically separating LYP from ALCL. The distinction must be made on clinical grounds alone. It

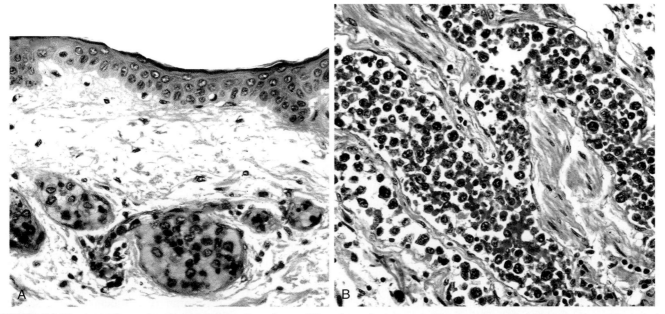

FIGURE 34-94 A peculiar and rare variant of cutaneous large cell lymphoma is represented by the lesion called *intravascular lymphomatosis*. **A** and **B,** The tumor cells are completely or largely confined to vascular lumina.

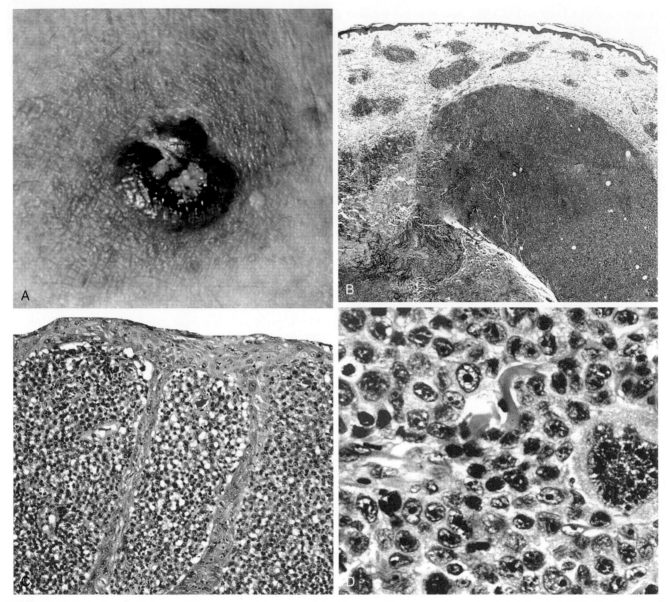

FIGURE 34-95   A, Anaplastic large cell lymphoma of the mammary skin, presenting as an ulcerated red-violet nodule. **B-D,** The tumor cells efface the corium and demonstrate a high level of nuclear pleomorphism.

is generally believed that LYP is a peculiar subtype of ALCL that can be controlled immunologically by the host and confined to the skin. Thus, the favored diagnostic label in such cases is *CD30+ lymphoproliferative disease*.[236,239–241]

Panniculitis-like T-cell lymphoma (PLTCL) is a rare tumor that infiltrates the subcuticular fat but does not involve the dermis or epidermis. As such, it clinically simulates panniculitides such as erythema nodosum.[242] Lesions of PLTCL are deeply seated, indurated, red-violet nodules that may ulcerate. Microscopy shows a predominantly deep dermal perivascular lymphoid infiltrate that permeates into the subcutaneous tissue (Figure 34-98). The lesional cell population is heterogeneous; it includes lymphocytes with variable nuclear atypia, macrophages, plasma cells, neutrophils, and eosinophils.[243] A characteristic finding in PLTCL is that lymphoid cells tend to encircle individual adipocytes (Figure 34-99). In

addition, one often observes subendothelial permeation of blood vessels by atypical lymphocytes, zonal en masse necrosis in the panniculus, and the presence of karyorrhectic fragments (nuclear dust) throughout the lesion.[244]

Immunohistochemically, PLTCL demonstrates reactivity for pan-T-lymphocyte markers, but may show aberrant antigenic patterns such as coexpression of CD4 with CD8 in the same cell population. CD68 and CD163 are seen in monocytic-type cells in the infiltrate, and these often contain phagocytosed erythrocytes or cellular debris. Histochemical stains for microorganisms are negative.[243]

T-cell receptor gene (TCRG) rearrangement analysis is often pursued in cases of PLTCL. In the author's experience, despite the undeniable biologic malignancy of this process, no clonal rearrangements are seen in approximately 30% to 40% of cases. Therefore, the ultimate diagnosis must rest on morphologic evaluation

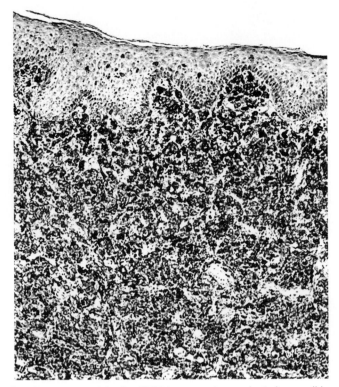

FIGURE 34-96   Diffuse immunoreactivity for CD30 is present in anaplastic large cell lymphoma of the skin.

and clinical correlation in those instances. Put another way, one should never exclude PLTCL diagnostically simply because of negative TCRG studies.

Mycosis fungoides (MF; cutaneous T-cell lymphoma [CTCL]) is a peculiar T-cell malignancy that, by definition, begins in the skin and is confined to it for long periods of time.[229,244] Patients with this condition are usually adults older than 20 years, who develop multiple reddish patches, plaques, or annular lesions in many skin areas (Figure 34-100). Diffuse erythroderma is another potential manifestation, with or without intense pruritus. Over several years, the lesions of MF usually become more numerous and tumefactive. Eventually, a proportion of patients develop visceral involvement, often after a morphologic transformation of their tumors into large cell lymphomas. If atypical lymphocytes are present in the peripheral blood as well, patients with CTCL are said to have *Sézary's syndrome*.[227]

A definite histologic distinction between early MF and subacute or chronic spongiotic dermatitis is often impossible.[245–247] Features favoring the former diagnosis include grouped lymphocytes in the epidermis, especially with little or no associated spongiosis; a linear arrangement of lymphoid cells at the base of the epidermis; folded nuclear membranes and increased nuclear-to-cytoplasmic ratios in lesional lymphocytes; "halos" around intraepidermal lymphoid cells; and "wiry" change in the collagen of the upper dermis (Figures 34-101 and 34-102).[248] When these findings are suboptimally visualized, an interpretation of "atypical epidermotropic lymphoid infiltrate" may be given. There is little to be gained by rushing to a diagnosis of MF because the treatments for chronic spongiotic dermatitides and early CTCL are essentially the same.

Immunohistochemical evaluation may provide data favoring an interpretation of MF if there is deletion of a pan-T-lymphocyte marker in the lesional cells and the lymphoid population is predominantly CD4+. Nonetheless, immunohistology is not a diagnostic panacea in this context and many cases of MF demonstrate no antigenic aberrations.[249]

As cited previously, the appearance of clinical tumor-stage MF may be accompanied by a histologic transformation of CTCL. In the late stages of that disease, tumoral lymphoid infiltrates strongly resemble the image of de novo ALCL, featuring a large cell, anaplastic, CD30+ population.[229,250] Survival is usually limited to approximately 18 months after this change occurs.

Granulocytic sarcoma (GS; extramedullary myeloid tumor, myeloid leukemia cutis) of the breast and mammary skin is a tumefactive manifestation of overt or "smoldering" acute myelogenous leukemia.[251–253] Strangely, it may appear before marrow changes or peripheral blood findings are diagnostic of the latter condition. In some cases, cutaneous GS is the first sign of "blast crisis" in patients with *chronic* myelogenous leukemia.[254] The skin lesions of GS are indistinguishable clinically from those of non-Hodgkin's lymphomas, typically being represented by red or violaceous nodules and plaques.

Microscopically, GS demonstrates effacement of the dermis by medium-sized, atypical mononuclear cells. They are often arranged in sheets or linear profiles in the corium (Figure 34-103) and may be accompanied

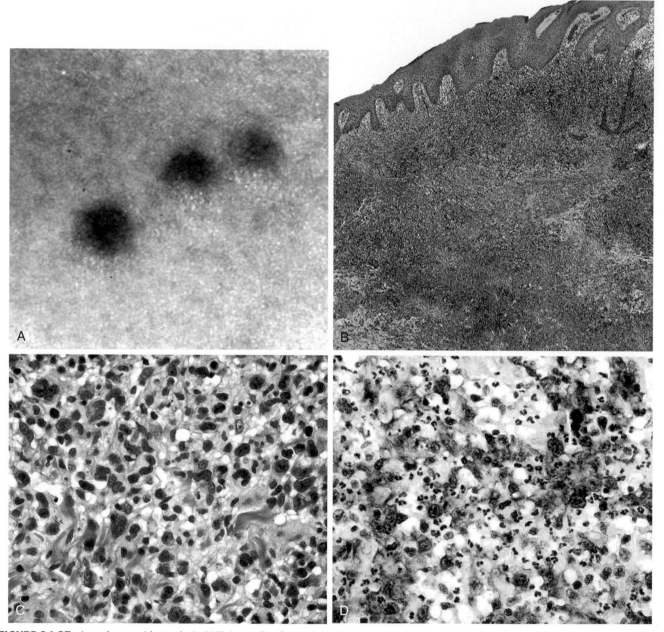

FIGURE 34-97 Lymphomatoid papulosis (LYP) is another form of CD30+ cutaneous lymphoproliferative disease. **A,** Unlike anaplastic large cell lymphoma (ALCL), LYP manifests as multiple, discrete, self-healing papules. **B** and **C,** In other respects, LYP and ALCL are virtually identical morphologically. **D,** The similarity includes immunoreactivity for CD30. Thus, a differential diagnosis between LYP and ALCL depends on the clinical details.

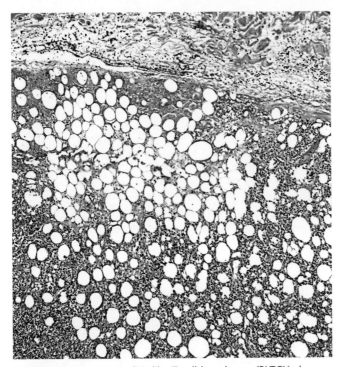

FIGURE 34-98 Panniculitis-like T-cell lymphoma (PLTCL) shows a polymorphous infiltration of variably atypical lymphoid cells in the subcutis. Karyorrhectic debris and areas of en masse fat necrosis may be present in PLTCL.

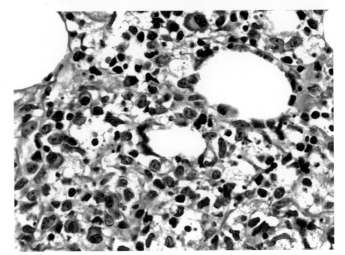

FIGURE 34-99 Another characteristic finding in PLTCL is the circumferential "ringing" of adipocytes by atypical lymphoid cells.

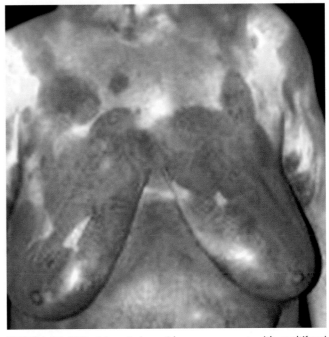

FIGURE 34-100 Mycosis fungoides may present with multifocal patches or plaques or with widespread erythroderma, as seen in this case.

by a subpopulation of immature eosinophils. A time-honored maxim concerning GS is that this lesion should be considered when one wishes to make a diagnosis of lymphoma but cannot decide which type of lymphoproliferation is the proper category.[255] Histochemical positivity for chloroacetate esterase—with Leder's method—or immunohistochemical reactivity for myeloperoxidase (Figure 34-104), CD15, CD34, or CD117 is characteristic of GS. CD45 is only variably present in that tumor.

In the absence of systemic disease, GS of the skin is treated with cutaneous irradiation. Patients must subsequently be followed closely for the possible development of peripheralized acute leukemia, which requires multiagent chemotherapy.

Lymphoblastic leukemia/lymphoma (LBLL) likewise may involve the mammary skin, sometimes as the presenting manifestation of this systemic disease. Affected patients are usually adolescents or young adults who develop one or more violaceous cutaneous nodules on the breasts.[256–258] Microscopically, LBLL shows effacement of the entire dermis by a monomorphic population of intermediate-sized lymphoid cells with dispersed chromatin and inconspicuous nucleoli. In roughly one half of cases, one observes complex convolution of the nuclear membranes (Figure 34-105).[258] Mitotic activity and apoptotic bodies are both numerous. Immunohistologically, LBLL of the pre-T-cell type is reactive for CD43, CD99, and terminal deoxynucleotidyltransferase (TdT). Pre-B-cell lesions label for PAX5, with or without CD99 and TdT.[256] Regardless of lineage, all examples of LBLL also

show a high proliferation index in immunostains with Ki-67.

Mastocytoma of the skin of the breast is represented by a solitary flesh-colored or pink plaque or nodule, often with an irregular surface (Figure 34-106). The skin around the lesion commonly urticates when the plaque or nodule is squeezed.[259,260] Histologically, one sees a discrete collection of monomorphic, oval cells arranged in sheets and nests, effacing part or all of the dermis but with no permeation of the epidermis. Nuclei are oval, with indistinct nucleoli and "smudgy" chromatin, and the cytoplasm is amphophilic and can be finely granular (Figure 34-107). Mitotic figures are rare.[261] Mastocytomas can be labeled histochemically with the Leder

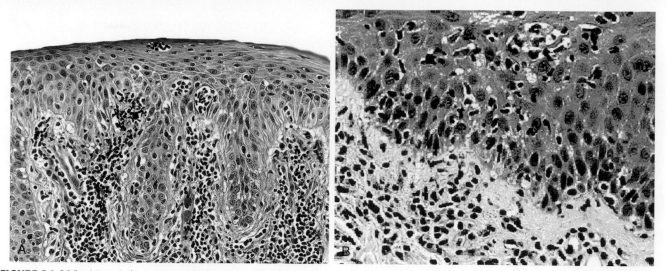

FIGURE 34-101 Mycosis fungoides (MF) shows variably dense lichenoid lymphoid infiltrates, comprising cells with convoluted nuclear contours ("Lutzner cells"). **A,** Small groups of such cells ("Pautrier microabscesses") are present within the epidermis, in the absence of significant spongiosis. **B,** Another common finding is that the atypical lymphoid elements of MF align themselves in single file at the epidermal base.

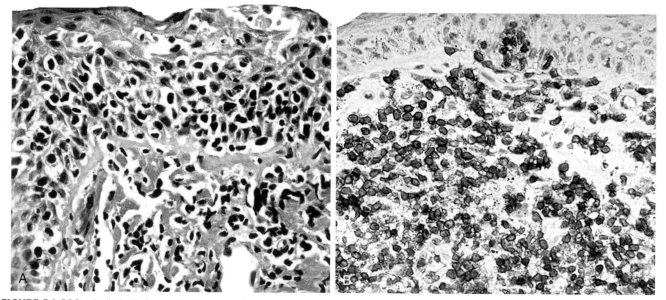

FIGURE 34-102 **A,** "Wiry" change in the upper dermal collagen may be present in MF as well. **B,** The lesional cell population is immunoreactive for CD4.

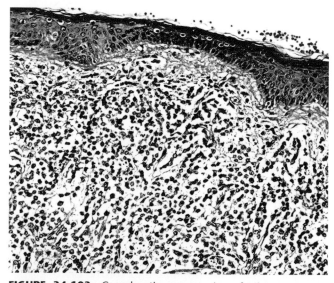

FIGURE 34-103 Granulocytic sarcoma (tumefactive acute myelogenous leukemia; leukemia cutis) often shows effacement of the dermis by aggregates of atypical mononuclear cells, which may be arranged in a linear fashion.

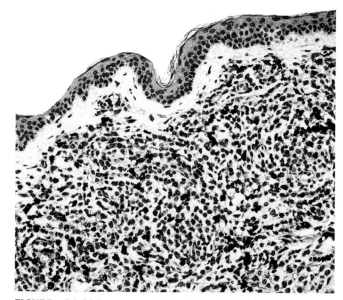

FIGURE 34-104 Immunostains for myeloperoxidase—shown here—and other granulocytic markers are positive in cutaneous granulocytic sarcoma.

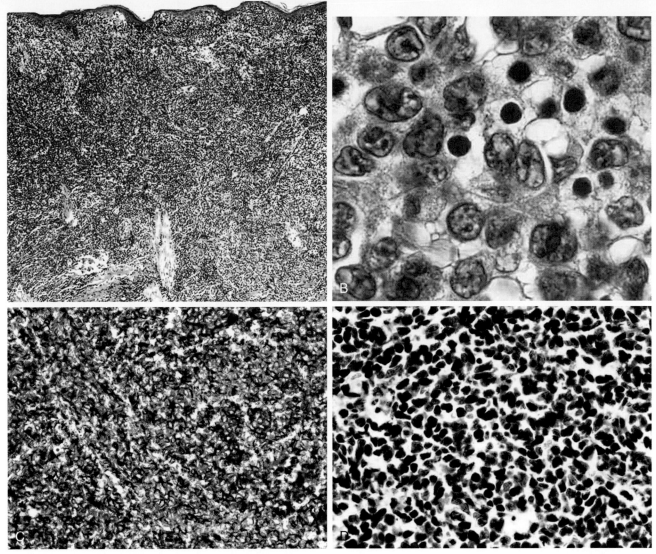

FIGURE 34-105 **A,** Lymphoblastic leukemia/lymphoma (LBLL) in the skin is represented by a dense round cell infiltrate that replaces the corium. **B,** Tumor cells in many cases of LBLL show convolutions of the nuclear membranes. LBLL is immunoreactive for CD10 (**C**) and terminal deoxynucleotidyl transferase (**D**).

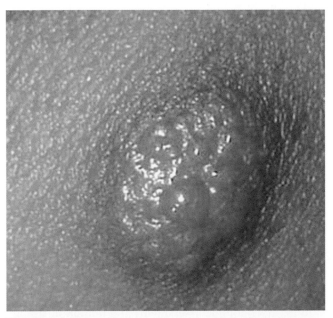

FIGURE 34-106 Solitary mastocytoma of the skin presents as a "juicy" flesh-colored plaque or nodule. The surrounding skin often urticates when the lesion is squeezed.

stain (Figure 34-108) and the Giemsa method or other Romanowsky dyes. Immunohistologically, they are reactive for CD117, calretinin, and tryptase.[261]

METASTATIC TUMORS OF THE MAMMARY SKIN

It is true that any malignancy of the deep tissues *could* metastasize to the skin of the breast, but that statement is more hypothetical than real. In actual practice, cutaneous metastatic lesions have a marked tendency to affect skin areas that are near to their sites of origin. In other words, those that are seen in the mammary skin have usually arisen either *in* the breast or in the thorax—particularly in the lungs.[262,263]

Another relatively common source of metastasis to the breast is cutaneous melanoma, even if the primary tumor was originally far away from the chest. Both the skin of the breast and the deeper mammary parenchyma may play host to metastatic melanoma.[264]

In children and adolescents, metastatic rhabdomyosarcoma must be considered to account for a malignant small cell neoplasm of the breast and mammary skin (Figure 34-109). Secondary deposits of neuroblastoma,

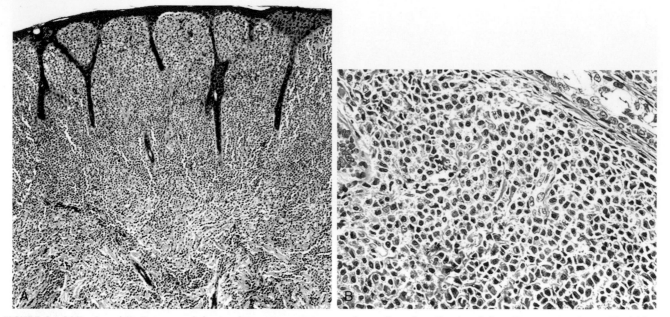

FIGURE 34-107 A and **B,** Groups and sheets of monotonous mononuclear cells replace the dermis in solitary mastocytoma. Nuclei have regular, oval contours, and dispersed chromatin. The cytoplasm may be finely granular.

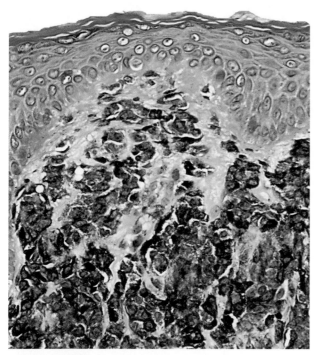

FIGURE 34-108 Strong reactivity is seen in the cells of solitary mastocytoma with the Leder (chloroacetate esterase) stain.

melanoma, or PNET represent additional possibilities in that specific context.[262,265] Immunophenotypic findings in this general group of tumors are summarized in Table 34-1.

Breast carcinomas account for most metastatic mammary skin tumors in adults, by far. Moreover, several clinical presentations can be associated with such lesions. The most common is the appearance of one or several reddish plaques or nodules, in or around a prior mastectomy scar (Figure 34-110). *Inflammatory* carcinoma and *carcinoma erysipelatoides* are terms used when the breast is diffusely erythematous and warm (erysipelas-like) (Figure 34-111). This appearance is caused by the presence of metastatic mammary carcinoma deposits in dermal lymphatic spaces,[266,267] a finding that can be corroborated with a podoplanin immunostain (Figure 34-112). *Carcinoma en cuirasse* is still another presentation—and a hideous one at that—of metastatic breast cancer involving the mammary skin, in which the thoracic integument becomes greatly thickened and discolored. Its name derives from the likeness that early observers drew to a breastplate of armor.[268] Finally, metastases from breast carcinoma—and other tumors as well—may assume a linear and pseudovesicular appearance, imitating the image of Herpes zoster infection (Figure 34-113).[269,270] The clinical evolution of most cases after cutaneous metastases appear is distinctly adverse. The great majority of patients with such neoplasms are expected to die within 12 months, regardless of the anatomic origins of the tumors.[262,266]

SUMMARY

This chapter focuses on neoplasms that affect the mammary skin. The take-home message for the diagnostician is to be keenly aware of the lesions that affect the mammary skin versus the mammary parenchyma. In certain instances, there is substantial overlap of these disease entities, and only careful clinical information, imaging studies, morphologic assessment, and immunohistology may be able to critically define them.

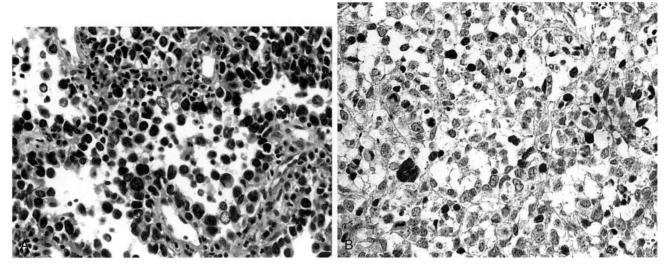

FIGURE 34-109 A, Metastatic rhabdomyosarcoma is a strong consideration when one encounters multinodular lesions in the breast skin, parenchyma, or both in patients younger than 25 years. **B,** This lesion shows nuclear immunoreactivity for myogenin as well as other myogenous markers.

TABLE 34-1	Immunohistologic Differential Diagnosis of Metastatic Small Cell Neoplasms in the Skin of the Breast							
Tumor Type	**Age**	**CK**	**NB84**	**MM**	**CD43/45**	**CD99**	**FLI-1**	**S100**
SCC	A	+*	0	0	0	±	±	0
NBL	C	0	+	0	0	0	0	0
RMS	C	0	0	+	0	±	0	0
PNET	C	0	±	0	0	+	+	0
MM	E	0	0	0	0	±	0	+
NHL	E	0	0	0	+	±	0	0
GS	E	0	0	0	+†	0	±	0

*Keratin reactivity is often "dotlike" and paranuclear in small cell neuroendocrine carcinomas.
†GS may also be reactive for myeloperoxidase, CD34, CD117, and lysozyme.
A, adult; C, child; CK, cytokeratin; E, either child or adult; FLI-1, friend leukemia virus–related nuclear antigen; GS, granulocytic sarcoma; MM, malignant melanoma; NB84, neuroblastoma-related antigen 84; NBL, neuroblastoma; NHL, non-Hodgkin's lymphoma; RMS, rhabdomyosarcoma; PNET, primitive neuroectodermal tumor; S100, S100 protein; SCC, small cell carcinoma.

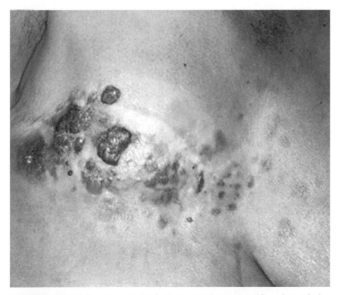

FIGURE 34-110 Metastatic breast carcinoma in the skin of the chest, represented by multiple nodules that surround and involve a mastectomy scar.

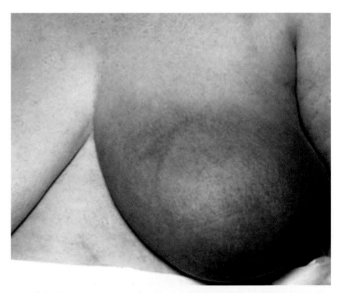

FIGURE 34-111 "Inflammatory" carcinoma (*"carcinoma erysipelatoides"*) is caused by diffuse involvement of dermal lymphatic spaces by metastatic breast carcinoma.

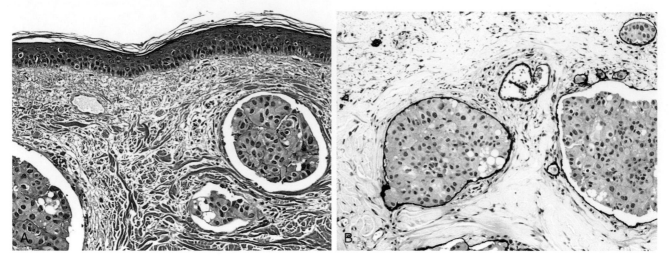

FIGURE 34-112 A, Tumor cell groups of metastatic breast carcinoma are present in dermal lymphatics in "inflammatory" carcinoma. **B,** They are further delineated with an immunostain for podoplanin, a lymphatic-endothelial marker.

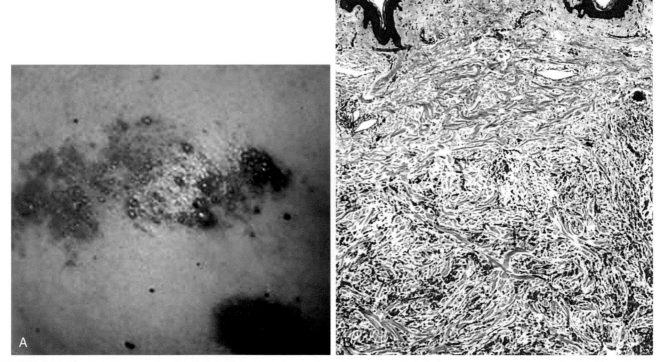

FIGURE 34-113 A, This example of metastatic breast carcinoma has a "zosteriform" clinical appearance, simulating the eruption of Herpes zoster. **B,** Histologically, nests and cords of metastatic tumor cells are present in the deep dermis.

REFERENCES

1. Hurwitz S. Epidermal nevi and tumors of epidermal origin. Pediatr Clin North Am 1983;30:483-494.
2. Su WPD. Histopathologic varieties of epidermal nevus: a study of 160 cases. Am J Dermatopathol 1982;4:161-170.
3. Young R, Jolley D, Marks R. Comparison of the use of standardized diagnostic criteria and intuitive clinical diagnosis in the diagnosis of common viral warts (verrucae vulgaris). Arch Dermatol 1998;134:1586-1589.
4. Steigleder GK. Histology of benign virus-induced tumors of the skin. J Cutan Pathol 1978;5:45-52.
5. Genc M, Yavuz M, Cimsit G, et al. Radiation port wart: a distinct cutaneous lesion after radiotherapy. J Natl Med Assoc 2006;99:1193-1196.
6. Yeatman JM, Kilkenny M, Marks R. The prevalence of seborrheic keratoses in an Australian population: does exposure to sunlight play a part in their frequency? Br J Dermatol 1997;137:411-414.
7. Brownstein MH, Fernando S, Shapiro L. Clear-cell acanthoma: clinicopathologic analysis of 37 new cases. Am J Clin Pathol 1973;59:306-311.

8. Laur WE, Posey RE, Waller JD. Lichen planus-like keratosis: a clinicohistopathologic correlation. J Am Acad Dermatol 1981;4:329-336.

9. Prieto VG, Casal M, McNutt NS. Lichen planus-like keratosis: a clinical and histological reexamination. Am J Surg Pathol 1993;4:329-336.

10. Frigy AF, Cooper PH. Benign lichenoid keratosis. Am J Clin Pathol 1985;83:439-443.

11. Long CC, Marks R. Increased risk of skin cancer: another Celtic myth? A review of Celtic ancestry and other risk factors for malignant melanoma and nonmelanoma skin cancer. J Am Acad Dermatol 1995;33:658-661.

12. Robinson JK. Risk of developing another basal cell carcinoma: a 5-year prospective study. Cancer 1987;60:118-120.

13. Okun MR, Blumenthal G. Basal cell epithelioma with giant cells and nuclear atypicality. Arch Dermatol 1964;89:598-602.

14. Geisse J, Caro I, Lindholm J, et al. Imiquimod 5% cream for the treatment of superficial basal cell carcinoma: a double-blind, randomized, vehicle-controlled study. J Am Acad Dermatol 2002;47:390-398.

15. Kao GF. Carcinoma arising in Bowen's disease. Arch Dermatol 1986;122:1124-1126.

16. Strayer DS, Santa Cruz DJ. Carcinoma in-situ of the skin: a review of histopathology. J Cutan Pathol 1980;7:244-259.

17. Garijo MF, Val D, Val-Bernal JF. Pagetoid dyskeratosis of the nipple epidermis: an incidental finding mimicking Paget's disease of the nipple. APMIS 2008;116:139-146.

18. Weedon D. Skin Pathology. 2nd ed. New York: Churchill-Livingstone; 2002:1158.

19. Rocamora A, Badia N, Vives R, et al. Epidermotropic primary neuroendocrine (Merkel-cell) carcinoma of the skin with Pautrier-like micro abscesses: report of three cases and review of the literature. J Am Acad Dermatol 1987;16:1163-1168.

20. Hashimoto K, Lee MW, D'Annunzio DR, et al. Pagetoid Merkel cell carcinoma: epidermal origin of the tumor. J Cutan Pathol 1998;25:572-579.

21. Traest K, De Vos R, van den Oord JJ. Pagetoid Merkel cell carcinoma: speculations on its origin and the mechanism of epidermal spread. J Cutan Pathol 1999;26:362-365.

22. Wick MR, Scheithauer BW. Primary neuroendocrine carcinoma of the skin. In Wick MR, ed. Pathology of Unusual Malignant Cutaneous Tumors. New York: Marcel Dekker; 1985:107-180.

23. Wick MR, Patterson JW. Merkel cell carcinoma and the Azzopardi phenomenon. Am J Dermatopathol 2007;29:315.

24. Miettinen M. Keratin-20: immunohistochemical marker for gastrointestinal, urothelial, and Merkel cell carcinomas. Mod Pathol 1995;8:384-388.

25. Chan JKC, Suster S, Wenig BM, et al. Cytokeratin-20 immunoreactivity distinguishes Merkel cell (primary cutaneous neuroendocrine) carcinomas and salivary gland small cell carcinomas from small cell carcinomas of various sites. Am J Surg Pathol 1997;21:226-234.

26. DeLellis RA, Shin S. Diagnostic immunohistochemistry of endocrine tumors. In Dabbs DJ, ed. Diagnostic Immunohistochemistry. New York: Churchill-Livingstone; 2002:209-240.

27. Brinkschmidt C. Immunohistochemical demonstration of chromogranin-A, chromogranin-B, and secretogranin in Merkel cell carcinoma of the skin: an immunohistochemical study suggesting two types of Merkel cell carcinoma. Appl Immunohistochem 1995;3:37-44.

28. Rossi S, Orvieto E, Furlanetto A, et al. Utility of the immunohistochemical detection of FLI-1 expression in round cell and vascular neoplasms using a monoclonal antibody. Mod Pathol 2004;17:547-552.

29. Goepfert H, Remmler D, Silva E, Wheeler B. Merkel cell carcinoma (endocrine carcinoma of the skin) of the head and neck. Arch Otolaryngol 1984;110:707-712.

30. Marrogi AJ, Wick MR, Dehner LP. Pilomatrical neoplasms in children and young adults. Am J Dermatopathol 1992;14:87-94.

31. Booth JC, Kramer H, Taylor KB. Pilomatrixoma—calcifying epithelioma (Malherbe). Pathology 1969;1:119-127.

32. Cazers JS, Okun MR, Pearson SH. Pigmented calcifying epithelioma: review and presentation of a case with unusual features. Arch Dermatol 1974;110:773-774.

33. Pfaltz M, Bruckner-Tuderman L, Schnyder UW. Type VII collagen is a component of cylindroma basement membrane zone. J Cutan Pathol 1989;16:388-395.

34. Brucker-Tuderman L, Pfaltz M, Schnyder UW. Cylindroma overexpresses collagen VII, the major anchoring fibril protein. J Invest Dermatol 1991;96:729-734.

35. Mentzel T, Requena L, Kaddu S, et al. Cutaneous myoepithelial neoplasms: clinicopathologic and immunohistochemical study of 20 cases suggesting a continuous spectrum ranging from benign mixed tumor of the skin to cutaneous myoepithelioma and myoepithelial carcinoma. J Cutan Pathol 2003;30:294-302.

36. Mambo NC. Eccrine spiradenoma: clinical and pathologic study of 49 tumors. J Cutan Pathol 1983;10:312-320.

37. Kersting DW, Helwig EB. Eccrine spiradenoma. Arch Dermatol 1956;73:199-227.

38. Johnson BL Jr, Helwig EB. Eccrine acrospiroma: a clinicopathologic study. Cancer 1969;23:641-657.

39. Helwig EB. Eccrine acrospiroma. J Cutan Pathol 1984;11:415-420.

40. Diaz NM, Palmer JO, Wick MR. Erosive adenomatosis of the nipple: histology, immunohistology, and differential diagnosis. Mod Pathol 1992;5:179-184.

41. Miller L, Tyler W, Maroon M, Miller OF 3rd. Erosive adenomatosis of the nipple: a benign imitator of malignant breast disease. Cutis 1997;59:91-92.

42. Rosen PP. Cutaneous neoplasms. In Rosen's Breast Pathology. Philadelphia: Lippincott-Raven; 1997:789-799.

43. Henner MS, Shapiro PE, Ritter JH, et al. Solitary syringoma. Report of five cases and clinicopathologic comparison with microcystic adnexal carcinoma of the skin. Am J Dermatopathol 1995;17:465-470.

44. LeBoit PE, Sexton M. Microcystic adnexal carcinoma of the skin: a reappraisal of the differentiation and differential diagnosis of an underrecognized neoplasm. J Am Acad Dermatol 1993;29:609-618.

45. Goldstein DJ, Barr RJ, Santa Cruz DJ. Microcystic adnexal carcinoma: a distinct clinicopathologic entity. Cancer 1982;50:566-572.

46. Cooper PH. Sclerosing carcinomas of sweat ducts (microcystic adnexal carcinoma). Arch Dermatol 1986;122:261-264.

47. Ward BE, Cooper PH, Subramony C. Syringomatous tumor of the nipple. Am J Clin Pathol 1989;92:692-696.

48. Foschini MP, Krausz T. Salivary gland-type tumors of the breast. Semin Diagn Pathol 2010;27:77-90.

49. Lloyd J, Flanagan AM. Mammary and extramammary Paget's disease. J Clin Pathol 2000;53:742-749.

50. Sitakalin C, Ackerman AB. Mammary and extra mammary Paget's disease. Am J Dermatopathol 1985;7:335-340.

51. Sakorafas GH, Blanchard DK, Sarr MG, Farley DR. Paget's disease of the breast: a clinical perspective. Langenbecks Arch Surg 2001;386:444-450.

52. Kohler S, Smoller BR. A case of extramammary Paget's disease mimicking pemphigus vulgaris on histologic examination. Dermatology 1997;195:54-56.

53. Wolf R, Berstein-Lipschitz L, Rothem A. Paget's disease of the nipple resembling an acantholytic disease on microscopic examination. Dermatologica 1989;179:42-44.

54. O'Malley FB, Baue A. An update on apocrine lesions of the breast. Histopathology 2008;52:3-10.

55. Murray JC, Pollack SV, Pinnell SR. Keloids: a review. J Am Acad Dermatol 1981;4:461-470.

56. Wick MR, Mills SE, Ritter JH, Lind AC. Postoperative/posttraumatic spindle-cell nodule of the skin: the dermal analogue of nodular fasciitis. Am J Dermatopathol 1999;21:220-224.

57. Kang SK, Kim HH, Ahn SJ, et al. Intradermal nodular fasciitis of the face. J Dermatol 2002;29:310-314.

58. Fitzpatrick TB, Gilchrest BA. Dimple sign to differentiate benign from malignant pigmented cutaneous lesions. N Engl J Med 1977;296:1518.

59. Gonzalez S, Duarte I. Benign fibrous histiocytoma of the skin: a morphologic study of 290 cases. Pathol Res Pract 1982;174:379-391.

60. Marrogi AJ, Dehner LP, Coffin CM, Wick MR. Benign cutaneous histiocytic tumors in childhood and adolescence, excluding Langerhans cell proliferations: a clinicopathologic and immunohistochemical analysis. Am J Dermatopathol 1992;14:8-18.

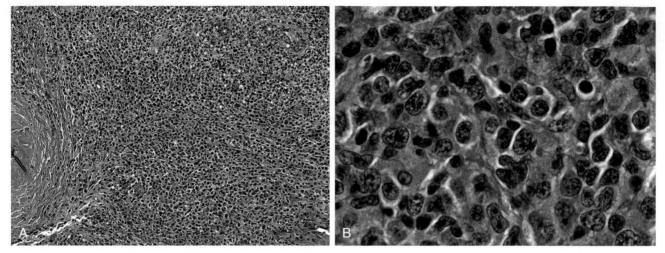

FIGURE 35-1 Diffuse large B-cell lymphoma. Architectural effacement by sheets of large lymphoid cells (**A**) with high magnification showing large cells with irregular nuclear contours, vesicular chromatin and prominent nucleoli (**B**).

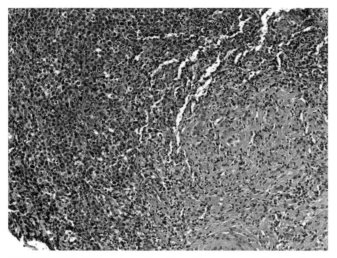

FIGURE 35-2 Diffuse large B-cell lymphoma. Areas of sclerosis can accompany the neoplastic infiltrate.

(1) centroblastic, with oval to round vesicular nuclei, fine chromatin, and several nucleoli and (2) immunoblastic, characterized by a single prominent nucleolus and sometimes plasmacytoid features. Centroblastic morphology appears to predominate in both localized and disseminated breast DLBCL, but this distinction is not considered an important one.[8] Areas of background sclerosis may also be seen, especially in disseminated cases of DLBCL (Figure 35-2).[8] Lymphoepithelial lesions have been reported in DLBCL without a coexisting MALT component.[18] Distinction from carcinoma can be difficult on morphologic grounds alone. Although the lack of cellular cohesion and absence of an in situ component may be useful histologic features favoring lymphoma, the presence of in situ carcinoma does not exclude the possibility of a lymphoma because epithelial and hematopoietic neoplasms may rarely coexist.[23]

The large lymphoid cells are immunoreactive for B-cell markers such as CD20, CD79a, and PAX5 (Figure 35-3), have variable expression of germinal center–associated and other B-cell subset markers, are negative for T-cell markers such as CD3, and are negative for epithelial markers such as cytokeratin. The nuclear proliferation marker Ki-67 can be used to assess the proliferation fraction as well as nuclear size and morphology (Figure 35-4) and may be particularly useful in distorted or small biopsies. If fresh tissue is available, flow cytometric studies can be used to look for a more detailed lymphoid phenotype and monotypic light chain restriction, although a subset of DLBCLs are surface light chain–negative (24% in one study).[24] In addition, a negative flow cytometric evaluation would not preclude involvement by lymphoma if the involved area was not sampled or if insufficient viable tumor cells are present for evaluation, issues that may arise in small biopsies or high-grade tumors.

DLBCL, NOS, has been divided into two molecular subgroups (germinal center B-cell–like [GCB] and activated B-cell–like), and three immunohistochemical subgroups: CD5 positive DLBCL, GCB, and non–germinal center B-cell–like (non-GCB).[22] CD5 is a T-cell–associated antigen that is uncommonly seen in primary breast DLBCL (13% in one series of 15 cases).[18] The 2 patients with CD5+ breast DLBCL in this study were both still alive without relapses after 35 and 171 months of follow-up, although CD5 expression has been reported to be associated with an unfavorable prognosis in de novo DLBCL.[25] The absence of cyclin D1 expression would distinguish DLBCL from the vast majority of aggressive variants of mantle cell lymphoma (MCL), which are also CD5+ lymphoid neoplasms. The other two immunohistochemical categories (GCB and non-GCB) are related to the molecular subgroups, although this information is not required for diagnosis and currently does not affect treatment planning.[26] The GCB versus non-GCB distinction, which is most commonly performed using three antibodies and the "Hans algorithm," follows from gene expression studies that identified a germinal center type of DLBCL that had a better prognosis than the activated B-cell type of DLBCL.[27,28] This algorithm defines GCB origin as demonstrating

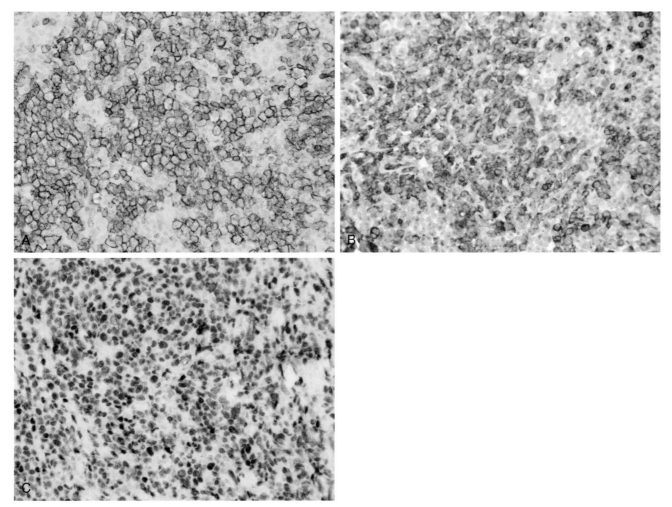

FIGURE 35-3 Diffuse large B-cell lymphoma. Diffuse large B-cell lymphoma is typically positive for the B-cell markers CD20 (**A**), CD79a (**B**), and PAX5 (**C**), which is particularly useful to highlight nuclear size.

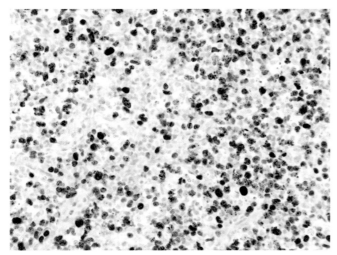

FIGURE 35-4 Diffuse large B-cell lymphoma. Ki-67 shows many proliferating cells that would not be expected in an indolent lymphoma.

greater than 30% CD10+ cells or, if CD10 is negative, greater than 30% *bcl6*+ cells and less than 30% *IRF4/MUM1*+ cells. All other cases are considered non-GCB type. Whether the immunohistochemical-defined subgroups also demonstrate a better survival among the GCB group is controversial; however, the GCB type appears to have an equivalent or better prognosis than the non-GCB type.[28,29] Using the Hans algorithm, primary breast DLBCL predominantly shows a non-GCB phenotype (Figure 35-5).[8,18,30] This finding is consistent with the lack of ongoing somatic hypermutation in DLBCLs of the breast.[18]

TREATMENT AND PROGNOSIS

Treatment includes limited surgery, with no increased benefit for mastectomy, together with anthracycline-based chemotherapy such as CHOP (cyclophosphamide, doxorubicin, vincristine, and prednisone) and radiation therapy (RT).[16,26,31] Currently, addition of the anti-CD20 monoclonal antibody is part of the standard therapy for both limited and advanced-stage DLBCL.[26] However, one small prospective study of 32 breast DLBCL patients found that the addition of rituximab did not improve the response rate, event-free survival, or overall survival (OS) compared with those in historical controls in early-stage disease.[32] Further prospective studies will be important in determining the efficacy of rituximab and other targeted therapies in primary breast DLBCL. One study of PBLs that included 17 breast lymphoma; however, it may identify at least a rare MALT lymphoma.[2]

On mammogram, the masses may have irregular, partly defined or well-defined borders. Doppler sonography reveals heterogeneity and the strong vascularization of MALT lymphomas. By contrast-enhanced breast MRI, MALT lymphomas are hyperintense on T2-weighted images and isointense on T1-weighted images with strong and rapid contrast enhancement.[46] Computed tomography (CT) has been reported to show homogenous attenuation and moderate enhancement of well-marginated masslike lesions.[47] Although PET is less sensitive in indolent lymphoma, MALT lymphomas demonstrated 54% ^{18}F-FDG avidity with 97% ^{18}F-FDG avidity seen with DLBCL, and 100% ^{18}F-FDG avidity seen with HL, BL, MCL, anaplastic large cell lymphoma (ALCL), nodal marginal zone lymphoma, lymphoblastic lymphoma, angioimmunoblastic T-cell lymphoma, NK/T-cell lymphoma, and plasmacytoma.[21] Interestingly, ^{18}F-FDG/PET may be more sensitive in MALT lymphomas with plasmacytic differentiation owing to significantly increased uptake.[48]

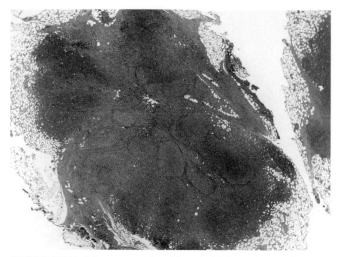

FIGURE 35-7 Mucosa-associated lymphoid tissue (MALT) lymphoma. The lymphoma forms a mass lesion that, on low magnification, could mimic an intramammary lymph node. However, note the associated bands of sclerosis and absence of a lymph node capsule.

KEY CLINICAL FEATURES

Extranodal Marginal Zone Lymphoma of Mucosa-associated Lymphoid Tissue (MALT Lymphoma)

- **Definition:** Extranodal lymphoma composed of neoplastic marginal zone cells with occasional plasmacytic differentiation.

- **Incidence/location:** Second most common PBL

- **Imaging features:** Variable appearance by mammography, heterogeneity and strong vascularization by Doppler sonography; by PET, overall lower ^{18}F-FDG avidity as compared with more aggressive lymphomas, although MALT lymphomas with plasmacytic differentiation show significantly more avidity

- **Prognosis:** Tend to remain localized for long periods of time. Relapses may occur late in the disease course or in other extranodal mucosal sites.

- **Treatment:** Surgery/radiation therapy, with or without chemotherapy, rituximab.

^{18}F-FDG, ^{18}F-fluorodeoxyglucose; MALT, mucosa-associated lymphoid tissue; PBL, primary breast lymphoma; PET, positron-emission tomography.

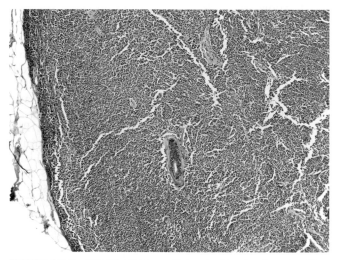

FIGURE 35-8 MALT lymphoma. Entrapped benign breast epithelium is found within the infiltrate.

HISTOLOGY, PHENOTYPE, GENOTYPE, AND CYTOGENETIC FINDINGS

MALT lymphomas usually form a discrete mass, with a well-circumscribed lymphoid infiltrate and occasional bands of sclerosis (Figure 35-7). The low-magnification appearance may resemble an intramammary lymph node; however, entrapped epithelium is present and a well-defined nodal architecture is lacking (Figure 35-8). In other cases, the infiltrate is less well circumscribed.[8] The lymphoid cells are predominantly small with clumped chromatin. Although a "monocytoid" appearance is typical with a moderate amount of pale cytoplasm (Figure 35-9), some MALT lymphomas have only scant

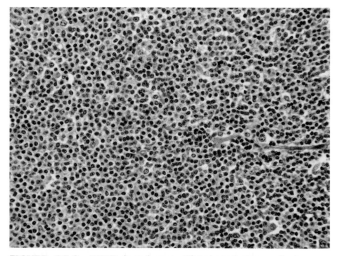

FIGURE 35-9 MALT lymphoma. The lymphoma cells have a "monocytoid" appearance with abundant cytoplasm.

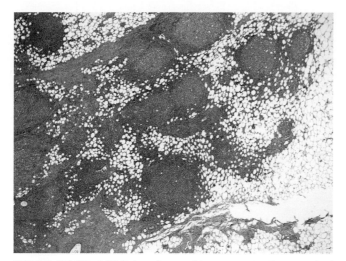

FIGURE 35-10 MALT lymphoma. Numerous reactive germinal centers are seen associated with this MALT lymphoma.

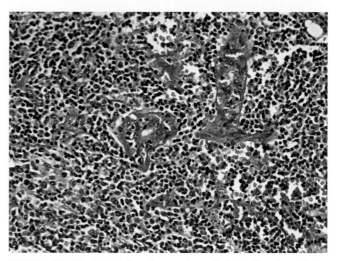

FIGURE 35-12 MALT lymphoma. Lymphoid infiltration of the breast epithelium with formation of lymphoepithelial lesions.

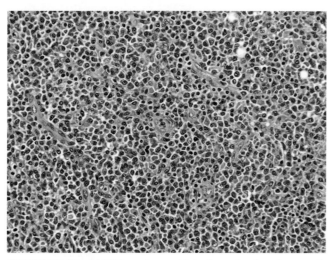

FIGURE 35-11 MALT lymphoma. Note the extensive plasmacytic differentiation with sheets of mature-appearing plasma cells.

cytoplasm. Numerous reactive germinal centers may be present within or at the periphery of the mass, with or without infiltration by the MALT lymphoma (follicular colonization) (Figure 35-10). Plasmacytic differentiation may be present (Figure 35-11). In one series, a monoclonal plasma cell component was identified in 72% of breast MALT lymphomas, with 36% of breast MALT lymphomas showing greater than 20% plasma cells within the infiltrate.[49] In some cases, plasmacytic differentiation may be so marked that plasma cell myeloma or plasmacytoma could be considered in the differential diagnosis. Lymphoepithelial lesions may be present (Figure 35-12), but unlike gastric or salivary gland MALT lymphomas, they are infrequent. Although scattered larger transformed-appearing cells may be seen, sheetlike proliferations of large lymphoid cells are not, and if identified, a separate diagnosis of DLBCL should be rendered.

The neoplastic cells are monoclonal B cells that express pan-B-cell markers such as CD20, Pax5, and CD79a, and often demonstrate coexpression of *bcl2*.

Most, but not all, cases are CD5−, and CD10 expression is not seen.[50,51] Expression of CD43 has been reported in 30% to 50% of breast MALT lymphomas.[2,49] Unlike most MCLs, MALT lymphomas lack cyclin D1 expression.

When reactive follicles accompany the neoplastic infiltrate, immunostains can be helpful in delineating the *bcl6+*, CD10 usually positive, and *bcl2−* reactive germinal center cells from the *bcl6−*, CD10−, usually *bcl2+* MALT lymphoma cells that surround and infiltrate follicles (Figure 35-13). Follicular dendritic cell (FDC) markers (CD21, CD23, CD35) may also be useful in highlighting expanded FDC meshworks (Figure 35-14). Although a Ki-67 immunostain will typically show a low proliferation index among the neoplastic B-cell population, this stain will highlight numerous proliferating germinal center cells in the reactive follicles that should not be interpreted as areas of transformation (Figure 35-15). Particularly in cases with plasmacytic differentiation, immunohistochemical and/or in situ hybridization (ISH) studies for kappa and lambda can establish light chain restriction (Figure 35-16). If eosinophilic amorphous extracellular material is noted, a Congo red stain may be useful to evaluate for amyloid.

Trisomies 3, 12, and 18 may be seen in breast MALT lymphomas, although the frequency of trisomy 3 is lower than in MALT lymphomas of the stomach, parotid, and thyroid (33% vs. 60%).[52] *MALT1* gene rearrangements [t(11;18)(q21;q21), t(14;18)(q32;q21)], which are frequent among some MALT lymphomas at other sites, have not been identified in breast MALT lymphomas.[53,54] Other MALT lymphoma–associated cytogenetic abnormalities not identified in localized breast lesions include *bcl10* [t(1;14)(p22;q32)] and *FOXP1* [t(3;14)(p14.1;q32)] translocations.[52,54–58]

TREATMENT AND PROGNOSIS

In contrast to DLBCL, patients with localized MALT lymphomas may be managed with local therapy alone, and the role of chemotherapy in this group is

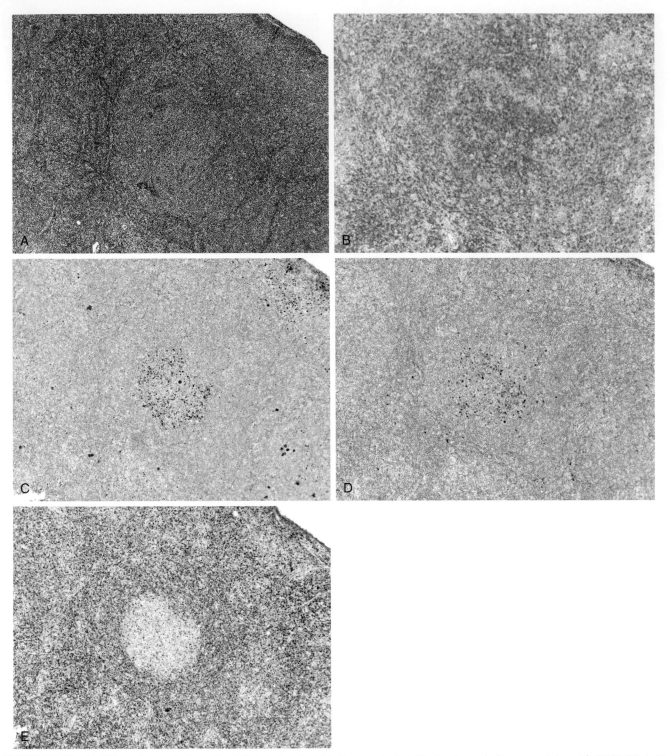

FIGURE 35-13 MALT lymphoma. **A,** A reactive follicle is found within the neoplastic infiltrate. A panel of immunostains with CD20 (**B**), bcl6 (**C**), CD10 (**D**), and bcl2 (**E**) is helpful in delineating the CD20+ BCL6– BCL2+ MALT lymphoma cells surrounding the CD20+ BCL6– BCL2– reactive germinal center. Note the down-regulated CD10 expression that may be seen when MALT lymphomas colonize reactive follicles.

unclear.[3,26,59] Surgical excision with RT provides excellent local control.[3] Observation may also be considered for some patients, especially if the diagnostic biopsy was excisional, although locoregional RT should be considered in the setting of positive margins.[26] Chemotherapy may be recommended for advanced stages (III or IV). Immunotherapy with rituximab has also been shown to

be safe and efficacious in MALT lymphoma.[60] If MALT lymphoma coexists with DLBCL, the tumors should be treated as DLBCL.[26]

Breast MALT lymphomas are typically indolent and patients have an excellent overall survival. In the largest series examining clinical outcomes of indolent breast lymphomas, the OS was 92% at 5 years and 65% at 10

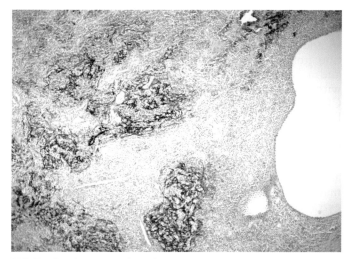

FIGURE 35-14 MALT lymphoma. A CD21 immunostain shows the expanded follicular dendritic cell meshworks due to follicular colonization.

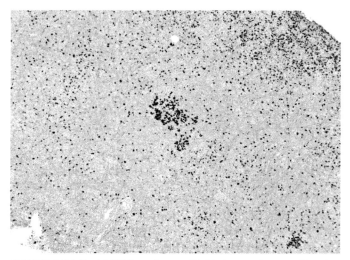

FIGURE 35-15 MALT lymphoma. Ki-67 shows a low proliferation index within the MALT lymphoma. Note the reactive germinal center with more numerous proliferating cells.

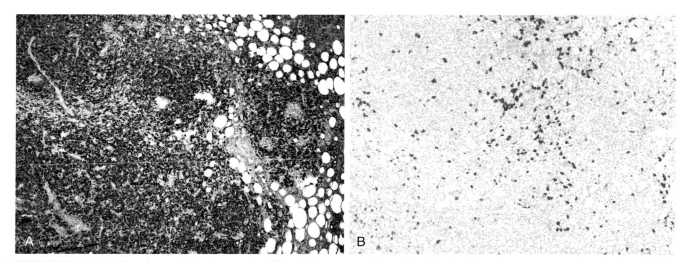

FIGURE 35-16 MALT lymphoma with plasmacytic differentiation. Kappa (**A**) and lambda (**B**) light chain immunohistochemical stains demonstrate cytoplasmic kappa light chain restriction.

years. However, the 5-year and 10-year progression-free survival (PFS) were 56% and 34%, with up to half of relapses occurring within the first 5 years of follow-up.[45]

PROGNOSTIC FACTORS

There is a higher risk of relapse if the management includes only surgery.[45] Most of the relapses are again responsive to treatment and do not affect OS. Late relapses are known to occur with extranodal MALT lymphomas, including breast MALT lymphomas, necessitating long follow-up periods.[45,61,62]

DIFFERENTIAL DIAGNOSIS

The differential diagnosis includes both specific and nonspecific benign infiltrates as well as other small B-cell lymphomas. Reactive lymphoid proliferations may form tumor-like lesions with a dense inflammatory infiltrate and simulate lymphoma, termed "pseudolymphoma" in the older literature. Although some of the histologic features of "pseudolymphoma," such as the presence of germinal centers, a polymorphous lymphoid infiltrate, and a predominance of mature lymphocytes,[63] are now recognized as classic features of MALT lymphoma, some specific benign clinicopathologic entities, such as immunoglobulin G_4 (IgG_4)–related sclerosing mastitis, have also probably been included within this category.[64] Generally, reactive infiltrates are composed of a heterogeneous admixture of T and B cells, without overt destruction of the underlying architecture. Although sheets of B cells outside follicles are not generally seen in extranodal locations, they may be seen in some benign breast processes, including lymphocytic mastitis/diabetic mastopathy and cutaneous lymphoid hyperplasia of the nipple (see details later). Flow cytometric, cytogenetic, and/or molecular studies may be useful ancillary studies to identify and characterize clonal lymphoid populations.

Lymphocytic mastitis/diabetic mastopathy is an uncommon mass-forming lesion that most frequently

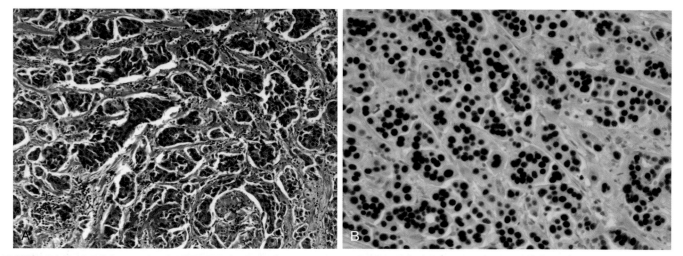

FIGURE 36-5   **A,** High-power magnification of primary breast micropapillary carcinoma. **B,** Tumor is strongly positive for ERs (and negative for CA125), supporting the clinical impression of primary breast carcinoma.

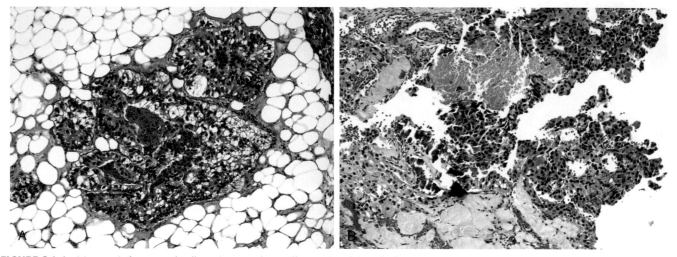

FIGURE 36-6   Metastasis from renal cell carcinoma, clear cell type, involving the breast parenchyma. **A,** Island of metastatic renal cell carcinoma involving the breast parenchyma with low-grade nuclei and clear cytoplasm, lying in fibrovascular stroma. **B,** Occasionally, metastatic renal cell carcinoma shows focal tumor calcifications, an uncommon finding of metastatic tumor involving the breast.

appearance with focal areas of adenosquamous differentiation.[9,12,82] The histomorphology of the metastatic endometrial carcinoma depends on the tumor grade, whereas a solid growth pattern can mimic poorly differentiated breast carcinoma. Endometrioid adenocarcinoma is positive for CK7, ER, PAX8 and PgR but usually negative for GCDFP-15. A few cases of metastatic cervical and vulvar squamous cell carcinoma to the breast have been reported.[2,5,13,83,84] In all cases, breast metastasis usually indicates disseminated metastatic disease and a poor prognosis. An uncommon cause of metastatic tumor in postpartum breast is choriocarcinoma.[58,85]

GENITOURINARY TRACT TUMORS

There are only isolated case reports documenting RCC metastasizing to the breast. Metastatic RCC to the breast has been reported 16 times with 8 cases representing the initial presentation of metastatic disease.[16,17,86–89] Although metastases were present in approximately 30%

of patients with RCC, the breast was rarely involved.[88,89] Metastatic RCC in the breast may precede the diagnosis of the occult RCC or metastasis may occur decades later (≤18 yr) after initial resection of the tumor.[89] Conventional RCC is the most common renal malignancy that metastasizes to breast. The abundant clear or granular cytoplasm with a relatively low nuclear-to-cytoplasmic ratio and prominent fine vessels are useful clues to the correct diagnosis (Figure 36-6).

While RCC antigen is helpful to identify renal cell carcinoma, up to 33% of breast carcinomas may be positive for RCC.[89a] PAX2 is more helpful in this situation, as it is positive in more than 75% of clear cell and papillary renal carcinomas.[89b]

Benign breast lesions with foam cells, such as fat necrosis or benign neoplasms, such as granular cell tumors, adenomyoepithelial lesions, or lactating adenoma can be confused with this neoplasm.[89] Primary breast carcinomas such as secretory carcinoma, glycogen-rich carcinoma, histiocytoid carcinoma, and lipid-rich carcinoma

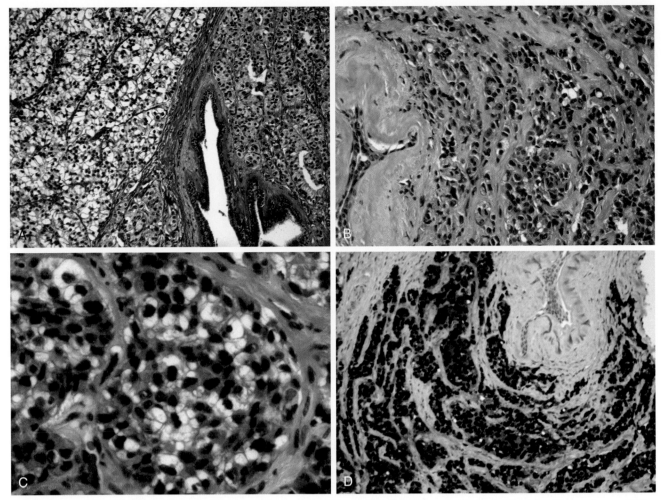

FIGURE 36-7 Primary breast carcinoma with clear cytoplasm. **A,** Primary breast carcinoma, glycogen-rich type, shows clear cytoplasm, mimicking metastatic renal cell carcinoma. **B** and **C,** Core biopsy of a breast mass in a patient with a history of renal cell carcinoma. Biopsy shows poorly differentiated carcinoma with occasional clear cytoplasm. **D,** Tumor cells are strongly and diffusely positive for ERs (and negative for other renal carcinoma markers), reinforcing the diagnosis of primary breast carcinoma.

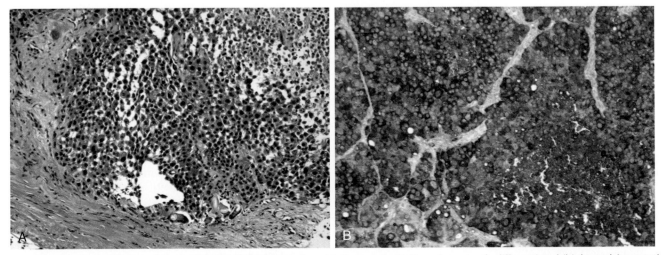

FIGURE 36-8 Metastasis from the prostate seen in the breast of an elderly man. **A,** Sections show poorly differentiated (high-grade) prostatic adenocarcinoma. **B,** Tumor cells are positive for prostate-specific antigen.

are also among the main entities considered in the differential diagnosis[86] (Figure 36-7). An unusual case of metastatic RCC to the breast from an occult renal primary in a woman who had previous lumpectomy owing to mammary carcinoma in the same breast has been reported.[89]

Prostate carcinoma is one of the most common primary sites that metastasizes to the male breast.[77] Prostatic carcinoma may have columnar cells with relatively bland nuclei with nucleoli, with overlapping histology with breast carcinoma (Figure 36-8). In men, involvement of the breast

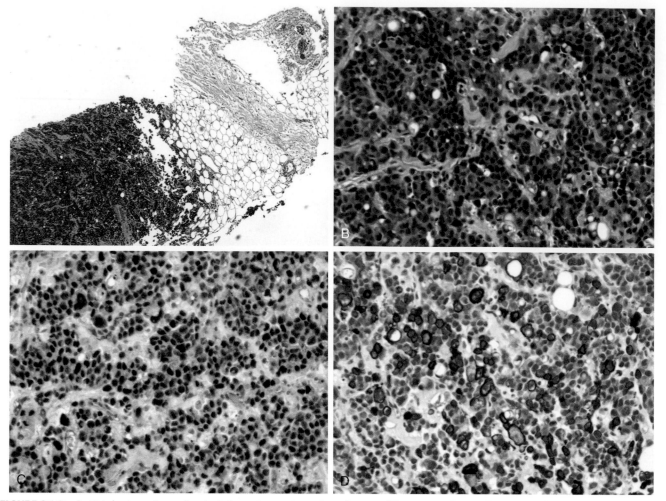

FIGURE 36-9 **A,** Histologic sections of metastatic gastroesophageal carcinoma, diffuse type to breast. **B,** Tumor cells show poorly differentiated adenocarcinoma with signet-ring cells. Tumor cells are positive for CDX-2 (**C**) and cytokeratins 20 and 7 (**D**).

by metastatic prostatic adenocarcinoma has been a frequent finding at autopsy.[11] Breast involvement was identified in 26% of patients with prostatic adenocarcinoma with microscopic examination.[10,13] Charache in 1953[90] reported metastatic prostatic carcinoma initially presenting as a breast mass, and the primary site was not detected until autopsy. Several authors have described patients with bilateral breast metastases from prostatic adenocarcinoma.[91–93] Although any breast mass in a patient with a history of prostatic carcinoma should raise the question of metastases, rare reports have described independent synchronous or metachronous primary carcinomas of the prostate and breast.[94] A collision tumor consisting of metastatic prostatic carcinoma in a solid papillary carcinoma of the male breast has also been described.[95] Transitional cell carcinoma of the urinary bladder has also been reported to metastasize to the breast.[9,96]

Immunohistochemistry is crucial in the differential diagnosis between primary and metastatic carcinoma in the male breast. Conventional RCC is usually positive for the RCC marker (90%), whereas up to 33% of breast cancers are positive.[89b,97] CD10 is present in a high proportion of conventional and papillary RCCs (90%), but it is rarely expressed in breast cancer (5%).[98] ER, GCDFP-15, and CK7 are rarely expressed in conventional RCC,[99] although CK7 is usually expressed

in the papillary type of RCC.[99,100] PSA and prostatic acid phosphatase are excellent markers of prostatic carcinoma because both are expressed in nearly 100% of tumors.[101] One report suggests that PSA is not a specific marker because it stains 15% of primary mammary carcinoma.[102] ER, GCDFP-15, and CK7 positivity are uncommon in prostatic carcinoma.

GASTROINTESTINAL TUMORS

The intestinal type of gastric carcinoma may resemble invasive ductal carcinoma of the breast, and diffuse gastric carcinoma may resemble invasive lobular carcinoma of the breast (Figure 36-9). Gastric carcinomas are reported to be the most common metastatic malignancy to the breast in the Korean population.[2] Metastatic gastrointestinal mucinous carcinoma is histologically indistinguishable from primary mucinous carcinoma of the breast.[13] In 1936, Dawson[103] described a woman with diffuse lymphatic invasion of both breasts from signet-ring cell gastric adenocarcinoma. Later, Yeh and coworkers[2] reported additional cases with a similar presentation.

ER and GCDFP-15 are rarely expressed by gastric carcinoma, whereas CK20 and CDX2 are usually positive in gastric carcinoma (see Figure 36-9).

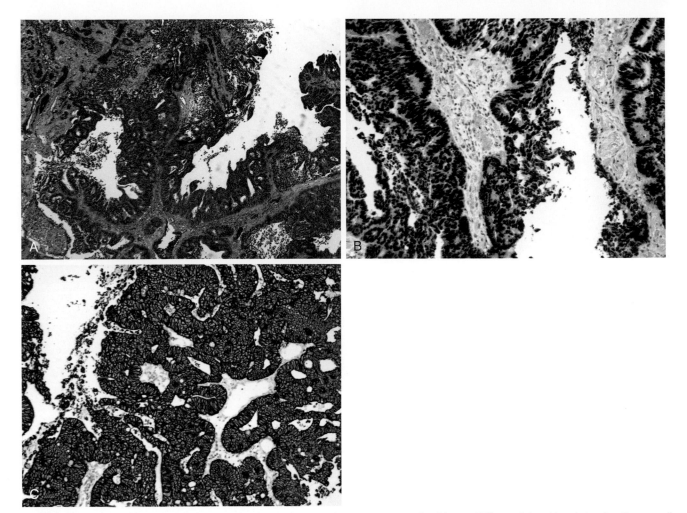

FIGURE 36-10 Metastasis from colorectal carcinoma. **A,** Sections show tumor necrosis with pencil-like nuclei and brush border. Tumor cells are strongly positive for CDX-2 (**B**) and cytokeratin 20 (**C**).

Despite being the most common gastrointestinal tract tumor among adults, colorectal carcinomas are rarely reported to metastasize to the breast (Figure 36-10). Only a few cases have been reported in the literature, three of which were seen in men, including one case of rectal small cell carcinoma.[2,104–108] Metastatic breast colorectal carcinoma and the primary tumor can present as synchronous lesions, or breast metastases may follow the primary by months to years. Immunohistochemistry shows that the majority of colorectal carcinomas are usually CK7– and CK20+ and CDX2+.[109] In contrast, primary breast carcinomas are CK7+ and CK20– and CDX2–. Metastases to the breast are usually associated with disseminated metastases and a poor prognosis. Yeh and coworkers[2] reported three cases of hepatocellular carcinomas metastatic to the breast. Gallbladder carcinoma and esophageal squamous cell carcinoma have also been reported to metastasize to breast, progressing from asymptomatic lesion to death within 3 weeks.[110–112]

NEUROENDOCRINE TUMORS (CARCINOID TUMORS)

Well-differentiated neuroendocrine neoplasms (carcinoid tumors) are slow growing with a tendency for late metastases (<19 yr).[113] Upalakalin and colleagues[113]

estimated that 41% of all carcinoid tumors in the breast were metastases from extramammary sites. Patients with metastases to the breast present an average 10 years younger than patients with primary breast carcinoids and have a worse prognosis.[114]

In carcinoid syndrome, an enlarged liver and multiple metastatic nodules in both breasts are possible presenting manifestations.[20,114] Although the presence of carcinoid syndrome is highly suggestive of metastases from a gastrointestinal origin, its absence does not rule out the possibility of an extramammary origin.[20,114] A breast mass may be the first indication of an occult carcinoid tumor.[20,96,113,115,116] The majority of primary occult carcinoid tumors are located in the lung and ileum/ileocecum, followed by the appendix and ovary.[5,20,113,115] Fishman and associates[117] have reported a breast metastases from an occult ovarian carcinoid tumor. The lesion was diagnosed and treated as a lobular carcinoma for 1 year before the ovarian primary was identified.

A carcinoid tumor of the breast may be misdiagnosed as an epithelial malignancy even when the patient has a known history of a carcinoid tumor elsewhere. Immunohistochemical analysis can provide some clues to the primary site of carcinoid tumors. Expression of CDX2 and CK20 favors gastrointestinal origin, whereas TTF-1 and CK7 expression favors pulmonary origin.[118]

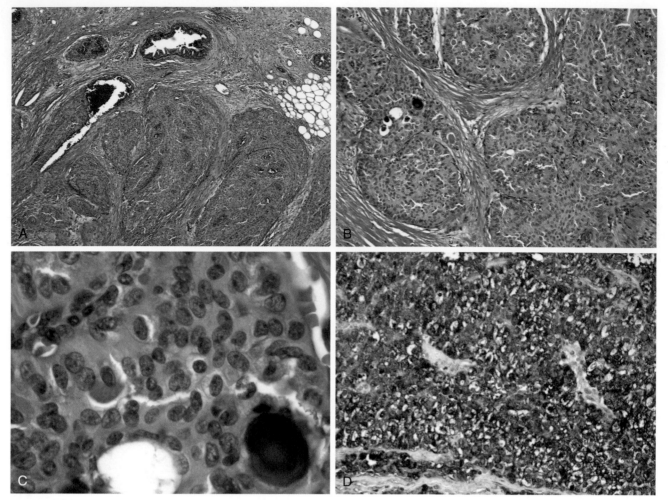

FIGURE 36-11 Metastasis from thyroid papillary carcinoma. **A,** Tumor infiltrates the breast parenchyma and is intermixed with benign breast tissue. **B,** Tumor shows papillary architecture, vascular stroma, and occasional psammoma body formation. **C,** Tumor cells show nuclear features of papillary carcinoma such as intranuclear inclusions and multiple nuclear grooves. **D,** Thyroglobulin and TTF-1 are positive in tumor cells, reinforcing the diagnosis of metastatic thyroid carcinoma.

ER, PgR, and GCDFP-15 are often expressed by mammary neuroendocrine carcinomas. However; PgR can be expressed in some pancreatic endocrine tumors.[119]

THYROID TUMORS

Medullary thyroid carcinoma (MTC) is an uncommon thyroid cancer and has been reported to metastasize to the breast.[120] All patients were women with persistent elevated calcitonin level after treatment and the failure of other imaging modalities to detect residual disease.[120] Distant metastasis occurred late, usually to the breast. Metastatic MTC gland can have an infiltrating pattern that mimics infiltrating lobular carcinoma of breast.[121] Immunohistochemical studies showed that the neoplastic cells were positive for CK7, neuroendocrine markers, calcitonin, and TTF-1 but negative for ER and PgR.

Papillary and follicular carcinoma of the thyroid may rarely metastasize to the breast.[24] Only a few reports of metastatic papillary thyroid carcinoma to the breast have been published.[122–125] The majority of the cases showed conventional morphology; however, one case showed the histologic features of tall cell variant[125] (Figure 36-11). An anaplastic component arising within papillary carcinoma

metastatic to the breast was also reported.[124] Thyroid carcinoma is positive for TTF-1 and thyroglobulin, effectively excluding a diagnosis of breast carcinoma.

OTHER CARCINOMAS

Salivary gland carcinomas such as mucoepidermoid and acinic cell carcinomas, neoplasms not often considered as a source of metastatic tumor, have been rarely reported to metastasize to the breast.[12,108,126] Metastases from medulloblastoma[126] and neuroblastoma[127] have been reported in children and adults.

SARCOMAS

Both primary and metastatic sarcomas in the breast are rare. Sarcoma is more commonly seen as a component of metaplastic carcinoma or phyllodes tumor.[128] Metastatic sarcoma to the breast includes rhabdomyosarcomas,[12,129,130] uterine leiomyosarcoma,[2,31,131] synovial sarcoma,[132] hemangiopericytoma, alveolar soft part sarcoma,[133] Ewing's sarcoma,[5,134] low-grade endometrial stromal sarcoma,[135] and malignant fibrous histiocytoma. These tumors may be difficult to distinguish

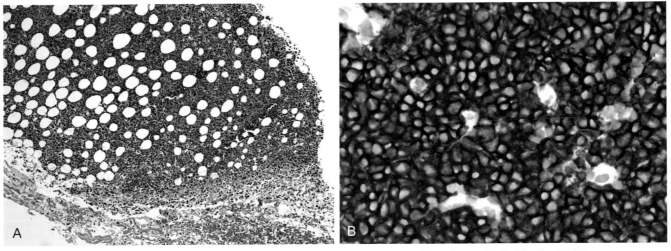

FIGURE 36-12   A, Histologic section of metastatic breast large B-cell lymphoma. **B,** Positive for CD20.

from primary mammary sarcomas and some metaplastic mammary carcinomas.[128] Given the known limitations of a CNB, accurate diagnosis becomes very difficult unless there is a prior history of the sarcoma.

HEMATOPOIETIC MALIGNANCIES

Secondary spread of lymphomas to the breast is reported to account for approximately 0.07% of all breast malignancies (see also Chapter 35). However, these secondary lymphomas compose the largest group (17%) of tumors that can involve the breast.[4,89,136] Wiseman and Liao[137] defined the clinical criteria for the diagnosis of primary breast lymphoma when the breast is the clinical site of the first major manifestation of the lymphoma: there is no history of previous lymphoma or widespread lymphomatous disease and the lymphoma is demonstrated with close association to breast tissue in the pathologic specimen. They also state that ipsilateral lymph nodes may be involved if they develop simultaneously with the primary breast tumor. Previous reports document a right-sided predominance. However, one study has shown equal involvement of the right and left breast.[138] The presence of B symptoms (fever, night sweats, and weight loss) is uncommon.

The most common histologic type reported in the literature when primary and secondary cases are grouped together is diffuse large B-cell lymphoma (Figure 36-12), which represents 45% to 90% of all cases.[4] Burkitt's-type lymphoma and mucosa-associated lymphoid tissue–type lymphoma have also been documented.[7,136–138] Secondary involvement of the breast with a T-cell lymphoma has been reported in only a few cases.[7] Immunohistochemistry and polymerase chain reaction (PCR) for immunoglobulin heavy chain clones or translocations are often helpful.

Leukemia occasionally involves the breast. The morphology of the blasts or more differentiated cells may give a clue to the diagnosis, but a high index of suspicion may be needed to make the correct diagnosis if there is no clinical history. Myeloma rarely involves the breast.[58,82] The plasmacytic morphology and pattern of infiltration around lobules can suggest the diagnosis. Demonstration of light chain restriction is important in establishing the correct diagnosis. CD38 and CD138 are especially useful markers of plasma cell differentiation, but neither is specific.

Prognosis

The appropriate treatment option can be challenging in metastatic breast carcinomas. There is little information in the literature regarding what is considered the best practice. In the study by Vaughan and coworkers,[25] 61% of patients underwent some form of resection but only 22% of these patients had their resection with curative intent. Surgical debulking or excision for palliative purposes may be appropriate in widely metastatic disease. Metastases to the breast have been associated with poor prognosis, with most patients dying within 1 year of diagnosis.[89,120] Vaughan and coworkers[25] reported a mean survival time of 17.8 months after the diagnosis of a breast metastasis of nonhematologic origin. Median survival in a review of 27 cases of melanoma metastases to the breast was 12.9 months.[56] Metastatic disease in the breast is a marker for disseminated metastatic spread and, therefore, indicates a poor prognosis.[30,135] Mastectomy may be performed to obtain local control of bulky, ulcerated metastatic lesions. Wide excision can be supplemented by radiotherapy to the breast for radiosensitive neoplasms and axillary dissection may be performed, especially if the lymph nodes appear to be grossly involved.[13] Patients with smaller metastasis not causing problems with local control and not having clinical evidence of axillary metastases may be treated with extensive surgical resection.

SUMMARY

The correct identification of metastatic tumors in the breast is of vital importance to proper patient management. Recognition depends on the pattern of breast disruption, lack of an in situ component, unusual tumor cell morphology, and disseminated lympangitic spread. The analysis begins with patient history, in most instances, and generally will follow the workup of tumors of unknown origin when patients lack a history of a prior neoplasm.